MW01230838

WITHDRAWN
LIFE UNIVERSITY
LIBRARY

THE
ABDOMINAL PLAIN FILM

Stephen R. Baker, MD
Professor and Acting Chairman
Department of Radiology
Albert Einstein College of Medicine
Bronx, New York

LIFE COLLEGE-LIBRARY
1269 Barclay Circle
Marietta, GA 30060

APPLETON & LANGE
Norwalk, Connecticut/San Mateo, California

0-8385-7896-9

Notice: Our knowledge in clinical sciences is constantly changing. As new information becomes available, changes in treatment and in the use of drugs become necessary. The author and the publisher of this volume have taken care to make certain that the doses of drugs and schedules of treatment are correct and compatible with the standards generally accepted at the time of publication. The reader is advised to consult carefully the instruction and information material included in the package insert of each drug or therapeutic agent before administration. This advice is especially important when using new or infrequently used drugs.

Copyright © 1990 by Appleton & Lange
A Publishing Division of Prentice Hall

All rights reserved. This book, or any parts thereof, may not be used or reproduced in any manner without written permission. For information, address Appleton & Lange, 25 Van Zant Street, East Norwalk, Connecticut 06855.

90 91 92 93 94 / 10 9 8 7 6 5 4 3 2 1

Prentice Hall International (UK) Limited, *London*
Prentice Hall of Australia Pty. Limited, *Sydney*
Prentice Hall Canada, Inc., *Toronto*
Prentice Hall Hispanoamericana, S.A., *Mexico*
Prentice Hall of India Private Limited, *New Delhi*
Prentice Hall of Japan, Inc., *Tokyo*
Simon & Schuster Asia Pte. Ltd., *Singapore*
Editora Prentice Hall do Brasil Ltda., *Rio de Janeiro*
Prentice Hall, *Englewood Cliffs, New Jersey*

Library of Congress Cataloging-in-Publication Data

Baker, Stephen R., 1942—
     The abdominal plain film / Stephen R. Baker.
        p.   cm.
     ISBN 0-8385-7896-9
     1. Abdomen—Radiography. I. Title.
     [DNLM: 1. Abdomen—radiography.   WI 900 B168p]
   RC944.B344   1990
   617.5'507572—dc20
   DNLM/DLC
   for Library of Congress   90-9
                                                                        CIP

Acquisitions Editor: Stephany S. Scott
Production Editor: Lauren Manjoney
Designer: Janice Barsevich

PRINTED IN THE UNITED STATES OF AMERICA

To my children, Amelia, Elizabeth, Catherine, and Nina.

Contributors

Milton Elkin, MD
Distinguished University Professor Emeritus
Department of Radiology
Albert Einstein College of Medicine
Bronx, New York

Harry Delany, MD
Professor
Department of Surgery
Albert Einstein College of Medicine
Bronx, New York

Contents

Preface

The plain film of the abdomen is a neglected area of radiology. Although its clinical relevance in the evaluation of many abdominal disorders persists today, even with the wide use of powerful cross-sectional techniques such as computed tomography and ultrasonography, it continues to receive scant attention in the current diagnostic imaging literature. All too often, its study has been relegated to a peripheral position in radiology residency programs, treated with diffidence by trainees and attending roentgenologists alike.

Is the abdominal film outmoded, a fit topic merely for those with an antiquarian bent? It is my contention that it remains an important examination providing pathognomonic signs for some disorders and pertinent information for many others. The plain film is also readily available, easy to obtain, and relatively inexpensive. Moreover, its interpretation can be a real challenge and, therefore, compelling to the diagnostician because of its intellectual fascinations.

It is surprising that such a worthy subject has never been treated exclusively in a single textbook. Frimann-Dahl's epochal monograph, *Roentgen Examinations in Acute Abdominal Diseases* was a pathfinding analysis that is still germane today. Its focus was narrow, however, and it did not concern itself with chronic conditions or with the wide range of abnormal abdominal calcifications. An excellent work of recent vintage, *Abdominal Radiology*, edited by McCort, et al, emphasized plain films in both the adult and pediatric presentation but also included radiological findings observed by intravenous pyelography and barium contrast studies of the GI tract.

This book employs a pattern approach to the interpretation of plain films. The descriptions and discussions are based on reasoning from radiological observation to diagnosis. The first two chapters comprise an overview of the subject. The initial chapter considers uses, limitations, and technical considerations of the plain film. It is followed in chapter 2 by a discussion of the principles of the evaluation of abdominal gas, mass, and calcification. Chapters 3 through 9 apply these principles to specific organs and abdominal regions. The last chapter, on the roentgenographic appearance of surgical clips and staples, can be regarded as an appendix. It considers the interpretations of the appearances of metallic artifacts a subject not previously presented elsewhere as a coherent topic. This book is devoted solely to abnormalities of adults; the range of pathology in the pediatric age group is so vast and often so distinct from diseases of the fully grown that it deserves separate discussion.

Although I have borrowed widely from many contributors, the vast majority of cases were culled from files in my own hospital—a large teaching center with an active emergency ward. Most of the entities depicted here, including both classical appearances of uncommon entities and unusual manifestations of common abnormalities, should be encountered on a recurring basis in similar institutions. Even for radiologists based in smaller hospitals and clinics, it is important to be aware of the plain film configurations of rare diseases, especially if prompt recognition results in effective treatment.

This book owes its life to the assistance of numerous individuals. I appreciate particularly the efforts of my residents and colleagues who alerted me to each new interesting case. Without their cooperation I could not have proceeded. Special thanks go to Donna Chinea for patiently typing draft after draft and for finding things after I lost them, a very frequent occurrence. Louis Mendez made most of the prints for the book, a herculean task he performed with skill and good cheer. And, most of all, I wish to acknowledge the perseverance of my wife and daughters who put up with my absences and distractions while this book was in gestation.

CHAPTER ONE

Uses, Limitations, and Technical Considerations

In recent years, two continuing trends in radiology have tended to diminish the importance of the plain film of the abdomen. Sophisticated modalities such as ultrasonography and computed tomography have been applied with great success to the investigation of a range of abdominal conditions. Used singly or in sequence, they have extended our ability to evaluate and monitor many diseases. With their aid, many diagnoses hitherto determined only at operation or autopsy can now be achieved with markedly decreased patient risk. The plain film, limited in scope and sensitivity, often seems irrelevant in the presence of such powerful imaging procedures.

In the present climate of cost consciousness and risk management, the notion of efficacy has emerged as a strong consideration in medical decision making. Customary examinations are now placed under careful scrutiny to ascertain if their diagnostic value justifies their pertinence for specific clinical presentations. The abdominal film has not fared well in many of these studies. Several assessments of its efficacy have questioned its role either as a definitive examination or as a preliminary radiograph prior to contrast studies.

However, it would be misguided to neglect or dismiss the information that plain films often provide. The interpretation of cross-sectional images is frequently enhanced by an inspection of scout radiographs. Occasionally, unexpected but crucial observations about solid organs or unopacified hollow structures can be made before and during contrast examinations of the gastrointestinal or genitourinary tracts. It is therefore necessary to be familiar with the plain film appearances of many types of abdominal pathology so that the appropriate corroborative studies can be done. Moreover, there remains a large group of frequently encountered entities for which the plain film is either pathognomonic or at least highly characteristic. Many of these are acute and life-threatening diseases requiring expeditious diagnosis and prompt treatment.

Despite its partial eclipse by newer modalities, the plain film retains a position in the imaging firmament. Its exact place has not been fully settled, as new signs and applications for it are still being discovered just as traditional uses for the plain film have come under critical surveillance. Any physician interested in abdominal diseases should be aware of its capabilities. Radiologists, especially, must have a comprehensive understanding of its virtues and limitations.

Plain films are obtained for two reasons—as a separate examination for the evaluation of abdominal disorders and as a preliminary X-ray as part of a more complex radiographical procedure. In the past, abdominal plain films have been requested as survey roentgenograms in a search for abnormal findings even in the absence of signs and symptoms of disease. In this context, the yield is generally very low. Rosenbaum and colleagues, in a study of 500 routine abdominal plain films obtained on patients older than 40 years, reported unsuspected findings in 7%, but in only three individuals were the observations of clinical importance. The majority of clinically silent abnormalities were gallstones and renal calculi.[1] Gillespie analyzed the survey roentgenogram of the abdomen in a series of 4517 men who received periodic health examinations.[2] He also demonstrated a low rate of positive results with a majority of radiographic findings related to the lumbar spine. Next most frequent were prostatic calculi and arterial calcification—two findings that by themselves do not call for treatment or additional tests.[2]

It is clear that plain films of the abdomen should only be done if there is a heightened expectation of abnormality. The yield of abdominal roentgenographs depends on the type and the severity of the disease. One indication for radiographic evaluation is abdominal pain. Eisenberg and colleagues showed that plain films are only helpful if the pain is moderate to severe or if there is also significant abdominal tenderness.[3] In their study of 1780 emergency room patients, more than half of the requested abdominal plain films need not have been done because the patient's complaints were either mild or minimal pain or tenderness. Such a reduction in X-ray use would not have been accompanied by a failure to diagnose even one significant abnormality.[3] A review of 1000 patients with acute abdominal pain by Brewer and colleagues also revealed limitations in the usefulness of plain films.[4] However, 40% of the patients in their series were between 15 and 24 years of age and the two most common diagnoses in this group were appendicitis and pelvic inflammatory disease.[4] There are specific plain film findings for appendicitis but they occur in a minority of cases and in most instances the diagnosis is usually made on clinical grounds. Pelvic inflammatory disease rarely exhibits diagnostic abnormalities on plain films. It is probable that in an older patient population the diagnostic yield of abdominal radiographs would be higher.

Many conditions are not amenable to diagnosis on plain radiographs unless their clinical presentation is exceptional. Gastrointestinal bleeding has few manifestations on preliminary films. Han and colleagues described a characteristic appearance of massive amounts of blood clots in the stomach and colon.[5] However, this unusual roentgenographic finding occurs in only a small fraction of cases and in most patients only substantiates what has already been established through history and physical examination. Smaller hemorrhages have no distinguishing plain film manifestations and therefore abdominal radiographs are superfluous in the determination of the cause or extent of gastrointestinal bleeding. Aside from calcified gallstones common hepatobiliary diseases have few plain film features. Acute cholecystitis is better diagnosed by ultrasonography or technetium-99m cholescintigraphy, the best initial imaging test for obstructive jaundice is ultrasonography, and cholangitis and acute hepatitis are not detected by radiographic modalities.[6] Masses in the liver are not seen on plain films unless there is marked hepatomegaly or intrahepatic calcifications. In a minority of cases, distinctive plain films manifestations of pancreatitis can be observed.[7] Nonetheless, in most cases the diagnosis is made from history, clinical appearance, and laboratory tests.

Two common conditions for which abdominal films are of great value are perforated viscus and intestinal obstruction. The upright chest X-ray can demonstrate as little as 1 to 2 mL of free air[8] and is the most sensitive view (Fig 1–1). The supine radiograph of the abdomen, however, not only reveals massive effusions of intraperitoneal gas (Fig 1–2) but also small collections localized anterior to the liver, in Morison's pouch or in the lesser sac (Fig 1–3). In obtunded and otherwise debilitated patients who

cannot assume the erect position, the recognition of subtle signs of free air on recumbent views assumes crucial diagnostic importance. The supine film alone is frequently diagnostic for gastric, small bowel, or large bowel obstruction. For patients with renal colic, plain films are essential to determine the presence and number of stones. Noncontrast radiographs of the abdomen can often detect the presence of an abscess if not measure its extent. Several investigations have demonstrated that there is at least one sign of abdominal abscess on 65% to 87% of preliminary supine abdominal films (Fig 1–4).[9,10] Bowel infarction produces a range of radiographic findings most of which are nonspecific but the production of streaks of gas in the wall of the small and large bowel or in the portal venous systems are unusual but diagnostic roentgenographic findings that can help direct prompt management (Fig 1–5).

In obese patients for whom physical examination may be unrewarding, the plain film can differentiate between fat and ascitic fluid. Palpation of the spleen and abdominal masses may be difficult in patients of all body shapes and supine films of the abdomen can be a useful adjunct to physical examination. Also, there are several infrequently encountered acute conditions for which plain films are highly informative, including emphysematous cholecystitis (Fig 1–6) and gallstone ileus (Fig 1–7).

Scout films of the abdomen have been advocated as part of intravenous urography, oral cholecystography, and barium enema examinations. There is no debate about the value of preliminary films for contrast investigation of the urinary tract as small or faintly calcified stones in the renal pelves, ureters, and bladder can be obscured by iodinated contrast material. Scout films have little utility in oral cholecystography studies. Preliminary radiographs have been advocated because of the apprehension of missing a faintly calcified gallstone that could be obscured by contrast collecting in a nonobstructed and functioning gallbladder.[10] However, recent reports have shown that this possibility is too uncommon to justify the inconvenience and radiation dose occasioned by an additional visit to the radiology department for a preliminary film before the ingestion of oral cholecystography tablets.[11–13]

The value of a scout film prior to barium enema examination is more controversial. Thoeni and Margulis surveyed radiology departments across the country and found the respondents equally divided about the need for a preliminary film before barium evaluation of the colon.[14] Opponents of the routine scout view argue that it is not helpful in assessing the adequacy of bowel preparation.[15] Although extracolonic abnormalities can be observed in prelim-

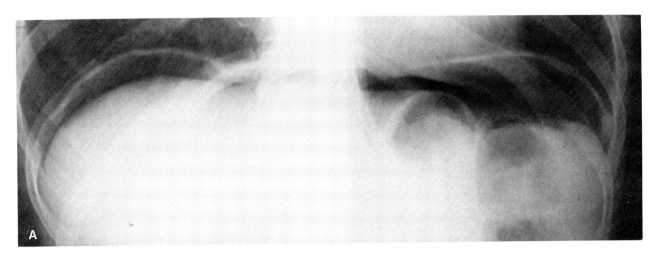

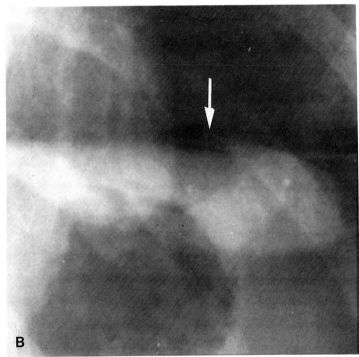

Figure 1–1. A. Upright chest film. Large pneumoperitoneum. Air collects below the domes of both hemidiaphragms. **B.** Very small pneumoperitoneum. A sliver of gas is present on the upright chest film just below the dome of the left hemidiaphragm (*arrow*).

inary views, most of these findings will also be discerned on films with barium filling the colon. The incidence of unsuspected findings outside the colon is low, ranging from 4.5% to 8.5%.[15,16] A single plain film of the abdomen imparts an average ovarian dose of approximately 200 mrad in women, which is about 25 times the gonadal dose of a chest X-ray.[17] For younger patients at least, the radiation burden and low yield outweighs the small likelihood of discovering clinically valuable information on preliminary plain films.

The elimination of the scout radiograph seems appropriate for outpatients, who are usually healthier and better prepared than hospitalized patients. To proceed with the barium enema in the absence of a preliminary abdominal film may not be cost effective for inpatients, however, as they would have to endure a second enema examination if the first study were incomplete because of poor preparation.[18] Although small amounts of feces cannot be demonstrated with accuracy, the plain film can recognize massive amounts of fecal residue as well as

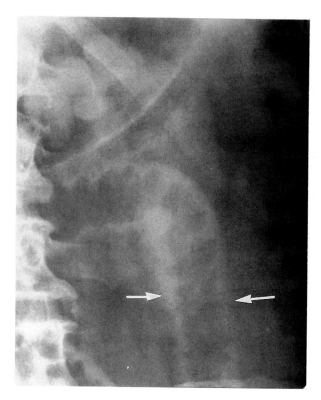

Figure 1–2. Massive intraperitoneal air permits visualization of the wall of a segment of the small bowel (*arrows*), making it appear to stand out in relief.

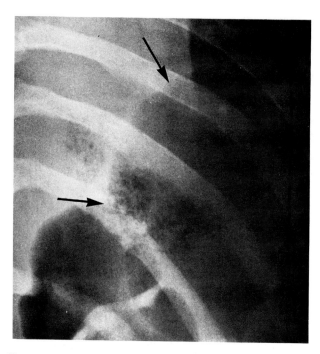

Figure 1–4. Splenic abscess. Bubbles of gas (*lower arrow*) and large unilocular lucency that does not conform to bowel (*upper arrow*) are two plain film findings of intraperitoneal abscess.

small collections of contrast material from previous gastrointestinal studies (Fig 1–8).[19] The typical population in a general hospital includes patients with neurological diseases, many elderly and enfeebled individuals, and varying numbers of newly admit-

ted patients who have received narcotic medications either illicitly or by prescription. Any of these inpatients are apt to have a large bowel filled with feces at the time a barium enema is requested—an observation that plain films can easily acknowledge.

There are other reasons for not abandoning the plain film before barium enema. Diverticulitis is a common indication for contrast evaluation of the co-

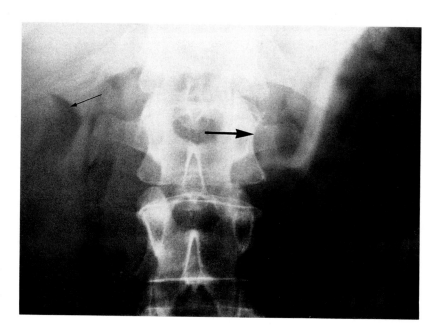

Figure 1–3. Perforated ulcer. A moderate amount of intraperitoneal gas has collected in Morison's pouch (*small arrow*) and in the lesser sac (*large arrow*).

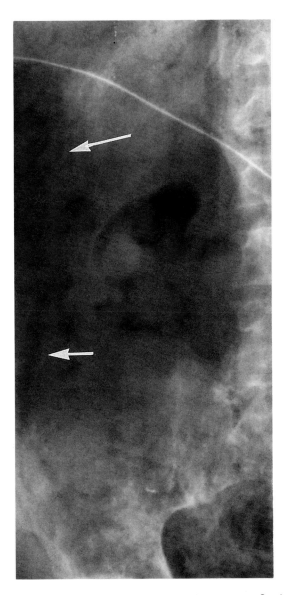

Figure 1–5. Mesenteric ischemia with portal venous gas. Gas has entered the wall of infarcted bowel, appearing as encircling streaks (*lower arrow*). The linear lucencies (*upper arrow*) represents gas in the branches of the portal vein.

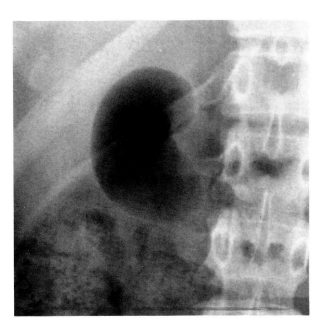

Figure 1–6. The spontaneous formation of gas in the lumen of the gallbladder is a hallmark of emphysematous cholecystitis.

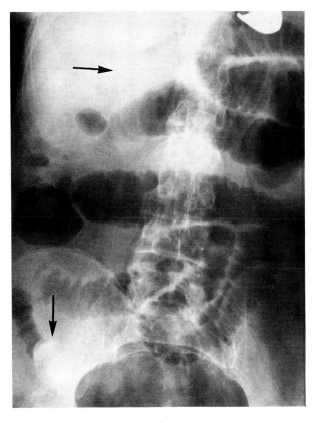

Figure 1–7. The plain film triad of gallstone ileus is seen here: (1) Faint gas in the biliary tree (*upper arrow*); (2) bowel obstruction with gas in the distended small intestine; (3) obstructing gallstone in the distal small bowel (*lower arrow*). (*Courtesy of Dr. John Adler*).

lon in older people. Occasionally the inciting cause is an inadvertently swallowed foreign body, usually a chicken bone, which makes its way through the gut before penetrating a sigmoid diverticulum where it can then cause acute and recurrent infections (Fig 1–9). If no scout film is done, diverticulitis may be recognized but the foreign body that caused it will be obscured by barium and the underlying abnormality will go undetected.

The scout film also is an aid to the completion of a successful fluoroscopic examination. The transverse colon almost always contains gas when the patient is in a supine position. The location of this

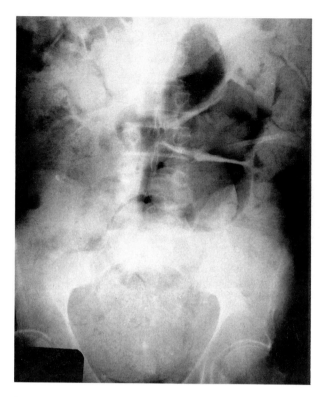

Figure 1–8. Fecal impaction in a narcotics abuser. Scout film of the abdomen. The barium enema was delayed and active purgation begun to remove the fecal residue.

colonic segment can help direct the performance of the barium enema. A low-lying transverse colon, a frequent normal finding in older patients, can obscure other large bowel segments on barium enema. Similarly the cecum may extend into the pelvis and overlie the sigmoid colon. Observing these anatomic variants on scout film before the passage of contrast material can enable the fluoroscopist to choose a technique of bowel opacification that allows clear visualization of all sections of the colon.[20]

TECHNICAL CONSIDERATIONS

The supine view is the mainstay of the plain film abdominal examination. In order to best appreciate subtle differences in contrast, the voltage should be near 60kV for thin patients.[21] Such a setting permits good penetration and contrast at relatively short exposure times and allows visualization of the thin fat planes that surround solid organs and muscles.

The importance of maintaining the lower edge of the supine film at the level of the obturator foramen cannot be overemphasized. A higher positioning will exclude observation of the inferior extension of the peritoneal cavity. Incarcerated inguinal or femoral herniae, which are often the cause of small bowel obstruction, can be missed by an improperly centered supine film (Fig 1–10). Also, pelvic tumors

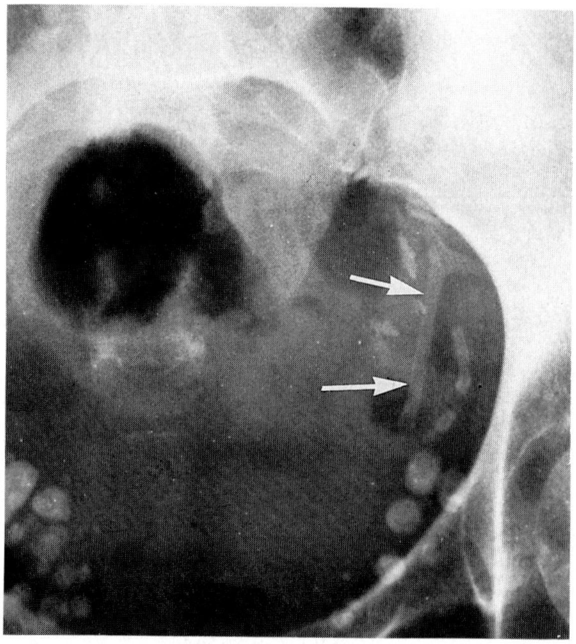

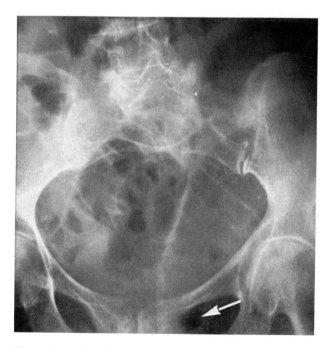

Figure 1–9. A patient with diverticulitis. The scout film reveals a chicken bone fragment (*arrows*) that has perforated through a sigmoid diverticulum producing an abscess.

Figure 1–10. Small bowel obstruction due to an incarcerated femoral hernia (*arrow*).

and abnormal calcifications may not be revealed if the supine radiograph does not extend below the upper margin of the symphysis pubis (Fig 1–11A). In patients with a long trunk, a coned-down film of the pelvis may be necessary to ensure that all of the abdomen is seen (Fig 1–11B).

In the majority of patients with intestinal obstruction or adynamic ileus, a supine plain film is sufficient for diagnosis. However, intraperitoneal gas may go undetected with this view alone. A single abdominal film may not encompass the right upper quadrant and the domes of both hemidiaphragms. The additional view that provides the most information about bowel perforation is the upright chest X-ray.

The central beam of an upright chest X-ray should pass just above the diaphragmatic domes, almost parallel with the gas–liquid interface resulting from small amounts of free air in the peritoneal cavity. Thus, this view is more sensitive for the determination of pneumoperitoneum than an upright abdominal film in which the radiographic beam passes through the interface obliquely. The chest X-ray, of course, can reveal pleural and pulmonic abnormalities, both of which can have a bearing on

diagnosis for patients with abdominal complaints. Pleural effusion may be an intrathoracic manifestation of upper abdominal abscess or a concomitant of metastatic disease from an abdominal source. Pneumonia in the lower lobes of the lung can first present with pain referred below the diaphragm.

Most textbooks of radiology favor a routine three-view plain film examination, including a supine film and upright radiographs of the chest and abdomen.[21–23] The predominant advantage of the erect abdominal projection is the demonstration of fluid levels, which had been thought to be critical in the differentiation of mechanical obstruction of the bowel from adynamic distension of the large or small intestine. Doubt has since been cast on the specificity and reliability of fluid levels as a sign of obstruction,[24,25] so that the value of the upright abdominal film for routine use has been questioned.

Mirvis and colleagues found that erect films added little to the roentgenographic evaluation of abdominal pain. They studied 252 consecutive patients, each of whom had a three-view study of the abdomen.[26] Of 51 patients whose plain films suggested a specific diagnosis in 30 both the supine and erect films revealed the same abnormality. In an ad-

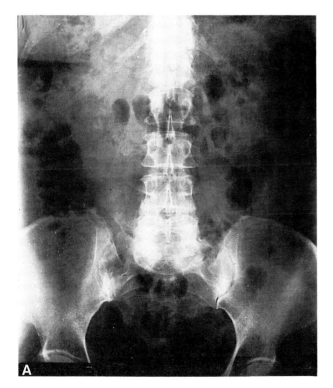
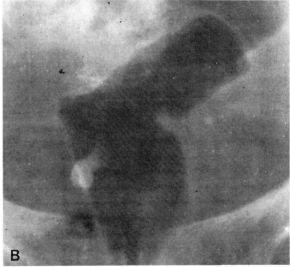

Figure 1–11. A. The initial film of the abdomen was interpreted as normal. It was centered too high, with its lower margin above the symphysis pubis. **B.** Coned-down view of the pelvis shows a tooth. The patient had a cystic teratoma of the right ovary.

ditional 13 cases, a finding was observed on supine films but not on the erect view. In only eight was the upright abdominal film more diagnostic than the supine film and in three of these the erect chest X-ray showed the pertinent observation more clearly. In the remaining five cases, the erect abdominal film findings did not alter patient management.[26] Simpson and colleagues evaluated 87 patients with bowel obstruction. Each had a recumbent and erect abdominal film.[27] In 69% the diagnosis was made on supine films alone and in an additional 7% the erect film added unique diagnostic information.[27] In 24% of cases, obstruction could not be seen on either film, an observation consistent with previous reports.[28] Simpson and colleagues concluded that the erect films should not be requested routinely. In another series of 100 consecutive emergency room abdominal studies, de Lacey and colleagues found the upright film to be unnecessary in almost every case.[29]

Is there still a place for the upright projection in the evaluation of abdominal pain? Supine films are limited in the diagnosis of intestinal obstruction if the bowel is filled with fluid. The "string of pearls" sign produced by small amounts of intraluminal small bowel gas situated between the bowel wall and hypertrophied valvulae conniventes is highly suggestive of mechanical obstruction and can be seen more easily on erect films than on supine views (Fig. 1–12). If there is a paucity of bowel gas and obstruction is a likely possibility, the erect view should then be a part of the plain film examination.[24]

At times, patients are too sick to assume the upright position, and erect radiographs of the abdomen or chest are contraindicated. The cross-table lateral projection with the right side elevated is an excellent substitute. Not only does it demonstrate free air under the diaphragm as it projects over the upper liver shadow, it can also reveal the string of pearls sign and other evidence of intestinal obstruction. Miller maintains that it is even more sensitive than the erect chest film for the diagnosis of pneumoperitoneum in patients with upper abdominal adhesions.[30] An additional advantage is its ability to reveal duodenal ileus, which is one of the more specific plain film findings of pancreatitis (Fig 1–13).[31] In general, however, the right-side-up lateral decubitus view should not be done routinely and should only be requested when supplementary information is needed after the standard supine film has been obtained.

In the evaluation of large bowel distention, the prone view can often be decisive in distinguishing adynamic ileus from obstruction. In the supine position gas collects in the transverse colon and liquid feces moves to more dependent locations in the ascending colon, descending colon, and rectum. Turning the patient from the supine to the prone position redistributes colonic gas away from the transverse colon and towards the proximal and descending colon. Distension of the transverse colon is a feature of both ileus and left-sided colon mechanical obstruction. In this clinical situation the prone view can be

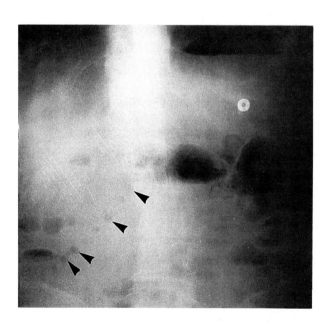

Figure 1–12. Erect view. String of pearls sign (*arrowheads*). The supine film contained little gas and was not diagnostic for intestinal obstruction.

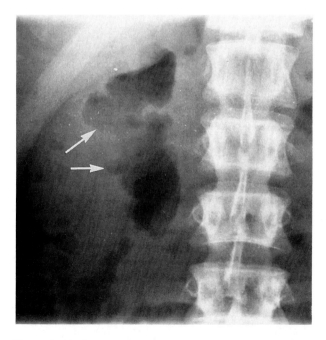

Figure 1–13. Acute pancreatitis has produced a duodenal ileus with gas in the distended proximal duodenum (*arrows*). Right-side-up decubitus view.

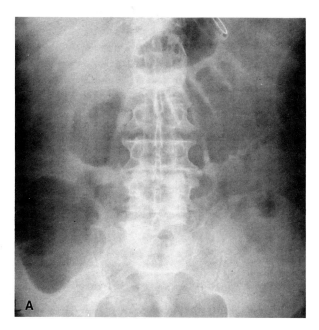 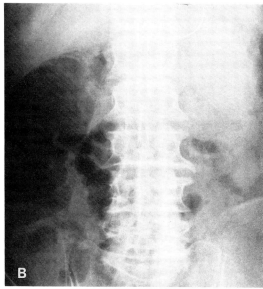

Figure 1–14. A. Obstructing carcinoma of the mid-descending colon. The supine film shows gas in the ascending colon and transverse colon. **B.** On the prone film the transverse colon contains fluid only and there is gaseous distention of the right colon and the proximal descending colon.

very helpful (Fig 1–14). It is important to remember that obstruction can be intermittent, incomplete, or recent and the distal colon may still contain gas at the time of plain X-ray. Digital examination of the rectum does not introduce air from outside, but enemas, sigmoidoscopy, and colonoscopy may allow air to gain entry into the large intestine, thereby confusing the interpretation of both supine and prone radiographs.[32]

Assessment of the sigmoid colon and rectum can also be aided by a right-side-up view with a vertical beam.[33] This projection favors the passage of gas to the distal colon and permits a differentiation of ileus from obstruction. It also enables evaluation of contour abnormalities of the colonic wall caused by mural lesions and extensive masses.

A supine view of the abdomen with a horizontal beam should be considered in patients who have had surgery and now present with acute abdominal pain and distension. In addition to intraperitoneal adhesions, bowel obstruction after abdominal operation may be due to an incarcerated incisional hernia which, if air filled, can be demonstrated with this view (Fig 1–15). Oblique and coned-down projections have as their chief advantages a clear depiction of abdominal calcification. The left posterior oblique view is particularly valuable in assessing the length and width of abdominal aortic aneurysms (Fig 1–16).

For many acute conditions, the passage of time is a key component in the selection of a correct di-

agnosis. The temporal pattern of pain and its relation to other signs and symptoms are often crucial determinants. Over a several-hour period patients can swallow significant amounts of gas and evacuate large volumes of fluid from the gut. Bowel dis

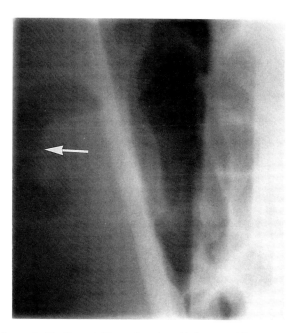

Figure 1–15. Cross-table supine view. Air is trapped in an incarcerated incisional hernia, which is the site of bowel obstruction (*arrow*).

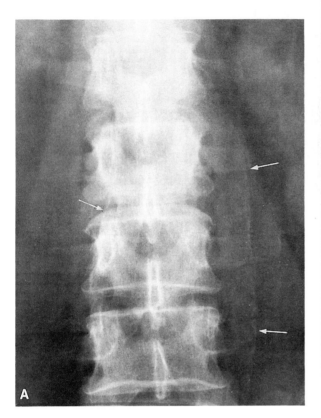
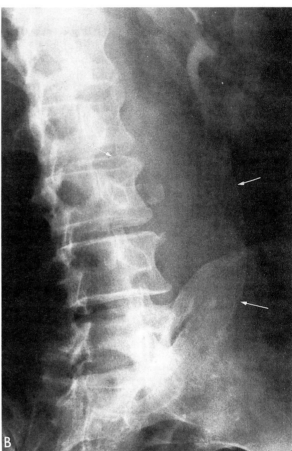

Figure 1–16. A. Supine film demonstrates a calcified abdominal aortic aneurysm. **B.** The oblique view better demonstrates the dimensions of the aneurysm.

tension as a response to adjacent or generalized inflammation may appear rapidly. Ureteral stones can move distally and even be discharged from the bladder in a short time. Quickly evolving pathological processes mandate the importance of serial films. Especially for the assessment of bowel obstruction and renal lithiasis the repeat supine view of the abdomen may be the definitive radiological examination.

REFERENCES

1. Rosenbaum HD, Lieber A, Hanson DO, et al. A routine survey roentgenogram of the abdomen on 500 consecutive patients over 40 years of age. *Am J Roentgenol.* 1964;91:903–904.
2. Gillespie HW. Routine abdominal radiology in periodic health examinations. *Acta Radiol (Diagn).* 1970;10:299–304.
3. Eisenberg RL, Heincken P, Hedgcock MV, et al. Evaluation of plain radiographs in the diagnosis of abdominal pain. *Ann Surg.* 1983;197:464–469.
4. Brewer RJ, Golden GT, Hitch DC, et al. Abdominal pain: An analysis of 1,000 consecutive cases in a university hospital emergency room. *Am J Surg.* 1976; 131:219–224.
5. Han SY, Witten DM, Prim HS. Plain film findings in massive gastrointestinal bleeding. *Am J Roentgenol.* 1977;128:437–439.
6. Simeone JF, Novelline, RA, Ferrucci JT Jr. Comparison of sonography and plain films in evaluations of the acute abdomen. *Am J Roentgenol.* 1985;144:49–52.
7. Millward S, Breatnach E, Simpkins KC, et al. Do plain films of the chest and abdomen have a role in the diagnosis of acute pancreatitis? *Clin Radiol.* 1983;34:133–137.
8. Miller, RE, Nelson, SW. The roentgenographic demonstration of tiny amounts of free intraperitoneal gas: Experimental and clinical studies. *Am J Roentgenol.* 1971;112:574–585.

9. Lundstedt C, Hederstrom E, Holamin T, et al. Radiologic diagnosis in proven intraabdominal abscess formation: A comparison between plain films of the abdomen, ultrasonography and computerized tomography. *Gastrointest Radiol.* 1983;8:261–266.

10. Twomey B, deLacey G, Gajjar B. The plain radiograph in oral cholecystography: Should it be abandoned? *Br J Radiol.* 1983;56:99–100.

11. Connell TR, Stephens DH, Carlson HC, et al. Upper abdominal abscess a continuing and deadly problem. *Am J Roentgenol.* 1980;134:759–765.

12. Andersen JF, Madsen PER. The value of plain radiographs prior to oral cholecystography. *Radiology.* 1979;133:309–310.

13. Harned R, Leveen RF. Preliminary abdominal films in oral cholecystography: Are they necessary? *Am J Roentgenol.* 1978;130:477–479.

14. Thoeni RF, Margulis AR. The state of radiographic technique in the examination of the colon: A survey. *Radiology.* 1978;127:317–323.

15. Eisenberg RL, Hedgcock MW. Preliminary radiographs for barium enema examination: Is it necessary? *Am J Roentgenol.* 1981;130:115–116.

16. Harned RK, Wolf BL, Williams SM. Preliminary abdominal films for gastrointestinal examination: How efficacious? *Gastrointest Radiol.* 1980;5:343–347.

17. Penfil RL, Brown ML. Genetically significant dose to the United States population from diagnostic medical roentgenology, 1964. *Radiology.* 1968;90:209–216.

18. Schwab FJ, Glick SN, Teplick SK, et al. The barium enema scout film: Cost effectiveness and clinical efficacy. *Radiology.* 1986;160:615–622.

19. deLacey B, Wilkins R, Cramer B, et al. The accuracy of plain film radiography in assessing colonic faecal contamination. *Clin Radiol.* 1983;34:73–74.

20. Baker SR. Preliminary abdominal film before barium enema examinations. *Am J Roentgenol.* 1981;137:183. Letter.

21. McCort JJ. Examination technique. In: McCort JJ, ed. *Abdominal Radiology.* Baltimore. Williams & Wilkins Co. 1984:1–8.

22. Samuel E, Laws JW. The acute abdomen. In: Sutton P, Grainger RG, eds. *A Textbook of Radiology.* London: Churchill-Livingstone; 1975:806–818.

23. Mindelzun RE, McCort JJ. Acute abdomen. In: Margulis AR, Burhenne HJ, eds. *Alimentary Tract Radiology.* St. Louis, Mo:CV Mosby Co.;1983:391–480.

24. Gammill SL, Nice CM Jr. Air fluid levels: Their occurrence in normal patients and their role in the analysis of ileus. *Surgery.* 1972;71:771–780.

25. Donahue JK, Hunter C, Balch LT. Significance of fluid levels in x-ray films of the abdomen. *N Engl J Med.* 1958;259:13–15.

26. Mirvis SE, Young JWR, Keramati B, et al. Plain film evaluations of patients with abdominal pain: Are three radiographs necessary? *Am J Roentgenol.* 1986;147:501–503.

27. Simpson A, Sandeman D, Nixon SJ, et al. The value of an erect abdominal radiograph in the diagnosis of intestinal obstruction. *Clin Radiol.* 1985;36:41–42.

28. Tibblin S. Diagnosis of intestinal obstruction with special regard to plain roentgen examination of the abdomen. *Acta Chir Scand.* 1969;135:249–252.

29. deLacey BO, Wignall BK, Bradbrooke S, et al. Rationalizing abdominal radiography in the accident and emergency department. *Clin Radiol.* 1980;31:453–455.

30. Miller RE. The technical approach to the acute abdomen. *Semin Roentgenol.* 1973;8:267–279.

31. Balthazar EJ, Lutzker S. Radiological signs of acute pancreatitis. *CRC Crit Rev Clin Radiol Nucl Med.* 1976;7:199–242.

32. Golden DA, Gefter WB, Gohel VK. Digital examination of the rectum as a source of rectal gas. *Radiology.* 1981;141:618.

33. Laufer I. The left lateral view in the plain film assessment of abdominal distension. *Radiology.* 1976;119:265–269.

CHAPTER TWO

Principles of Abdominal Plain Film Interpretation

INTRODUCTION

The abdomen is composed primarily of soft tissues similar to water in density. Plain radiographs cannot distinguish two soft tissue structures if they abut on each other. This is true for both solid or liquid-containing masses and organs because all share with water the same capacity to absorb X-ray photons. The demonstration of anatomic information depends upon the arrangement of soft tissues with respect to fat or gas collections that lie next to, around or within them. Functional, metabolic, and mechanical diseases of the stomach and intestines can be recognized by the presence, location, extent, and contour of gas. Enlargement of organs and masses are ascertained by their effect on nearby bowel loops and their displacement or obliteration of adjacent normal fat. Moreover, in many conditions, distinctive patterns of calcification provide useful and sometimes definitive diagnostic evidence on abdominal films. Understanding the interrelationships of the four radiographic densities, namely gas, fat, water, and calcium, is fundamental for plain film interpretation. The purpose of this chapter is to consider the radiographic features of each of these densities in detail, emphasizing both the range of normal configurations and the appearance of pathological entities.

GAS

Unlike the lung, in which air in the tracheobronchial tree and in the pulmonary alveoli provide a background, abdominal gas is usually relatively meager and highly variable in concentration and location. However, the sharp black contrast of gas in comparison to the gray shading of denser structures allows recognition of very small lucencies. Normally, gas may be seen in the stomach, small intestine, colon, and occasionally in the vermiform appendix. If a lucency appears to reside outside the lumen of the tubular gastrointestinal tract, it should be viewed with suspicion because it is most often indicative of a significant abnormality such as an intra-abdominal perforation, abscess, ulceration, or fistula.

The Constituents of Intestinal Gas

The predominant source of stomach and small bowel gas is swallowed air. As the transit time through the mouth and esophagus is usually no more than a few seconds and the absorption of gas through the gastric wall takes several minutes, the chemical constituents of stomach gas are nearly identical to air. More distally, the composition of intestinal gas depends upon the differing rates of absorption of ingested atmospheric gases and gas produced by the digestion of food. Carbon dioxide is so rapidly absorbed in the stomach and in the small intestine that sustained distension of the bowel by this gas alone is impossible. Oxygen is slightly less soluble than carbon dioxide but nitrogen is especially resistant to absorption and thus remains the major component of upper intestinal gas.

In both the small and large intestine, very little gas can enter the lumen from the bloodstream. Thus in closed loop obstructions, gas is slowly absorbed and will decrease in volume if no swallowed air can pass into it. The main constituents of flatus are nitrogen, carbon dioxide, hydrogen, and methane, with oxygen a minor component. Bacterial metabolism is the source of hydrogen and its production depends on the amount of fermentable, nonabsorbable substrate (usually oligosaccharide) delivered to the large intestine. Carbon dioxide formation usually parallels hydrogen production. Methane is constantly generated throughout the day but the average amount of gas produced is genetically influenced, with some individuals more able to accommodate methane-forming bacteria. As in the upper gastrointestinal tract, nitrogen from swallowed air contributes more to the extent of colonic gas than endogenously created gas from bacterial fermentation.[1,2]

Normal Gas—Appearance

Stomach. Each section of the gastrointestinal tract has a particular "signature"—a distinctive pattern of luminal gas accumulation that allows it to be identified even when there has been displacement of the gut by a mass or through a hernial orifice. The slightly undulating gastric rugae helps to identify the stomach (Fig 2–1). The rugae are submucosal ridges that are directed roughly parallel to the long axis of the body and the antrum of the stomach. In the gastric fundus, they are often sparse and tend to have diverse orientations. The rugae always maintain a slightly wavy outline but can become effaced if the stomach becomes increasingly distended (Fig 2–2). In the nearly empty gastric lumen, the only identifying lucency may be a small amount of air trapped between two rugal folds. It is important not to confuse this normal appearance with the fixed narrowing of a scirrhous carcinoma or other infiltrating lesions of the stomach (Fig 2–3). The normal stomach is highly distensible and successive films usually reveal a change in the configuration of intraluminal gas. Infiltrating lesions, on the other

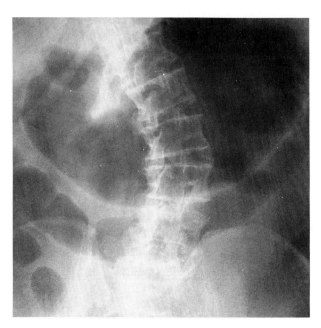

Figure 2–2. Distended stomach. Dilatation of the gastric lumen has effaced the rugae.

hand, produce a consistently constricted gastric air shadow.

The appearance of the gastric bubble is modified by the addition of liquid and solid material. Gastric juices and ingested liquids fill in the valleys

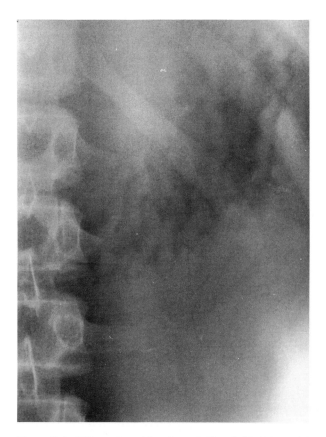

Figure 2–1. Oblique view of the stomach. The air-filled stomach is identifiable by the slightly waxy rugae.

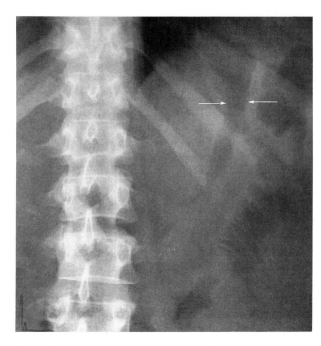

Figure 2–3. A narrowed stomach due to fibrosis from lye ingestion. No rugae are seen in the diffusely constricted lumen (*arrows*).

between the rugal ridges, obscuring these indentations. At the same time, the overall density of the gastric bubble becomes less black. If liquid retention continues, the gastric air shadow is no longer discernible on supine films. If even a few cubic centimeters of gas remains, however, decubitus or upright views can still reveal a fluid level indicating the location of the gastric lumen (Fig 2–4B). Retained solid food mixed with gas and liquid imparts a mottled or smudgy appearance to the stomach (Fig 2–5).

Small Intestine. It has been stated that the presence of more than a few milliliters of gas in the small intestine is an abnormal finding.[3] This supposition is based on the fact that air is rapidly absorbed in the normal small bowel and thus its continued presence could indicate mechanical obstruction or adynamic ileus. However, in many people, rapid swallowing of air is a habitual activity and, during stressful periods, it may become even more pronounced (Fig 2–6A). Ingestion of a highly carbonated beverage will also introduce air into the jejunum and ileum. Rapid transit to the proximal small bowel of large quantities of air can exceed temporarily the intes-

tines' absorptive capabilities and an abdominal film obtained at that moment may demonstrate a gas-filled but normal small bowel. Consequently, pathological small bowel distension should only be diagnosed in the appropriate clinical context and not solely by the interpretation of a single supine abdominal film.

Small intestinal loops are recognized by the encircling valvulae conniventes. Also known as Kerckring's folds or the plicae circulares, these intraluminal projections consist of intestinal epithelium, muscularis mucosa, and submucosal layers, all of which are continuous with the small bowel wall. Since they contain muscle fibers, their appearance is labile, becoming more prominent in the distended bowel proximal to a mechanical obstruction (Fig 2–7). In hypotonic conditions, muscle relaxation makes them less conspicuous (Fig 2–8). Valvulae conniventes are most obvious in the duodenum and jejunum, becoming less frequent more distally, and in the terminal ileum they may be very scarce (Fig 2–9). A minimal amount of air gives them a serrated appearance and yet, with increasing distension, they appear thinner but more elongated. Nonetheless,

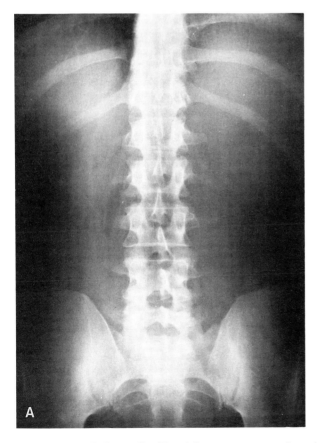
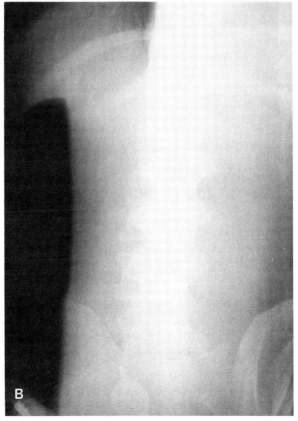

Figure 2–4. A. Supine film. The abdomen appears nearly gasless. No evidence of air in the stomach. **B.** Decubitus view. Left side down. A large air–fluid level in the right abdomen reveals a markedly distended stomach filled with liquid and air.

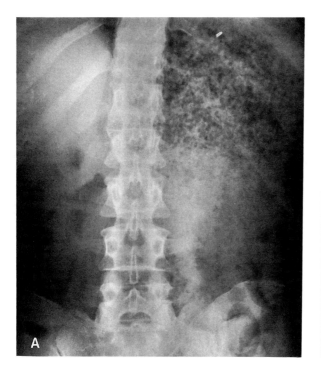
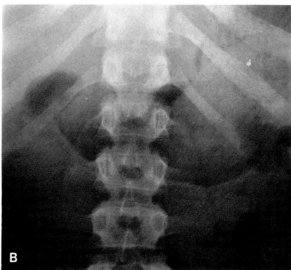

Figure 2–5. A. Gastric obstruction. Dilated stomach containing food particles. **B.** Nonobstructed stomach. Semisolid gastric contents within the lumen. This radiograph was obtained soon after a meal.

even with marked dilatation of the lumen, the folds remain visible.

Each valvulae is nearly identical to its immediate neighbor in thickness, length, and in orientation perpendicular to the long axis of the bowel. Nor-

mally, the intervening bowel wall forms a right angle with each fold but an oblique course of a series of valvulae suggests tethering of the small bowel wall by intramural or extraintestinal masses or tumors. In small intestinal segments proximal to a mechan-

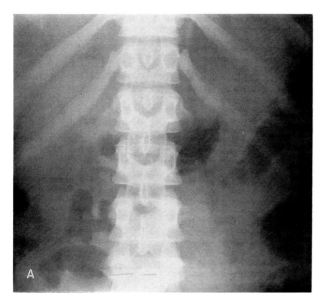
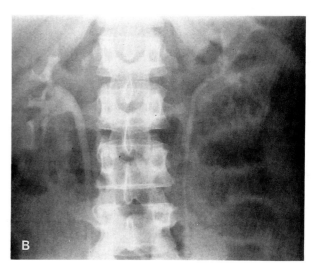

Figure 2–6. The rapid accumulation of small bowel air in a normal person. **A.** A scout film for an intravenous urography. There is little gas in the small bowel. **B.** Ten-minute film. Swallowed air now fills the jejunum.

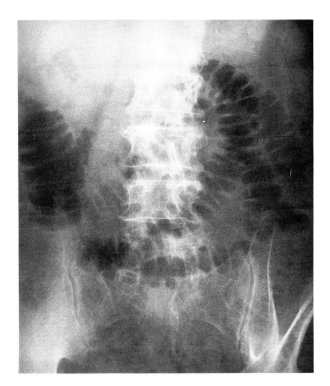

Figure 2–7. Distal small bowel obstruction. The small bowel is distended and the valvulae conniventes are prominent.

ical obstruction, the valvulae thicken and, as fluid accumulates in the small intestine, the clear definition between the folds and the lumen is gradually lost. Moderate amounts of succus entericus become trapped between folds and the residual gas assumes

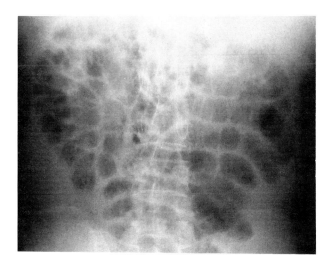

Figure 2–8. A patient with ascites. There is mild dilatation of the small bowel but no obstruction. The valvulae are preserved but not prominent.

a slitlike configuration (Fig 2–10). With further accretions of liquid, the remaining gas appears as bubbles which are best seen in upright or decubitus films as a chain of rounded lucencies. This has been termed the "string of pearls" sign (Fig 1–12).

Colon. The gas-containing large intestine can be recognized by the bulging of the haustral outpouchings. In order to accommodate the tenia coli, the three longitudinal muscles that extend from the cecum to the rectum, the tethered colonic wall forms three rows of sacculations, which are most prominent in the ascending and transverse colon but are regularly present in the left colon as well. Each haustrum is delimited by a plica semilunaris, a crescentic fold of colonic wall that projects into the lumen. The plicae and the haustra contain muscle and are influenced by the contractions of the tenia coli. Thus, they are not fixed in appearance but are dynamically dependent on bowel tone. Like the valvulae conniventes, the plicae and haustra can efface if the colonic wall becomes hypotonic. The haustra can also be flattened by adjacent structures such as the left lateral peritoneal wall, which abuts on the outer surface of the descending colon. In the partially distended colon the plicae appear to extend entirely across the lumen, but with increasing distension, these localized indentations are seen as incomplete septations rather than as encircling rings (Fig 2–11). The plicae are also more widely spaced than the valvulae, another feature that helps distinguish the large bowel from the small bowel.

Perhaps the most important difference between the colon and the small intestine is the presence of intraluminal solid material in the large bowel. Rarely, intestinal parasites, undigested foreign matter, or ectopic gallstones are recognized within a loop of air-filled jejunum or ileum. Almost always, however, the small intestine contains only liquid and gas. Solid feces conclusively identify the colon. The fecal consistency can vary from liquid to scybalous concretions that are dry and hard (Fig 2–12). Most fecal masses have irregular borders and a mottled internal architecture resulting from the trapping of small bubbles of gas within them. Because feces are surrounded or at least bordered by colonic gas, they are readily visible on plain films.

Occasionally, the "signatures" of large or small bowels are not distinct and a tubular gas loop that has features of both intestinal segments may be observed. When it is important to identify that loop without the administration of opaque contrast material a helpful and simple maneuver is to fill the colon with air (Fig 2–13). If the questionable segment is part of the colon, it will distend with air in

18

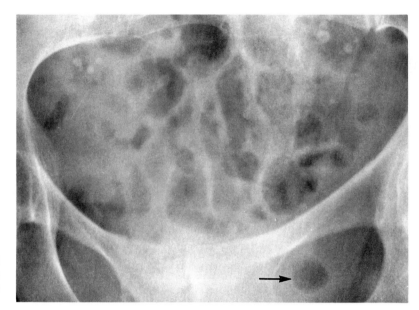

Figure 2–9. A patient with a nonobstructing left inguinal hernia (*arrow*). There are numerous ileal loops containing gas in the pelvis. None contain recognizable valvulae conniventes.

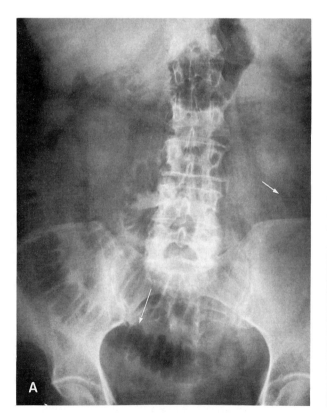

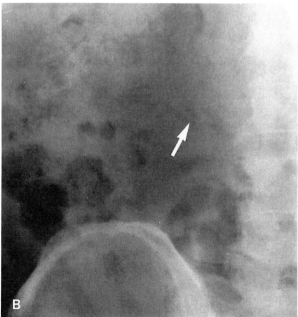

Figure 2–10. A. Distal small bowel obstruction. The lower arrow points to distended small bowel filled with air. The upper arrow is directed towards small bowel filled with fluid and air. The air appears as slits of radiolucencies. **B.** Another patient with an obstructed small intestine. The only clue to the diagnosis are several slits (*arrow*) indicating a distended small bowel loop with prominent valvulae conniventes. The loop is filled with succus entericus and a little gas.

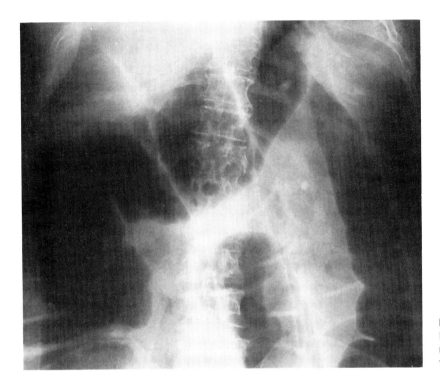

Figure 2–11. Dilated colon in a patient with Parkinson's disease. The plicae indent the lumen. Note their wide spacing compared to the valvulae conniventes of the small bowel.

continuity with the large bowel lumen. If it remains separate and unaffected after colonic insufflation, however, it must be a small bowel loop or extraintestinal gas.

Appendix. Air in the appendix is neither rare nor necessarily abnormal. It appears as a homogeneous tubular lucency that usually makes one or more bends along its course from cecal orifice or appendiceal tip. The length of the gas-filled lumen depends upon the orientation of the appendix to the radiographic beam. If the appendix is directed primarily in the anterior–posterior plane, the lumen appears foreshortened. On the other hand, it is surprising how long some normal appendices can be with their tip situated quite far from the proximal ascending colon. Air tends to collect in retrocecal appendices that extend superiorly from the cecum (Fig 2–14).

The inconstant location of the right colon and the variable length of the appendix allows the tubular lucency of the appendiceal lumen to occupy any portion of the right colon, even sometimes reaching across the midline (Fig 2–15). An abnormal appendix containing gas is an unusual finding. It almost always occurs in association with clinical evidence of appendicitis. Typically, the lumen is distended, straightened, and shortened, often lacking the gentle curves of the disease-free, gas-filled appendix (Fig 2–16).

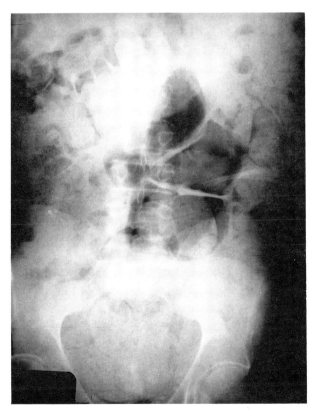

Figure 2–12. Massive fecal impaction. The distended colon is filled with many discrete fecal masses, some of which are clearly outlined by gas.

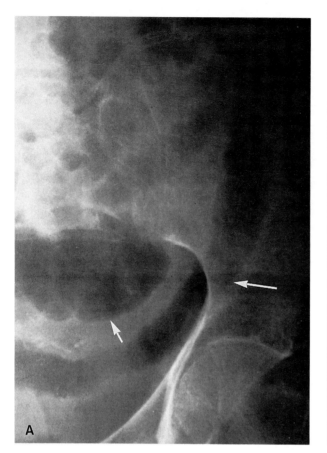
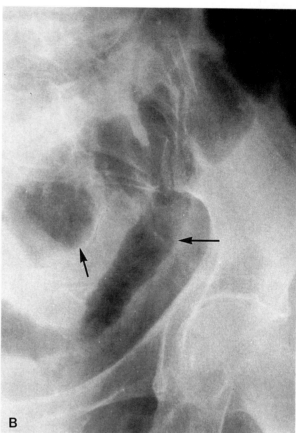

Figure 2–13. A. A long segment of bowel is gas filled (*long arrow*). It is not clear if it is small or large intestine. Above it is a wider amorphous loop (*short arrow*). **B.** After colonic air insufflation, the more superior loop is shown to be the colon (*shorter arrow*). The lower loop contains even less gas now and therefore must be part of the small bowel (*long arrow*).

Normal Gas—Location

Location is as crucial as shape in the characterization of intra-abdominal lucencies. In the normal gastrointestinal tract, the fixed points of reference are the gastric fundus, the ligament of Treitz, the hepatic and splenic flexures, and the rectum. All other gastric and bowel regions including the cecal pouch exhibit great variability in position (Fig 2–17). It is not enough to be familiar with the most frequent location of anatomic landmarks, one must also consider the range of sites the bowel may occupy.

Stomach. Several factors influence bowel position and length. Body habitus is strongly predictive of the orientation of the stomach. Asthenic patients often have elongated J-shaped stomachs with the greater curvature located in the left mid to left lower abdomen. In these individuals, the air-filled duodenal bulb appears above the antrum (Fig 2–18). In the aged, there is a tendency for the stomach to become ptotic, with the gastric body descending to the level of the pelvis. This is often observed in osteoporotic elderly women who frequently suffer from dorsal kyphosis and multiple vertebral compression fractures. The kyphosis tends to project the anterior stomach more inferiorly and the compressed vertebrae shorten the trunk.

The stomach of thick-set patients is typically oriented horizontally. Frequently, the air-filled duodenal bulb is situated lateral to the antrum but it may be posteriorly placed and hidden within the larger lucency of the distal stomach. Occasionally, the antrum extends far to the right of the mid line and may overlie the right renal shadow (Fig 2–19). Horizontal stomachs are often associated with a pseudotumor in the gastric fundus or proximal body evident on supine radiographs. The "mass" is produced by fluid collecting posteriorly in the dependent portions of the stomach (Fig 2–20).

The direction and position of the central radiographic beam may create the impression that a transversely directed stomach is located above the diaphragm. This illusion can occur when the beam is centered below the umbilicus; the divergent superior rays then pass through both the anteriorly situated stomach and the posterior lung fields (Fig 2–21).

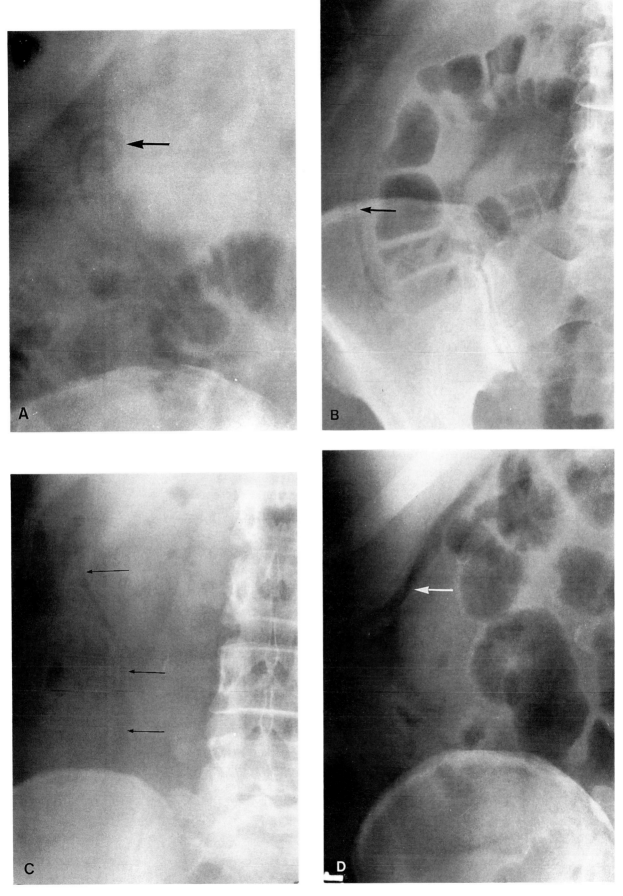

Figure 2–14. The range of appearances of a normal air-filled appendix. **A.** Curvilinear tubular lucency (*arrow*). **B.** Air-filled appendix lateral to the cecum (*arrow*). **C.** Elongated air-filled appendix ascending medial to the cecum (*arrow*). **D.** Air in an appendix superimposed on the inferior margin of the liver (*arrow*).

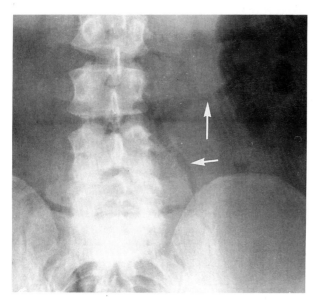

Figure 2–15. Air in the appendix situated to the left of the midline (*arrows*). The large bowel is malrotated with the cecum on the left.

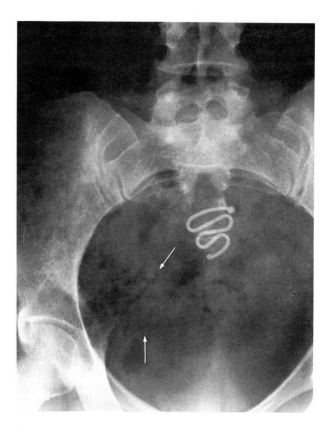

Figure 2–17. Low-lying cecum. The feces-filled cecum is situated in the pelvis extending almost to the midline (*arrows*). This is a normal variant of colonic position.

Stomach and Transverse Colon. A spatial relationship of great value for plain film interpretation is the close association of the stomach and the transverse colon. Connected by the gastrocolic ligament, displacement or distension of one affects the position of the other. The course of the transverse colon is very variable. It can be horizontally oriented (Fig 2–21) or may describe a wide convex downward arc suspended between the hepatic and splenic flexures (Fig 2–22). Occasionally, it takes a redundant, some-

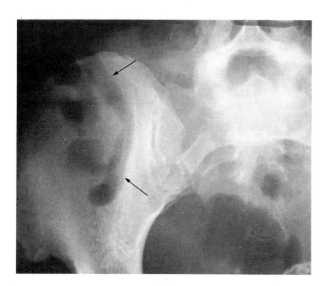

Figure 2–16. A distended gas-filled appendix (*arrows*). This patient has a perforated cecal carcinoma with an abscess at the appendiceal orifice.

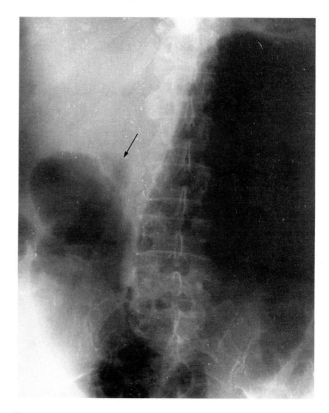

Figure 2–18. Gastric dilatation in a J-shaped stomach. The duodenal bulb is also filled with air (*arrow*).

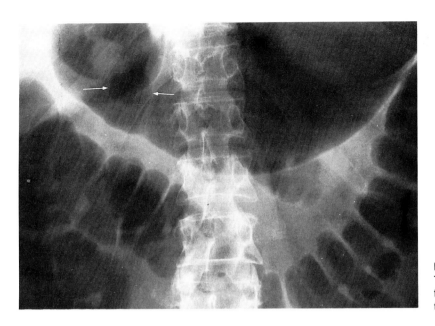

Figure 2–19. Distended horizontal stomach. The antrum overlies the right kidney. The air-filled duodenal bulb is superimposed on the distal stomach (*arrows*).

what serpentine course across the abdomen. In nearly every case, the configuration of the transverse colon is determined by the orientation of the stomach. An elongated stomach occurs in conjunction with a convex downward, transverse colon whereas a straight, transverse colon usually signifies a horizontal stomach.

The length and degree of laxity of the gastrocolic ligament is also variable. In some patients, the superior margin of the transverse colon and the inferior edge of the stomach appear in close approximation. In others, there may be a gap of 10 to 15 cm between them (Fig 2–23). A wide space between these two hollow structures is normal; a mass in the gastrocolic ligament should be diagnosed only if it creates an extrinsic impression on the lumen of one or both.

Recognition of the transverse colon should be the first step in the evaluation of plain films of the abdomen. Normally, the large intestine contains at least a small amount of gas. In the supine position, the least dependent segment is the transverse colon. As such, it should nearly always be seen because colonic gas will flow into it. The identification of the transverse colon also allows unequivocal recognition of the stomach, which lies above it. Following

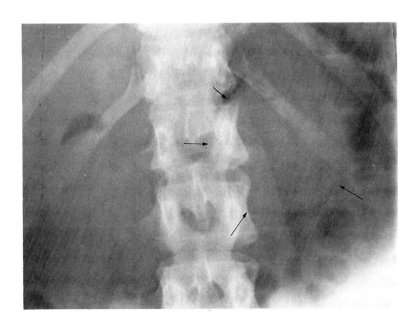

Figure 2–20. Pseudotumor of the stomach. Arrows outline a soft tissue density occupying the gastric lumen. It represents fluid in the dependent posterior portion of the proximal body of the stomach.

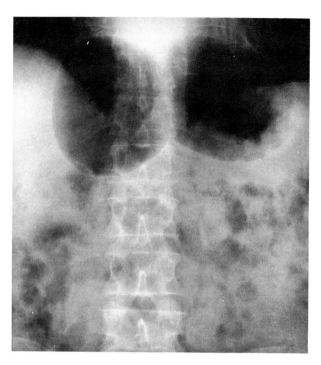

Figure 2–21. Angle of beam illusion. The air-filled transversely oriented stomach is, in fact, within the abdomen. The radiograph is centered too low, projecting the anterior stomach over the lower thorax. Observe also the horizontally directed feces-filled transverse colon.

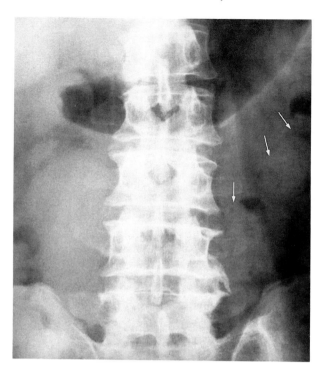

Figure 2–23. The feces-filled distal transverse colon (*arrows*) is parallel to but separated from the stomach.

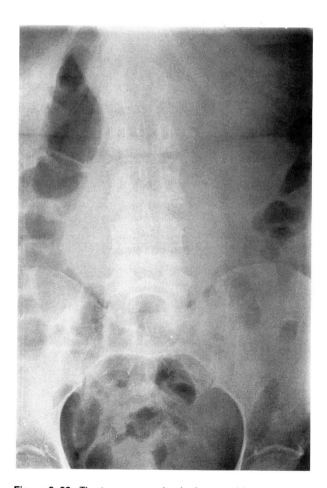

Figure 2–22. The transverse colon is depressed by a distended stomach filled with liquid.

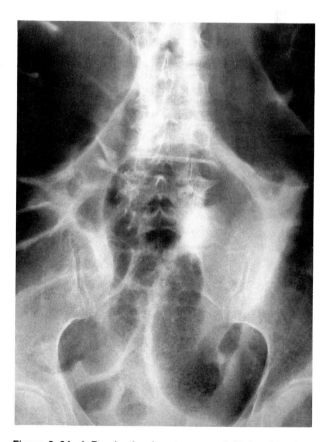

Figure 2–24. A Russian immigrant woman. A lifetime high-fiber diet has lengthened her colon. The dilated sigmoid colon rises out of the pelvis.

24

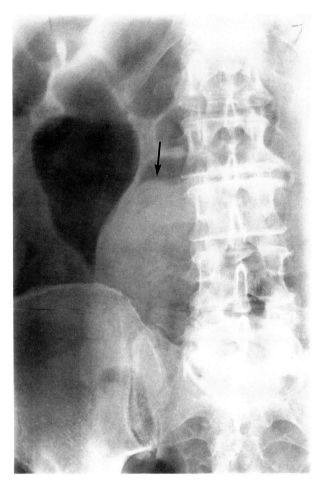

Figure 2–25. Redundant sigmoid colon. A fluid-filled sigmoid loop (*arrow*) causes extrinsic impression on the gas-filled cecum.

preciated, it can be mistaken for distended small bowel and even for nonintestinal gas collections.

Intestinal Displacement. The stomach and the intestines can be displaced from their expected location in several ways. A large mass may push bowel away from it as it grows. Volvulus of the bowel involves obstruction, torsion, and intestinal migration. For example, in cecal volvulus, a typical appearance is isolated dilatation of the cecum, which rotates around its mesenteric attachments and comes to lie in the left upper quadrant (Fig 2–26).

Herniation through abdominal orifices allows bowel to enter other body regions. Hiatus hernia is the most common and can be recognized on plain films by the appearance of gastric rugae in the mediastinum. In the lower abdomen, inguinal and femoral hernias are frequent. If gas-containing bowel accompanies the hernial sac it can be observed on abdominal radiographs as long as care is taken to include the inguinal region, at least to the level of the obturator foramen, above the lower edge of the film (Fig 2–27). Bowel migration may occur laterally through a Spigelian hernia, anteriorly through the umbilicus or at a point of postsurgical weakness, superiorly across a diaphragmatic rent or through

the transverse colon antegrade and retrograde leads to the hepatic and splenic flexures and from there the ascending and descending colons can be traced. Once the transverse colon is seen, the identity of nearby small bowel loops becomes clearer.

Sigmoid Colon. The normal sigmoid colon is also very variable in length and location. In middle-aged and elderly individuals who have consumed a lifetime diet high in fiber, the large bowel in general and the sigmoid segment in particular lengthen considerably. The redundant loops of sigmoid colon extend out of the pelvis and may occupy any position in the lower and mid abdomen (Fig 2–24). Usually, they are located to the left of the abdomen but may lie next to the cecum (Fig 2–25) and even extend more laterally, insinuating themselves between the ascending colon and the peritoneal wall. Frequently, the redundant sigmoid colon contains gas. If this normal variation of bowel configuration is not ap-

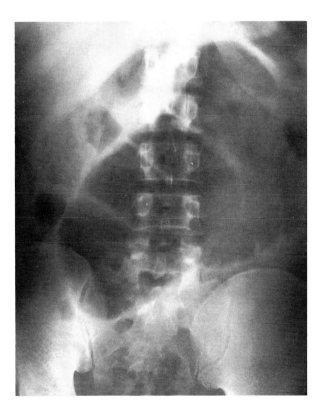

Figure 2–26. Cecal volvulus. The markedly dilated cecum extends from the right lower abdomen to the left upper quadrant. The plicae semilunares identify colonic gas.

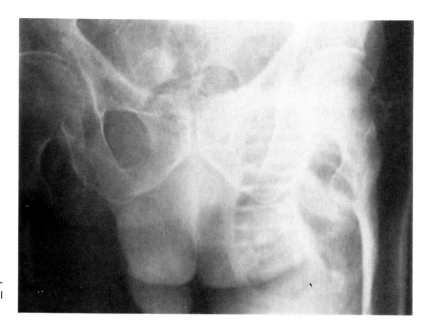

Figure 2–27. Large inguinal hernia. The appearance of valvulae conniventes reveals small intestine within the left inguinal hernia sac.

the foramina of Bochdalek or Morgagni, and posteriorly through an internal hernia that permits the retroperitoneal displacement of intestinal loops.

Congenital malrotations, either generalized or limited to the small bowel, are also diagnosable on plain radiographs. The key to the detection of small bowel malrotation is the presence of gas-filled intestine in the right upper quadrant of the abdomen.

Normally, the jejunum is situated in the left mid abdomen and the ileum occupies the right and the left lower abdomen and the pelvis. The right upper quadrant should not contain small bowel unless the intestine is incompletely rotated or displaced by a mass (Fig 2–28). Inasmuch as gas in the transverse colon should be seen in nearly every supine film of the abdomen, its absence in patients with no history

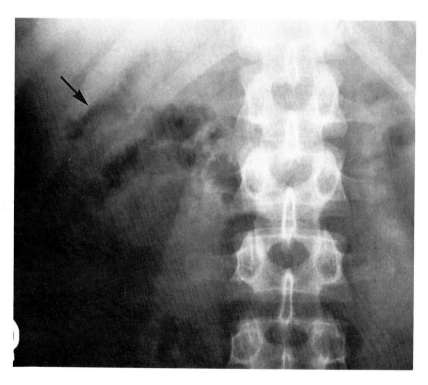

Figure 2–28. Malrotation of the intestines. The arrow points to a section of small bowel with serrated margins. The sawtooth pattern represents the valvulae conniventes, indicating a partially filled jejunal loop. Normally, small intestine does not occupy the right upper quadrant. Also, there is no transverse colon shadow. Contrast studies demonstrated the small intestine on the right side of the abdomen and the colon entirely on the left.

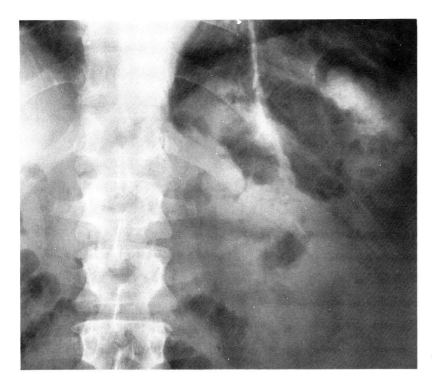

Figure 2–29. Postgastrectomy. Billroth II anastomosis. Three gas containing structures in the left upper quadrant. The most lateral is the splenic flexure containing feces. Its medial neighbor is the gastric pouch. Most medial is the jejunum which was pulled upward to create the gastrojejunostomy anastomosis.

of bowel surgery is also consistent with malrotation.

Surgical resection of the tubular gastrointestinal tract often rearranges the position of remaining bowel. After a Billroth II anastomosis, the jejunum is elevated and attached to the gastric remnant (Fig 2–29). The proximal small bowel will then be seen more superiorly than normal. Colonic resections shorten the length of the remaining bowel, and often the transverse colon is either removed or displaced (Fig 2–30). Hence, this otherwise dependable landmark may be lost.

Luminal Abnormalities. Abnormalities of the gastric and intestinal walls are suggested by distortions of the bowel gas pattern. Polypoid lesions form rounded intraluminal indentations that may have a smooth or lobulated contour (Fig 2–31). The persistence of such filling defects in a constant location in the bowel lumen is necessary to substantiate the diagnosis. Almost always, a follow-up radiograph is required because food particles in the stomach or adherent feces in the colon may simulate a mass. At a point of angulation of bowel, a pseudo-filling defect can be created that resembles a polypoid density (Fig 2–32). Constricting lesions are detected by a fixed narrowing of the stomach or intestine. There must be sufficient distension of the lumen near the point of narrowing to avoid confusion with an undiseased segment of bowel that is merely devoid of

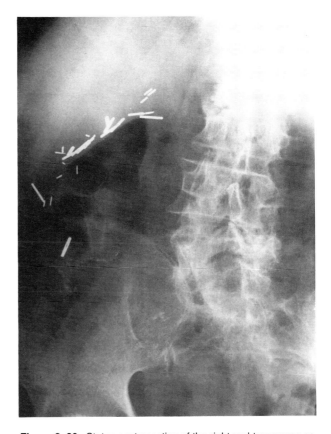

Figure 2–30. Status postresection of the right and transverse colon for an extensive carcinoma of the hepatic flexure. Surgical clips, sutures, and gas in the ileum and colon are seen at the site of anastomosis. There are no gas shadows along the expected course of the transverse colon, however.

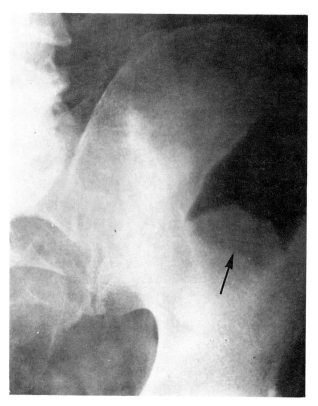

Figure 2–31. Lipoma of the sigmoid colon. The arrow points to an intraluminal mass intermediate in density between gas and soft tissue. It persisted on several films. Its smooth margins and relative lucency enabled a preoperative diagnosis of lipoma to be made.

gas at the time the film is obtained (Fig 2–33).

Another indication of a constricting lesion is the double-lucency sign. The normal lumen tends toward a cylindrical configuration. If the lumen is completely gas filled there is usually little difference in the degree of lucency between the periphery and the center of the lumen. On supine views, as liquid enters the lumen, the homogeneous blackness of gas is replaced by a gradual increase in grayness. If two clearly defined lucencies are superimposed on each other, it frequently indicates gas within two separate bowel loops. However, it may also represent a pathological outpouching such as gas within a diverticulum that lies immediately above or below the bowel loop from which it arises. Yet another possibility is that the roughly cylindrical contour of the lumen has been disrupted by an irregular tumefaction growing into it. As the mass enlarges, it produces crevices and small recesses that contain gas. Usually, the double lucency created by a constricting tumor has sharp contours punctuated by angular promontories. The double lucency sign is unusual but its appearance is often dramatic and strongly suggestive of a rapidly growing mass (Fig 2–34).

On plain radiographs, ulcerations are difficult to recognize en face unless they are very large. Smaller excavations are not sufficiently deep to pro-

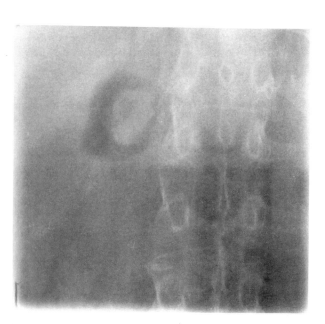

Figure 2–32. The duodenal bulb is distended by gas. The gastric antrum projects into it, simulating a filling defect. Both the antrum and duodenum were normal.

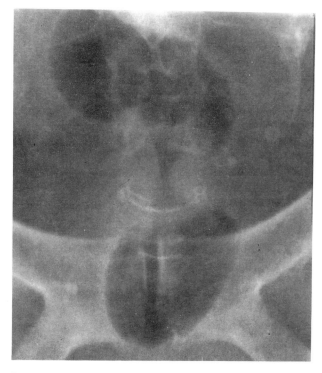

Figure 2–33. Constricting carcinoma of the rectum. The marked narrowing of the lumen persisted on successive films.

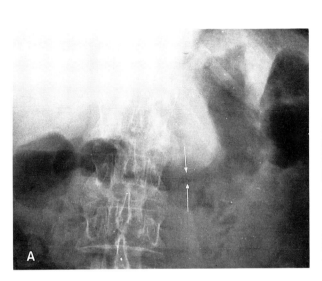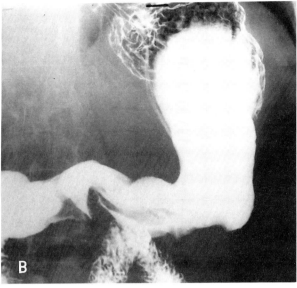

Figure 2–34. Gastric lymphoma. The double-lucency sign. **A.** Arrows indicate a tapering of part of the gastric air shadow within the larger lucency of the lumen of the stomach. **B.** Barium contrast confirms the constricting lesion in the corpus of the stomach.

duce a double lucency sign. In profile, they are slightly easier to discern as they project from the adjacent lumen (Fig 2–35). However, if the lumen is primarily fluid filled, even extensive ulcerations will not be seen on radiographs without contrast material. Diffuse infiltration of the wall of the stomach and intestines can also be seen on plain films. Thick-

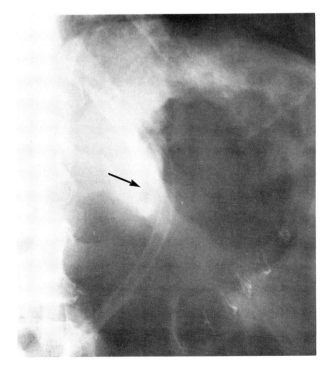

Figure 2–35. Benign gastric ulcer protruding from the lesser curve of the stomach (*arrow*).

ening of the rugae in the stomach, widening of the small bowel valvulae conniventes, effacement of haustra, and nodularity of the wall of all sections of the gastrointestinal tract are important signs (Fig 2–36). Both intrinsic and extrinsic diseases can replace the smooth, arcuate haustral contour with an irregular serrated appearance. In diffuse diseases of the large intestine, the transverse colon is frequently the best place to look for infiltrating lesions because it is nearly always gas filled and, like the rest of the wall, becomes atonic when inflamed. Careful evaluation of the transverse colon is particularly important in the recognition of toxic megacolon, which occurs as an acute exacerbation of ulcerative colitis and other acute inflammations of the large bowel. Characteristically, the bowel is distended and the plicae and haustral contours are obliterated (Fig 2–37).

Diverticula occur throughout the gastrointestinal tract with varying incidences depending upon location. They are infrequent in the stomach, where they are confined primarily to the posterior margin of the fundus. Duodenal diverticula are common and usually innocuous findings on barium contrast studies. More distally in the small bowel, diverticula are only occasionally seen. Colonic diverticula are found in more than 50% of patients older than 60 years who are referred for barium enema examination. They are especially plentiful in the sigmoid colon but very rare in the rectum. For the most part, diverticula are small, and, except for the sigmoid colon, where they can appear as circular lucencies alongside the lumen, they are not detected on plain films. In the duodenum and the sigmoid colon,

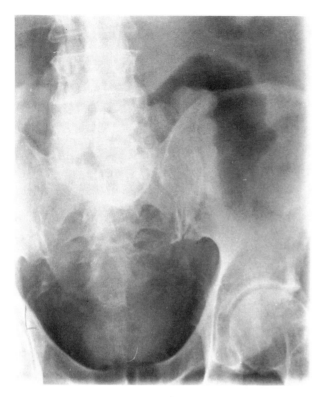

Figure 2–36. Thumbprinting of the wall of the sigmoid colon. Submucosal accumulations of blood produce nodular impressions on the lumen. The plicae and haustra are effaced.

however, unusually large diverticula can appear as round, featureless gas collections. Unlike abscesses, they have smooth walls and are not associated with an adjacent or surrounding mass. As they usually contain much bowel gas and relatively little liquid, they appear homogeneously black, often more lucent than an intestinal loops of similar diameter (Fig 2–38).

Bubbles and Streaks. Within the small intestinal lumen a linear array of bubbles suggests the string of pearls sign, which is a hallmark of mechanical obstruction (Fig 1–12). In the bowel wall, innumerable bubbles characterize pneumatosis cystoides intestinalis. These intraluminal air deposits are of varying size and occasionally have straightened borders where they come into contact with adjacent bowel loops. They occur most frequently in the large intestines but are also found in the small bowel and even in the stomach. Typically, they tend to outline the course of the bowel wall that contains them (Fig 2–39). Pneumatosis, by itself, is usually a benign condition whose major complication is spontaneous pneumoperitoneum. Infrequently, these cysts can be seen extending into the nearby mesentery.

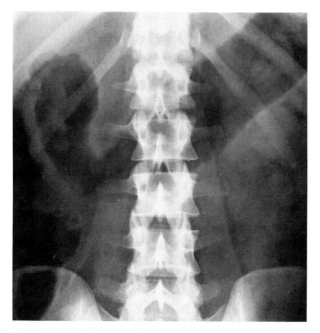

Figure 2–37. Toxic megacolon in a patient with ulcerative colitis. The transverse colon and right colon are distended and gas-filled. No haustra or plicae are present. Nodularity and wall thickness are suggested by the irregular contour of the ascending and proximal transverse colon.

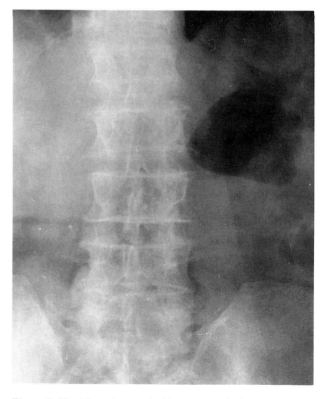

Figure 2–38. A large lucency lacking rugae, valvulae conniventes, or haustra superimposed over the stomach. It is a diverticulum of the fourth portion of the duodenum.

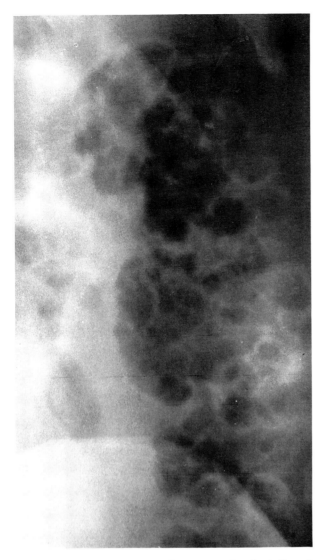

Figure 2–39. Bubbles of varying diameters conforming to the outline of the descending colon. A typical example of pneumatosis cystoides intestinalis.

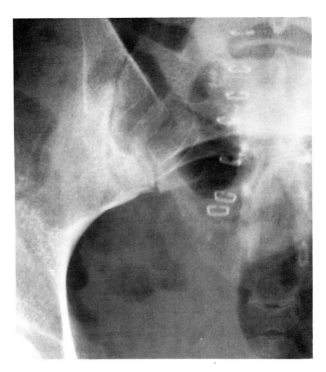

Figure 2–40. Postoperative abscess. This patient had a colon resection 5 days previously. She has a high fever and right lower quadrant tenderness. Myriad bubbles of varying size identify a large pelvic abscess.

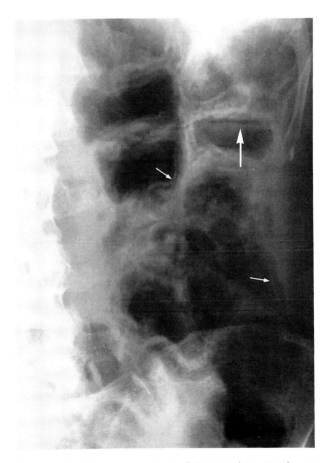

Figure 2–41. Mesenteric ischemia. Submucosal gas streaks are seen throughout the left colon. (*small arrows*). The larger arrow indicates a streak within a plica semilunares.

Outside the bowel, "bubbles are bad" is an apt slogan because they almost always mean abscess or necrotic tumor. Characteristically, abscess bubbles are uniformly small and often appear to be associated with a mass. When situated near the colon, extraintestinal bubbles may resemble feces, and it is not always possible to distinguish between the two on plain films. Solid feces tend to have at least part of their perimeter well defined by surrounding intestinal gas whereas abscess bubbles have a smudgy consistency with no well-demarcated edges (Figs 1–4, 2–40).

If bubbles are bad, streaks are sinister. In the bowel wall, they suggest ischemia. There should be no confusion between intramural streaks and the slitlike appearance of intraluminal gas, which is delimited by valvulae conniventes in a partially liquid-filled small bowel loop. Generally, mural streaks follow the contour and length of an intestinal loop.

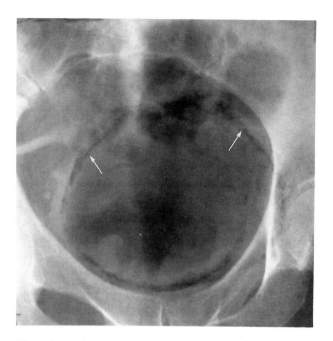

They can also extend into the plicae, as these partial septations indent the lumen (Fig 2–41). On the other hand, intraluminal gas slits are oriented perpendicular to the axis of the bowel and are arrayed in a series of parallel lines. Streaks in the wall of other hollow structures also indicate disease, being diagnostic of cystitis in the urinary bladder (Fig 2–42) and emphysematous cholecystitis in the gallbladder (Fig 2–43). Retroperitoneal gas usually appears as a series of streaky lucencies. In the upper abdomen, they are best seen just lateral to the vertebra, as they often parallel the long axis of the psoas muscle (Fig 2–44). Laterally and in the lower abdomen, the orientation of retroperitoneal streaks is less regular. A single streak may be the only plain finding of retroperitoneal gas and should not be misinterpreted as an inconsequential artifact (Fig 2–45).

Tubular Lucencies. Aside from gas in the appendix, all tubular lucencies are abnormal. Gas can enter the ureters from a fistula with the bowel or may

Figure 2–42. Emphysematous cystitis in a diabetic. Streaks in the vesical wall outline the bladder (*arrows*).

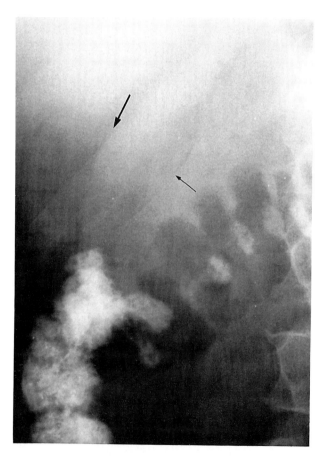

Figure 2–43. Emphysematous cholecystitis. The contrast in the colon is unabsorbed Telepaque. A faint streak outlines the medial border of the gallbladder wall (*small arrow*). The large arrow points to air in the gallbladder lumen.

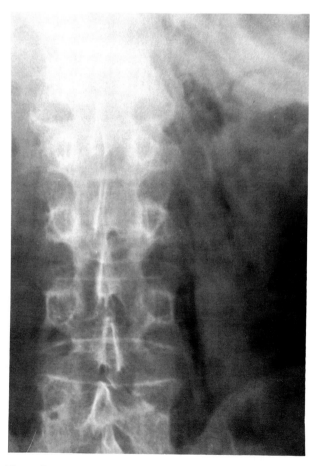

Figure 2–44. Perforated carcinoma of the sigmoid. Gas entered the retroperitoneum, appearing as streaks of lucency overlying the left psoas muscle.

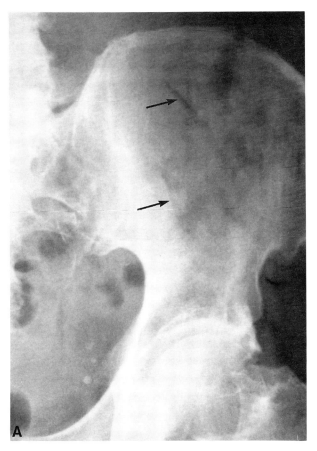

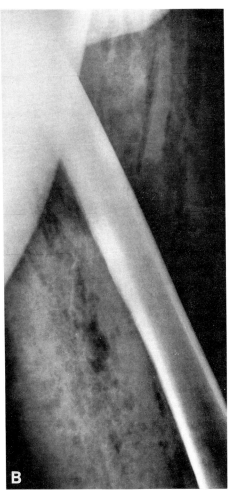

Figure 2–45. A diabetic patient with perforated sigmoid diverticulitis and gas gangrene of the left lower extremity. **A.** The only finding on this abdominal film is retroperitoneal streaks of gas in the left lower quadrant (*arrows*). **B.** Lateral film of the left femur—gas extends from the abdomen to the muscles of the thigh. Amputation was necessary.

be produced by gas-forming organisms residing in the urinary tract. In the right upper quadrant, a sparsely branching and obliquely oriented lucent conduit is a plain film evidence of air or gas in the biliary tree (Fig 2–46). A finely arborizing lucency extending more peripherally is pathognomonic for portal vein gas (Fig 1–5).

Large Lucencies. Hollow organs outside the tubular gastrointestinal tract may become gas filled. Typically, they appear as featureless lucencies whose shape conforms to the configuration of the organ itself. Thus, gas in the gallbladder is oblong or pear shaped (Figs 1–6, 2–47) whereas air in the urinary

bladder is round or elliptical with a lateral diameter greater than the width of the rectum (Fig 2–48). Air can be trapped in a vaginal tampon appearing as a broad, slightly curving band (Fig 2–49). Gas in the uterine corpus is most often in the form of large bubbles whose extent depends upon the size and orientation of the uterus (Fig 2–50).

A large extraintestinal gas lucency of amorphous configuration is most likely an abscess cavity. Often, smaller bubbles are situated close to the larger collections of pus. Even large abscesses appear surprisingly gray on plain films, not black like giant diverticula, because they usually contain much fluid as well as gas. They have irregular contours

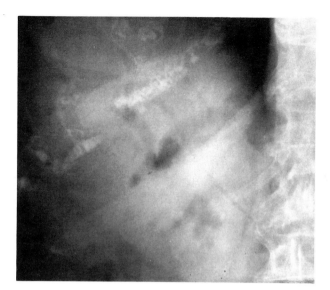

Figure 2–46. Gas in the biliary tree. The branching pattern of the gas-filled right and left hepatic ducts and the common bile duct is seen. The patient had a cholecystoduodenal fistula.

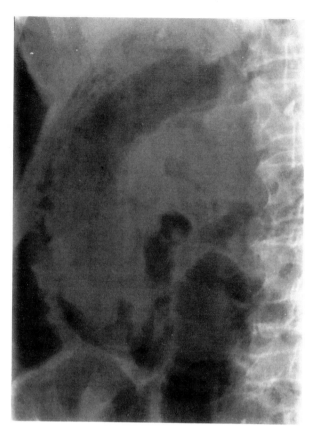

Figure 2–47. Emphysematous cholecystitis. Sausage-shaped gas in the gallbaldder lumen. Gas is also present in the gallbladder wall and in pericholecystic tissues (*Courtesy of Dr. Jutta Greweldinger*).

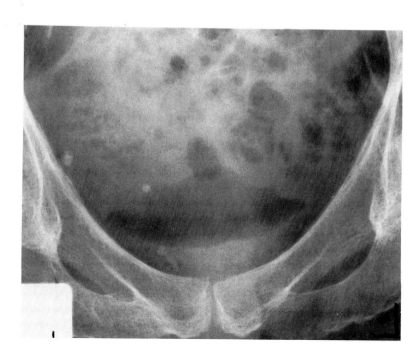

Figure 2–48. Air in a partially filled urinary bladder appears as a featureless, elliptical gas collection.

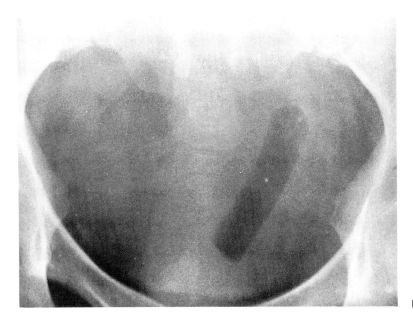

Figure 2–49. Air within a vaginal tampon.

and sometimes a poorly defined mass can be seen adjacent to or surrounding them (Fig 2–51). When abscesses form in solid organs such as the spleen or the kidney, they are frequently multilocular, with a complex inner architecture representing the destroyed parenchyma within them. Confined to peritoneal recesses such as Morison's pouch, abscesses tend to be more homogeneous. It is sometimes difficult to distinguish a large abscess from free interperitoneal air. Plain films in the erect and decubitus positions can reveal the extensive movement of free air whereas in an abscess, gas is confined to the focus of infection. Occasionally, large abscesses are undetected because they produce a localized intestinal ileus. The overlying gas-filled intestinal loops can shroud small bubbles and even obscure a single larger lucency. Moreover, an abscess cavity itself may mimic a segment of normal bowel (Fig 2–52). Necrotic tumors and ulcerated masses connecting to the gastrointestinal tract may also appear as large irregular lucencies and can be mistaken for abscesses (Fig 2–53).

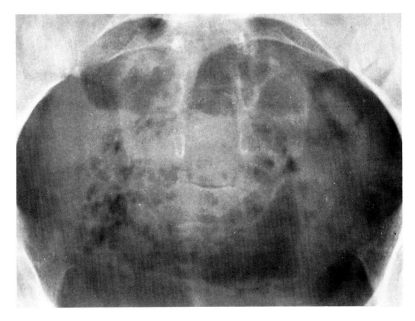

Figure 2–50. Mottled lucencies with small bubbles and larger air collections conform to the shape of an enlarged uterus. This patient had a septic abortion and the gas is confined to the uterine wall.

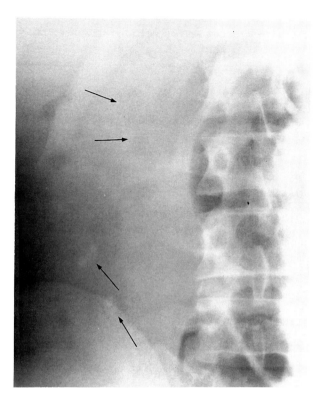

Figure 2–51. Subhepatic abscess secondary to perforated appendicitis. The lower arrows point to two calcified appendicoliths. The upper arrows identify a large abscess cavity partially filled with fluid. Smaller gas filled cavities are also present laterally and inferiorly.

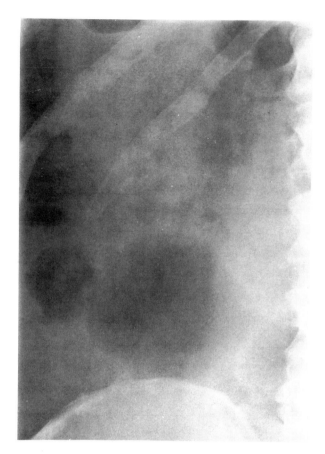

Figure 2–52. Periappendiceal abscess. A single large lucency resembles gas in the cecum.

Skin-based Lucencies. Ulcerations and surgical defects of the skin are additional causes of single amorphous lucencies. Similar to the gas collections of intra-abdominal abscesses, they may have a homogeneous appearance with irregular contours. Because they contain air and no liquid, they are almost always very sharply defined. Decubitus ulcers in the pelvis often overlie the course of the ileum and rectum and may be confused with bowel gas. These skin lesions lack valvulae conniventes or haustra, which help identify the small and large intestines (Fig 2–54).

In elderly patients with poor skin turgor and redundant dermal folds, air can be trapped between the abdominal wall and the surface of the radiographic table. Although the air is outside the patient, it is nevertheless within the path of the radiographic beam and therefore appears as an extensive featureless black shadow that conforms to no anatomic structure. If it is superimposed over the flanks, it is sharply marginated medially at its interface with the skin but it fades imperceptibly into the ambient air laterally. Often, several parallel lines are found within the large lucency demarcating a series of skin folds surrounded by air (Fig 2–55). A striking lucency that straddles the mid line in the lower abdominal region may occur in elderly indi-

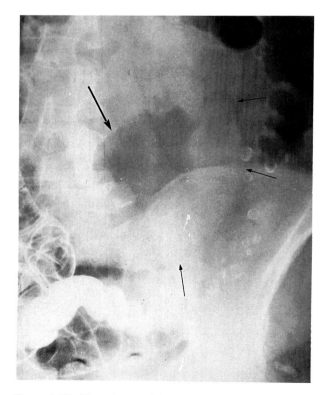

Figure 2–53. Ulcerating small bowel leiomyosarcoma communicating with the intestinal lumen. The irregular lucency is a large ulceration (*long arrow*). The surrounding mass can also be seen (*short arrows*).

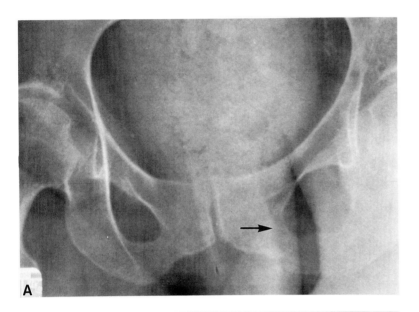

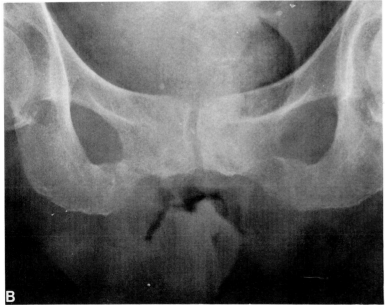

Figure 2–54. A. This oblong lucency (*arrow*) represents air in a decubitus ulcer in a paraplegic patient. **B.** Irregular lucency below the symphysis pubis is air trapped in an ulcer in a patient with a necrotic vaginal carcinoma.

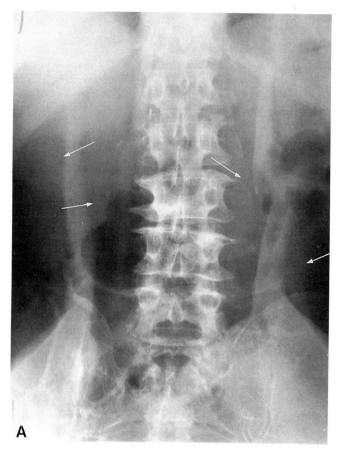

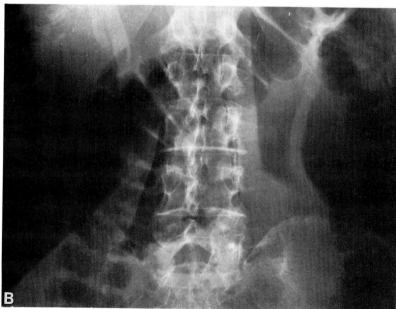

Figure 2–55. A. Each arrow points to a separate air pocket outside the patient delimited by folds of skin. **B.** Another patient with angulated collections of air bordered by skin folds. Superimposed on bowel gas, they create a confusing pattern of lucencies.

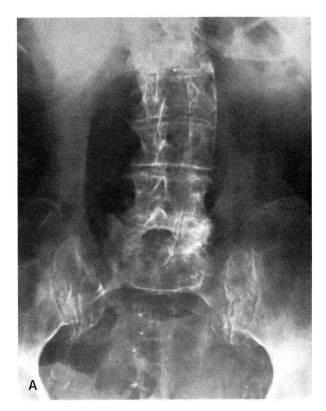
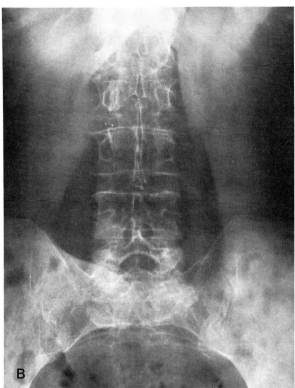

Figure 2–56. Two different patients **(A)** and **(B)** with central skin fold lucencies. Lumbar lordosis allows air to collect beneath the spine and above the table top.

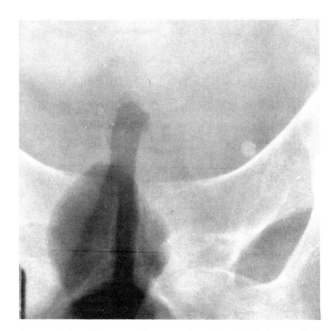

Figure 2–57. Air trapped between the gluteal folds in a patient who has had a recent loss of weight. There was no skin ulceration or other abnormality.

viduals who have an accentuated lumbar lordosis. In the supine position, a hollow is created between the spine and the table top. Its inferior border is the point of contact between the supporting surface and the skin overlying the sacrum (Fig 2–56). Air may also be trapped between the buttocks, creating peculiar patterns of decreased density (Fig 2–57). These skin fold lucencies are often persistent on successive supine films but changing position will reveal their true nature as they disappear on prone, erect, or decubitus views. Typically, they have a bizarre and unmistakable appearance, and yet, on occasion, they can closely mimic pathological intra-abdominal lucencies and should always be considered in the differential diagnosis of extraluminal gas.

FAT

Fat casts a faintly lucent shadow, not quite as black as air but much less bright than solid structures or liquid-filled organs and masses. Especially in the pelvis and retroperitoneal spaces, accumulations of fat are variable in abundance but relatively constant in location. The intimate and predictable spatial relationship between adipose tissue and muscle permits the recognition of two well-known landmarks on plain films of the abdomen—the properitoneal fat line and the lateral margin of the psoas major muscle.

Normal Fat

Normal deposits of fat adjacent to solid organs outline the visceral contours. The appendices epiploica are lipid-laden bodies affixed to the wall of the large intestine. In some patients, they are scanty but in others are so ample that they encircle the wall of the large bowel. Occasionally, fat can be found in the omentum and in mesenteric leaves. Also, aggregations of adipose tissue are distinctive plain film markers of intra-abdominal fat-containing tumors.

The Properitoneal Fat Stripe

On supine radiographs, fat is arrayed in strips that outline the muscles of the lateral abdominal wall. Additional fat planes separate the muscles from the skin and from the peritoneal cavity. In the dermis, epithelial, and connective tissue it can usually be distinguished from the broader subcutaneous layer, which is often heavily invested by fat. Thinner and more sharply defined lucent bands are interposed between the external oblique, internal oblique, and transversalis muscles. The properitoneal fat line is the lateral extension of the posterior pararenal retroperitoneal space (Fig 2–58). As such, it is in continuity with the continuous circumferential band of fat that connects the subcutaneous tissue around the umbilicus with the retroperitoneum.

The lucent properitoneal fat line can be obliterated by retroperitoneal effusions, pus, and blood. Occasionally, focal loss of the properitoneal fat line is caused by lateral extension of an intraperitoneal tumor or abscess. The properitoneal fat line can vary considerably in width depending upon the extent of body fat. It becomes more prominent in patients who are on long-term, high-dose corticosteroid medications, which cause truncal obesity. In overweight individuals, it appears as a broad band of lucency oriented vertically in the mid abdomen but curving medially as it descends in the pelvis. On the right side, the properitoneal fat is continuous with the retroperitoneal fat that defines the inferior angle of the liver. A more slender fat line extends superiolateral to the caudal hepatic margin. In thin persons, extraperitoneal fat may be too limited to produce a clearly defined lucent stripe. Focal narrowing of the properitoneal fat line can be caused by gaseous distention of the colon. Diffuse narrowing of the fat line with lateral displacement occurs in mas-

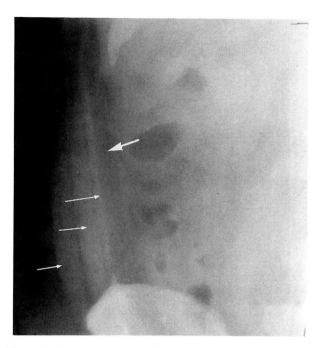

Figure 2–58. The lateral abdominal wall. From lateral to medial the three small arrows are placed on the external oblique, internal oblique, and transversalis muscle, respectively. Fat is interposed between the muscles. Between the transversalis muscle and the bowel is the properitoneal fat line.

sive ascites (Fig 2–59). On overpenetrated films, the technical reduction of contrast tends to diminish differences in density between soft tissue structures. Thus, the loss of the properitoneal fat line should only be relied upon in films of adequate quality obtained in well-nourished or obese patients.

Loss of the properitoneal fat stripe should be regarded as an auxiliary sign occasionally helpful along with other findings of retroperitoneal inflammation or hemorrhage. It should never secure a diagnosis by itself, however. The great variability of properitoneal fat along with its frequent lack of symmetry, restricts its effectiveness as an indicator of disease.

Widening of the distance between an intact properitoneal fat line and the wall of the ascending or descending colon suggests intraperitoneal disease. Ascitic fluid, abscess, and hemoperitoneum may all displace the large bowel medially (Fig 2–59).

Not all lucencies immediately lateral to the properitoneal wall are fat. Massive amounts of extraperitoneal air can infiltrate the properitoneal fat stripe, often widening it as it dissects anteriorly (Fig 2–60). This is an important, but rarely emphasized, sign of pneumoretroperitoneum. Moreover, the presence of focal collections of gas peripheral to the well-defined properitoneal fat line suggests a local-

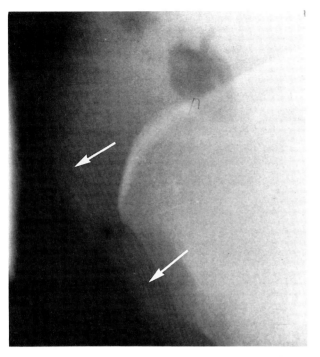

Figure 2–59. Lateral displacement and compression of the pro-peritoneal fat line by ascites (*arrows*). The gas-filled bowel has been displaced medially.

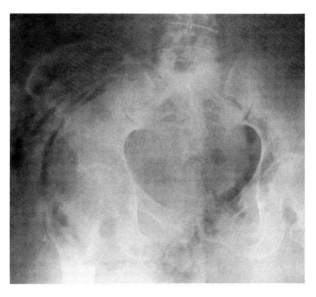

Figure 2–61. Gas outside the expected position of the properitoneal fat line. This patient has a large ventral hernia that has incarcerated. The streaks represent gas in the tissue plane in an infarcted abdominal wall.

ized abscess, herniation of bowel loops through a defect of the abdominal wall, or necrosis of the wall itself (Fig 2–61).

The Psoas Sign

Fat in the posterior pararenal retroperitoneal space is situated adjacent to the lateral edge of the psoas

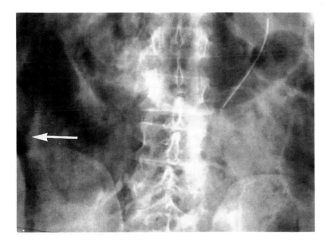

Figure 2–60. Pneumoretroperitoneum. Air entered the retroperitoneum after perforation of a duodenal diverticulum at endoscopy. In addition to mottled lucencies overlying the right kidney, air has penetrated the right properitoneal line (*arrow*).

muscle. It is this intimate juxtaposition of fat and water density that enables the psoas muscle to be seen on supine radiographs. The search for the psoas margin is part of the ritual of plain film interpretation. In most clinical circumstances, however, it is a sign of limited value.

The psoas originates from the transverse processes of the upper lumbar vertebrae and joins the iliacus muscle in the pelvis before inserting on the lesser trochanter of the femur. Its lateral margin describes a straight line oblique to the vertebral axis as it extends from the upper abdomen inferiorly.

Inflammation, tumor, or abscess confined entirely to the psoas muscle should not affect the interface between it and adjacent retroperitoneal fat. If the edge of the psoas is overlain by distended, gas- or feces-filled colonic segments, however, it will not be well seen. Moreover, a slightly oblique film can obscure the psoas line because abundant retroperitoneal fat may not extend as far forward as the anterior surface of the muscle. Hence, if the supine patient turns slightly toward one side, the radiographic beam may not pass through a sharp muscle–fat interface (the fat is now posterior rather than lateral to the muscle), thus causing the ipsilateral psoas line to be lost (Fig 2–62). With these limitations in mind, absent psoas shadows, even if unilateral, have little clinical significance.

An intact psoas line is more valuable because preservation indicates intact retroperitoneal fat lateral to the muscle. Moreover, a unilateral convexity

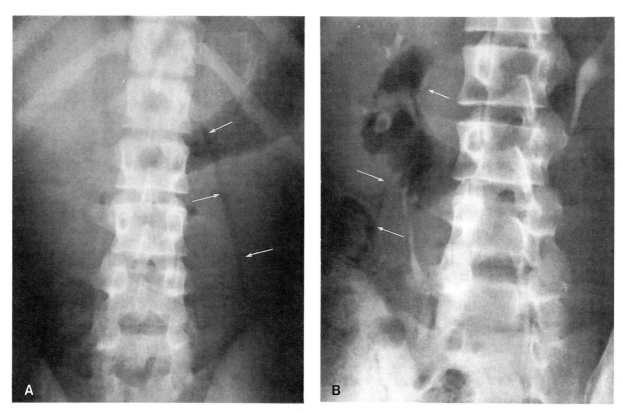

Figure 2–62. A. Scout film for an intravenous urography. The left psoas line is well seen (*arrow*). The right psoas margin is indistinct. **B.** Ten-minute film. Now the right psoas line is sharp and the upper left psoas is obscured. Slight obliquity of the patient can markedly affect visualization of the psoas line.

of the psoas muscle contour suggests an intramuscular mass or abscess (Fig 2–63). Bilateral psoas muscle convexity is found in well-developed men and is almost always a normal finding (Fig 2–64). An increase in brightness of one psoas without a change of its size is a helpful sign of a separate mass superimposed on the muscle shadow (Fig 2–65).

Occasionally, fat outlines the lateral margin of the quadratus lumborum muscle (Fig 2–66). As this structure is much thinner than the psoas major, the fat line demarcating it is usually more faint. Furthermore, the quadratus lumborum muscle extends more lateral than the psoas and should not be mistaken for it.

Pelvic Fat

A generous accumulation of fat in the pelvis can be an aid in differentiating masses in that region. At times, it is difficult to clearly distinguish bladder distension from ovarian tumors or uterine enlargement. Usually, a layer of fat accompanies the vesical dome (Fig 2–67). Recognition of this thin lucent stripe will define the superior border of the bladder and help separate it from other masses situated above.

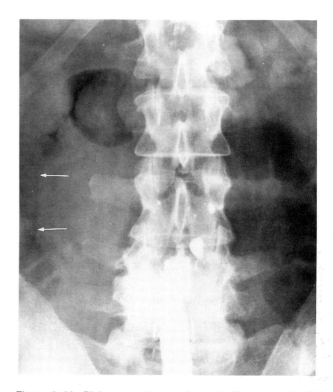

Figure 2–63. Right psoas abscess (*arrows*). The enlarged right psoas is convex laterally but the fat plane is intact. The left psoas is normal.

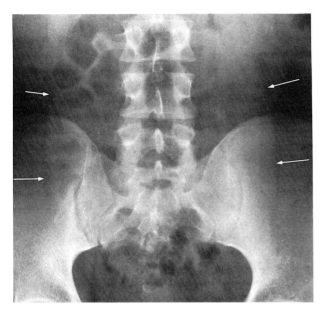

Figure 2–64. A weightlifter with hypertrophied psoas muscles, both of which bulge laterally (*arrows*).

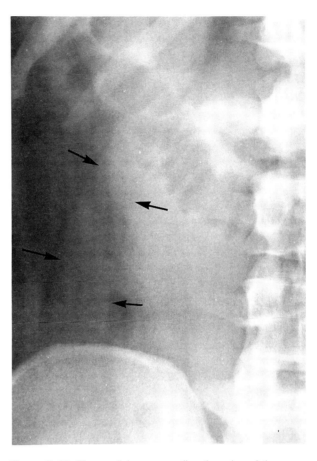

Figure 2–66. The medial arrows outline the edge of the psoas muscle. The lateral arrows point to the quadratus lumborum muscle.

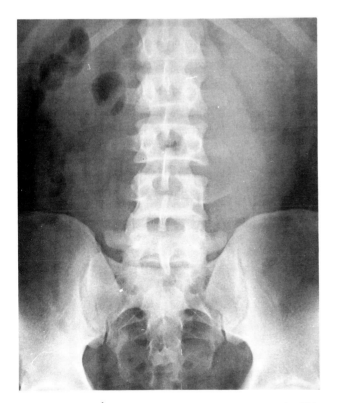

Figure 2–65. Increase in density of the left psoas muscle. This was the only plain film finding of a large lymphomatous mass in the left anterior pararenal space. The psoas was uninvolved by the mass.

Fat also abuts on the rectum and on the perineal muscles. In patients who have lost muscle mass, fat may interdigitate between the obliquely oriented fibers of the levator ani muscle. Sometimes, intramuscular strips of fat simulate stripes of gas in retroperitoneal tissues. The localization of fat in the course of the levator ani and its frequent bilateral appearance identify this innocuous finding, however. (Fig 2–68). Elsewhere in the pelvis, the displacement of fat by water density masses occasionally allows recognition of tumors or abscesses on plain films.

Retroperitoneal Fat

Fat is a major constituent of the posterior pararenal space and the perirenal space. It is contiguous with the posterior edge of the liver, helping to outline the caudal hepatic edge. Often, there is sufficient fat around the kidneys to permit delineation of the lateral, superior, and inferior renal margins. Masses in the kidney can be seen on plain films, primarily because they are separable from other retroperitoneal structures by perirenal fat. Although the adrenal

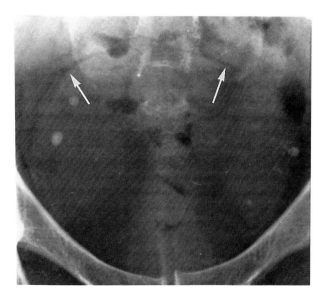

Figure 2–67. A well-defined strip of fat caps the dome of the distended bladder (*arrows*). There is extensive fat throughout the pelvis.

glands lie in a bed of adipose tissue, their small size limits plain film identification. The pancreas is almost never seen on scout radiographs of the abdomen because there is insufficient fat surrounding it. Occasionally, fat can extend lateral to the spleen and even beneath the left hemidiaphragm, where it can simulate a pneumoperitoneum (Fig 2–69).

Retroperitoneal adipose tissue usually imparts a homogeneous lucency. If the fat is infiltrated by blood, pus, or pancreatic juices, however, the retroperitoneum may have a mottled appearance on

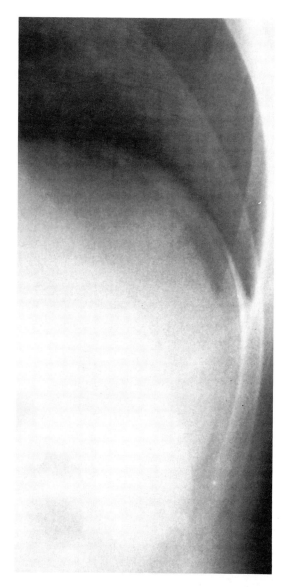

Figure 2–69. A curvilinear band of fat around the posterior spleen lies just below the left hemidiaphragm and mimics free air in the peritoneal cavity.

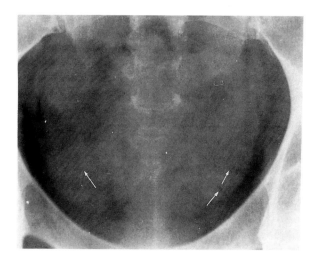

Figure 2–68. Faint, obliquely oriented strips of fat can be seen in both the right and left levator ani muscles (*arrows*). A normal finding.

plain films, as the water density of retroperitoneal fluid insinuates itself in the connective tissue planes in this region. The radiographic evidence of these effusions can resemble the irregular lucencies and densities of a gas-containing abscess. In such situations, a definitive diagnosis is not achievable by plain films and computed tomography is necessary for further evaluation.

Intraperitoneal Fat

In patients with large and numerous appendices epiploica, fat may virtually envelop the bowel wall. On plain films of the abdomen, aggregations of these normal fatty bodies permit visualization of the colonic wall even though there may be no gas within its lumen (Fig 2–70). On films of excellent quality, the margin of much of the ascending, transverse, and descending colons can be seen in obese patients. Moreover, the outer surface of small bowel loops can be discernible if they border pericolic fat (Fig 2–71).

Fat-Containing Tumors

Cystic teratoma of the ovary is the most common abdominal tumor recognized by its fat content on plain films. The adipose tissue in these lesions should never be confused with normal pelvic fat. Almost always, the faint lucency within the tumor is clearly demarcated and appears less black than nearby bowel gas. It may resemble gas within an abscess but there is rarely a gas–fat level on upright films in cystic teratomas of the ovary, whereas gas–fluid levels should be expected in abscesses manifested by a large, single lucency on supine films (Fig 2–72). Cystic teratomas frequently contain teeth or bone along with fat, the combination of which is pathognomonic on plain films.

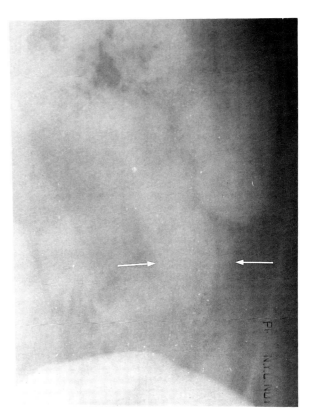

Figure 2–71. The walls of fluid filled small bowel loops can be seen as they abut pericolic and properitoneal fat (*arrows*).

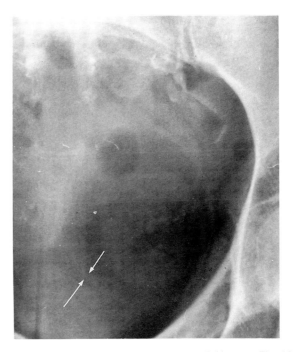

Figure 2–72. A large cystic teratoma of the (left) ovary. The thin ovoid line delimiting the tumor is the water density cyst wall (*arrows*). It can be seen because it is situated between fat within the tumor and pelvic fat outside of it.

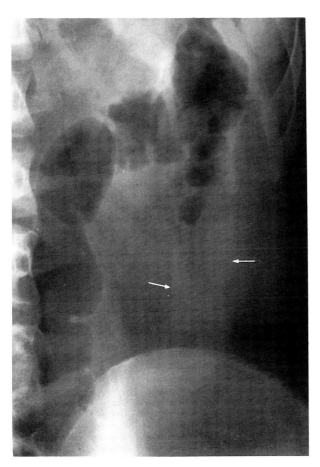

Figure 2–70. Pericolic and properitoneal fat bring into relief the wall of the descending colon (*arrows*).

Benign lipomas of the flank or back appear as well-delimited lucencies. Liposarcomas have a predilection for the retroperitoneum. They may contain only scattered fragments of fat and thus a definitive diagnosis is often not apparent on plain films even if a large mass is seen. If both lucencies and streaky calcifications are present, however, the diagnosis can be suggested. In actuality, the characteristic plain film findings of liposarcoma are unusual and the tumor is detected by the displacement of adjacent organs rather than the observation of fat within it.

Retroperitoneal teratomas also contain fat but their typical appearance depends upon the formation of teeth or bone. The fat in these tumors is rarely a major roentgenologic feature.

SOFT TISSUE DENSITIES

The abdomen is occupied by organs whose predominant chemical constituent is water. These viscera, both solid and hollow, along with their feeding and draining vessels, lie in close proximity to one another, often with their surfaces in direct contact. Since the X-ray beam cannot discern the contour of two structures of similar density along the plane at which they abut, enlargement of organs and the presence of masses may often go undetected on plain abdominal roentgenographs. Visualization is aided by the displacement of adjacent gas or fat. On the skin and near the lumen of the colon and stomach even small lesions are recognizable as they project into the lucent background provided by ambient air or intestinal gas. Renal masses can be suggested by their effect on fat in the perirenal space. In other abdominal locations, however, such as the lower abdomen and pelvis, the frequent absence of normal low-density landmarks makes it more difficult to diagnose masses or organ enlargements on plain films. Thus, clinically silent tumefactions may attain a large size before they are recognized radiographically. It is important, therefore, to appreciate subtle signs of displacement of contiguous structures on plain films so that appropriate decisions about more definitive imaging tests can be made.

Skin-Based Masses

Masses that lie upon or project through the skin can be very clearly defined on plain radiographs because they are nearly surrounded by ambient air. Almost always, the patient and referring physician are aware of these lesions because they are obvious at inspection of the abdominal wall. The problem on plain films is not detection but correct interpretation because they may be erroneously considered to be located intra-abdominally rather than superficially.

A criterion of these lesions is their sharp margination, which allows even relatively small epidermal excrescences to be seen. It is crucial not to assign these rounded densities to the wall or the lumen of the gastrointestinal tract even though they may overlie the lumen of the colon, small intestine, or stomach on a single plain radiograph. In neurofibromatosis, skin protuberances are usually multiple and although some seem to lie within the bowel, others are clearly situated outside intestinal lumens (Fig 2–73).

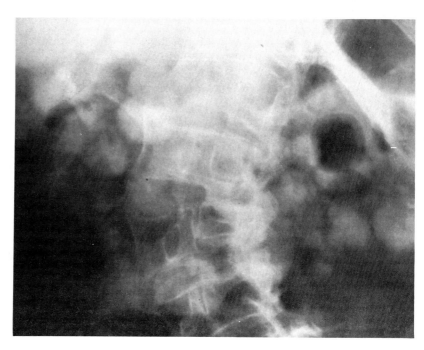

Figure 2–73. Neurofibromatosis. Numerous round masses of varying size stand out clearly because they protrude from the skin.

A large ventral hernia can extend far from the anterior abdominal wall. The intensely sharp contrast between ambient air and the water density of the sac and its intraperitoneal contents makes the lumen appear even denser than the rest of the abdomen (Fig 2–74). The sign of heightened brightness is also a characteristic feature of protruding masses. Evisceration of small bowel loops is an extreme example of a mass extending beyond the contour of the trunk. The abrupt difference between air and bowel is so marked that the intestinal loops seem to be opacified by contrast material whereas, in fact, it is the surrounding lucency that makes them appear so opaque (Fig 2–75).

Another clue to the location of these projecting lesions is the incomplete border sign. If the mass protrudes at right angles from the normal skin surface with its long axis oriented along the path of the beam, it will be sharply marginated throughout its circumference because at all points air is interposed between the skin and the mass. If its long axis is in profile or oblique to the radiographic beam, however, its border will be indistinct at the site of anchorage to the skin because both the mass and the

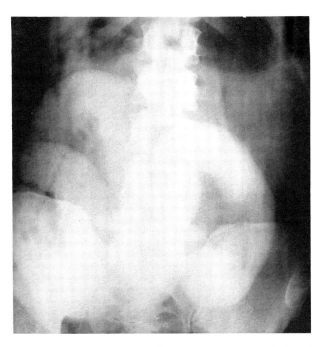

Figure 2–75. This patient received no contrast material. Bowel loops are sharply delimited because they lie on the abdominal wall. The patient suffered an eviscerating stab wound.

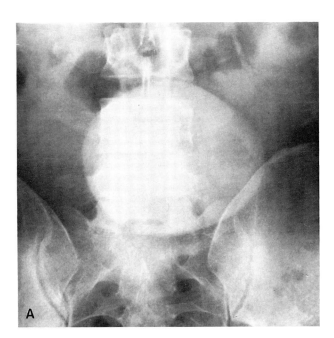

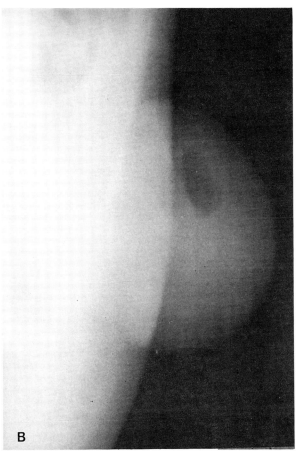

Figure 2–74. Protuberant ventral hernia. **A.** Supine view demonstrates very clear definition because the hernia is encircled by air. **B.** Cross table lateral view clearly shows the projecting hernia with bowel gas within it.

contiguous skin are of similar density (Fig 2–76).

In an obese person, redundant fat rolls may trap air between them. This is seen just above the buttocks. Large, subcutaneous, soft tissue masses in overweight patients can distort the symmetry of fat folds, enabling them to be detected on plain films (Fig 2–77).

Marked stretching of the panniculus by subcutaneous fat can be recognized by a wide convex downward arc overlying the pelvis. The panniculus is broader than the peritoneal cavity and extends lateral to the properitoneal fat line. In most patients, it appears as a smooth, uninterrupted interface, but after a lower abdominal operation, scar formation retracts the skin and causes a focal indentation or puckering (Fig 2–78).[4]

Organomegaly and Masses

Plain film delineation of organomegaly and intra-abdominal tumors depends upon a careful analysis of displacement of adjacent structures. Most solid and hollow organs can be pushed by enlarging masses. The stomach and transverse colon are particularly mobile. In general, structures closer to a mass are more profoundly displaced than those further away. For example, marked relocation of the transverse colon suggests a lesion that extends an-

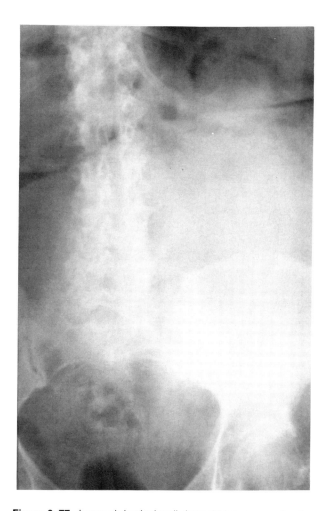

Figure 2–77. Large abdominal wall desmoid tumor occupies the left side of the abdomen. Its superficial location is evidenced by the asymmetric sharp superior edge where it is bordered by ambient air.

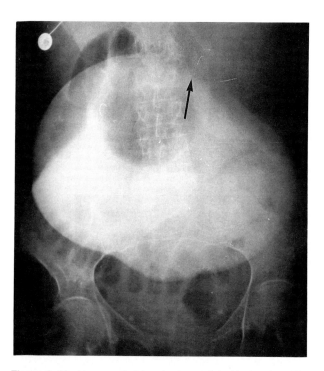

Figure 2–76. Huge ventral hernia. Incomplete border sign. The margins of the hernia are distinct except for a site of attachment to the abdominal wall that is oblique to the radiographic beam (*arrow*).

teriorly whereas repositioning and reorientation of the kidney indicates a posteriorly situated tumefaction. Since most plain films are obtained with the patient in the supine position, medial–lateral or superior–inferior displacements are easier to recognize than anterior–posterior displacements, which are directed along the path of the radiographic beam.

More distant consequences of abscesses and tumors are occasionally encountered as well. The spread of pus, blood, or tumor along the transverse mesocolon from pancreas to colonic wall or along the small bowel mesentery to the air-filled cecum are classic examples of the dissemination of disease within selected routes in the peritoneal cavity.

In the upper abdomen, the vector principle first described by Whalan and colleagues is an important means of localization of masses of water density.[5,6]

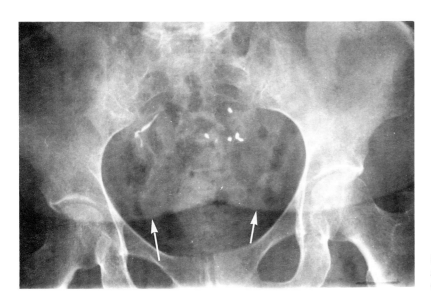

Figure 2–78. The puckered panniculus sign. An indentation of the panniculus (*arrows*) indicates previous abdominal surgery.

It relates the direction of movement of normal structures as they accommodate themselves to the growth of organs or masses. On plain films, the gas-filled stomach, transverse colon, hepatic and splenic flexures, and renal outlines are frequently used in vector analyses. This means of evaluation of organ displacement is particularly valuable for the localization of small to moderate-sized masses. Very large lesions cause such marked disruption that a site of origin is often not ascertainable by measuring organ displacement alone.

Hepatomegaly can be focal or diffuse. An enlarging liver often pushes the hepatic flexure downward. This finding may be difficult to determine because there is a wide range of normal locations for the hepatic flexure. Usually, the proximal transverse colon passes over the lower pole of the right kidney. If the hepatic flexure appears low and the transverse colon is also located below the right renal shadow, enlargement of the anterior liver should be considered. An additional finding of hepatomegaly is extension of the hepatic shadow across the right psoas margin (Fig 2–79). Posterior hepatomegaly may depress the right kidney inferiorly. Masses in the left lobe of the liver can deviate the stomach laterally (Fig 2–80) and depress the gas-filled lesser curvature. Hepatomegaly as well as subphrenic masses can elevate the right hemidiaphragm. Gallbladder enlargement is occasionally seen on plain films. Characteristically, it causes inferior displacement and depression of the proximal transverse colon (Fig 2–81).

The spleen can enlarge medially, inferiorly, or in both directions (Fig 2–82). Inferiorly oriented

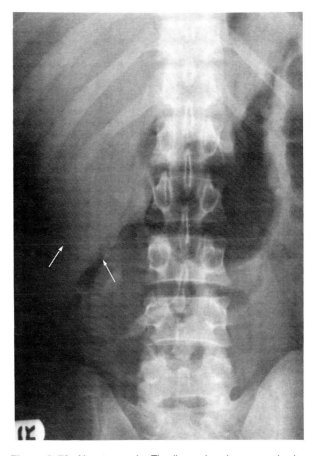

Figure 2–79. Hepatomegaly. The liver edge depresses the hepatic flexure below the lower margin of the right kidney (*arrows*). The liver also extends across the superior right psoas margin.

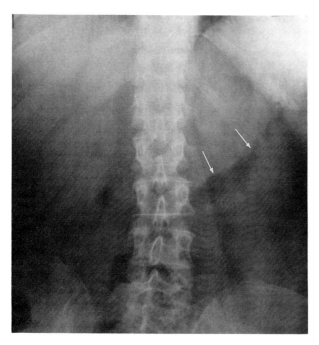

Figure 2–80. Marked hepatomegaly. Deviation of the stomach laterally and inferiorly (*arrows*).

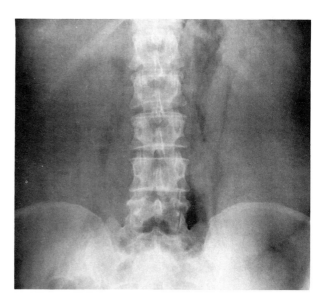

Figure 2–82. A large spleen pushes the stomach medially. Its inferior edge extends below the left iliac crest.

splenomegaly most markedly affects the splenic flexure, which is depressed downward. It can also displace the left kidney inferiorly as well as alter its axis or it can grow anteriorly, leaving the kidney undisturbed (Fig 2–83). Medial splenic enlargement can be appreciated on plain films by a lateral impression on the greater curvature of the stomach and by medial displacement of the air-filled gastric lumen. Unlike hepatic enlargement, splenomegaly rarely elevates the left hemidiaphragm.

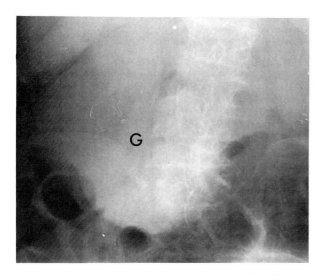

Figure 2–81. Hydrops of the gallbladder. A very big gallbladder (G) depresses the superior wall of the proximal transverse colon.

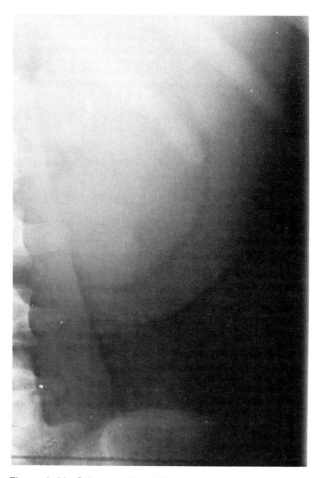

Figure 2–83. Splenomegaly. A large spleen extends anterior to the left kidney and left psoas muscle.

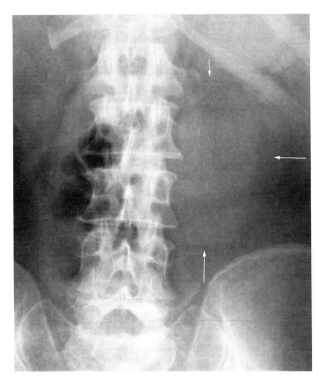

Figure 2–84. Left renal mass (*arrows*). The mass extends anterior to the left psoas muscle. Barium enema revealed depression of the distal transverse colon.

Gastric distension is usually recognized by air within its dilated lumen. At times, however, the stomach may be completely fluid filled and the key to its enlargement is the downward depression of the transverse colon (Fig 2–22). A large exogastric tumor of the stomach can push the transverse colon and sometimes even displace the right or left kidney. It may cause no disruption in the position of the stomach but typically it narrows the gastric lumen.

Tumors in the peritoneal recesses and their mesenteric attachments also produce predictable rearrangements of adjacent structures. A mass in the gastrocolic ligament is recognized by its upward impression on the greater curvature of the stomach and its downward impression on the transverse colon. Moreover, lesser sac abscesses, which often contain gas, may displace the stomach laterally.

Diffuse pancreatic enlargement is usually not seen on plain films because there is insufficient fat around the pancreas. Moreover, in pancreatitis, adjacent retroperitoneal fat is infiltrated by fluid. Pancreatic pseudocysts can form almost anywhere in the upper abdomen, thereby simulating masses arising from the adrenal glands, kidney, spleen, liver, stomach, and intestines. The unequivocal diagnosis

of a pseudocyst is not often made on the basis of plain film recognition of a water density mass. Almost always, a confirming test such as computed tomography or ultrasound is required.

In the right kidney, large masses in the lower pole often elevate the proximal transverse colon. Upper pole masses do not usually affect the colon, but a very large lesion may depress it (Fig 2–84). Left renal tumors generally displace the colon inferiorly. Straightening of the axis of the kidney may be caused by retroperitoneal, adrenal, or renal masses or by splenomegaly. Extension of the renal shadow across the psoas muscle suggests a horseshoe kidney. An adrenal mass often first comes to attention by rotation and downward deviation of the subadjacent kidney (Fig 2–85). Adrenal enlargement rarely influences the position of the transverse colon. Small retroperitoneal tumors are not detected on plain films unless they contain calcium. If they arise near the kidney, they can displace it anteriorly or laterally.

An area of paucity of intestinal gas may be the only plain film indication of an intraperitoneal tumor. Caution must be exercised before relying on this finding. It should only be used if there is extensive small bowel gas elsewhere in the abdomen (Fig 2–86). It has limited value in the right upper quadrant, where the small bowel is not usually located. In the left mid abdomen and left lower quadrant, the paucity of gas sign can be especially valuable as a clue to intestinal, mesenteric, or even retroperitoneal masses. It must be remembered that distended but gasless loops of small or large bowel can appear as a mass of water density. Simple obstruction, closed loop obstruction, and small bowel volvulus may all first appear as a soft tissue density, with normal or distended gas-filled loops displaced away from it.

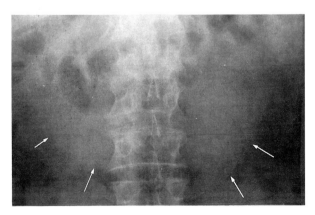

Figure 2–85. Horseshoe kidneys. The faint inferior right and left renal margins pass medially over the psoas muscles and the renal axes are strengthened (*arrows*).

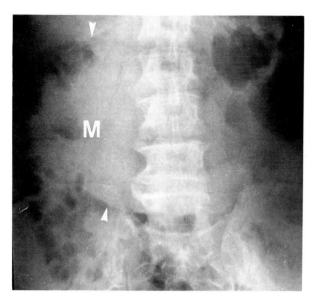

Figure 2–86. Paucity of gas in the right mid abdomen. The hepatic flexure is elevated. The superior and inferior extent of the mass (*arrowheads*) is delimited by intestinal gas. The mass (M) was a peritoneal cyst surrounding a retained lap pad.

The most common pelvic mass is a distended urinary bladder. As this is an anterior structure, vesical enlargement may occur without impingement on the air-filled small intestine, sigmoid colon, or rectum. It can appear as a diffuse haziness in the pelvis and lower abdomen with no other evidence of a mass (Fig 2–87). The presence of a fat stripe above the bladder distinguishes the normal vesical contours from uterine and adnexal masses. A characteristic feature of pelvic masses is their extension far into the abdomen (Fig 2–88). In the absence of calcification, which is a common feature of uterine leiomyomata, it is not possible to differentiate ovarian from uterine lesions with certainty. Other causes of pelvic masses include diverticula of the bladder, colonic tumors, small bowel tumors, and abscesses. Here too, plain film differentiation is limited unless gas, fat, or calcium are present. A cautionary note with any pelvic mass is to look closely at the integrity of the bony pelvis because osseous

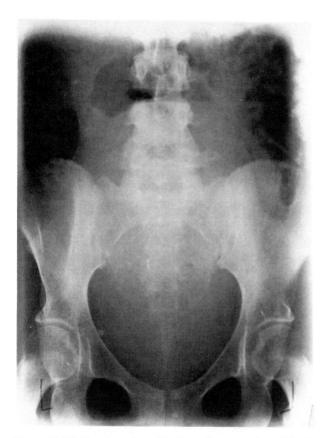

Figure 2–87. Massive urinary bladder enlargement in a diabetic patient. There is a homogeneous increase in opacity in the pelvis without evidence of a discrete mass. The bladder distends high up in the abdomen. Its superior extent is suggested by extrinsic pressure from below on a mid-abdominal gas loop.

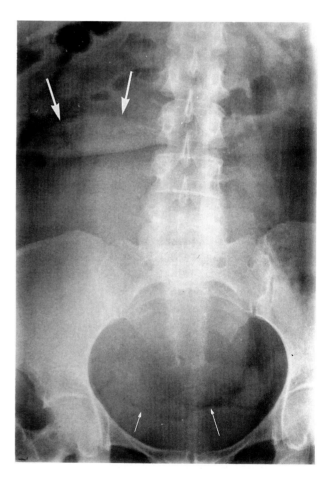

Figure 2–88. Serous cystadenoma of the ovary. This pelvic mass extends into the right abdomen (*upper arrows*). Its extravesical origin is indicated by the fat stripe above the bladder (*lower arrows*).

lesions emanating from the medial pelvic wall can extend into the pelvis, mimicking a soft tissue mass originating from the genitourinary or gastrointestinal tract.

CALCIFICATIONS

Numerous diseases can produce calcifications in the abdomen. Calcium deposition may occur in the walls of blood vessels and other conduits, within solid organs and tumors, and in the lumen of nearly every hollow structure. A systematic evaluation of the morphology, location, and mobility of any abnormal opacity can help narrow the etiologic considerations to a few very likely possibilities. In most cases, plain films offer sufficient information to permit a definitive diagnosis. At the very least, a careful assessment of appearance, position, and migration of a calcific density can direct the choice of subsequent imaging examinations.

Physiology

Calcification can be induced by marked and rapid elevations in serum calcium and phosphorous. The precipitation of calcium salts is also favored by an alkaline medium. Metastatic calcification refers to calcium deposition in normal tissues subjected to hypercalcemia and an elevated pH. It affects the kidney and stomach most often but the degree of parenchymal calcification is usually too limited to be seen on plain films. Radiographically, demonstrable metastatic calcification is infrequent, occurring in renal tubular acidosis, hyperparathyroidism, chronic renal failure, and occasionally with rapid bone destruction.[7] Far more common is dystrophic calcification, which occurs in vascular walls and in the stroma of solid organs in patients with normal serum calcium and phosphorous measurements. The histological disruption may be caused by trauma, ischemia, or necrosis. Hyaline collagen degeneration, a consequence of tissue damage, is particularly associated with calcium deposition. In tumors, rapid catabolism of lipids release fatty acids, which have an avidity for ionic calcium. Some mucin-producing tumors possess a glycoprotein that is biochemically similar to ossifying cartilage and thus a binder of calcium salts.[8] Although it is not always possible to single out the predominant factor that favors dystrophic calcification, the final common pathway leading to calcification is local tissue damage.

New bone formation in devitalized or degenerating tissue also occurs, but its incidence is much rarer than dystrophic calcification. It can appear as an isolated finding or in association with nonos-

seous calcium deposition. Factors that predispose to dystrophic calcification also promote bone production in previously normal tissue. It can be found in abdominal scars, retroperitoneal neoplasms, ovarian tumors, and occasionally in gastrointestinal malignancies. A less common form of calcium deposition, and one that occurs almost exclusively in ovarian serous cystadenocarcinoma, is psammomatous calcification. In dystrophic calcification, the deposition of calcium salts appears extracellularly. In psammomatous calcification, calcium is found intracellularly in growing tumor masses.[9]

Both local and systemic factors regulate stone formation in the liquid medium occupying the lumens of conduits and hollow organs. Hypercalcemia increases the possibility of renal, ureteral, and bladder stones. In the intestine, the gradient in pH from the duodenum to the ileum explains why calcified enteroliths occur in the distal small bowel but are not found in the more acidic duodenum. Additionally, local factors such as infection, debris formation, and obstruction with stasis also favor the growth of calculi. Stones may form in any blocked lumen, but their formation is enhanced if calcium concentration and pH are increased.

The mechanics and kinetics of calcium deposition still remain largely unknown. For example, it is not certain how and at what rate damaged tissues take up calcium. In most instances, however, calcification is a consequence of the interplay of recognizable local conditions and general factors.

Morphology

The formulation of a classification scheme for the morphology of abdominal calcification is difficult. Criteria that apply to a particular group of densities may be overly general to allow an explanation of a specific example or excessively detailed for practical application. Most previous surveys of abdominal calcifications have been descriptive and have avoided the issue of morphological differentiation of abdominal densities. The emphasis has been on the demonstration of the uniqueness of a number of individual densities. For example, the term "staghorn" is a description of a renal calculus occupying the pelvicalyceal system. As such, it serves to differentiate the appearance of that stone from other abdominal radiodensities. However, only a few calcifications are so easily identifiable by characteristic contours.

The features of value for a classification by morphology include shape, border sharpness, marginal continuity, and internal architecture. Consideration of these factors permits a grouping of abdominal calcification into four major morphological categories, each possessing a particular set of features. The four categories are concretions, conduit wall calcification, cystic wall calcification, and solid mass calcification. In the following sections, this classification scheme is discussed in detail. Mention is made of notable exceptions and potential pitfalls.

Concretions. A concretion is a calcified mass formed in the lumen of a vessel or hollow viscus. Concretions can be brightly or faintly calcified; the radiographic density depends upon the size of the opacity and the amount of calcium per unit volume. There are many sites at which concretions may form. The most common are the pelvic veins, the gallbladder, and the urinary tract. Concretions are created by the precipitation of calcium salts, as in renal calculi, or by calcium deposition in pre-existing venous thrombi with the development of phleboliths. Prostatic calculi occur predominantly in elderly males while appendicoliths are usually encountered in younger patients. Some concretions, such as pancreatic stones, appear to be influenced by inflammation but enteroliths and other densities have a more obscure etiology.

Concretions do not have a common shape. Small stones tend to be rounded or oval (Fig 2–89) whereas multiple gallstones are frequently faced (Fig 2–90) and urinary tract stones in a dilated pelvicalyceal system may also be faceted on at least one side of their perimeter. Calculi in the ureter are often angular but bladder stones are most often smooth. Occasionally, a unique form such as the

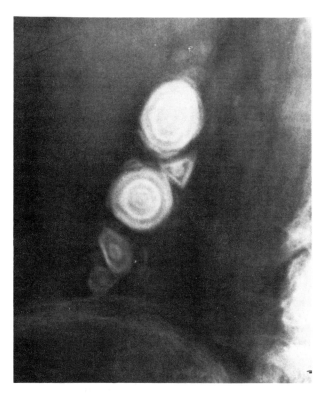

Figure 2–90. Calcified gallstones of varying shapes and sizes. Several of the stones are sharply faceted at points of interface with adjacent stones.

star-shaped bladder calculus is seen (Fig 2–91).

Concretions almost always exhibit a sharp, clearly defined external margin but occasionally may have irregular bulges (Fig 2–92). Stones are typically calcified throughout the entirety of their perimeter and almost always there are no discontinuities in

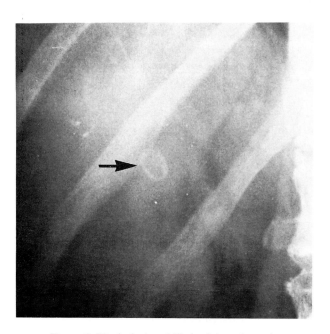

Figure 2–89. A single calcified gallstone (*arrow*).

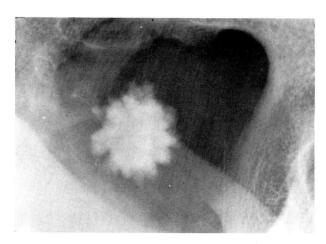

Figure 2–91. Oblique film of the pelvis. The star-shaped bladder calculus has symmetrically radiating projections, giving it a characteristic appearance.

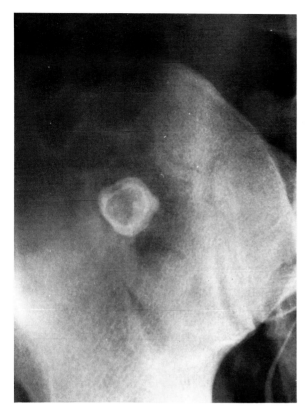

Figure 2–92. Appendicolith with a continuous margin of calcification and a small medial bulge of radiopacity.

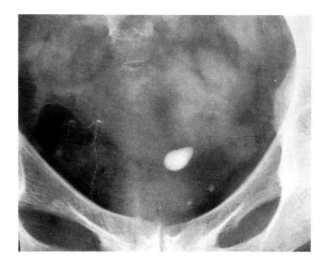

Figure 2–93. A stone in a ureterocele. Observe its homogeneous density and smooth contour.

their external margin. This is an important characteristic, especially if the interior of the concretion is radiolucent, because it helps to distinguish large stones from calcified cysts. If the outer ring of calcification is incomplete, it is unlikely to be a stone.

The internal architecture of concretions also encompasses a range of possibilities. They can be homogeneously dense, a pattern often encountered in urinary calculi (Fig 2–93), or they may have a slightly eccentric single lucency, an appearance that is typical of many phleboliths. Multiple laminations are an unequivocal indication of concretion morphology. Circumferential laminations are frequently encountered in gallstones, vesical calculi, and appendicoliths. Alternating bands of encircling lucency can be found within a concretion (Fig 2–94) or there may be a single dense band at or close to the external rim (Fig 2–95).

Each of these various internal patterns is quite distinctive. Laminations have a predictable parallel appearance. Usually, central lucencies are single. When there is only a marginal rim of calcification, its width is continuous with a minimally varied thickness throughout its circumference. The inner pattern of stones rarely assumes a mottled, whorled, or

patchy appearance. Even less common is the deposition of calcium on only one surface of a stone, which can be seen on plain radiographs as a streaky or amorphous focus of calcification (Fig 2–96). These exceptions notwithstanding, almost all stones exhibit geometric outlines and continuous contours.

Stones form within the lumens of preexisting conduits or hollow viscera. Unlike solid lesions or cysts, which are pathological masses that distort or displace normal organs, stones tend to remain within vessels or hollow viscera. When multiple cal-

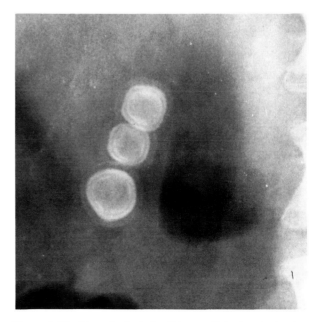

Figure 2–94. Three laminated gallstones. Note that the laminations are of varying density, with the outer ring the most faint.

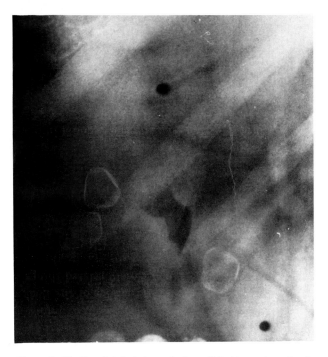

Figure 2–95. Two faceted stones in the gallbladder and another in the common bile duct. Calcification occupies only the margins of the calculi. Although the calcification is faint, it is circumferential in all three stones.

cific densities seem to be arrayed in a line, this indicates a common location in a hollow tube (Fig 2–97). Concretions are seldom seen outside expected locations. Examples are gallstones in the ileum or colon, appendicoliths in the peritoneal cavity or multiple phleboliths in a hemangioma (Fig 2–98). Generally, concretions do not pass through vascular or visceral walls and are seen in association with anatomic structures.

Conduit Wall Calcification. Conduits are hollow tubes through which fluids pass. In the abdomen, conduits include the components of the urinary tract, the pancreatic ducts, the vas deferens, the biliary ductal system, and the arteries and veins. Almost all conduit wall calcification in the abdomen involves the aorta and its branches. The tubular appearance of conduits is readily appreciated if the calcification is circumferential (Fig 2–99). En face, a ringlike density is often observed (Fig 2–100). In contrast to stones, discontinuities in the opaque ring are not rare or atypical. Since calcification in conduit walls is not uniform, lucent and radiodense areas are irregularly arrayed along the course of the vessel (Fig 2–101). However, calcification is confined only to the tubular walls. The presence of internal radi-

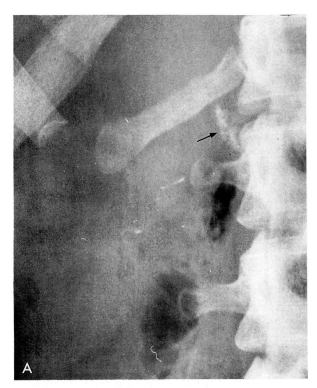
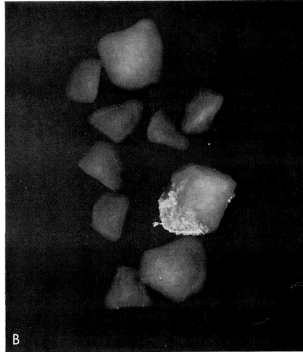

Figure 2–96. A. Irregular calcification in a cystic duct stone (*arrow*). **B.** The gallbladder was removed and radiographs of the stones were made. Note the dense calcification on only one side of the cystic duct stone (*arrowhead*) while the other calculi are only minimally calcified.

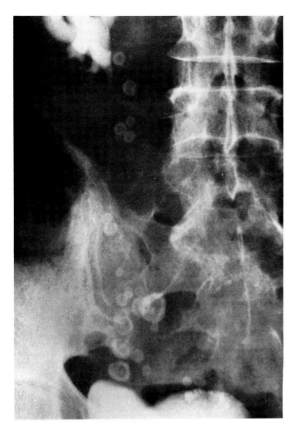

Figure 2–97. Multiple round densities adjacent to but outside the right ureter. All are phleboliths and the superior ones are in the right gonadal vein.

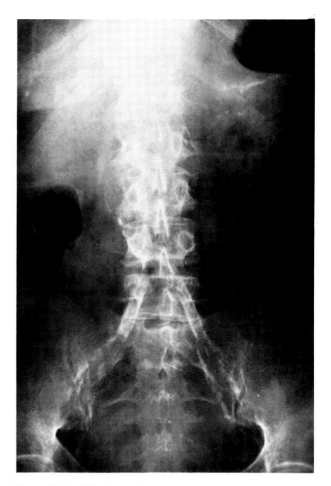

Figure 2–99. Tubular calcification characteristic of conduit morphology seen in both common iliac arteries and their branches.

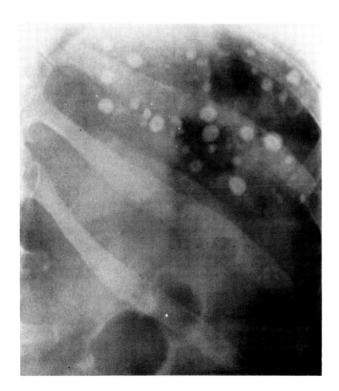

Figure 2–98. Multiple rounded concretions in the spleen. Some have central lucencies and most are greater than 5 mm in diameter. These are calcified phleboliths in a splenic hemagioma.

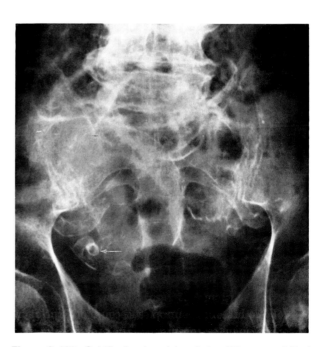

Figure 2–100. Calcification in pelvic arteries. Where a calcified vessel is seen en face it appears as a circle of radiopacity (*arrows*).

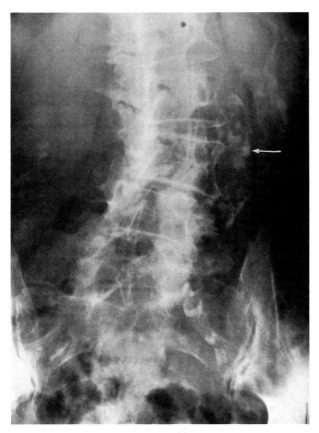

Figure 2–101. Plaques of calcification (*arrow*) in the abdominal aorta. Dense calcification may be seen in localized areas even if the X-ray beam does not pass through them tangentially.

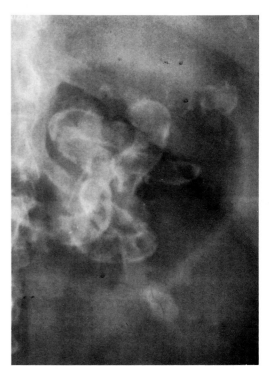

Figure 2–102. Calcification in the walls of a markedly convoluted splenic artery. Note the maintenance of parallel tracks of calcification despite the tortuosity of the vessel.

opacity suggests another morphological category.

As calcium deposition can occur throughout the circumference of a conduit, when the radiographic beam is directed perpendicular to the vessel, the margin presenting with the greatest wall thickness will appear most markedly calcified. Hence, in profile, conduit wall calcification is seen as parallel tracks of increased opacity (Fig 2–102). Although less common, a branching pattern is also characteristic of vessel wall calcification. This can be observed often at the bifurcation of the abdominal aorta and in intrarenal arterial classification (Fig 2–103). When a vessel of narrow caliber becomes densely calcified, it can have a stringlike appearance (Fig 2–104). In female pelves, a horizontal or a slightly undulated line of density often represents uterine artery calcification.

Conduit wall calcification is not always clearly recognizable, however. If there is only a single fleck of density, differentiation from a small calculus or from cortical bone is often difficult. This is especially true when it occurs in the region of the renal pelvis. Occasionally the question arises whether a linear

density signifies a calcification in the renal artery or the lateral margin of a vertebral transverse process (Fig 2–105). Since calcification within the vessel wall is not homogeneous, the margins of focal density may be indistinct or irregular.

Usually, conduit wall calcifications are found close to the expected location of a vessel. Hence, it

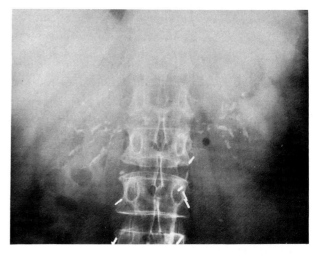

Figure 2–103. Bilateral calcification of the main renal arteries and the branching intrarenal arteries.

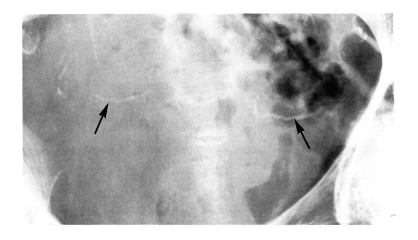

Figure 2–104. Bilateral uterine artery calcification (*arrows*). The lines of radiopacity represent calcification in these narrow vessels as they traverse the broad ligament.

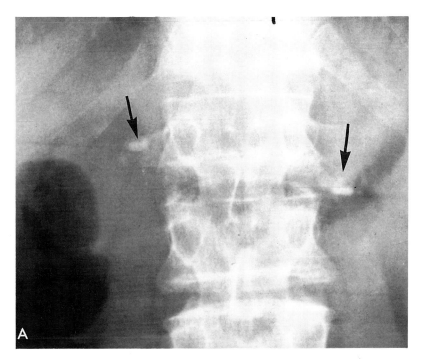

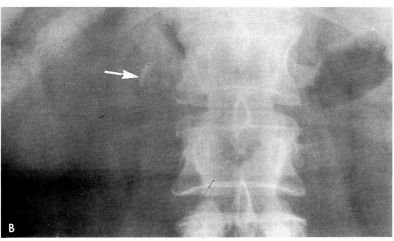

Figure 2–105. A. Bilateral focal renal artery calcification (*arrows*). Observe the horizontal orientation in the flecks of calcification in both arteries. **B.** A single linear density directed vertically cannot be a renal artery because of its orientation (*arrow*). In patients with bony demineralization, the ossified margin of a vertebral transverse process can be mistaken for arterial calcification.

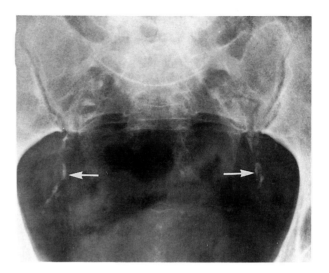

Figure 2–106. Calcification of the internal iliac arteries. Irregular plaques of the calcification are aligned in the direction of the internal iliac arteries (*arrows*).

would be unusual for conduit calcifications to be located at the lateral margin of the liver or spleen or in other peripheral locations. Dilated arteries, as well as those of normal caliber, may lengthen and become tortuous, however, residing several centimeters away from their expected location. For example, the abdominal aorta below the renal arteries may extend to the right side of the lumbar spine or far from the spine to the left and caudal to its normal bifurcation at L3 and L4.

Calcification can occur in either the medial or the intimal layer of the artery and both types have specific radiographical and pathological features. Intimal calcification results from deposition of calcium in arteriosclerotic plaques. Its presence indicates significant arterial disease and suggests the likelihood of vascular narrowing, especially in medium and small arteries. Arteriosclerotic plaques are patchy and the calcium deposits within them are focal and irregular in appearance. Almost all cases of asymmetric vascular calcification, whether in renal arteries, iliac arteries (Fig 2–106), or aorta, represent intimal calcification. Calcified plaques can be very extensive, resulting in thick, rough, amorphous calcification aligned along the course of the artery.

Medial calcification, first described by Monckeberg, is found entirely within the tunica media of the arteries, sparing both intimal and external elastic membranes. Medial calcification occurs primarily in the small and medium-sized muscular arteries and is most frequently seen in the pelvis, particularly in the iliac artery and its branches. In and near the kidneys, renal calcification is detected by smooth, continuous accumulations of calcium without focal irregularities or disruptions. The width of the band of calcification is unvarying and the density of de-

posits is uniform throughout the extent of the vessel (Fig 2–107).

The recognition of arterial calcification is usually easy if the calcification is extensive. However, if calcium deposition is focal and limited, it may often be missed or misinterpreted. Vascular calcification is oriented along the course of a vessel, and a single calcific deposit reflects that orientation. Commonly, it appears as a thin line or streaks of density, but in the internal or common iliac arteries focal calcification may be more irregularly shaped. Limited vascular calcification can occur in any vessel but is most common in the aorta, internal and common iliac arteries, renal arteries, and splenic artery.

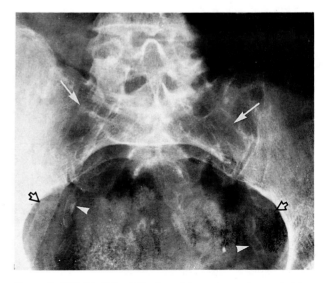

Figure 2–107. Medial calcification of the common (*arrows*), internal (*white arrowheads*), and external iliac arteries (*open black arrowheads*). Note the smooth, uniform linear calcification.

Cystic Calcification. In this discussion, a cystic calcification is any calcium deposition in the wall of an abnormal fluid-filled mass. Included in this category are epithelial-lined true cysts, pseudocysts that have a fibrous integument, and spherical and ovoid aneurysms. Although cysts are of varying types with differing histological appearances and etiologies, they all share readily recognizable patterns of calcifications. Crucial for the cystic pattern is the presence of a smooth, curvilinear rim of opacity (Fig 2–108). Although arcuate linear radiopacities can be seen in both conduits and cyst walls, the calcific rim of a cyst usually has a larger diameter than that of a conduit. However, the calcific rim need not be complete. Occasionally, only a portion of the wall may be radiodense (Fig 2–109). This is in sharp distinction to concretions where a complete rim of calcification is a hallmark. Since cysts usually have one encircling wall, they are rarely laminated. An incompletely calcified single margin indicates the presence of a cystic density, rather than a concretion.

Cysts are not always exquisitely round. They may be compressed on one side or they may have an oval configuration (Fig 2–110). The shape of a

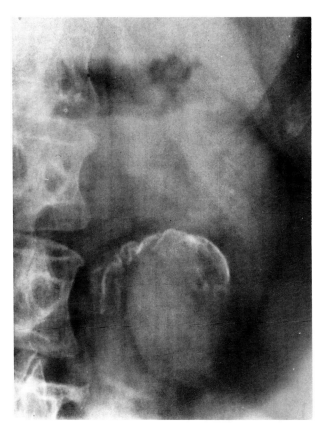

Figure 2–109. Calcified mesenteric cyst. Only a part of the cyst wall is calcified. Occasionally sections of a cyst wall may be non-curvilinear.

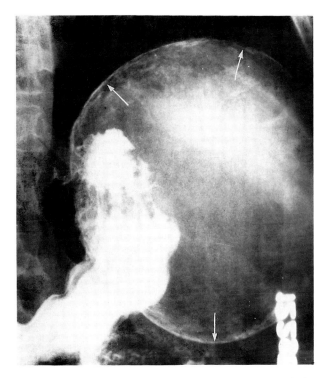

Figure 2–108. A large splenic cyst in a patient with barium in the stomach. The arrows point to its smooth outer margins.

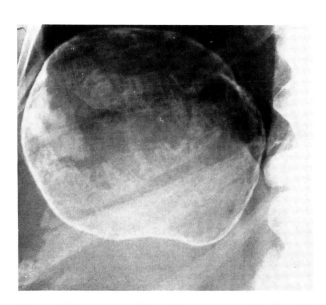

Figure 2–110. Large calcified echinococcal cyst of the liver. It is compressed on its inferior surface.

cyst depends greatly on its location. Cysts can displace and distort organs or vessels, or they can be confined by adjacent solid structures. Most cysts appear only with rim calcification. Occasionally, there appears to be central calcification as well, but this is seen when calcium deposition is so extensive that even surfaces that are not tangential to the X-ray beam are sufficiently dense to be visible (Fig 2–111). In such cases, the "interior" of a heavily calcified cyst has a smudgy and indistinct appearance, less radiopaque than the wall.

At times, it is difficult to differentiate calcification in cyst walls from that in solid masses. The outer surface of a cyst is usually smooth, whereas the transition between the inner surface of these calcifications and the liquid medium contained within it may be roughened and irregular. In solid mass calcification, the outer margin of opacity is often poorly defined. In general, the calcific rim of cysts are well-demarcated and arcuate, whereas in solid densities, smooth lines of calcification are much less common. Infrequently, leiomyomas of the uterus will have regularly arrayed curvilinear calcifications at their margins simulating cystic calcification.

The cystic pattern of calcification can be found almost anywhere in the abdomen whereas a peripheral density is unlikely to be a concretion or conduit. Common abnormalities with the radiographic appearance of the cystic type are aneurysm of the ab-

dominal aorta and the splenic artery. Aortic aneurysms are often associated with conduit calcification in the contiguous aorta and iliac vessels (Fig 2–112). Splenic aneurysms frequently occur in conjunction with calcification in adjacent portions of the splenic artery (Fig 2–113). Cystic calcification of the genitourinary tract includes renal cysts, renal artery and intrarenal aneurysms, echinococcal cysts, perirenal hematomas, multicystic kidneys, parapelvic cysts, and adrenal cysts. Solid neoplasms of the kidney and adrenal gland occasionally show calcification simulating that of cyst walls. In North America, calcified splenic and hepatic cysts occur much less frequently than calcified renal cysts. In other parts of the world, such as, the Mediterranean Basin and the Middle East, calcified cysts of the spleen and liver are common because of the high incidence of *Echino-*

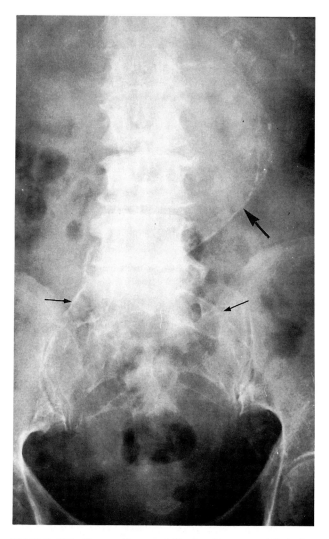

Figure 2–112. The curvilinear calcification (*large arrow*) is in the wall of an aortic aneurysm. Smaller arrows indicate calcification extending into the common iliac arteries.

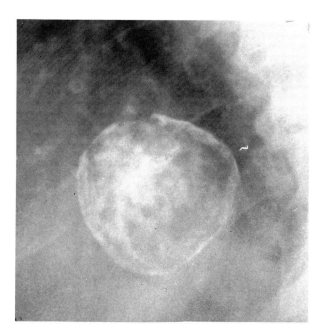

Figure 2–111. Heavily calcified hepatic echinococcal cyst with curvilinear opacities at the margin and poorly defined central calcification.

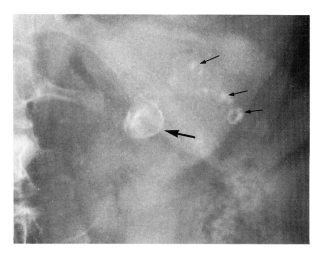

Figure 2–113. The large arrow points to a small splenic artery aneurysm. The smaller arrows are directed to calcifications in non-dilated portions of the artery. Coincident conduit calcification elsewhere in this vessel makes splenic artery aneurysm a strong diagnostic consideration.

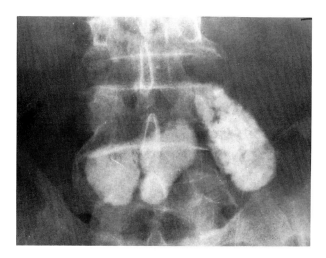

Figure 2–114. Mottled interior and slightly irregular margins are typical of mesenteric node calcification.

coccus granulosus infestation. Retroperitoneal tumors such as pheochromocytomas may assume a cystic appearance. In the lower abdomen, calcified cysts are more rare. Some of the entities found in this location are calcified mesenteric cysts, calcified mucoceles of the appendix, and calcified benign lesions of the ovary.

Solid Mass Calcification. The fourth category, solid mass calcification, encompasses the most diverse assemblage of radiological appearances. However, in almost all cases, this morphological type can be identified by its irregular calcified border and its complex inner architecture. Solid masses may appear as mottled densities, with scattered radiolucencies within calcified background. This is a typical appearance of calcified lymph nodes (Fig 2–114). A whorled pattern with incomplete bands and arcs of calcification around poorly defined lucent foci is a hallmark of uterine leiomyoma (Fig 2–115). Irregular flecks and streaks of radiodensity may occupy the substance of a mass (Fig 2–116). Another common pattern is flocculent calcification superimposed on a lucent background (Fig 2–117). Despite the dissimilarities in interior patterns, solid calcifications share the unifying feature of a nongeometric inner architecture. There is no regularity in the distribution of calcium deposition. In most instances, the interior calcification is more prominent than the marginal radiopacity. Frequently, calcification does not extend to the edge of the mass and the outer aspect of solid mass opacities may be discontinuous. At times, the mass contains several islands of amorphous den-

sity (Fig 2–118). Occasionally, the border of a solid mass is more densely calcified than the interior. Although this appearance resembles cystic calcification, only rarely are the margins smoothly arcuate. Most often they appear crenated or slightly angulated.

Solid masses can appear anywhere in the abdomen. They may be central or peripheral, adjacent to or within organs, or in the intraperitoneal or the retroperitoneal spaces. Most common are calcified mesenteric lymph nodes, which occur anywhere along a broad arc extending from the left upper quadrant to the right lower quadrant of the abdomen along the course of the small bowel mesentery. They can be multiple and of varied sizes. Tubercu-

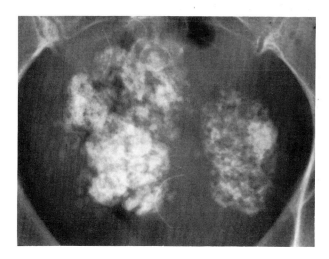

Figure 2–115. Two uterine leiomyomas in the pelvis show poorly defined calcification admixed with irregular lucencies.

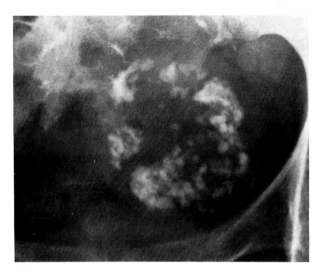

Figure 2–116. A leiomyoma of the uterus. There is dense flocculation of calcium in the mass.

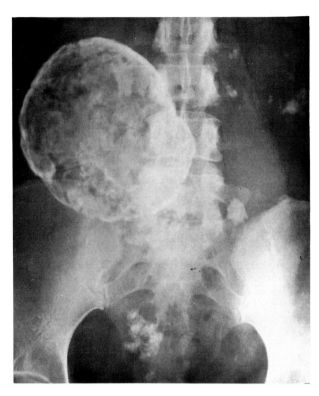

Figure 2–118. Multiple leiomyomas. Scattered foci of flocculent calcification in the pelvis and left upper quadrant. In the right upper quadrant there is a large calcific density resembling a cyst, but the marginal calcification is slightly irregular and the interior is very radiodense.

lous infection has been invoked as the cause of these densities. In most cases, there is no other evidence of granulomatous disease in the abdomen.

In women, the most frequent calcified solid masses in the pelvis are uterine leiomyomata. They are often multiple and may become very large. Leiomyomas of the uterus are not necessarily confined to the pelvis but can be seen almost anywhere in the abdomen. Usually, they have a whorled type of a calcification, but occasionally a prominent bordering rim may be seen. Solid mass calcification can occur in renal malignancies, adenomas, and hamartomas, as well as in tuberculous and chronic pyogenic abscesses. Splenic calcification of the solid mass type is uncommon and pancreatic mass calcifications are very rare. More frequent but still distinctly uncommon are calcified metastatic deposits in the liver. Both benign and primary malignant hepatic neo-

plasms containing calcified foci are rare, as are calcification in tumors originating from the hollow organs of the genitourinary tract. Aside from adrenal adenomas, other solid retroperitoneal tumors seldom calcify.

Psammomatous calcification is a type of solid mass opacification so specific that it merits separate discussion. Psammoma bodies are calcified concretions that occur intracellulary within the substance of ovarian serous cystadenocarcinomas. Individual calcifications are microscopic and cannot be discerned as distinct entities on a radiograph. Only masses of psammoma bodies, when sufficiently calcified and numerous, may be detected. Faint psammomatous calcification appears as a poorly localized, finely granulated pattern. Dense psammomatous calcification may be so intense that other structures will be obliterated if they are overlain by the mass. Psammomatous calcification appears as a cloudlike agglomeration without internal lucency or distinct borders (Fig 2–119). It occurs in primary lesions of the peritoneal cavity, metastatic deposits to the liver, and retroperitoneal lymph nodes. The amorphous calcification occasionally found in carci-

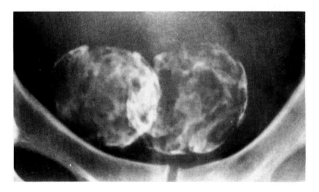

Figure 2–117. Two pelvic leiomyomas with both marginal curvilinear calcification and dense internal streaks and plaques.

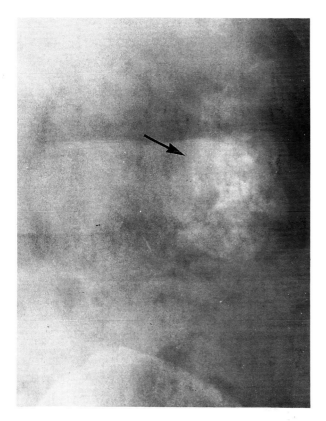

Figure 2–119. Psammomatous calcification. A film of the left lateral abdomen reveals a poorly defined area of increased density (*arrow*), representing an intraperitoneal metastasis from ovarian serous cystadenocarcinoma. Psammomatous calcification can easily be missed if not carefully sought.

nomas of the stomach, colon, and liver simulates psammomatous calcification, but in these malignancies, calcium deposition occurs in extracellular sites rather than in growing tumor.

Caveats. A classification of abdomen calcifications according to radiographical morphology can be helpful in the analysis of an unknown opacity. However, several limitations need to be emphasized. If a calcification is very small, it is difficult, if not impossible, to categorize. If it is too faint to have a definable inner pattern or margin, morphological analysis is not feasible.

The distinction between solid mass calcification and ossification may sometimes be difficult. Ossified structures contain trabecula, which appears as long thin strands of radiodensity oriented along a straight line or smooth arc. Parallel trabecula are usually of equal width in contrast to the varying width and direction of solid mass calcification. If a cortex has a thickened rim with smooth external and internal margins, the presence of bone is established (Fig 2–120). Dermoid cysts in the ovary are common pel-

vic masses in young females. Often, calcified teeth are observable within the lesion (Fig 2–121). Generally, it is not difficult to differentiate a calculus in the distal ureter from a tooth in a dermoid cyst. At times, however, the two densities may resemble one another and proper identification rests on the relationship of the calcification to an accompanying mass. Teeth are found within or at the margins of the dermoid cyst whereas stones will either be unassociated with a soft tissue mass or deviated away from it.

Occasionally, there are calcifications that have the radiographic characteristics of more than one morphological type. Calcification in the gallbladder wall is not rare (Fig 2–122) and sometimes can resemble a single, large gallstone. However, gallbladder wall calcification usually has a dense rim of variable width that may be continuously radiopaque whereas large gallstones almost always calcify uninterruptedly along their margins. Pancreatic stones are often dissimilar in size and configuration. They can appear to extend diffusely without evidence of placement within a closed space even though they are confined to the pancreatic ducts (Fig 2–123). Although these examples point out the possible pitfalls apparent in this classification scheme, in most cases it is still possible to ascribe a specific abdominal calcification to one of the four major categories with a reasonable measure of assurance.

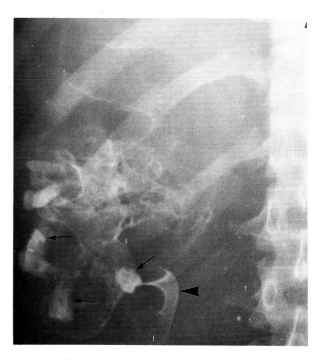

Figure 2–120. Retroperitoneal teratoma. Plain film of the abdomen reveals a complex density in the right mid-abdomen. Teeth are present (*small arrows*) along with bone (*arrowhead*). (*Courtesy of Dr. C. Y. Park*).

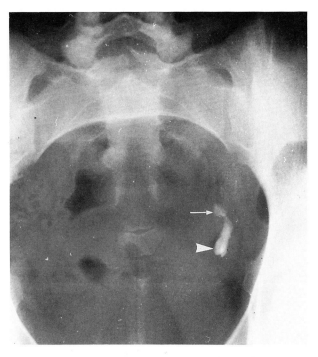

Figure 2–121. Teeth in an ovarian dermoid. Well-defined tooth in the left pelvis, consisting of crown (*arrowhead*) and root (*small arrow*).

Mobility

Movement in Hollow Structures. The movement of abdominal radiopacities, either during one examination or over a period of time, provides additional information that can lead to a plain film diagnosis. Gravity, respiration, peristaltic activity, and the growth of masses can all cause changes in the location of abdominal densities. An aid in the detection of stones within a fluid medium is the recognition of layering on films obtained in the upright position (Fig 2–124). With the X-ray beam directed horizontally, stratification of freely moving calcified concretions in a liquid medium can be appreciated. This is most often seen with gallbladder stones and calculi in hydronephrotic sacs. Very striking is the layering in milk of calcium, which is most common in the gallbladder and in calyceal diverticula in the kidney. Radiodensities lying free in the peritoneal cavity may demonstrate great mobility. These are rare lesions but their dramatic changes in position on sequential films aid in recognition. Mesenteric nodal calcification also exhibits movement but to a lesser extent than free intraperitoneal opacities. Opacities within fluid-filled structures, such as the lumen of the gastrointestinal tract, and the pelvicalyceal system may also move on successive films. Generally, calcification within solid organs does not move with change in patient position.

Effect of Respiration. Alterations in position with respiration may help to segregate retroperitoneal densities from intraperitoneal masses. Retroperitoneal calcifications are usually fixed and do not migrate significantly with phase of respiration. Intraperitoneal calcifications, especially in the upper abdomen, may be displaced by diaphragmatic excursion. Also, costal cartilage and soft tissue calcifications in the upper abdomen move with the ribs and thus will be at different locations in inspiration and expiration.

Migration. The migration of urinary calculi on successive examinations is frequently observed. This is due to propulsion toward the bladder by ureteral contractions and the flow of urine. Similarly, peristaltic activity in the intestinal tract causes movement of intraluminal densities (Fig 2–125).

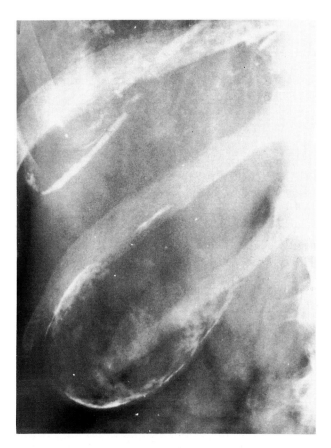

Figure 2–122. Calcified gallbladder. The presence of discontinuous linear calcifications describing an ovoid or pear-shaped mass is characteristic of a calcified gallbladder on plain films.

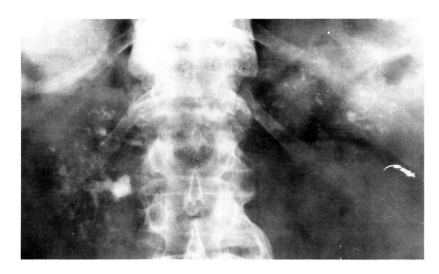

Figure 2–123. Diffuse pancreatic calcification. The intraductal calculi are of varying size, shape, and density.

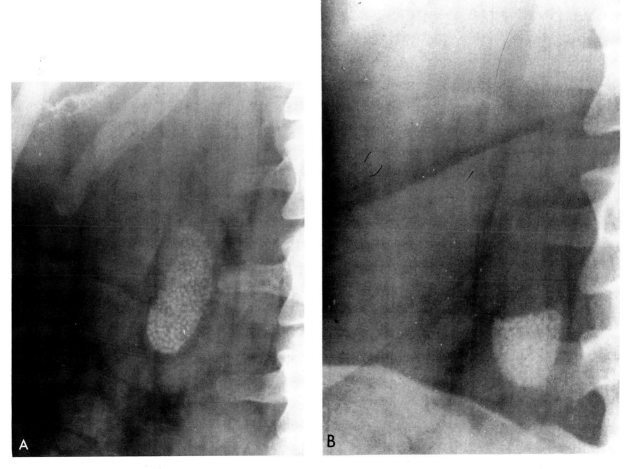

Figure 2–124. Supine **(A)** and upright **(B)** views of the abdomen in a patient with gallstones. Note the change in appearance when the patient is placed erect. The calculi sink to the fundus of the gallbladder.

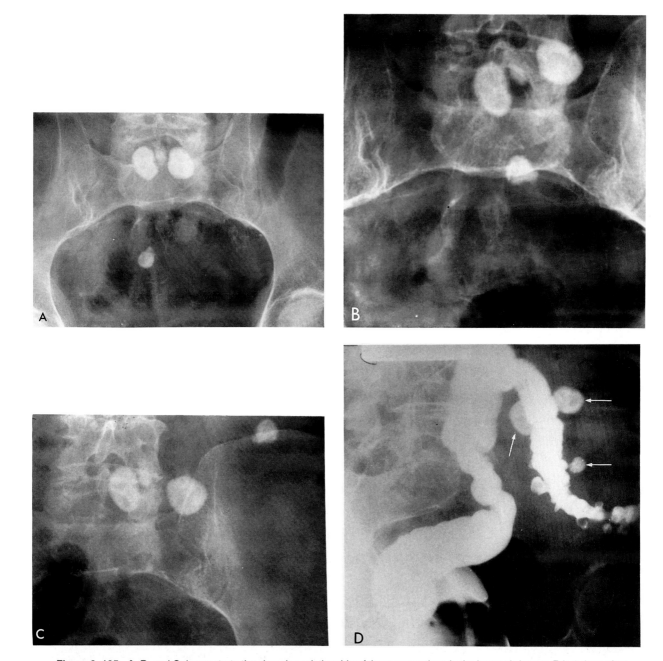

Figure 2–125. A, B, and **C** demonstrate the changing relationship of three concretions in the lower abdomen. **B** is 3 days after **A,** and **C** is 3 years later. Not only do the densities move in respect to fixed structures such as the sacrum, but the spatial relationships of each to the others also change. **D** is a film from a barium enema that reveals that all calculi are within diverticula in the sigmoid colon on a long mesentery (*arrows*). Peristalsis in the sigmoid continually changes the position of the stones.

Growth of Masses. Enlargement and contraction of calcium-containing masses may be evaluated by changes in the positions of calcification on serial radiographic studies. The size of aortic aneurysms can be ascertained on lateral films by the separation of calcification in the anterior wall of the vessel from the vertebral body. Any increase in this distance suggests enlargement of the aneurysm. The growth of noncalcified masses is suggested by displacement of adjacent fixed densities. Phleboliths will move very little in the pelvis, except when pushed by an adjacent mass. The phlebolith displacement sign is a neglected but valuable aid in the evaluation of pelvic masses (Fig 2–126).[10]

Fistula. The mobility of abdominal calcifications may be the result of processes not fully explainable by the effects of gravity, respiration, peristalsis, or local enlargement. Gallstone ileus is an intestinal obstruction caused by a gallbladder calculus that has

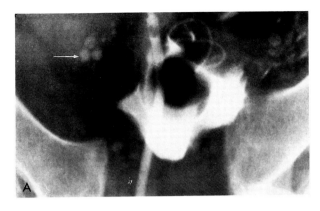

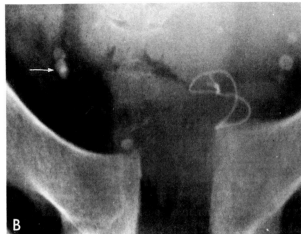

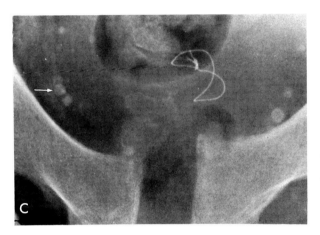

Figure 2–126. The phlebolith displacement sign. **A.** Three phleboliths (*arrow*) are displaced medially by a right pelvic hematoma, secondary to trauma. Note the diastasis of the symphysis pubis. **B.** Three weeks later, the hematoma is resolving and the phleboliths migrate laterally. Also, the phleboliths are now arrayed linearly. **C.** Three weeks later the hematoma has fully resolved and the phleboliths have returned to their normal position.

eroded through the gallbladder wall and then progressed through the lumen of the small bowel only to be restricted by the caliber of the terminal ileum or by narrowings in the large bowel. The initial observation of a calculus in the right upper quadrant calculus and the later demonstration of the same calculus in the pelvis or left lower quadrant points to this possibility.

REFERENCES

1. Andersen K, Ringsted A. Clinical and experimental investigations in ileus with particular reference to the genesis of intestinal gas. *Acta Chir Scand.* 1943;88:475–502.
2. Levitt MD, Bond JH Jr. Volume, composition and source of intestinal gas. *Gastroenterology.* 1970;59:921–929.
3. Rennell C, McCort JJ. Bowel gas and fluid. In: McCort JJ, ed. *Abdominal Radiology.* Baltimore, Williams and Wilkins Co.: 1984.
4. Bray JF. The puckered panniculus—A sign of previous surgery. *J Can Assoc Radiol.* 1983:34:75–76.
5. Whalen JP, Evans JA, Meyers MA. Vector principle; Right upper quadrant *Am J Roentgenol.* 1972;115:318–333.
6. Whalen JP, Evans JA, Shansea J. Vector principle in differential diagnosis of abdominal masses. I. Left upper quadrant. *Am J Roentgenol.* 1971;113:104–116.
7. Hilbish TF, Bartter FC: Roentgen findings in abnormal deposition of calcium in tissues. *Am J Roentgenol.* 1962; 87:1128–1129.
8. Kurturna P. A contribution to the problem of calcifications in malignant tumors. A case of late calcified retroperitoneal metastasis of an ovarian carcinoma. *Neoplasma.* 1964;11:633–642.
9. Widmann BF, Ostrum AW, Fried H. Practical aspects of calcification and ossification in the various body tissues. *Radiology.* 1938;30:598–609.
10. Steinbach HL. Identification of pelvic masses by phlebolith displacement. *Am J Roentgenol.* 1960;83:1063–1066.

LIFE COLLEGE-LIBRARY
1269 Barclay Circle
Marietta, GA 30060

CHAPTER THREE

Plain Film Radiology of the Peritoneal and Retroperitoneal Spaces

INTRODUCTION

The peritoneal cavity, with its numerous recesses and ligamentous attachments, and the retroperitoneal space, incompletely divided into perirenal and pararenal compartments, are involved in many serious abdominal conditions. Frequently, manifestations of disease in these regions are visible on plain films. Some of the signs of peritoneal and retroperitoneal pathology are readily apparent but others are much more subtle and require a detailed understanding of abdominal anatomy.

The plain film examination is often performed for the evaluation of air or gas within the peritoneal cavity. In most cases, spontaneous pneumoperitoneum is a surgical emergency requiring prompt diagnosis and undelayed operative intervention. The detection of small amounts of free air can be achieved by plain films if careful attention is given to proper technique (Fig 1–3B). Initially, at least, gas in the extraperitoneal space can appear with minimal signs and symptoms. Here, too, conventional radiography may provide the first clue to the presence of a potentially lethal extension of air from the gastrointestinal tract or the formation of gas within the urinary tract. Intraperitoneal and retroperitoneal effusions are characterized more fully with cross-sectional imaging techniques. Nevertheless, the plain film findings of fluid accumulation within these spaces may help direct the choice of subsequent diagnostic studies. Tumors unrelated by location or cell type to primary organs or blood vessels are rare within the peritoneal or retroperitoneal boundaries. Calcification is seldom seen in the peritoneal or retroperitoneal spaces unless confined to the mesenteric nodes, the walls of major arteries or as concretions in the lumen of pelvic veins.

PNEUMOPERITONEUM

Air in the peritoneal cavity has many causes. Table 3–1 provides a list of the diverse entities associated with pneumoperitoneum. Undoubtedly, this roster will continue to lengthen as new techniques and procedures, having pneumoperitoneum as a potential complication, gain widespread use. Intraperitoneal gas may be an expected and innocuous finding requiring no treatment or a sensitive indicator of a sudden and life-threatening perforation of a hollow viscus. In most instances, the reason for the entry of gas into the peritoneal cavity is clear but in some conditions such as jejunal diverticulosis, the mechanism for the passage of air across the intact small bowel wall is more obscure.

By far the most common cause of pneumoperitoneum is recent abdominal operation. After laparotomy, air will usually be present for 3 to 7 days, gradually decreasing in volume daily.[1] Prolongation of free air beyond 1 week is not necessarily abnormal and it has been reported to remain for 4 weeks before complete resorption. The type of anesthesia, the presence of drains, the development of peritonitis, and the coexistence of postoperative pulmonary complications do not influence the duration of pneumoperitoneum. The pace of the disappearance of air is age related, with resorption faster in young adults than in the elderly. Another important factor is the amount of air present in the peritoneal cavity at the conclusion of the operation as the time to ultimate removal of air is directly dependent on initial volume.[2] Felson and Wiot maintain that pneumoperitoneum is more extensive after pelvic or abdominal operations than postappendectomy.[3] Others have shown, however, that the type of incision has little effect on the persistence of free air after surgery.[4]

Body habitus appears to correlate well with

TABLE 3–1. CAUSES OF PNEUMOPERITONEUM

A. Trauma
   1. Penetrating wounds
   2. Postcolonoscopy
   3. Percutaneous endoscopy gastrostomy
   4. Postlaparotomy
   5. Postperitoneoscopy
   6. Postperitoneal tap
   7. Postculdoscopy
   8. Post barium enema
   9. Post upper GI tract endoscopy
B. Perforated viscus
   1. Gastric ulcer
   2. Gastric carcinoma
   3. Duodenal ulcer
   4. Colonic perforation
   5. Appendiceal perforation
   6. Ileocolonic perforation post renal transplantation
   7. Small bowel perforation
C. Communication through the female genital tract
   1. Diagnostic procedures for tubal patency
   2. Inadvertent cannulation of the endocervical canal
   3. Postpartum
      a. Abnormal position
      b. Cunnilingus
D. Extension from the chest
   1. Posterior communication
      a. Pneumomediastinum via retroperitoneum
      b. Pneumomediastinum via mesentery
   2. Anterior communication
   3. Pneumothorax via diaphragmatic rents
E. Pneumoretroperitoneum
F. Pneumoperitoneum—obscure physiology
   1. Neuromuscular disorders of the GI tract
   2. Jejunal diverticulosis
   3. Gastroscopy without obvious perforation
   4. Pneumatosis cystoides intestinally
   5. Therapeutic splenic embolization

clearance of intraperitoneal air. Bryant and colleagues found that pneumoperitoneum resolved more quickly in the obese than in individuals with asthenic habitus. Moreover, at any time in the postoperative period, overweight patients had less free air than their thinner counterparts.[4] Harrison and colleagues observed similar findings and offered the explanation that slender people have a more relaxed abdominal wall, creating a larger cavity to be filled by air introduced at surgery.[2]

Until 2 weeks after laparotomy, a small residue of free air should give no cause for alarm unless it is seen to increase in volume on successive films. In that case, perforation of a viscus should be considered strongly. However, in general, the plain film of the abdomen need not be obtained routinely after abdominal operation and should be interpreted with caution. Small to moderate increases in intraperitoneal air cannot be ascertained with certainty unless two consecutive films are obtained in the same pro-

jection. The view most sensitive for the detection of pneumoperitoneum is the upright chest film, but in many cases the patient may not be able to assume the erect position early in the postoperative period.[5] Thus, perforation occurring soon after surgery is a difficult diagnosis by plain films unless it produces a marked increase in free air.

Massive pneumoperitoneum is a feature of diagnostic studies such as peritoneoscopy and culdoscopy. It may also result from perforation of the colon during double-contrast barium enema or with colonoscopy.[6] Percutaneous endoscopic gastrostomy frequently produces a benign, self-limited pneumoperitoneum. For example, Gottfried et al observed free air in 11 of 29 patients undergoing this procedure.[7] Spontaneous colon perforation often allows a huge volume of gas to enter the peritoneal cavity, especially if the affected colonic segment has been distended at the time of mural disruption. The possibility of a large intraperitoneal deposition of gas is greatest if there has been acute or persistent dilatation of the proximal colon. In elderly or debilitated patients, cecal dilatation with fecal impaction promotes the formation of a stercoral ulcer that may then perforate. Ileocolonic perforation is an important complication of renal transplantation.[8] In such patients, the combination of fecal impaction and high-dose steroid use contributes to the heightened risk of intestinal rupture.

Interestingly, appendiceal perforation rarely appears with free air despite the fact that a communication is created between the appendiceal lumen and the peritoneal cavity. In most cases, inflammation has obstructed the appendix, restricting migration of bowel gas to it from the cecum. At the moment of perforation, only gas within the lumen (no more than 1 or 2 mL)[9] can be transferred to the peritoneal cavity. Assuming there is no barrier to flow by adjacent adhesions or omental coverage, the volume of gas contributed by the appendix is usually too small to be detected on plain films even with optimal radiographic technique.[10]

The most frequent cause of spontaneous pneumoperitoneum is perforation of a gastric or duodenal ulcer. The magnitude of free air is variable, being related to the size and site of the ulcer. A large perforation allows more rapid passage of air. if the perforation occurs near preexisting adhesions, gas is likely to be enclosed within a small area rather than dispersed widely. Anterior perforation is more likely to communicate with the greater peritoneal cavity while a posterior perforation is directed to and often first contained by the lesser sac or Morison's pouch. In upper gastrointestinal perforations, the volume of air in the peritoneal cavity is also related to the extent of aerophagia—the more air swallowed, the larger the pneumoperitoneum.

A feature distinguishing upper gastrointestinal ulceration from other types of perforated visci with pneumoperitoneum is the initial absence of generalized ileus. Keeffe and Gagliardi observed that few patients with perforated ulcer had dilated air filled intestine when the abdominal film was obtained soon after the onset of symptoms.[11] On the other hand, colonic perforation is almost always associated with dilated large and small bowel. It has been maintained that the chemical peritonitis produced by the perforation of the stomach or duodenum elicits no bowel atony at first but the bacterial peritonitis of colonic origin leads to an immediate reflux ileus. However, within 6 to 12 hours after gastric or duodenal perforation, microbial contamination ensues, resulting in an ileus of delayed onset.[11]

In women, the potential communication between the peritoneal cavity and ambient air can become a pathway for gas accumulation under exceptional circumstances. The Rubin test, in which carbon dioxide is introduced into the uterus, depends upon the establishment of a pneumoperitoneum to determine patency of the fallopian tubes. Air may also pass through the fallopian tubes during a pelvic examination. Cass et al reported a patient whose cervix was inadvertently cannulated by a bulb syringe during the performance of a Papanicolaou smear.[12] Through the aspirating tip of the syringe, air was introduced into the uterus from which it entered the peritoneal cavity. Vaginal douching with a carbonated beverage is another cause of pneumoperitoneum.[6] In the postpartum period, air may traverse the cervix, uterus, and fallopian tubes if the patient assumes the knee–chest position.[13] After childbirth, the widely patent cervix permits the retrograde movement of air that may be introduced by cunnilingus.[14,15]

Thoracic diseases and their treatments occasionally produce pneumoperitoneum. Air in the mediastinum can occur spontaneously in asthmatics during an acute attack and in normal patients undergoing strenuous physical activity, especially after the performance of the Valsalva maneuver. Alveolar rupture causes air to dissect along the peribronchial interstitial space that communicates with the mediastinum.[16,17] Mechanical ventilation and other types of barotrauma therapy may also force air into the mediastinum by the same mechanism.[18] The mediastinum is in direct continuity with the retroperitoneal space. Thus, if sufficient air is present, a pneumomediastinum can become a pneumoretroperitoneum. Gas may then penetrate the

peritoneal cavity by one of two mechanisms. The higher pressure in the retroperitoneal space can lead to direct perforation of the posterior peritoneal wall, or gas may dissect along the course of the mesenteric vessels, eventually reaching the peritoneal cavity.

Gas or air makes its way from the chest to the abdomen through small openings in the diaphragm at or near the midline anteriorly.[19] Hence, a pneumoperitoneum can have a thoracic origin without simultaneous air in the retroperitoneal space. Fataar and Schulman reported nine patients who developed air in the peritoneal cavity following spontaneous pneumothorax.[20] They postulated that there are potential rents in the diaphragm so minuscule that they may not be seen even at postmortem examination. With increased intrapleural pressure these transdiaphragmatic communications permit air and fluid to pass into the peritoneal space.[20] Such a pathway can explain the coexistence of a pleural effusion in a patient with ascites. However, in adults, a pneumothorax resulting from a pneumoperitoneum has not yet been described.[21] Intraperitoneal free air is an infrequent complication of cardiac surgery performed through a median sternotomy incision.[22] Apparently, the pericardial cavity can also communicate with the peritoneal space through small openings in the anterior medial insertion of the diaphragm.

There remains a heterogeneous group of unusual abdominal conditions associated with spontaneous pneumoperitoneum. Neuromuscular disorders of the gastrointestinal tract, which comprise a wide spectrum of diseases manifesting as chronic adynamic bowel distension, are occasionally complicated by pneumoperitoneum, even in the absence of a demonstrable mural tear.[23] A frequent concomitant of jejunal diverticulosis is recurrent intraperitoneal air that appears without warning and usually resolves without treatment. The cause of the leakage of air is not clear in these patients. It has been suggested that the epithelial lining may not be airtight in a jejunal diverticulum. Under special circumstances such as intermittent bowel obstruction there may be transient and minute disruptions of the diverticular wall, permitting gas to enter the peritoneal cavity. Another explanation is that these diverticula act as semipermeable membranes, allowing the transmural diffusion of gas across intact mucosa.[8,24,25]

Gastroscopy can produce pneumoperitoneum even without perforation of the stomach in patients with gastric ulcer. Perhaps with sudden and marked gastric dilatation air is forced into the wall of the stomach at the ulcer site. This leads to the formation of submucosal blebs that then burst, discharging gas into the peritoneal cavity.[2,6] In pneumatosis cystoides intestinalis, pneumoperitoneum may be recurrent, most probably caused by the perforation of one of the numerous thin-wall air cysts that line the bowel wall. Benign, self-limited pneumoperitoneum has been noted after therapeutic embolization of the spleen. The gas appears too rapidly to be a consequence of the replication of gas-forming microorganisms within the spleen but may be related to the liberation of nitrogen gas produced by the iatrogenic splenic infarction.[27]

TECHNIQUE

The formulation of an optimal technique for the plain film demonstration of free air in the peritoneal cavity owes much to the seminal studies of Miller and colleagues.[28] In order to detect very small amounts of free air they have recommended that a full radiographic evaluation include views of the abdomen in the left lateral decubitus, upright and supine positions. These projections should be taken in the radiographic suite, as portable films are usually inadequate for the demonstration of subtle collections of free air.

The left lateral decubitus film should be performed first. This projection offers several advantages. As free air assumes the least dependent position in the peritoneal cavity, in most patients it rises to the right upper quadrant just below the diaphragm, where it situates itself between the abdominal wall and the liver. The homogeneous hepatic density affords sharp contrast to even small volumes of gas (Fig 3–1). The major exception to this direction of flow occurs in women with wide hips in whom the least dependent intraperitoneal region projects over the iliac bone (Fig 3–2). Elevation of the right side enhances passage of swallowed air into the peritoneal space through a duodenal or distal gastric perforation. At the same time, gas in the lesser sac can escape through the foramen of Winslow to enter the greater peritoneal cavity. Soilage of the peritoneal space by pus, blood, food, or gastric acid is minimized when the right side is elevated.[28,29]

The patient should be placed in the left lateral decubitus position for 10 or 20 minutes to permit gas to percolate into the right upper quadrant. It is important to center this projection superiorly enough so that the lower right lung field is included in the film because free air will usually collect just below the right costophrenic angle. Chest technique is preferable to a standard abdominal technique be-

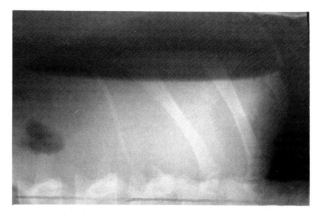

Figure 3–1. Left lateral decubitus view. A large collection of gas collects beneath the right border of the peritoneal cavity. Observe the shadow of the lateral edge of the liver within it.

cause an overpenetration of the right edge of the upper abdomen may miss the sliver of lucency that identifies a small pneumoperitoneum. For best results the film should be obtained during the expiratory phase of respiration. Generally, the left lateral decubitus film approximates the upright chest X-ray in its ability to detect minimal amounts of free air. If there has been a previous laparotomy, however, it may be the superior view because upper abdominal adhesions retard the movement of free air towards a subdiaphragmatic location.

The patient is then placed in a sitting or standing position. After a wait of 5 to 10 minutes to permit air to migrate superiorly, an upright view is obtained. This film should be positioned at the level of the apex of the diaphragm so that the central beam is parallel to a possible free air level that is usually situated just below the diaphragmatic dome (Fig 1–3A). If the beam is centered too low, small pockets of gas may not be appreciated. The midexpiratory or midinspiratory phase of respiration is best for the demonstration of free air.[30] The pneumoperitoneum series concludes with the standard supine film of the abdomen.

Such a comprehensive plain film series, with each film obtained at measured intervals, in proper order, and with appropriate technique, is highly sensitive for the recognition of free air. However, for acutely ill patients presenting with severe abdominal pain in a busy emergency room, it is not always possible to achieve an optimal radiographic assessment. Including the time required in preparation for the left lateral decubitus and upright views, the ideal study takes 30 to 35 minutes to perform, with nearly half the time spent with the patient on a radiograph table in the left lateral decubitus posi-

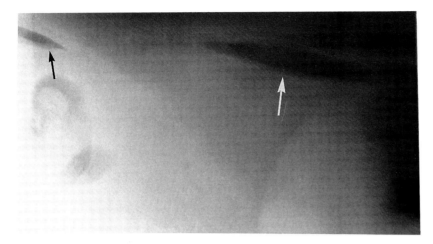

Figure 3–2. Pneumoperitoneum in an obese female. Left lateral decubitus view. Two collections of free air. The white arrow points to air below the right hemidiaphragm. The black arrow is directed to another pocket of air overlying the iliac crest.

tion. A diagnostic radiography room is thus occupied for one study for more than half an hour as the plain film evaluation runs its course. Many patients cannot rest on their side for an extended period and others may be too ill to stand or sit up for the erect view. All the while, the referring physician is eager to make a prompt diagnosis and may interfere with the correct sequence or timing of films as he or she observes the patient, obtains further history, repeats the physical examination and removes samples of blood or urine for laboratory tests. Moreover, the three views series is usually sought when pneumoperitoneum is strongly suspected. In many patients that diagnosis may be only remotely considered or even unsuspected at first and a complete plain film examination may not be requested.

For this reason, it is crucial that the radiologist become familiar with the signs of pneumoperitoneum that can be discerned on the supine film of the abdomen because that may be the only radiograph available for interpretation (Table 3–2). An expeditious and definitive diagnosis is possible in most instances from this view alone if careful attention is given to sometimes subtle but nonetheless reliable plain film findings.

In 1941, Rigler identified a sign for massive pneumoperitoneum that bears his name. Also known as the bas-relief or double-wall sign, it depends upon the observation that the wall of the bowel appears to stand out in "relief" when gas is present within the intestinal lumen and in the adjacent peritoneal cavity (Fig 1–1). Normally, only the interface between luminal gas and encircling bowel wall is seen; the serosal surface is not appreciated because it is of similar density to the peritoneal contents that abut it. If the peritoneal contents are displaced by air, however, the serosal margin of bowel now becomes clearly defined (Fig 3–3).[31] On occa-

sion, not only can free air be detected but mural thickening may also be demonstrated if the lumen is filled with gas (Fig 3–4). The double-wall sign requires a large volume of free air so that the bowel loops can be separated from each other. Schultz emphasized that ascitic fluid is also needed, often in excess of 1 L, so that gas-filled intestinal loops are displaced anteriorly. As they float on the fluid surface they are nearly surrounded by free air.[32]

However, Rigler's sign is insensitive and its presence only validates the presence of a pneumoperitoneum that is usually apparent on clinical grounds. Too often, it can be simulated by normal variations of intestinal configuration. Abundant fat in the omentum and appendices epiploicae may provide sufficient contrast to demarcate the serosal surface of the colon. Free air can be mimicked by contiguous loops of large or small bowel, as air within the lumen of an intestinal segment may appear to outline the wall of its neighbor (Fig 3–5). In actual-

TABLE 3–2. SIGNS OF PNEUMOPERITONEUM ON SUPINE ABDOMINAL FILMS

A. Mid and lower abdomen
  1. Rigler's sign (bas relief sign)
  2. Football sign (children)
  3. Visualization of the urachus
  4. Visualization of the lateral umbilical ligaments
  5. Pneumoscrotum sign
B. Right upper quadrant
  1. Inferior—the hepatic edge sign
  2. Posterior—Morison's pouch—doge's cap sign
  3. Anterior
    a. The lucent liver sign
    b. The falciform ligament sign
    c. The superior pocket of lucency sign
    d. Ill-defined extraluminal gas
C. Lesser sac gas

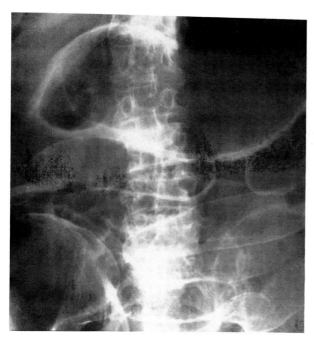

Figure 3–3. Bas-relief sign. Massive pneumoperitoneum from a perforated duodenal ulcer allows clear demarcation of the walls of many intestinal loops.

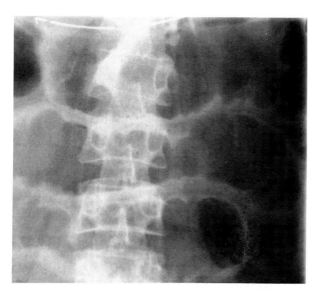

Figure 3–4. Bas-relief sign. Crohn's disease with intestinal obstruction and perforation. Free air outlines three distended small bowel segments. The two upper loops have thickened walls and the lower one is of normal caliber.

ity, it is the combined widths of two adjoining bowel walls that are highlighted. Intraperitoneal air is featureless whereas luminal gas bears the hallmarks of bowel, viz. the valvulae conniventes of small bowel or the haustra and plica semilunares of large bowel. In colonic distension, these intraluminal markers may not be well delimited and the double-wall sign can be suggested by two gas-filled loops lying next to each other.[33] If in doubt, the upright or left lateral decubitus films should be done to confirm the existence of free air with certainty.

In children, massive pneumoperitoneum can produce the football sign, so called because the distended air-filled peritoneal cavity looks like a football with its long axis directed vertically. The falciform ligament is often outlined and appears to bisect the peritoneal cavity, furthering the likeness to a football. However, such an appearance is seldom encountered in adults.[34] Jelaso and Schultz described the urachus sign, an elongated conical soft tissue density, which tapers superiorly near the midline.[35] The urachus, the intra-abdominal extension of the allantois, sometimes has a peritoneal reflection that can become visible in the presence of a large pneumoperitoneum. Attached to the urachus are the lateral umbilical ligaments, which form an inverted V as they diverge inferiorly and laterally from the midline. In some thin patients they can protrude slightly into the peritoneal cavity from their anterior abdominal attachments, becoming visible on supine films only if there is a large pneumoperitoneum. Either one or both ligaments may be seen, with a single ligament often closely resembling a colonic septation (Fig 3–6).[36] In most patients with a large rounded lucency projecting below the inguinal ligament, the gas collection is in an inguinal or femoral hernia sac. Rarely, in men and boys, free air can extend into the scrotum. The tunica vaginalis is a sheath of peritoneum surrounding the testes. The processes vaginalis is a peritoneal tube that passes through the inguinal ligament and connects the peritoneal cavity to the tunica vaginalis. In 60% of male infants and in 15% of men, it remains open, permitting peritoneal gas to enter the scrotum. Typically, the rounded density of the testes can be identified within the lucent, distended scrotum. It is the presence of the testes that distinguishes pneumoscrotum from gas within a hernia sac.[37,38] These unusual signs of a large pneumoperitoneum are anatomically interesting but are almost never crucial for the diagnosis, as other evidence of free air is always present.

On supine films, the findings of a large pneumoperitoneum are observed in the mid and lower

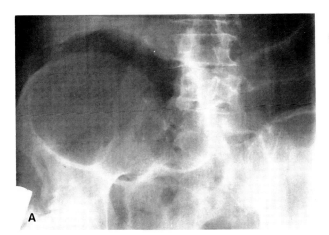
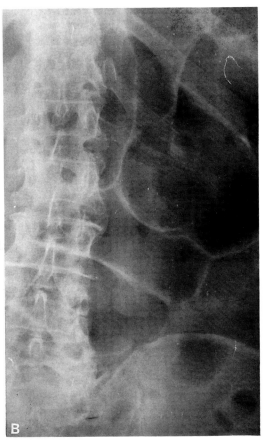

Figure 3–5. Two cases with a pseudo bas-relief sign. **A.** Small bowel loops adjacent to a dilated cecum simulate pneumoperitoneum. **B.** Several small bowel segments distended by gas abut each other, mimicking free air surrounding one intestinal segment.

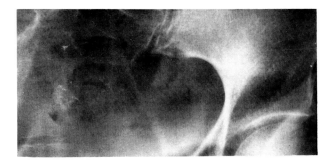

Figure 3–6. Massive pneumoperitoneum. Visualization of the left lateral umbilical ligament. The obliquely oriented linear density extending inferiorly from the left lateral sacrum is the ligament indenting the air-filled peritoneal cavity. It is straighter and longer than a colonic septation.

abdomen. It is also necessary to look at the upper abdomen, especially the right upper quadrant, where indications of free air are just as indisputable if often less immediately striking. Therefore, it is essential that no part of the abdomen be excluded from view during a plain film search for pneumoperitoneum. Inasmuch as the abdomen extends from the dome of the diaphragm to the inguinal region, a single film may not encompass the entire peritoneal cavity if the patient has a long trunk. An adequate examination may require two supine films, one centered in the lower abdomen and the other directed more superiorly.

The liver shadow provides a homogeneous density in the right upper quadrant. It should be at least as radiopaque as the spleen. A gas-containing right colon may be superimposed upon it, but the well-defined course of the large intestine and its identifying features of haustra, plica semilunares, and intraluminal feces are usually readily recognizable. Near the midline, the gas-filled distal stomach and

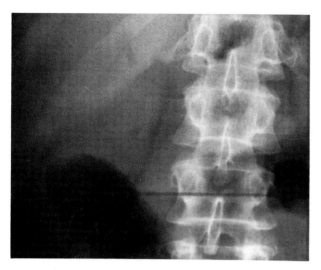

Figure 3–7. The liver shadow is not homogeneous. An irregular, faint lucency superimposed upon it is supine film evidence of pneumoperitoneum.

duodenal bulb are also normal lucent landmarks superimposed on the liver. Occasionally, malrotated proximal small bowel may overlie the liver shadow. In elderly and debilitated patients sharply marginated lucencies of air trapped in skin folds can be superimposed on the hepatic density, but they are almost always traceable beyond the peritoneal cavity (Fig 2–55). All other areas of decreased density, whether focal or diffuse in the right upper quadrant, must be suspected of containing extraluminal air.

Gas within the peritoneal cavity can be distributed ventral or dorsal to the liver. The ventral component is by far the larger and extends across the hepatic surface while the posterior extension or peritoneal space tapers medially and superiorly within the narrow confines of Morison's pouch. A large collection of air in front of the liver may make the hepatic shadow appear relatively lucent (Fig 3–7). For the most part, the diffusely lucent liver is an ancillary sign almost always appearing with other evidence of pneumoperitoneum. On supine films in patients with hydropneumoperitoneum or hemopneumoperitoneum, fluid tends to collect peripherally while air moves medially. An interface oriented in a craniocaudad direction and superimposed on the liver shadow strongly suggests combined intraperitoneal air and fluid. Often small gas bubbles are situated next to the sharp demarcation of fluid and air. The lateral extent of the central gas collection depends on the respective volumes of peritoneal effusion and free air.[34] Although this lucency crosses the midline it is most often best seen on the right side where the liver provides an excellent back-

ground (Fig 3–8). Occasionally, a distended stomach, a dilated colon, the large gas shadow of a cecal volvulus, a large subphrenic abscess, and air in skin folds can resemble a hydropneumoperitoneum. Differentiation from these other causes of a large lucency can be accomplished by upright or left lateral decubitus views.

A helpful sign of pneumoperitoneum or hydropneumoperitoneum involving the anterior superior peritoneal cavity is visualization of the falciform ligament. Extending slightly rightward and superiorly from the umbilicus to the liver, the falciform ligament and its rounded free edge, the ligamentum teres hepatis, merges with the visceral peritoneum at the anterior superior surface of the liver. The falciform ligament then plunges posteriorly into the porta hepatis, where it becomes continuous with the ligamentum venosum. The ligamentum teres is 6 to 14 cm in length and varies in width from 1 to 11 mm.[40] The wide range of thickness is dependent on the amount of fat within it. Harswell et al maintain that in 30% of cases, fat within the ligament can be seen on a plain film, an observation that has not been confirmed by others.[41] The course of the ligament is usually straight but it may describe a slightly concave or convex arc as it ascends from the umbilicus (Fig 3–9). It extends more inferiorly than the right crus of the diaphragm. The ligamentum teres hepatis is more vertically oriented than the obliquely positioned common bile duct, which also may be

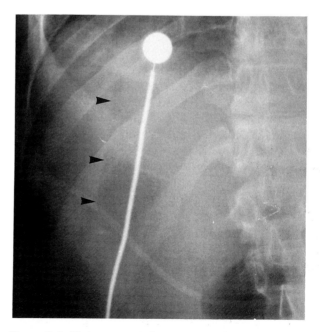

Figure 3–8. Hydropneumoperitoneum. The arrowheads are arranged along an interface with fluid laterally and a large collection of free air medially.

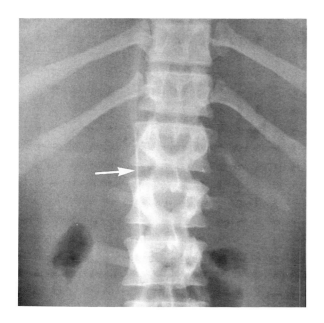

Figure 3–9. Free air in the anterior superior peritoneal cavity outlines a thin falciform ligament (*arrow*).

seen on plain films if invested with abundant fat.

Air in the upper peritoneal cavity collects on both sides of the ligamentum teres, bringing it into sharp relief. The ligament may be oblique to the radiographic beam or may be slightly folded near its umbilical end, causing it to appear widened inferiorly (Fig 3–10). Its characteristic location and sharp margins make for ready identification despite its wide variability in width.

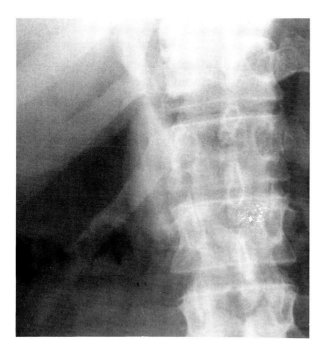

Figure 3–10. Visualization of the falciform ligament. Note its bulbous lower margin. Because the ligament need not be aligned parallel to the radiographic beam, sections of it may appear to be folded on itself. (*Courtesy of Dr. Murray Rosenberg.*)

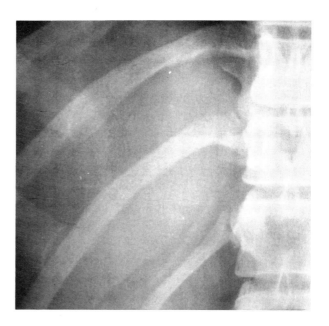

Figure 3–11. Perforated anterior duodenal ulcer. An isolated mitten-shaped lucency anterior to the liver was the only sign of pneumoperitoneum on supine films.

Smaller collections of anterior upper peritoneal free air, can be seen as rounded or oval pockets of lucency. Menuck and Siemers found an isolated focus of ventral air in 4 of 29 patients who had supine film demonstration of pneumoperitoneum. In our institution we have seen it even more frequently (Fig 3–11).[42] The focal lucency is located just below the apex of the right hemidiaphragm and may be missed if the supine film is improperly positioned (Fig 3–12). It can be confused with pneumoretroperitoneum or an interposed colon. Retroperitoneal gas tends not to reach the dome of the diaphragm and it

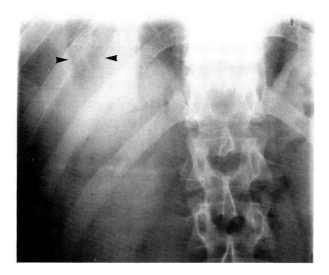

Figure 3–12. Perforated anterior ulcer. Another patient with an intraperitoneal air pocket anterior to the liver (*arrowheads*). This finding was nearly not detected because the film did not extend to the dome of the right hemidiaphragm.

rarely presents as a single large rounded lucency. An interposed colon almost always has the identifying mucosal features of the large intestinal lumen.

At times, the only manifestation of pneumoperitoneum is an agglomeration of bubbles visible over the liver surface, an appearance similar to a pneumoretroperitoneum from duodenal rupture or a gas-containing abscess. On supine films such minimal lucencies do not conform to the outline of any peritoneal recess and, therefore, an unequivocal diagnosis cannot be made on supine films (Fig. 3–13).

Left lateral decubitus or upright films are needed to establish the intraperitoneal position of such lucent collections.

Moving posteriorly, free air may reside under the liver edge. Occasionally the superior margin of such collections appears as a straight, obliquely oriented interface as free air comes in contact with the medial undersurface of the liver. Air in the inferior subhepatic space frequently has a distinctive conformation. The gas assumes an oblong appearance, with its long axis directed superiormedially (Fig 3–14).[43]

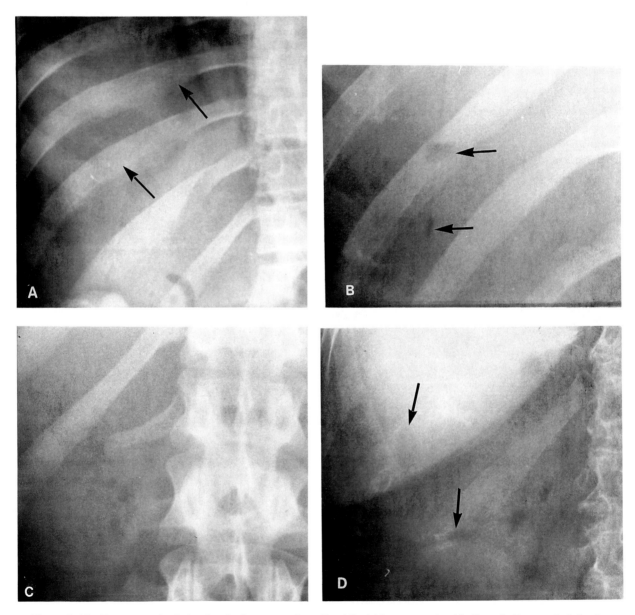

Figure 3–13.   Four cases of anterior air collections appearing with subtle right upper quadrant findings. **A.** Two poorly defined lucencies. Perforated gastric ulcer. **B.** Recent cecal perforation. Two small collections simulate gas in an abscess. **C.** Antral ulcer perforation. Bubbles of various sizes mimic retroperitoneal gas from a posterior perforation of the duodenum. **D.** Anterior duodenal ulcer perforation. A bubble and a streak are the only supine film signs of intraperitoneal air.

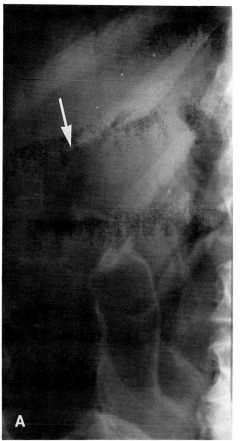

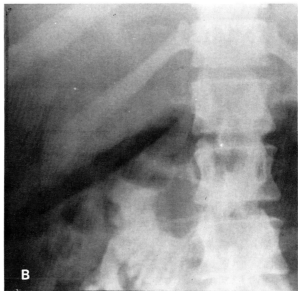

Figure 3–14. A. Massive pneumoperitoneum after rupture of the large bowel at colonoscopy. The bas-relief sign is seen. Also, gas is delimited by the inferior hepatic edge (*arrow*). **B.** Air introduced into the peritoneal cavity through a large rent in the duodenum which developed after biliary surgery. Air collects beneath the inferior liver margin as an elongated lucency with straight borders. The duodenum was opacified by contrast material through a nasogastric tube.

Morison's pouch, the superior extension of the subhepatic space, is interposed between the posterior edge of the liver and the anterior margin of the right kidney. Its dorsal location makes it the most dependent recess of the peritoneal cavity above the pelvis and thus a favored site for the formation of abscesses (Fig 3–15) and for the collection of air and gastric contents that have passed through perforations of the posterior wall of the distal stomach and duodenal bulb. Morison's pouch is situated just to the right of the midline, rarely extending more than 7 or 8 cm peripheral to the lateral border of the nearest vertebral body. Characteristically, it is situated no higher than the right 11th rib, where it is restricted above by the bare area of the liver. Occasionally, gas in Morison's pouch may have a rounded superior border. Much more typical is a crescentic lucency or a triangular configuration reminiscent of il corno, the ceremonial cap worn by the

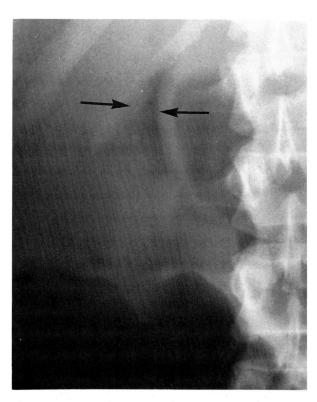

Figure 3–16. Doge's cap sign. The two arrows outline the apex of Morison's pouch filled by air from a perforated duodenal bulb ulcer.

doges of Venice (Figs 1–2, 3–16).[44] The hypotenuse of this triangle is oriented along the liver edge and parallels the right 11th rib. The geometric contour of the doge's cap distinguishes it from the rounded margins of other right upper quadrant lucencies, including a duodenal diverticulum, a gas-filled gallbladder, an intraperitoneal abscess, or a malrotated bowel.[45,46] However, it may be mimicked on plain films by a large, gas-filled duodenal bulb. The far posterior position of Morison's pouch can be appreciated on lateral films, where it is often superimposed on the body of the 11th or 12th dorsal vertebra.

LESSER SAC GAS

Communicating with the posterior subhepatic space through the foramen of Winslow, the lesser sac or omental bursa is another posterior peritoneal recess that when gas filled reveals distinctive plain film findings. The lesser sac occupies a central position behind the stomach in the upper abdomen and is delimited on the left by the gastrosplenic and gastrolienal ligaments. Posteriorly, it is defined by the posterior peritoneum as it crosses the pancreas, the left kidney, and the diaphragm. Its inferior extent is usually the transverse mesocolon, but there may be

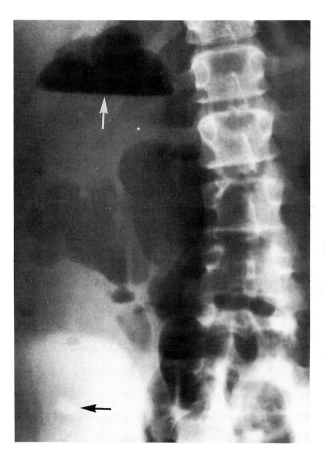

Figure 3–15. Upright film. Appendiceal abscess extending into Morison's pouch. The lower arrow points to an appendicolith. The appendix has perforated, producing a large abscess extending from the lower quadrant of the abdomen, where gas bubbles are seen, to Morison's pouch, which is occupied by a large collection of gas (*upper arrow*).

a caudal pouch that extends several centimeters below the transverse colon.[47,48] Goodwin and Lewicki reported gas in the lesser sac that entered from a perforated sigmoid colon in a patient with a capacious caudal pouch.[49] Most of the anterior border of the lesser sac is the stomach proper. Anteriormedially, the lesser omentum separates the lesser sac from the gastrohepatic recess. The caudate lobe of the liver borders the lesser sac on the right and the foramen of Winslow is located just cephalad to the duodenal bulb.[47]

Gas collections in the lesser sac create a homogeneous lucency that straddles the midline (Fig 3–17). Their right border is smooth, describing a slightly convex lateral curve usually in the same sagittal plane as the falciform ligament (Fig 3–18).[50] These lucencies are delimited superiorly by the left hemidiaphragm and inferiorly by the transverse colon. Even on upright views, lesser sac gas never ascends to the apex of the left hemidiaphragm, as it is confined by the left coronary ligament. A fold of parietal peritoneum containing the hepatic and left gastric arteries indents the left posterior border of the lesser sac, partially dividing it into right and left compartments. Small accumulations of gas may be confined to only one compartment whereas more extensive collections fill the sac entirely.[48] On cross-table lateral projections, lesser sac gas appears as a homogeneous lucency displacing the stomach ante-

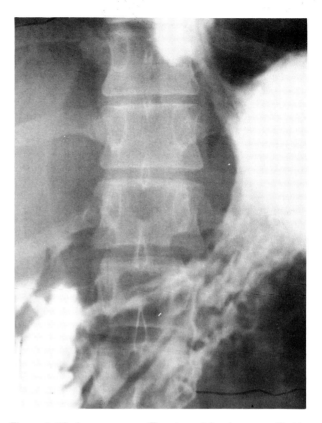

Figure 3–18. Lesser sac gas. The stomach has been opacified by contrast material. The featureless lucency is the lesser sac.

riorly. When the patient is placed in the right lateral decubitus position, the lucency extends to the hilum of the spleen. The left lateral decubitus position permits gas to traverse the foramen of Winslow and escape into Morison's pouch and the greater peritoneal cavity.

Air may enter the omental bursa whenever there is a massive pneumoperitoneum even if the source of free air is remote from it (Fig 3–19). The most common cause of an isolated lesser sac collection is perforation of a posterior gastric or duodenal ulcer.[51] Much less frequent is perforation of a neoplasm of the stomach, transverse colon appendix, or splenic flexure into this peritoneal recess.[52] In most instances of spontaneous rupture of the esophagus (Boerhaave's syndrome) the tear is situated in the intrathoracic portion of the esophagus, and pleural effusion and pneumomediastinum are the diagnostic plain film findings. Occasionally, the site of rupture is below the diaphragm and air enters either the retroperitoneal space or the lesser sac.[53] Perforation of the intraabdominal esophagus also occurs at gastroscopy. Almost always, it is the posterior wall of the esophagus that is affected, providing another cause of lesser sac lucency.[54]

However, ruptured viscus is not the only rea-

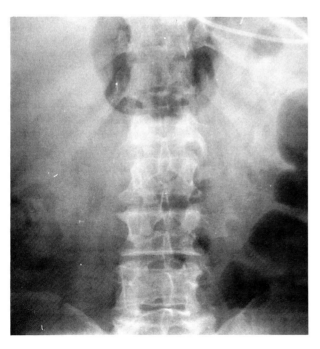

Figure 3–17. Air in the lesser sac from a posterior gastric ulcer perforation. A homogeneous upper abdominal lucency crossing the midline is a typical configuration.

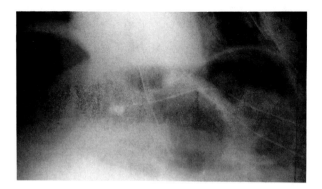

Figure 3–19. Perforated cecum. Intraperitoneal gas distends the greater peritoneal cavity represented by the lateral subdiaphragmatic lucencies. Gas also fills the lesser sac, which is the central lucency.

son for air to fill the omental bursa. Bowel may herniate through a patent foramen of Winslow or across a defect in the omentum. Primarily a disease of men (with a male-to-female ratio of 2.5:1), herniation into the lesser sac usually presents with epigastric pain made worse by extending the trunk and improved by bending forward.[55,56] Prompt plain film recognition can be crucial because immediate surgical correction is almost always the only treatment. Most often, small bowel loops occupy the lesser sac, appearing as multiple lucencies both medial and lateral to the stomach. Often the gastric air shadow is displaced medially, and lateral films reveal a complex array of densities and lucencies representing the displaced small intestinal segment deviating the stomach forward. Occasionally, the cecum migrates into the lesser sac. This rare condition is favored by a large right lobe of the liver, which helps direct a mobile cecum (ie, cecum on a long mesentery) towards the foramen of Winslow. Both a shortened or a very redundant transverse colon favor superior-medial migration of the cecum. An abnormally wide foramen of Winslow also appears to be a predisposing factor.[57,58] At first glance, a cecum in the lesser sac may be mistaken for a dilated transverse colon. Therefore, it is necessary to identify the transverse colon in continuity with adjacent large bowel segments before attempting to characterize any lucency that appears to overlie the stomach. The herniating cecum in the lesser sac can be identified by its characteristic haustra and plica semilunares. Not only will it deviate the stomach medially but it also displaces the duodenum to the left.

A gas-containing abscess is a third cause of lesser sac lucency. The typical features of intra-abdominal abscess, including poorly defined margins and numerous small bubbles with or without a single large lucency, help distinguish lesser sac abscess from pneumoperitoneum or bowel herniation. The recognition of the signs of abscess is crucial but localization to the lesser sac may not be possible on plain films alone. Mellins emphasized that lesser sac abscesses elevate the stomach, a distinctive finding that unfortunately cannot always be appreciated on supine abdominal films.[50] The gastric bubble may be displaced medially or laterally. Often, like the far more common left subphrenic abscess, the splenic flexure is depressed.[59] In lesser sac abscesses, lateral films usually demonstrate posterior pressure on and anterior deviation of the stomach, an appearance also encountered in large pus collections of the pancreas.

PSEUDOPNEUMOPERITONEUM

There are several conditions that mimic free air in the peritoneal cavity (Table 3–3). In some cases, the simulation of pneumoperitoneum on supine abdominal films is so close that a misleading diagnosis is made, eventuating in an unnecessary laparotomy. In the absence of clinical signs if the determination of free air rests solely on the observation of atypical lucencies that seem to be located below the diaphragm, the pseudopneumoperitoneum must be considered strongly.

The anterior–posterior course of the diaphragm need not describe one smooth curve. On frontal views of the abdomen, a faint decrease in density beneath one diaphragmatic dome may be caused by an undulation of that muscle. The lucency represents normally aerated lungs situated between two or more peaks of one hemidiaphragm. Similarly, localized eventration or herniation creates a double hump to the diaphragm with intrapulmonary air in the valley. On supine films, this normal lucency is usually poorly outlined below the diaphragm and lacks the sharp superior margins of free air (Fig 3–20). Almost always, such an appearance is confined to one hemidiaphragm while intraperitoneal air can often be seen bilaterally. Lateral and upright chest X-rays should be obtained to confirm the contour of the diaphragm and to demonstrate the absence of free air.

TABLE 3–3. CAUSES OF PSEUDOPNEUMOPERITONEUM

1. Irregular diaphragmatic contour
2. Basal platelike atelectasis
3. Chilaiditi's syndrome
4. Subphrenic fat
5. Upper abdominal abscesses containing gas
6. Pneumoretroperitoneum

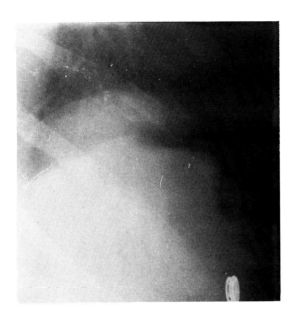

Figure 3–20. Pseudopneumoperitoneum due to diaphragmatic hernia. Posterior herniation projects above the left diaphragmatic dome. Air within the lung between the two muscular projections simulates subphrenic air.

When a single focus of platelike atelectasis appears just above the diaphragm and oriented parallel to it, a band of air-filled lung is seen between these two densities. It may be tempting to consider the atelectatic streak to be the diaphragm, with the subjacent lung as free intraperitoneal air. This form of pseudopneumoperitoneum is more common in patients with emphysema, in whom the diaphragms are flattened, but it may occur even in normal individuals. Most often, the atelectatic streak has a slightly irregular margin and is not as thick as the shadow of the diaphragmatic muscle (Fig 3–21).[60,61] Again, a lateral chest film can be helpful because the simulation of free air by atelectasis should not be seen simultaneously on frontal and lateral views.

Hepatodiaphragmatic interposition of the intestine, also known as Chilaiditi's syndrome, is a well-recognized but clinically innocuous variation of bowel position. It refers to an anterior insinuation of an intestinal loop between the liver below and the right hemidiaphragm above. It may be a temporary or permanent displacement that most often is a consequence of upward migration of the radiographic hepatic flexure. However, other segments of small or large bowel can occupy an anterior subdiaphragmatic location. Those factors that favor hepatodiaphragmatic interposition are a lifetime high-fiber diet, which elongates the colon, a small liver, and a widened thoracic cage, which creates space for the bowel below the diaphragm. Intermittent abdomi-

nal pain and intestinal distension have been attributed to hepatodiaphragmatic interposition, especially if the small bowel is involved. For the most part, however, Chilaiditi's syndrome is merely an incidental roentgenographic finding causing no symptoms. Its significance derives from its confusion with free air. Usually, it is easily distinguished by the identifying markers of bowel such as the valvulae conniventes of small bowel and the haustra and plica semilunares of the colon. Unlike free air, which most often rises to the apex of the diaphragm and is often bilateral, the position of the colon or small bowel is usually most obvious at the lateral margin of the right hemidiaphragm. Despite a sometimes large lucency on the right side, in Chilaiditi's syndrome there is almost never a parallel lucency below the left hemidiaphragm (Fig 3–22).[62,63]

A focal accumulation of fat just beneath the diaphragm is another cause of pseudopneumoperitoneum. Usually, affected individuals are neither obese nor receiving corticosteroid medications. Focal deposition of subphrenic adipose tissue is not a rare anatomic phenomenon, having been observed under the left leaf of the diaphragm in 7 of 600 patients in a study by Mokrohisky. In six of these, the crescent of lucency was seen laterally (Figs 2–6, 3–23).[64] On the other hand, the majority of patients in a review by Martinez and Raskin had a predominately medical accumulation of left-sided fat.[65] Lat-

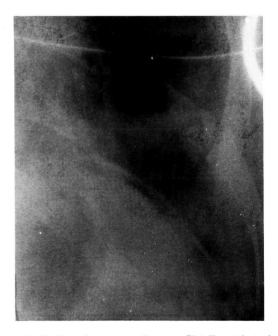

Figure 3–21. Pseudopneumoperitoneum. Platelike atelectasis in the left lower lung directed roughly parallel to the diaphragm resembles free intraperitoneal air if the atelectatic streak is mistaken for the diaphragmatic dome.

eral films may also reveal extensive fat both anteriorly and posteriorly. On the right side there appears to be a greater propensity for lateral and anterior localization. Occasionally, these adipose deposits may be extensive. In one report, subphrenic fat separated the liver from the diaphragmatic leaf by 2.5 cm.[66]

The differentiation of pneumoperitoneum from subphrenic fat can be difficult on plain films. Often, the fat deposit maintains a crescent appearance, unchanging with patient position, whereas free air migrates to the least dependent region of the peritoneal cavity and alters its configuration as the patient turns. Very small collections of intraperitoneal air can be seen on frontal and erect films but may not be discernible on lateral or supine views. Generally, extraperitoneal fat is recognizable on all projections. However, very small deposits may be seen on only one view, as visualization depends on the orientation of the radiographic beam with respect to the interface between fat and surrounding tissue. Free air tends to accumulate underneath the central portion of the diaphragmatic leaf whereas extraperitoneal fat is found in medial or lateral locations. On both sides, subphrenic fat agglomerations do not usually ascend to the summit of the diaphragmatic

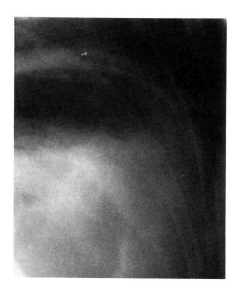

Figure 3–23. Pseudopneumoperitoneum. The sliver of lucency between the air-filled gastric fundus and the lateral left hemidiaphragm is extraperitoneal fat.

dome in its midzone. In this regard, extraperitoneal fat can mimic not only pneumoperitoneum but retroperitoneal air as well.

UPPER ABDOMINAL ABSCESSES

The most important condition to be distinguished from free air is upper abdominal abscess. Pus collections in the subphrenic and subhepatic spaces continue to be a very serious problem, with a recent report indicating a mortality of at least 30%. Subphrenic abscesses may arise spontaneously as a complication of pancreatitis, diverticulitis, or appendicitis, but more than half of them are the result of recent abdominal surgery.[67] In the postoperative interval, the earliest signs of upper abdominal abscess are often unrecognized by the patient or the physician.[68] Therefore, prompt demonstration of these potentially lethal infections is crucial for effective treatment and successful resolution.

There is little dispute that computed tomography is usually the definitive imaging investigation for the detection and delineation of upper abdominal abscesses. In the majority of cases, however, a survey film of the abdomen, an inexpensive and readily obtainable examination, can provide diagnostic clues that may hasten the decision to proceed with computed tomography. Lundstedt et al found plain film abnormalities of upper abdominal abscess in 13 of 20 patients studied. In another review of 77 patients, 87% had plain film evidence of an abscess.

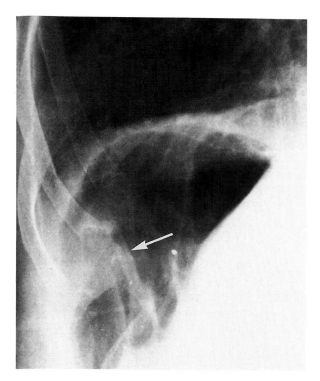

Figure 3–22. Chilaiditi's syndrome. Gas within the colon is interposed between the right hemidiaphragm and the liver. The arrow points to a thin plica semilunares that identifies the large bowel.

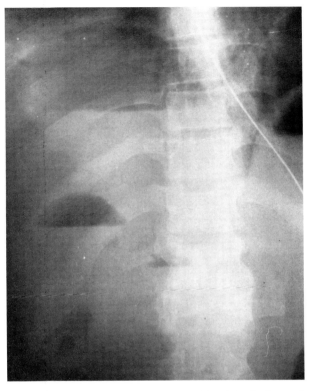

Figure 3–24. Right subphrenic abscess. The right diaphragm is elevated. A large gas and fluid collection, less lucent than the gastric fundus in the contralateral side, identifies the abscess on this upright film. There is also a smaller collection in the subhepatic space.

Gas within the pus collection was seen in 70%. Left-sided abscesses were more difficult to appreciate because the associated dilatation of the stomach, jejunum, transverse colon or splenic flexure obscured small and poorly defined extraluminal lucencies.[67] Simultaneous right and left bilateral subphrenic collections are rare, unlike the bilateral localization of moderate or large amounts of free air. With the exception of pancreatic and lesser sac abscesses, gas pockets are usually confined to one side of the midline. Manifestation of disease in the ipsilateral diaphragm and pleura occur in many upper abdominal abscesses, while pneumoperitoneum alone infrequently causes epiphrenic or pulmonary changes. Miller and Talman, in a retrospective analysis of 48 cases, observed elevation of the diaphragm in 95%, pleural effusion in 75%, and basal atelectasis in 47%.[70] It should be remembered, however, that these data were revealed on retrospective review and may not be appreciated as readily on prospective analyses of plain films of the abdomen. In general, the higher the index of suspicion, the greater the likelihood of discovering subtle abnormalities above and below the diaphragm.

A single large lucency in an abdominal abscess may appear as a well-defined, featureless gas deposit, or it may have irregular contours with indistinct borders (Fig 3–24).[71] Since most abdominal pus collections contain considerable fluid as well as gas, they are less lucent than an equal area of dilated bowel or free air. Unlike ulcer perforations that often do not induce prompt reflex bowel dilatation, abscesses almost always produce an adjacent ileus. Clusters of numerous small bubbles are a frequent concomitant of large abscess cavities.[72] On the other hand, bubbles are an uncommon feature of air in the peritoneal cavity unless accompanied by intraperitoneal fluid. Organ displacement and obliteration of fat planes are additional distinguishing findings of expanding and infiltrating abscesses. Lateral extension may cause loss of properitoneal fat stripe, which is always preserved in uncomplicated pneumoperitoneum.[73]

PNEUMORETROPERITONEUM

Air in the retroperitoneal space and in its lateral and anterior continuations in the abdominal wall may also be mistaken for free air on supine films. Adding to the possible confusion is the occasional coexistence of retroperitoneal and intraperitoneal air.[74,75] The importance of distinguishing between the two cannot be minimized, however, because retroperitoneal air differs markedly from pneumoperitoneum in etiology, clinical course, and treatment.

Trauma to the abdomen is the most common cause of pneumoretroperitoneum (Table 3–4). Ambient air may enter directly through the skin with penetrating wounds or after abdominal surgery. Perforation of the rectum or sigmoid colon during barium enema or endoscopy can result in a massive discharge of gas into the retroperitoneal tissues. Diagnostic pneumoretroperitoneum was performed

TABLE 3–4. CAUSES OF PNEUMORETROPERITONEUM

1. Postoperative
2. Post diagnostic procedure
3. Penetrating trauma
4. Blunt traumatic rupture of the duodenum
5. Pelvic trauma with perforation of the rectum
6. Spontaneous colon perforation
   a. Volvulus
   b. Diverticulosis
   c. Carcinoma
7. Extension from pneumomediastinum
8. Gas-containing retroperitoneal abscess

before the advent of computed tomography and ultrasonography to assess the size and shape of the adrenal glands. This technique took advantage of the ease of flow of gas through the retroperitoneal space during air insufflation accomplished by a needle placed in the retrorectal space. Blunt trauma may rupture the duodenum, resulting in a local accumulation of gas in the right perirenal or anterior pararenal space.[76] Also, with severe pelvic fractures, dislodged bony fragments can perforate the rectum, allowing bowel gas to escape into the retroperitoneal spaces. Spontaneous pneumoretroperitoneum is frequently a consequence of perforations of colonic diverticula or carcinomas. Usually, these patients have minimal symptoms at the time the retroperitoneal gas is discovered and they often seek attention complaining of painless fullness or crepitance in the flank. Volvulus of the sigmoid colon can rupture either within or posterior to the peritoneal cavity. The thorax and the extraperitoneal spaces communicate directly through the mediastinum posteriorly and, to a lesser extent, across small midline openings in the diaphragm anteriorly. Thus, any cause of pneumomediastinum may also produce a pneumoretroperitoneum. A chest X-ray should be done whenever retroperitoneal air is detected. Abscesses, produced by gas-forming organisms, may appear in any retroperitoneal compartment. Since the perirenal space is open inferiorly, an emphysematous renal abscess can involve the anterior and posterior pararenal spaces as well.

The retention of air in the retroperitoneum has not been studied extensively. Older et al obtained serial radiographs of patients who had undergone nephrectomy by an extraperitoneal approach and found that 92% had retroperitoneal gas on the initial postoperative film.[77] Approximately two thirds of these still had air revealed by supine radiographs obtained between 9 and 12 days after operation. In nearly every instance, the air was oriented along the course of the descending or ascending colon and had an elongated configuration or a bubbly pattern indistinguishable from an abscess.[77,78] Whether the natural course of the resolution of postoperative air is similar for other types of pneumoretroperitoneum has not yet been determined. It is likely that the persistence of air depends upon its initial volume in this space. A continued appearance of retroperitoneal lucency beyond 2 to 3 weeks also seems to be a normal finding in some patients.

The plain film manifestations of retroperitoneal emphysema are protean; to make sense of its diverse patterns it is helpful to consider its appearance in various locations. Beneath the diaphragm, it is often difficult to differentiate retroperitoneal from intraperitoneal air, but there are subtle but important distinctions between the two. Retroperitoneal air is usually crescentic, with curvilinear upper and lower borders. It moves little and maintains its shape in all projections. Free intraperitoneal air is highly mobile and on upright or lateral decubitus views it has a straight lower border. Subphrenic extraperitoneal air or gas tends to remain constant or increase slightly during expiration as the diaphragm ascends. During expiration, the compression of the retroperitoneal space by the diaphragm serves to decrease the area of retroperitoneal lucency. Pneumoperitoneum is responsive to the negative intraabdominal pressure during the inspiratory phase of respiration and tends to increase in area, with a corresponding decrease during expiration. Free air rises to the peak of the diaphragmatic dome whereas retroperitoneal air is usually positioned more inferiorly (Fig 3–25). Retroperitoneal air generally accumulates either medially or laterally rather than directly beneath the apex of the diaphragmatic leaf (Fig 3–26).[79] The central portion of the diaphragm is a smooth tendinous cupola connected more inferiorly to the prominent muscular fibers that help perform the work of breathing. Retroperitoneal air can indent the rough surface of the muscle, producing vertically oriented bands of lucency and density. The "visible muscle" sign is not seen with pneumoperitoneum because the posterior peritoneal wall separates free air from the irregular contours of the contractile surface of the diaphragm.[80]

Lucent streaks characterize small and moderate collections of retroperitoneal gas below the sub-

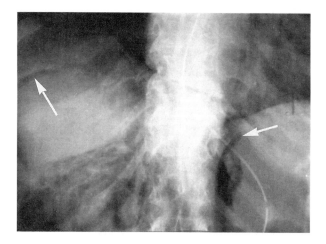

Figure 3–25. Pneumoretroperitoneum. On the right, the crescentic lucency does not reach the diaphragmatic dome (*arrow*). On the left, retroperitoneal air collects medially (*arrow*).

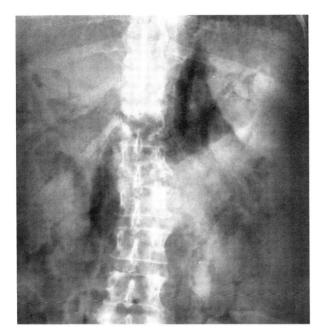

Figure 3–26. Retroperitoneal gas from perforated colonic stercoral ulcer. Streaks of lucency and a more homogenous medial subdiaphragmatic accumulation are seen.

phrenic region. They tend to respect the boundaries of the retroperitoneal compartments in which they arise. Perforation of the descending duodenum is confined to the right anterior pararenal space but less often the perirenal space is breached and air may dissect into it (Fig 3–27).[81,82] The posterior pararenal compartment is usually spared, however, and its lateral extension, the properitoneal fat stripe, remains uninvolved. Sigmoid (diverticular) and carcinoma perforation result in pneumoretroperitoneum initially limited to the left side of the abdomen (Fig 3–28). It can ascend over the psoas muscle while sparing the flank stripe, as it is usually enclosed in the anterior pararenal space (Fig 2–44). Sometimes it may preferentially seek the posterior pararenal

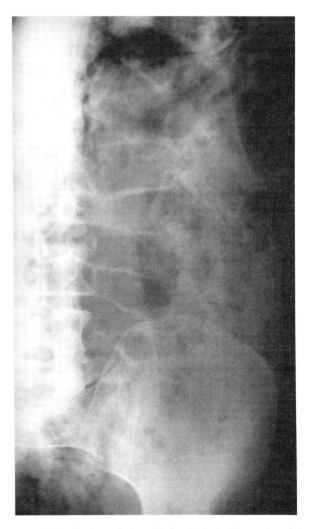

Figure 3–28. Perforated sigmoid diverticulosis. The patient felt well but complained of left flank crepitus. Bubbles point to gas collections in the subcutaneous tissue of the left flank. The streaks in the upper abdomen represent pneumoretroperitoneum. There is no gas in the flank stripe.

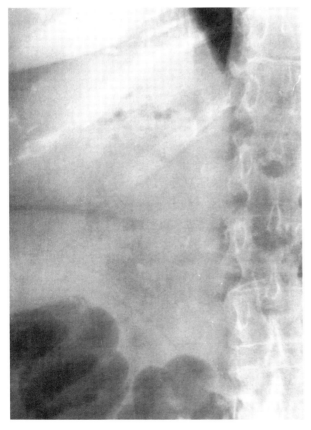

Figure 3–27. Perforated duodenum. A localized collection of bubbles and a fainter, more diffuse lucency below it indicate air in the anterior pararenal space.

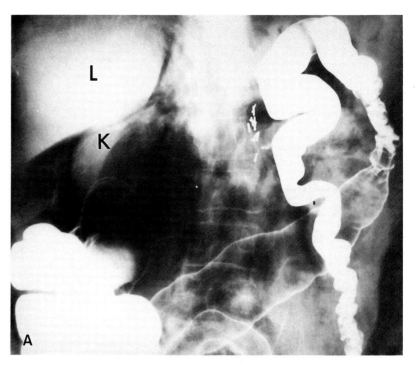

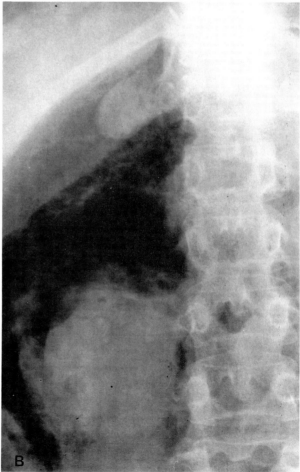

Figure 3–29. A. Massive retroperitoneal emphysema from perforated rectum during barium enema examination. Separate streaks have been replaced by a homogeneous lucency, which makes the right kidney (K) and the posterior liver edge (L) stand out. **B.** Retroperitoneal air insufflation. Gas introduced into the retroperitoneal space in sufficient volume has provided enough contrast to visualize a right adrenal adenoma.

space, where it penetrates the flank stripe while remaining lateral to the psoas muscle. Typically, rectal perforations are bilateral and displace the properitoneal fat lines on both sides.[79]

When a pneumoretroperitoneum becomes extensive, however, these well-defined distributions no longer apply. Large duodenal perforations can eventually extend into the posterior pararenal compartment (Fig 2–60), and a sigmoid perforation may produce bilateral retroperitoneal emphysema if enough gas passes through it. The extraperitoneal space is capacious and large quantities of gas can distend it with relatively little discomfort. Massive accumulations create a homogeneous lucency, outlining the posterior–interior liver edge, the renal shadows, and the adrenal surfaces (Fig 3–29).[83] Iatrogenic perforation often introduces a large volume of gas. It may first come to attention when a postprocedure chest X-ray reveals a pneumomediastinum that results from retroperitoneal gas escaping superiorly.

Enlargement of the retroperitoneal space by air or gas can disrupt the posterior peritoneal wall, producing a pneumoperitoneum. It is important then to look for signs of free air even if retroperitoneal emphysema is first identified. When infection complicates pneumoretroperitoneum, penetration of the soft tissue of flanks can ensue, with gas dissecting along facial planes to the back, buttocks, and lower extremities (Fig 2–45).[84–87]

PSEUDOPNEUMORETROPERITONEUM

There are numerous causes of streaks, bubbles, and amorphous lucencies that can simulate retroperitoneal air (Table 3–5). Occasionally, free air closely resembles retroperitoneal air both in subphrenic and midabdominal locations. Gas-forming abscesses confined within the liver, pancreas, spleen, or subphrenic space can mimic air or gas in the perirenal or anterior pararenal compartments. Fat in the right renal sinus is frequently suggestive of the localized gas collections resulting from perforation of the descending duodenum. Roentgenographically visible renal sinus fat, is a usually bilateral feature that may aid in its differentiation from the unilateral findings of duodenal rupture (Fig 3–30). In markedly obese patients, hemorrhage from the kidney or from a leaking abdominal aortic aneurysm can inflitrate abundant retroperitoneal fat, producing a mottled pattern of lucency and density similar to the appearance of diffuse accumulations of retroperitoneal air and fluid.[88] Rarely, excessive localized proliferation of retroperitoneal fat results in unusual distributions of lucent foci. This condition is well known in the pelvis but may also occur in the mid abdomen.[89] The streaks of pneumoretroperitoneum can be simulated by fat in the psoas muscle (Fig 3–31) or by gas in the soft tissues of the back in patients with gangrene (Fig 3–32). Another pitfall is the peculiar dimensions of air pockets trapped in skin folds that can look like the ribbons of lucency of massive retroperitoneal emphysema, especially when they extend over the properitoneal fat stripes. Finally, factitious pneumoretroperitoneum may have a iatrogenic etiology. Air introduced into the soft tissues of the back during attempts at epidural anesthesia can resemble extraperitoneal air.[90]

TABLE 3–5. PSEUDOPNEUMORETROPERITONEUM

1. Pneumoperitoneum
2. Abscesses within liver or spleen
3. Subphrenic abscess
4. Fat in the renal sinuses
5. Excessive retroperitoneal fat
6. Retroperitoneal hemorrhage
7. Fat in the psoas muscles
8. Spontaneous subcutaneous emphysema
9. Iatrogenic subcutaneous emphysema

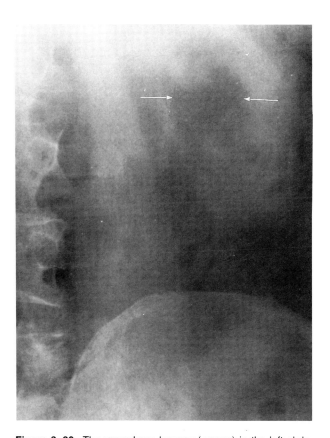

Figure 3–30. The amorphous lucency (*arrows*) in the left abdomen is not pneumoretroperitoneum but fat in the renal sinus.

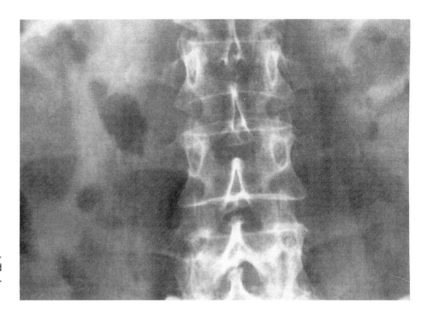

Figure 3–31. Pseudopneumoretroperitoneum. The thin streaks are confined within and aligned along the course of the psoas muscle and represent fat.

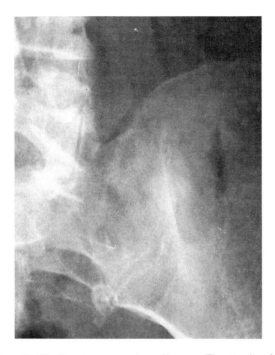

Figure 3–32. Pseudopneumoretroperitoneum. The streaks of lucency overlying and superior to the left iliac crest are in the subcutaneous tissue in a patient with gangrene.

ASCITES

The importance of plain films of the abdomen in the evaluation of ascites has diminished in recent years with the introduction of cross-sectional imaging techniques. Most plain radiographic signs of ascites have limited reliability whereas computed tomography and ultrasonography are able to de-tect small effusions with great accuracy. Moreover, they can quantify the extent of fluid and demonstrate coexistent masses within and near the peritoneal cavity.

Despite the restricted utility of plain films, it would be a mistake to completely neglect their contribution to the assessment of ascites. The supine radiograph is often the first imaging examination obtained in a patient with an enlarged abdomen. Frequently, it is difficult to differentiate between obesity and intraperitoneal fluid on clinical grounds alone. In most cases, the plain film can demonstrate a massive or moderate effusion even if it is relatively insensitive for the recognition of small fluid accumulations. The prompt determination of the absence of substantial ascites or intraperitoneal mass may obviate the need for an extensive diagnostic workup in a patient with expanding abdominal girth.

The best radiographic evidence for the lack of significant intraperitoneal fluid is preservation of the shadow of the hepatic angle. On the right side, the properitoneal fat stripe, which is in continuity with the posterior pararenal retroperitoneal compartment, lies just peripheral to the lateral edge of the liver. The inferior border of the liver abuts omental fat and adipose tissue surrounding the ascending colon and hepatic flexure, both of which are primarily intraperitoneal structures. Except in children and emaciated adults, omental fat is a constant anatomic feature whereas pericolic fat is more variable in abundance. Normally, the homogeneous mass of the liver stands out clearly against the lucent background of adjacent fat (Fig 3–33). However, if as-

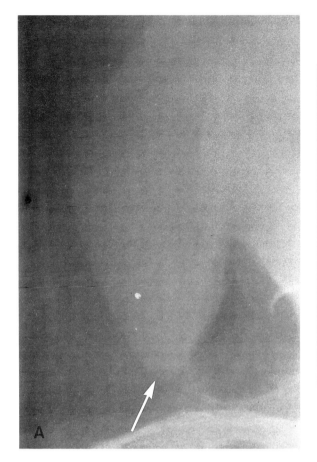
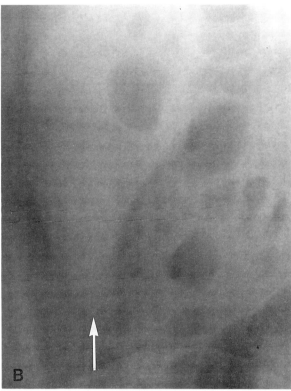

Figure 3–33. Two examples of preservation of the hepatic angle. In (**A**) the liver tip is rounded (*arrow*), and in (**B**) it is more angular. In both, abundant intraperitoneal fat surrounds the hepatic angle.

cites should displace the omentum and colon medially, the hepatic angle loses its clear demarcation even though the properitoneal fat is undisturbed. It must be emphasized that the hepatic angle corresponds to the inferior lateral tip of the liver. More medially, the hepatic edge is often obscured by fluid and gas in bowel loops.[91]

This sign has several pitfalls. Proper technique using low kilovoltage is essential for its demonstration. Adhesions in the lower abdomen may retard the flow of fluid along the right paracolic gutter. In such cases, the hepatic angle could be preserved even in the face of ascites.[92] Occasionally, intraperitoneal fluid accumulates in Morison's pouch preferentially without extending laterally and inferiorly adjacent to the liver. The hepatic angle sign is retained, giving no indication that fluid has collected elsewhere in the peritoneal cavity.[93]

Loss of the hepatic angle need not be the result of poor technique or ascites. Meyers et al have shown that the inferior liver edge may be lost with extraperitoneal effusions involving all three retroperitoneal compartments.[94] They maintain that ret-

roperitoneal fat is also border forming with the hepatic angle, and when it is replaced by fluid the liver edge cannot be discerned even if omental fat is unaffected. Excessive feces in the hepatic flexure can also obliterate the hepatic angle.[95] These caveats notwithstanding, in a study of the distribution of ascites, obscuration of the hepatic angle was found in 98% of patients and was seen to be a dependable indication of intraperitoneal fluid.[92]

Much has been written about the widening of the homogeneous density of the fluid-filled paracolic gutter in ascites and hemoperitoneum. Small effusions increase the distance between the flank stripe and gas in the colonic lumen beyond the normal distance of 2 to 3 mm.[96] With continuing accretions of fluid, the flank stripe narrows and the gas-filled bowel moves further away from it (Fig 3–34).[97,98] It has been claimed that as little as 25 mL of ascites can be detected along the right paracolic gutter if the films are obtained during the inspiratory phase of respiration with the patient supine and the knees flexed. Maximal distension of the right gutter can be achieved if the patient assumes the right lat-

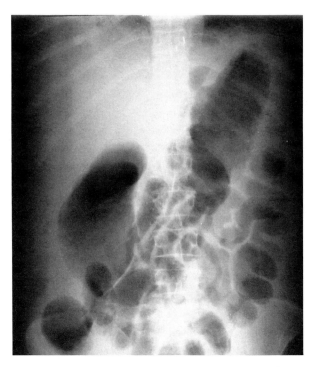

Figure 3–34. Malignant ascites from metastatic breast carcinoma. The descending colon is displaced from the lateral wall of the abdomen as fluid fills the paracolic gutter.

eral decubitus position for 1 or 2 minutes before the supine film is obtained.[92]

The widened paracolic gutter sign also has limitations. The small bowel may be normally interposed lateral to the colon on both the right and left side. Adhesions limit free flow of fluid from the pelvis and the upper abdominal peritoneal recesses.[96] The distended paracolic gutter sign is comparable in sensitivity to the loss of the hepatic angle for the plain film detection of ascites.[92]

Frimann-Dahl emphasized the pertinence of pelvic accumulation of intraperitoneal fluid.[99] One third of the volume of the peritoneal space [93] is in the pelvis, and the pouch of Douglas is a favored site for intra-abdominal malignant seeding.[100] The capacity and the conformation of the pelvic peritoneal space is variable, depending upon the distension of the bladder and rectum, the extent of extraperitoneal fat, the configuration of the sacrum, and the shape of the pararectal recesses.[92,96] A fluid-filled bladder or rectum may impinge upon pelvic peritoneal effusions, displacing them laterally.[101] Larger fluid collections can appear as symmetrical bulges somewhat resembling "dog ears" (Fig 3–35). The greater the amount of pelvic adipose tissue, the smaller the volume of the lower peritoneal cavity. Similarly, a capacious area created by a posterior angulated sacrum may limit the lateral extent of the pelvic peritoneal space as it lengthens its sagittal expanse. Fluid often collects in the dorsomedial pararectal recesses before involving the lateral recesses.[92]

All these anatomic variants lessen the dependability of the signs of pelvic accumulation of intraperitoneal fluid. Also, intestinal loops may mimic free fluid collections. The diagnostic value of rounded fluid densities in the pelvis has been vastly overrated. In our experience, it is seldom definitive and never occurs without evidence of ascites in the flank and at the hepatic angle.

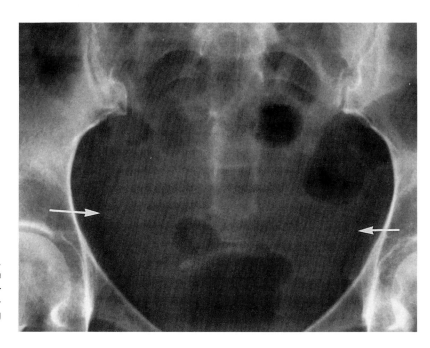

Figure 3–35. Pelvic accumulation of ascites. Situated above the bladder is a large collection of peritoneal fluid most prominent laterally (*arrows*). The bowing of peritoneal fluid peripherally occasionally suggests the contour of dog ears.

An interesting sign of intraperitoneal fluid, first reported by Hellmer in 1942, is visualization of the medially displaced lateral edge of the liver.[102] It is a radiological curiosity, rather than a helpful diagnostic finding, because marked ascites (usually in excess of 100 mL) is needed to visualize the liver edge.[103] Proto and Lane have shown that there is a 5% difference in density between the liver and ascitic fluid, which is enough to allow perception of a distinct interface between the two on plain films.[104] Hellmer's sign is more common in ascites of malignant disease than cirrhosis, probably because the fatty cirrhotic liver more closely approximates the density of intraperitoneal fluid. It is also not seen with hemoperitoneum because intraperitoneal blood is nearly isodense to the hepatic substance.[104] Wixson et al have demonstrated a displaced lateral edge of the liver as a result of a contiguous extraperitoneal fluid collection, indicating that Hellmer's sign is not pathognomonic for ascites.[105]

The lateral edge of the liver is best noticed if the patient is placed in the right posterior oblique position (Fig 3–36). A clearly demarcated right hepatic margin has also been seen with extensive retroperi-

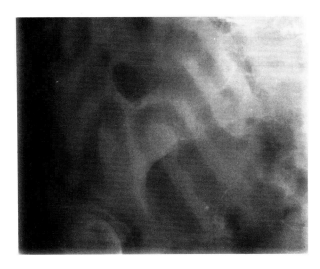

Figure 3–37. Tuberculous peritonitis. Coned-down view of the right lower quadrant. The gas-filled bowel loops appear rigid, as they are fixed in place by fibrosis, fluid, and peritoneal granulomas.

toneal fat (Fig 6–7) and in various diseases associated with increased storage of iron, such as hemolytic anemia treated by repeated transfusions and hemochromatosis. In all these conditions, not only the lateral but also the inferior and superior edges of the liver stand out, whereas in ascites, only the lateral hepatic surface is visible.

There are other plain film findings that have been associated with ascites, but all of them are either nonspecific or first observed when intraperitoneal fluid has reached massive proportions. Apparent separation of bowel loops may occur with intraperitoneal fluid but is more often evidence of the incidental radiographic juxtaposition of two bowel segments some distance from each other or increased fluid in adjacent intestinal lumens.[106] Absence of the lateral psoas margin has little relationship to intraperitoneal effusion and is more dependent on the degree of retroperitoneal fat adjacent to that muscle. An overall increase in density of the abdomen, the so-called ground glass sign, is often an artifact of poor technique. However, when it is a result of ascites there is always other radiographic evidence that intraperitoneal fluid is present.[95]

Finally, ascites can be complicated by masses and strictures in the peritoneal cavity. In metastatic carcinoma, lymphoma, radiation fibrosis, and peritoneal tuberculosis, bowel loops are tacked down and stiffened, often lacking the identifying markers of valvulae conniventes or haustra. The bowel loops are fixed in place rather than floating medially, as their location and appearance are influenced by a combination of tumoral or granulomatous masses, fluid, and fibrosis within the peritoneal cavity (Fig 3–37).

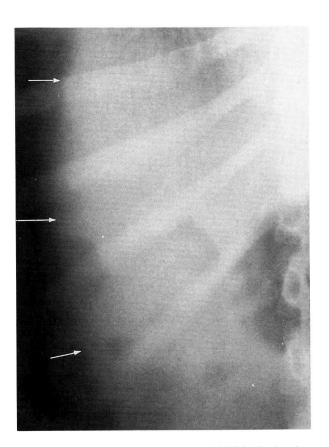

Figure 3–36. Hellmer's sign. The arrows highlight the interface between the denser lines medially and the more lucent ascitic fluid laterally.

CALCIFICATION IN THE PERITONEAL CAVITY

A heterogeneous group of radiodensities can be found within the peritoneal cavity and its mesenteric attachments. They include concretions of variable size, large cystic calcifications, and solid opacities.

The appendices epiploicae are fatty collections attached to the colon and are located along the anterior and posterior–inferior teniae coli. There are approximately 100 appendices epiploicae arrayed throughout the course of the colon.[107–109] They generally range between 0.5 and 5.0 cm in diameter but some can be as large as 10 cm.[110] Torsion of these bodies compromises blood flow and leads to infarction. A devitalized appendix epiploica may calcify and detach from its colonic moorings, becoming free in the peritoneal cavity.[111] Although torsion causes pain, mobile detached appendices epiploicae are asymptomatic.[112] Typically they are round or oval densities with radiolucent centers and thin calcified margins. When they are no longer attached to the colon they tend to migrate to the pelvis, the most dependent part of the peritoneal cavity.[113] Appendices epiplocae may be suspected on plain abdominal radiographs by their characteristic annular or elliptical marginal calcification, their movement on suc-

cessive films, and their location outside the gastrointestinal and genitourinary tracts (Fig 3–38). Rarely, omental fat deposits may calcify and come to lie free in the peritoneal cavity, where they look like appendices epiploicae (Fig 3–39).

Almost always, only one or two appendices epiploicae are visualized. In rare instances numerous large pericolic fat bodies may calcify, producing a remarkable pattern on plain films (Fig 3–40). Similar in appearance are the radiodense margins of lipid granulomas that form around exogenous oil within the peritoneal cavity (Fig 3–41). Synonyms for this entity include lipogranulomas, oil granulomas, and paraffinomas. Most often they are introduced directly by the surgeon during an abdominal operation. They can also enter the peritoneal cavity through the uterus and fallopian tubes if hysterosalpingography is performed with fat-soluble contrast material. Another port of entry is through a perforated rectum after mineral oil enema. In the past, some surgeons have advocated the use of mineral oil as a lubricant, but in many instances droplets of lipid have become nidi within the peritoneum for the formation of cystic masses with fibrous margins. Marginal calcification can occur within 4 months after the introduction of a liquid material, but in other cases these rounded opacities first appeared 30 years after operation.[114,115] Typically, the lipid

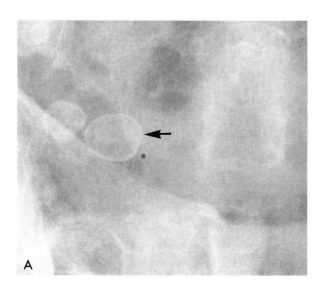

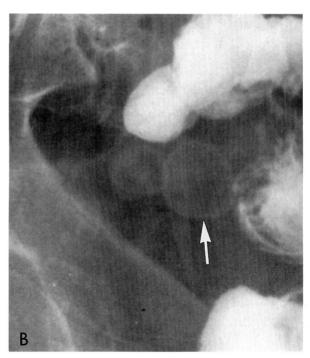

Figure 3–38. A. Two calcified appendices epiploicae (*arrow*). **B.** A film from a barium enema shows them to be outside the colon (*arrow*).

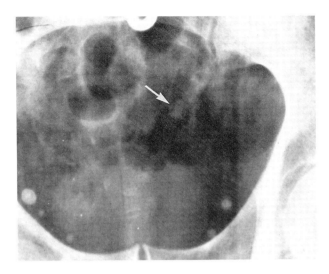

Figure 3–39. Faint rounded calcification above the bladder (*arrow*). The calcification was removed incidentally at bladder surgery and was found to be an intraperitoneal nodule of fat necrosis.

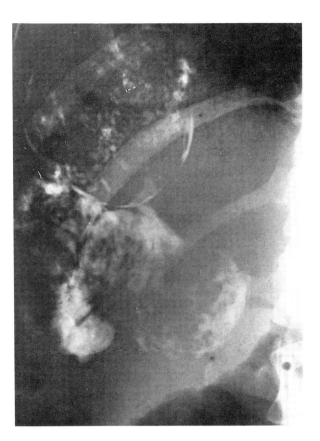

Figure 3–42. Mixed solid and cystic calcification in liver metastases from mucinous cystadenocarcinoma of the ovary. Often these tumors are associated with cystic calcification in the peritoneum. (*Courtesy of Dr. Paul Cohen.*)

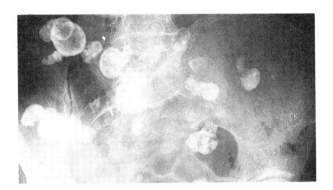

Figure 3–40. A patient with numerous calcified appendices epiploicae. (*Courtesy of Dr. Mariel Dulbey.*)

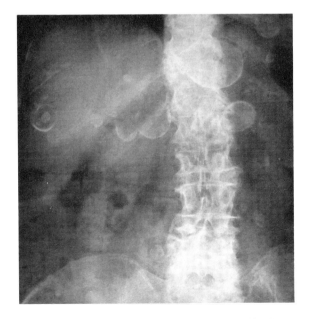

Figure 3–41. Numerous rounded intraperitoneal calcifications typical of intraperitoneal lipid granulomas.

granulomas have varying diameters and may be found in any location within the peritoneal cavity. Computed tomography investigations have revealed their true nature as they demonstrate both a radiopaque margin and a lucent center.[116,117]

In pseudomyxoma peritoneii, the peritoneal cavity is studded with mucin-containing globules varying from a few millimeters to several centimeters in width. They form with the rupture of an appendix containing carcinoma or with peritoneal seeding from an ovarian mucinous cystadenocarcinoma.[118–120] Although it has been stated that pseudomyxoma peritoneii can be a complication of benign lesions of the ovary and appendix, the only well-documented cases have been in patients with malignancy.[121] Characteristically, innumerable small rounded calcifications of varying diameter are seen. A few cysts may be irregularly marginated and some may contain central calcification.[122–124] There may also be small, solid collections of calcium interspersed between the cysts.[119] The calcific lesions of pseudomyxoma peritoneii may be diffusely situated throughout the peritoneum space or can be confined in localized collections often superimposed on the liver or spleen (Fig 3–42). Pseudomyxoma peritoneii simulates calcified lipid granulomas. These gelatinous tumefactions are rarely as dense as the sharply marginated opacities surrounding exogenous material, however.

Calcification can occur in the walls of cysts of the mesentery (Fig 3–43) and omentum (Fig 3–44). These cysts may be congenital or a result of inflammation or trauma. Typically, they resemble other cysts with curvilinear marginal calcification.[125,126] Mesenteric and omental cysts can move on sequential films but on a single abdominal radiography they may not be differentiable from cysts in adjacent organs. Lateral and oblique projections demonstrate that they are anterior to the pancreas, kidney, spleen, and adrenal glands. However, at times, retroperitoneal cysts, which can also displace the bowel, may be indistinguishable from intraperitoneal cysts on plain films (Fig 3–45).

Solid calcification within the peritoneum occurs in tuberculosis and metastatic tumors. Tuberculous foci vary in size and may remain separate or coalesce into thick plaques.[127–129] Fibrotic reaction

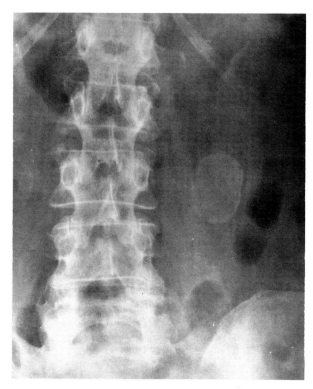

Figure 3–44. Calcified cyst in the gastrocolic ligament. The annular type calcification is typical for cysts of any type.

within the peritoneum mats down the mesentery and the intestines and helps to localize and isolate the infection into several pockets.[130] When the tuberculous lesions caseate, they can calcify, and the distribution of calcification reflects the extent of peritoneal involvement (Fig 3–46).[131,132] Sheetlike deposits or thick masses up to 10 cm in diameter may be seen along with smaller, scattered calcific conglomerations.[133] Because one of the sources of peritoneal infection is tuberculous mesenteric lymphadenopathy, radiodense nodes may be present as well.[134] Intraperitoneal calcification is usually more extensive and diffuse than nodal calcification and can be found at the periphery of the peritoneum.

Both primary and metastatic intraperitoneal neoplasms occasionally calcify. In the rare mesothelioma of the peritoneum diffuse calcifications sometimes occur.[135,136] More commonly, calcification is found in metastases to the peritoneum. Serous cystadenocarcinoma of the ovary and adenocarcinoma of the colon are the primary sites with the greatest predilection for peritoneal calcification (Fig 2–119). Usually, the metastatic deposits are faint densities with poorly defined margins. Denser calcifications are typical for intraperitoneal undifferentiated carcinoma.[137]

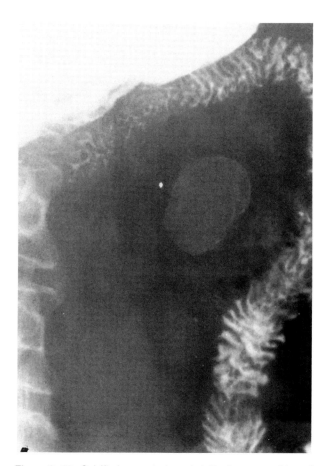

Figure 3–43. Calcified mesenteric cyst. A film from a small bowel series shows a cystic calcification in the mesentery.

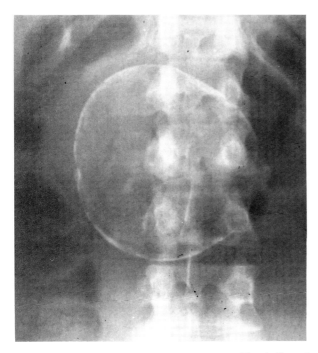

Figure 3–45. Calcified retroperitoneal hematoma. The rimlike calcification of this density mimics the appearance of intraperitoneal cysts.

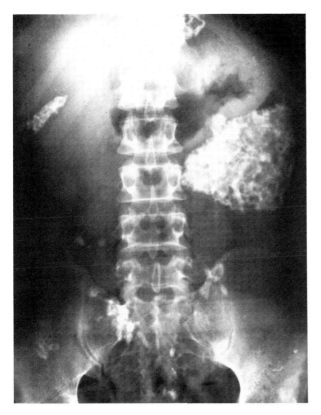

Figure 3–46. Tuberculous peritonitis. A large plaque in the left mid abdomen as well as multiple nodular densities scattered elsewhere in the peritoneal space. (*Courtesy of Dr. Robert Mindelzun.*)

LYMPH NODE CALCIFICATION

Abdominal lymph node calcifications are among the most frequently observed opacities on plain films of the abdomen. Most often, nodal calcifications are easily recognized, but at times they can be mistaken for other radiopacities such as ureteral stones, appendicoliths, and uterine leiomyoma. The appearance of nodal calcifications is variable, but they nearly always exhibit the morphological features of a solid mass.

Calcification can occur in any abdominal nodal chain, but by far the most common are mesenteric lymph nodes (Fig 3–47). In nearly every instance, mesenteric node calcification is caused by tuberculous mycobacteria.[138] Previously, when intestinal tuberculosis was common, involvement of mesenteric lymph nodes was nearly universal (Fig 3–48). With the elimination of bovine tuberculosis as a clinical problem in most developed countries, the incidence of lymph node calcification has decreased.[139,140] Nevertheless, calcified lymph nodes are still recognized on plain films of the abdomen in patients with no history of intestinal disease.[141,142] Mycobacteria enter intestinal lymphatics after passing through bowel mucosa and are deposited in mesenteric nodes.[143] Both animal and human studies have revealed that bacteria can pass through epithelial cells in the intestinal wall without residual damage.[141–146]

Today, most mycobacteria entering the gastrointestinal tract originate from pulmonary foci. Nearly everyone who has had a clinical or subclinical tuberculous infection has swallowed mycobacteria. Most of the bacilli pass through the intestinal tract, but some penetrate the mucosa and eventually collect in lymphoid tissue. Almost all patients with calcified mesenteric nodes have had a pulmonary tuberculous infection.[147] Some may have residual evidence of disease in the lungs but chest X-rays often do not reveal changes of tuberculosis, especially when the initial infection occurred early in childhood. Moreover, not everyone with calcified mesenteric lymph nodes is a positive reactor to tuberculin. It is well recognized that a response to tuberculin will diminsh with time.[148] In many patients with calcified mesenteric nodes, the first exposure of intestinal lymphoid tissue to mycobacteria may have occurred several decades previously.

Mycobacteria causes caseation necrosis and hyaline degeneration of lymphoid tissue. Both processes promote the deposition of calcium salts. Only a portion of a node may calcify, but usually most of it becomes radiodense. Typically, the calcification is sharply defined with a curvilinear margin that is no more opaque than the interior of the node (Figs 3–

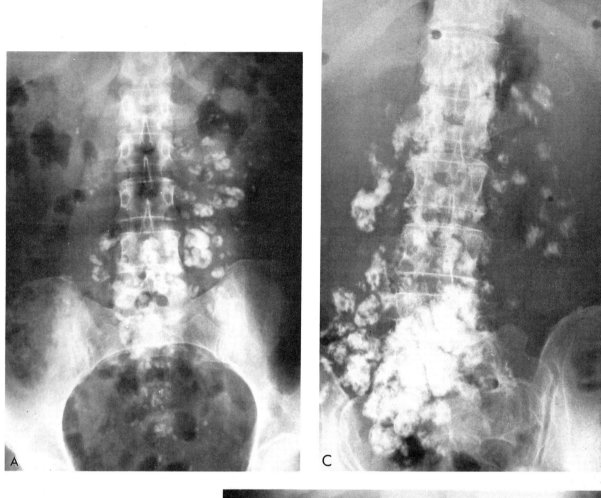

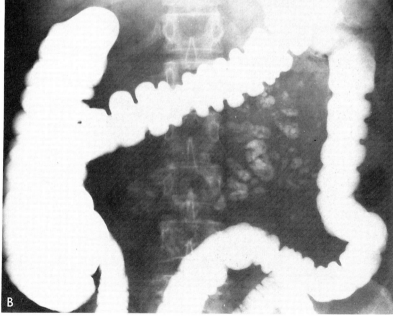

Figure 3–47. A. Widespread, predominantly mesenteric node calcification. **B.** Calcified mesenteric nodes. A film from a barium enema shows the relationship of mesenteric nodes to the colon. **C.** Another patient with extensive mesenteric node calcification.

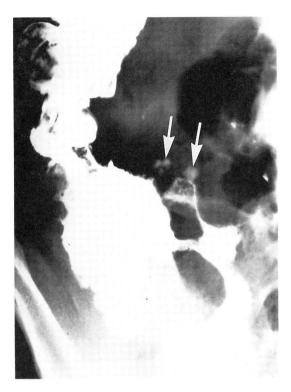

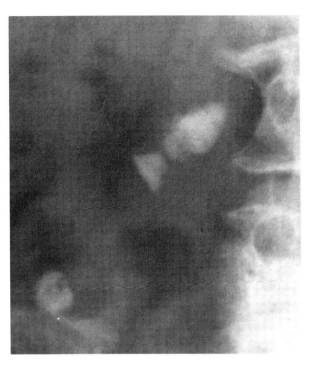

Figure 3–50. Triangular, ovoid, and rounded calcified mesenteric nodes.

Figure 3–48. Calcified nodes (*arrows*) in the mesentery of a patient with ileocecal tuberculosis. Note the strictures in the cecum and terminal ileum. Nowadays, most calcified mesenteric nodes are unassociated with active intestinal disease.

49). Occasionally, calcified nodes may appear as elongated, triangular, or roughly rectangular densities (Fig 3–50). If multiple nodes are seen, they may differ in the extent of opacity, with some brightly calcified nodes next to others that are more faint (Fig. 3–51). Minute, rounded lucencies are almost always present and are located in both the center and the periphery, giving the node a mottled appearance. Rarely, a lymph node will have a homogeneous lucent center and an annular rim of calcification.[149]

Calcified nodes vary greatly in size. A few may reach 7 cm in their longest axis, but usually they range between 1 and 3 cm in diameter (Fig 3–52).[150] The most frequent location of calcified mesenteric nodes is in the right lower quadrant because intestinal lymphoid tissue is most prominent there and bowel contents move slowly in the cecum, permitting more bacteria to penetrate the mucosa and enter draining lymphatics.[151] However, calcified lymph nodes may be seen elsewhere in the mesentery, even in the absence of right lower quadrant calcification. Mesenteric nodes can change in location on sequential examinations, the amount of movement related to the distance form the root of the mesentery.[147] To a limited extent, they can also change their position relative to each other (Fig 3–53).

Calcification in para-aortic nodes is uncommon. Occasionally it occurs in asymptomatic patients with

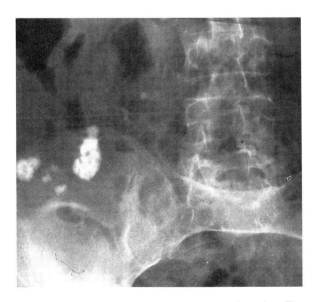

Figure 3–49. A typical appearance of mesenteric nodes. There are nodes of varying size with dense calcification. The larger nodes have curvilinear margins and multiple lucencies in the center and periphery.

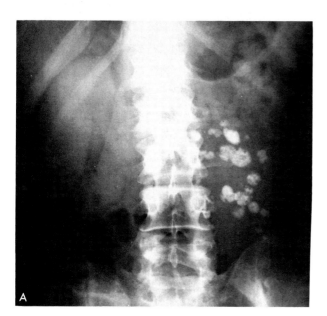
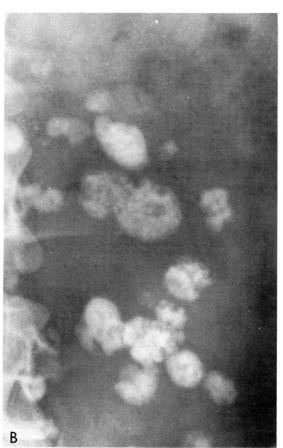

Figure 3–51. A. Many calcified mesenteric nodes but none are in the right lower quadrant. **B.** Detail of **A.** The nodes have differing degrees of radiopacity.

no history of therapy. When seen in conjunction with calcified mesenteric nodes, para-aortic node calcification may be an indication of active or healed disseminated tuberculosis (Fig 3–54).[152] When only the para-aortic nodes are radiodense, however, the etiology is often obscure. The most common cause of isolated para-aortic node calcification is infiltration by tumor. Metastatic adenocarcinoma of the colon and serous cystadenocarcinoma of the ovary are the two most common tumors associated with calcified nodes in this region.[153–160] In colon cancer, calcification appears in areas of degenerating tissue, but in serous cystadenocarcinoma of the ovary, calcification is laid down intracellularly in psammoma bodies in a growing tumor (Fig 3–55). In both malignancies, nodal calcification may occur before calcification in the primary site. Other carcinomas in which calcified para-aortic metastases have been demonstrated include cervix,[161,162] testes,[162] stomach,[163,164] breast,[162] thyroid,[162] and kidney.[153] Occasionally lymphomas calcify before therapy is

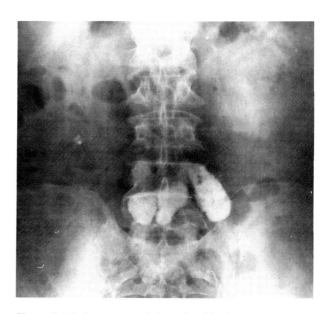

Figure 3–52. Large mesenteric nodes. The largest measures 7 cm.

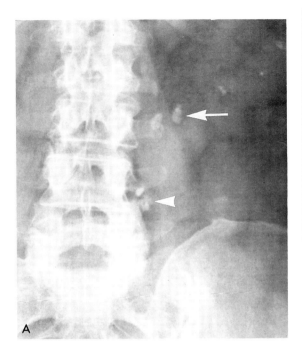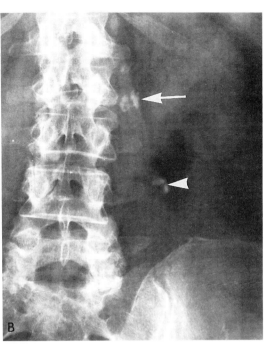

Figure 3–53. Calcified mesenteric node movement. The two upper nodes (*arrows*) move relative to each other on films taken at different times. The lower nodes (*arrowheads*) change their position also.

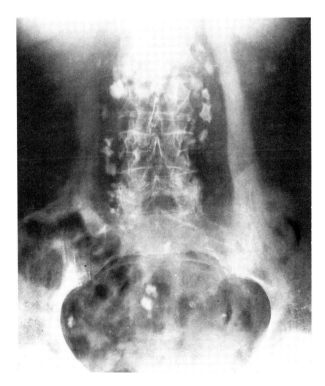

Figure 3–54. Calcification in mesenteric and para-aortic nodes in a patient with a history of tuberculosis.

instituted.[165,166] Bone formation in nodes occurs in metastatic osteosarcoma,[167] adenocarcinoma of the colon,[168] and testicular teratocarcinoma,[169] where nodes in the left renal hilus may also ossify (Fig 3–56), Rarely, calcification is found in para-aortic nodes in silicosis, almost always along with extensive mediastinal nodal calcification (Fig 3–57).

Calcified metastatic nodes tend to be larger than those involved with tuberculosis because of the enlargement of the node by the tumor.[170] Initially they are faintly calcified but later may increase in density and extent.[171] Usually they appear as speckled, stippled, or finely mottled opacities.[172,173] Occasionally ringlike or plaquelike calcification is seen.[174] Calcification may be found in nodes infiltrated with seminoma, Hodgkin's lymphoma, or cervical cancer after chemotherapy or radiotherapy has been instituted.[174–176] The alkaline pH within nodes containing metastasis, a consequence of cellular destruction, favors calcium deposition.[163] After therapy, roentgenographically visible calcification may ensue rapidly, sometimes as early as 5 weeks, and almost always within 1 year (Fig 3–58).[162] This is in contrast to intervals of between 10 and 36 months following exposure to mycobacteria before nodal opacification appears.[143]

Increased lymph nodes density is not always due to calcification or ossification. It can be simulated by contrast material remaining after lymphangiography. Residual contrast nearly always is confined to para-aortic and pelvic nodes (Fig 3–59).

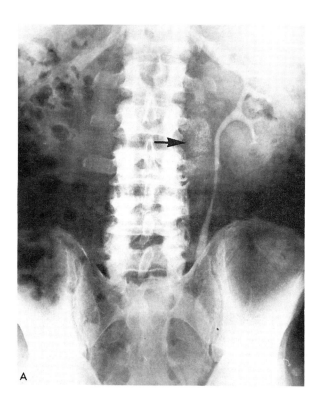
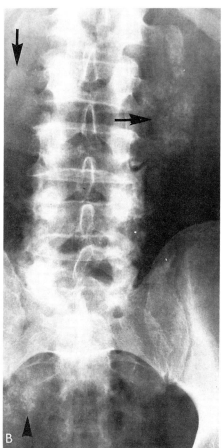

Figure 3–55. Lymph node calcification: metastases from rectal carcinoma. The primary tumor was removed but there was no history of radiotherapy of chemotherapy prior to the onset of calcification. **A.** Calcification of left para-aortic nodes (*horizontal arrow*) on film from an intravenous urography. **B.** Follow-up examination reveals right additional para-aortic nodal calcification (*vertical arrow*) and iliac node calcification (*arrowhead*). (*Courtesy of Dr. Ronald Schliftman.*)

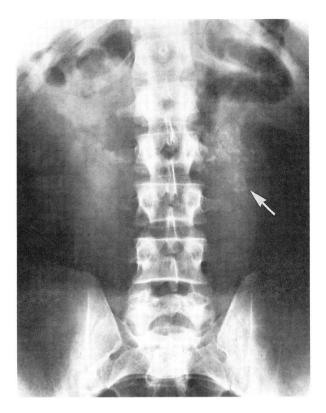

Figure 3–56. Metastatic teratocarcinoma of the testes. Only the mass adjacent to L2 (*arrow*) was seen on plain films; at surgery an ossified lymph node metastasis just below the left renal hilus was found. The patient had received no therapy prior to this film.

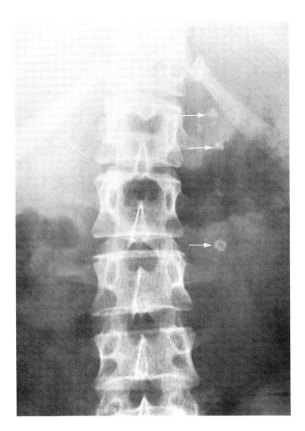

Figure 3–58. Calcified para-aortic nodes following radiotherapy for Hodgkin's disease (*horizontal arrows*). Calcified gallstones are present on the right (*oblique arrows*).

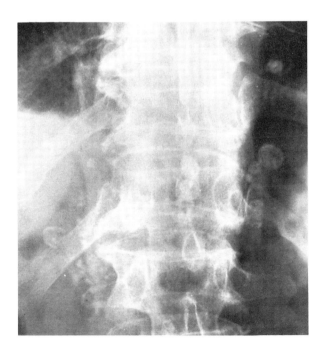

Figure 3–57. Bilateral eggshell calcification in para-aortic lymph nodes in a patient with silicosis. There were similar changes in mediastinal and hila nodes.

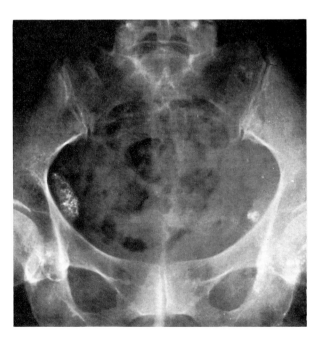

Figure 3–59. Remnants of lymphangiographic contrast material in pelvic nodes. Note the similarity of the nodal opacification to that seen in Figure 3–62.

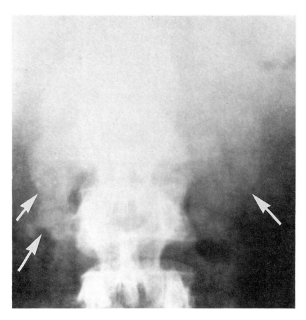

Figure 3–60. Hemosiderin-laden lymph nodes. Arrows point to enlarged para-aortic nodes infiltrated with iron. The nodes are enlarged.

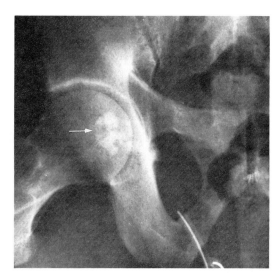

Figure 3–61. Inguinal node calcification (*arrow*) in a patient with gonorrhea.

Sometimes contrast in nodes resembles calcification secondary to treatment of Hodgkin's disease or other neoplasms. Contrast tends to diminish or even disappear over a period of time, and this may be a useful finding if a sequence of films is available. On occasion, however, lymph node calcification can also gradually disappear.[177]

Increased deposition of hemosiderin is sometimes visible on plain films as faint opacities in para-aortic nodes. Patients with thalassemia who have received multiple blood transfusions for a long time may have enlarged nodes in the upper lumbar and lower thoracic area, which can be seen on plain films. The nodes are generally moderately enlarged and only slightly more dense than the surrounding soft tissues. Almost always, the liver and spleen are also enlarged (Fig 3–60).[178]

Isolated calcification of inguinal nodes is rare but may be seen in tubercular or gonococcal infection (Fig 3–61). Pelvic node calcification is also very uncommon. Nodal opacification can occur in tuberculosis after extension from foci in the adnexa or adjacent muscle and bone (Fig 3–62),[179] in metastatic colon carcinoma, and after treatment of cervical malignancy. Lymphangiographic contrast can persist in pelvic nodes and may resemble calcification. An extremely dense pelvic node suggests bone formation in metastatic osteosarcoma (Fig 3–63).

Many of the radiodense entities discussed in this monograph may mimic calcification in lymph nodes. Among these are stones in the urinary, bil-

iary, and gastrointestinal tract and solid masses in the buttocks and uterus. Differentiation of these densities from lymph nodes is usually not difficult. The anatomic distribution of nodal calcification is generally readily discernible, employing either a supine abdominal film alone or in conjunction with oblique and lateral projections. Oblique films demonstrate the anterior position of gallbladder calculi as well as the posterior locations of urinary tract calcifications and the far posterior and lateral positions of opacities in the buttocks. The solid mass

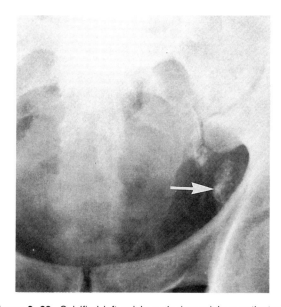

Figure 3–62. Calcified left pelvic node (*arrow*) in a patient with tuberculosis.

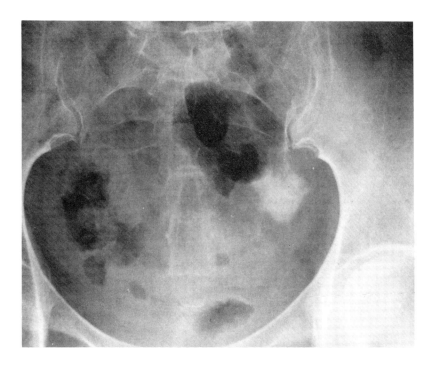

Figure 3–63. Metastatic osteosarcoma to the left adnexa simulating calcification in an inguinal node. (*Courtesy of Dr. C. Charnsangavej.*)

configuration of most lymph node calcifications can distinguish them from the ringlike or laminated appearance of concretions in the urinary tract, gallbladder, or appendix.

CALCIFICATION IN THE AORTA AND THE ILIAC ARTERIES

Arterial calcification is a frequently encountered finding on plain films of the abdomen. With advancing age, the probability of calcium deposition in vascular walls increases, and in the elderly, calcification is common. Usually, arterial calcification is easily recognized. However, difficulties in interpretation arise when the focus of radiopacity is faint, small, or displaced from its usual position. It is these circumstances that demand careful inspection of plain films because the observation of vascular calcification may avoid the need for further imaging procedures, or at least direct the workup to more definitive examinations. For example, the presence of calcification in the wall of an aortic aneurysm on plain abdominal films can readily indicate the location and size of the aneurysm. Appreciation of the conduit morphology of vascular calcification can help distinguish arterial densities from other radiodensities.

The appearance of calcification depends on three factors: (1) the orientation of the vessel wall with respect to the X-ray beam, (2) the degree of calcium deposition, and (3) the location of calcification in the vessel wall. When an artery is oriented perpendicular to the X-ray beam and is diffusely calcified, two parallel tracks of radiopacity can be observed (Fig 2–99). They represent calcification at the sites in the vessel wall where the radiographic beam is directed tangentially. X-rays passing through the vessel on a tangent must traverse the greatest thickness of vascular wall, and this section of the wall will appear more dense on radiographs. Hence, although the entire vessel may be calcified, often only marginal lines of calcification are appreciated. On the other hand, when the lumen is parallel to the X-ray beam, the artery is viewed en face and the radiographic beam then passes through a similar path along all parts of the calcified vascular wall of (Fig 2–100). In either case, calcification may be spotty and irregular, reflecting the inhomogeneous nature of calcium deposition in arterial walls.

The pattern of calcification in extensively calcified aneurysms is relatively independent of position with regard to the X-ray beam. This is particularly true in saccular aneurysms, which assume a spherical configuration and appear as arcuate lines of radiodensity. Usually, the curvilinear calcification of an aneurysm does not describe a complete circle, the area of absent calcification representing the orifice of the neck of the aneurysm (Fig 2 113). In fusiform aneurysms, two convex outward tracks of calcification are observed (Fig 2–112). Most often, aneurysms are larger than calcified vessels of normal caliber.

Dilated arteries as well as those of normal caliber may lengthen and become tortuous. Thus, although arterial calcification is most often found at an expected anatomic site, it may also be seen on plain films away from its usual position. For example, the abdominal aorta below the renal arteries can extend to the right side of the lumbar spine, or far from the spine to the left, or caudal to its normal bifurcation at L3–L4 (Fig 3–64).

The recognition of arterial calcification is usually easy if the calcification is diffuse and extensive. However, if calcium deposition is focal and limited, it may often be missed or misinterpreted. Vascular calcification is oriented along the course of vessel and a single calcific deposit reflects that orientation (Fig 2–104). Commonly, it may appear as a thin line or streaks of density, but in the internal or common iliac arteries focal calcification may be more irregularly shaped. Limited vascular calcification can occur in any vessel but is most common in the aorta, internal and common iliac arteries, renal arteries, and splenic artery.

Calcification of the Abdominal Aorta

Aortic calcification occurs mostly as a result of atherosclerosis.[180,181] It may be of little clinical significance, cause no symptoms, and not necessarily be associated with calcification in other arteries. Calcifications in the distal abdominal aorta and the common iliac arteries are often seen together, however.

The incidence of abdominal aortic calcification advances with age. Rare under 40, its presence increases steadily with each decade. In younger patients, calcification may be due to aortitis of various etiologies, renal failure, or hyperparathyroidism.[182–185] In one study of 610 consecutive patients aged 15 years and older seen in the emergency room at a university hospital, abdominal aortic calcification was found in 20% of all patients and 40% of those over age 45.[186] In a survey of garment workers over age 40 in New York City, Epstein et al found calcification in the abdominal aorta in 26% of patients.[187] This is similar to a finding from Iceland of a 33% incidence in individuals over 40.[188]

Calcification in the aorta may be more common in women, but the evidence is conflicting.[186,189,190] Some investigators point to a female preponderance, whereas others have found the same incidence in both sexes. Elkeles attributed the higher frequency of aortic calcification in elderly women to the increased presence of osteoporosis following menopause.[189] He proposed that calcium lost from osteoporotic bones could be deposited in the damaged intima of the aorta. Anderson et al noted a correlation between osteoporosis and aortic calcifications in both sexes and concluded that the appar-

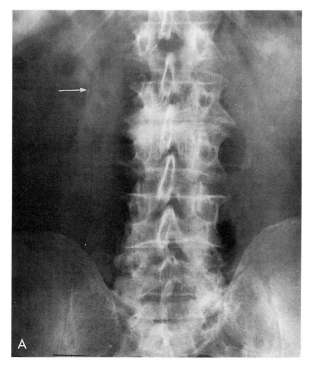
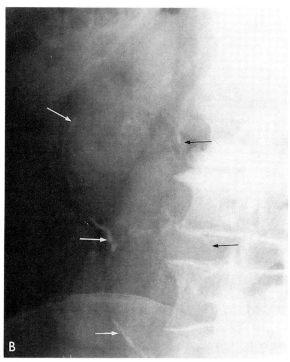

Figure 3–64. Multiple saccular aneurysms in the abdominal aorta. **A.** Anterior–posterior projection. A small linear calcification is identified (*arrows*) just medial to the right kidney hilus. **B.** Right posterior oblique projection. A saccular aneurysm of the abdominal aorta is clearly identified (*arrows*). The aneurysm is displaced to the right because of the tortuosity of the aorta.

ent association is largely accounted for by the accelerated occurrence of both conditions with aging.[190]

The percentage of patients with a calcified abdominal aorta varies with ethnicity and geography.[187,191,192] The greatest incidence has been found in Caucasians in North America and in Europe. It is less common in blacks residing in either North America or Africa, and very infrequent in some populations in Asia, South America, and Africa. Dietary and socioeconomic differences may explain the discrepancies in incidence, but no specific causes or factors have been isolated.

Tobacco consumption may play a role because atherosclerosis and calcification in the aorta occur more frequently in smokers.[193–195] Auerbach and Garfinkel found advanced calcification in the aorta in 85% of patients over 55 who smoked one pack or more per day in comparison to only 63% in nonsmokers of a similar age.[193] The precise mechanism by which smoking affects the aortic wall is not known. However, animal experiments suggest that a constituent of tobacco smoke may impede the normal migration of cholesterol from the intima into the vascular lymphatics, thereby promoting plaque formation.

There is an association between aortic calcification and some systemic diseases. The incidence of calcification in the aorta and iliac arteries is higher in hypertensive and diabetic patients.[194] Epstein et al found that individuals with diabetes had approximately twice as much aortic calcification as nondiabetics.[187] Unlike the pelvic vessels, aortic calcification in diabetics is mostly in the intima. Meema et al found a high incidence of aortic calcifications in patients aged 15 to 30 with chronic renal disease.[185] On the other hand, there may be a negative correlation between abdominal aortic calcification and carcinomas of the stomach, breast, and prostate.[196–199] The reason for the relative protection of the aorta in patients with these malignancies is unclear.

Radiographic Findings in Abdominal Aortic Calcification

The appearance of calcification in the abdominal aorta varies with the extent of the atherosclerotic process. Calcification is best detected when the X-ray beam hits the atherosclerotic plaque tangentially. Thus, on the anteroposterior projection of the abdomen, calcification in the lateral walls is demonstrated, whereas on lateral views the anterior and posterior walls can be seen (Fig 3–65). Calcification is more frequent below the renal arteries and may often extend into both common iliac arteries. In advanced cases, the calcification can outline the entire aorta. Almost always, the distribution of calcification is irregular and patchy in appearance. If calcification is focal, it may not be appreciated on an anteroposterior projection owing to the overlying lumbar vertebrae. Oblique or lateral views that separate the aorta from the spine may then be helpful in revealing calcified plaques. Rarely, calcification may be smooth and uniform, and in this instance one should consider Takayasu's aortitis, or aortitis due to connective tissue disorders.[182,183,199]

Rarely, clots within the lumen of the aorta can calcify (Fig 3–66).[200,201] Occurring either in aneurysms or in vessels of normal caliber, calcium may deposit through the entirety of a clot, causing it to appear on plain films as a uniform density with granular or mottled internal architecture. Since the aorta usually overlies the spine and clot calcification is almost never very dense, it may not be recognized on supine films. Steep oblique and lateral films are often required to demonstrate this phenomenon.

Calcification in Abdominal Aortic Aneurysms

Atherosclerosis is the most common cause of abdominal aortic aneurysms. The incidence of aneurysms in autopsy series is approximately 0.5%.[202] More than 95% of atherosclerotic aneurysms occur in patients between 60 and 80 years old, and their incidence is four times more common in men than in women. Steinberg and Stein found calcification on abdominal films in 55% of patients with documented aortic aneurysms.[203] The calcification may be of two types. In the majority, scattered plaques of calcification are noted (Fig 3–67), but in approximately 10%, long curvilinear lines are seen. Preliminary abdominal radiographs may not always reveal the extent of an aneurysm or delineate its size, but in many cases they can play an important role in first ascertaining the diagnosis.

The recognition of a calcified abdominal aortic aneurysm on plain films depends upon the size and configuration of the aneurysm, the extent of calcification, and the degree of tortuosity of the aorta. Large and extensively calcified saccular aneurysms are usually easily seen, and their size can be determined on plain films of the abdomen. Fusiform aneurysms can be diagnosed accurately when both walls of the aneurysms are identified. When only one wall of the aneurysm is identified, however, size may not be gauged on a single supine film. In this situation, oblique and lateral views of the abdomen are helpful in establishing the diagnosis. If the calcification is focal, faint, or obscured by bowel gas, tomography can be used to localize the aneurysm (Fig 3–68) and determine its size. Abdominal aortic aneurysms are frequently associated with tortuosity

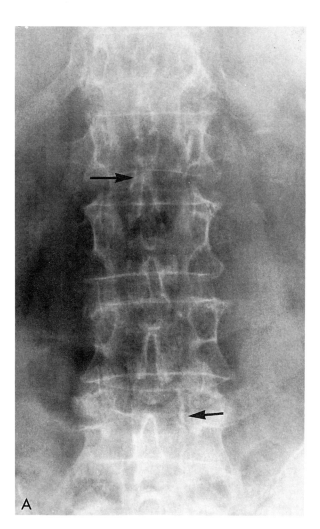
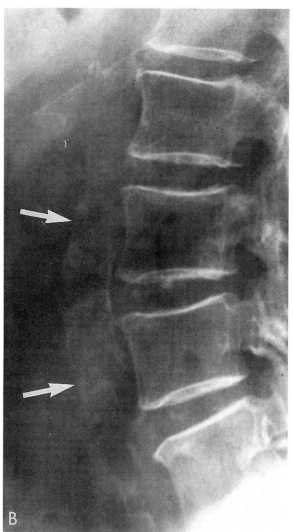

Figure 3–65. Calcification in the abdominal aorta. **A.** Anterior–posterior projection. The wall calcification (*arrows*) are seen only faintly because of overlying vertebrae. **B.** Lateral projection. The calcifications are better demonstrated.

and elongation of the abdominal aorta. Thus, calcification in these aneurysms can be identified far away from the midline on the left or on the right side of the lumbar spine. A ruptured aortic aneurysm should be considered if there is a marked change in the location of calcifications of two successive films.[204] Less reliable signs of rupture are an associated soft tissue mass and unilateral loss of the psoas shadow or renal outline.[205] Finally, a crescent of gas within a mycotic abdominal aortic aneurysm has been observed on plain radiographs, with confirmation by computed tomography.[206]

The common iliac arteries are the second most frequent site for abdominal arterial calcification, primarily a consequence of atherosclerosis and often associated with lower abdominal aortic calcification. Common iliac artery calcification, when extensive,

is usually easy to recognize because it presents as well-defined parallel lines of radiodensity following the expected direction of the artery (Fig 3–69). If calcification is limited, it may be mistaken for bony densities because the common iliac arteries overlie the lower lumbar vertebrae and sacrum. When there is tortuosity and elongation of the aorta and common iliac arteries, the course of the iliac arteries may assume a vertical or horizontal course rather than oblique orientation (Fig 3–70). Occasionally it may be difficult, if not impossible on one film, to distinguish between a focal calcification in the common iliac artery and a ureteral calculus, particularly when the calcification is projected over the sacrum. If the long axis of the calcification can be observed, it will most often point in the direction of the conduit with which it is associated. Thus, calcification in the com-

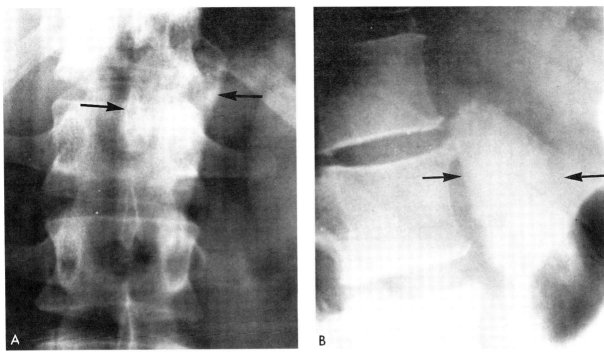

Figure 3-66. Calcification in a clot in the abdominal aorta. **A.** Supine film of the upper abdomen. Solid calcification in the area of the upper abdominal aorta (*arrow*), overlying the spine. **B.** Lateral projection. Intraluminal clot calcification is seen more clearly (*arrows*). (*Reprinted with permission of* Cardiovascular and Interventional Radiology.)

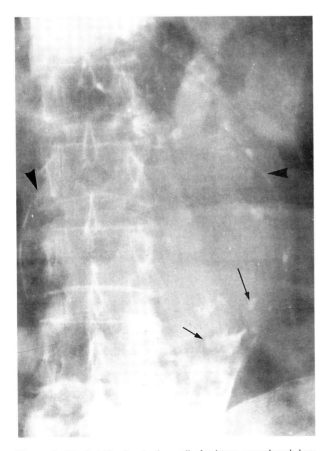

Figure 3-67. Calcification in the wall of a large saccular abdominal aortic aneurysm (*arrowheads*). Note the scattered plaques of more dense calcification (*arrows*) at the lower margin of the aneurysm.

mon iliac artery will tend to line up along an axis extending toward the aorta, while a ureteral calculus is more vertically aligned. Moreover, ureteral stones can move on successive films, whereas vascular calcifications are fixed.

After the aorta, the common iliac artery is the next most frequent site for aneurysmal dilatation in the abdomen. These aneurysms are usually fusiform and may be continuous with a dilated distal aorta. Most often, the aneurysms are elliptical, with the orientation of the ellipse along the expected axis of the artery (Fig 3-71). Calcified saccular common iliac artery aneurysms occur occasionally. At times, they can simulate cystic masses in the pelvis or lower abdomen. A helpful distinguishing feature of calcified aneurysms in the common iliac arteries is the accompanying presence of extensive vascular disease in the aorta and other iliac vessels.

The internal iliac or hypogastric artery is a common location for calcification in middle-aged and elderly individuals. Calcification is usually due to atherosclerosis and can be seen as irregular plaques of radiodensity. In diabetic patients, it can be of the medial type, presenting as smooth continuous parallel lines of radiodensity in both internal iliac arteries and their branches.

The internal iliac artery arises from the common iliac artery, courses vertically at the superior lateral portion of the pelvis, and then divides into posterior and anterior divisions. In the posterior division, the most frequently calcified vessels are the gluteal ar-

111

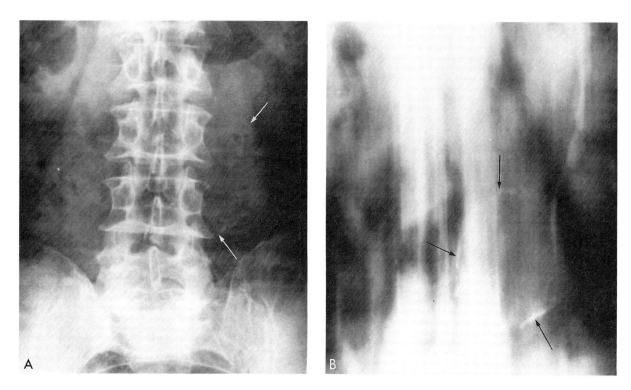

Figure 3–68. Saccular aneurysm of the abdominal aorta. **A.** Anterior–posterior projection. The calcification is faint and obscured by bowel gas (*arrows*). **B.** Tomogram of the abdomen. The calcified aneurysm (*arrows*) is clearly identified.

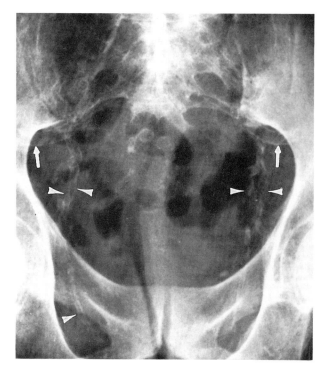

Figure 3–69. Internal iliac artery calcification. Multiple branches of the internal iliac artery are calcified. The superior gluteal artery (*arrows*) runs horizontally over the iliac bone. The obturator and internal pudendal arteries (*arrowheads*) follow a similar course and reach the obturator foramen.

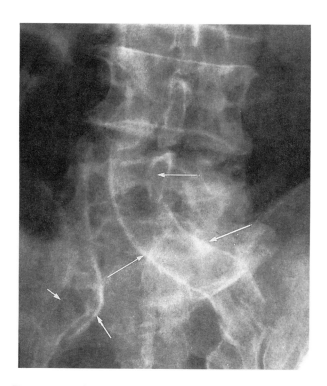

Figure 3–70. Calcified tortuous common iliac arteries. Parallel tracks of calcification (*arrows*) in both common iliac arteries.

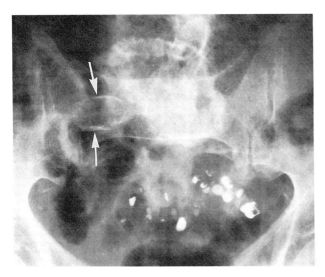

Figure 3–71. Calcified fusiform aneurysm of the common iliac artery. The elliptical lines of calcification (*arrows*) lie along the course of the right common iliac artery.

teries, which are easy to recognize because they extend laterally as they supply the gluteus muscles. Parallel linear tracks of calcification with multiple branches running across the iliac bone are characteristic of this vascular calcification. From the anterior division arise the internal pudendal, obturator, uterine, and cystic arteries. The internal pudendal and obturator arteries follow a similar path along the lateral wall of the pelvis and then turn medially and inferiorly. Calcifications in both vessels are rec-

ognized as tracks of density originating from the hypogastric artery, passing along the lateral wall of the pelvis, and branching in the region of the obturator foramen (Fig 3–69).

In males, opacification of the vas deferens may simulate calcification in arteries. Both structures are conduits and the pelvic portion of the spermatic cord has a caliber similar to that of the iliac arteries. Moreover, the pattern of calcification may be identical. The vas, however, follows a path different from that of either the internal iliac artery or its branches (Fig 3–73). If a section of a calcified pelvic conduit is long enough that its orientation can be determined, it is usually possible to distinguish between the vas deferens and nearby vessels.[207–209]

Aneurysms of the internal and external iliac arteries or their branches are rare. Because they are usually well-defined saccular aneurysms they may resemble other rounded calcifications in the pelvis such as mucoceles of the appendix, mesenteric cysts, benign ovarian cysts, and cystic-appearing leiomyomas of the uterus (Fig 3–72).

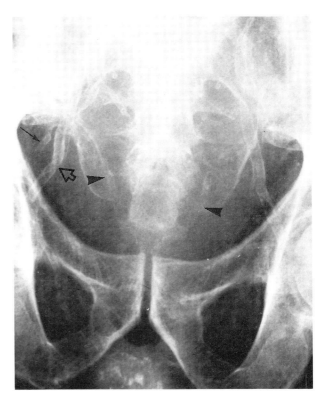

Figure 3–73. Internal iliac artery calcification and calcified vas deferens. The intrapelvic portion of the vas deferens runs laterally and superiorly from the seminal vesicles (*arrowheads*), then descends at the lateral pelvic wall (*arrow*) down to the scrotum. The descending portion of the vas may be mistaken for a branch of the internal iliac artery (*open arrow*), which runs in a similar direction.

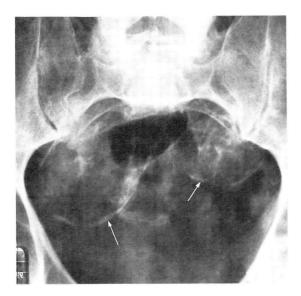

Figure 3–72. Saccular aneurysms of the internal iliac arteries. Curvilinear calcification convex outward in both internal iliac arteries (*arrows*). (*Courtesy of Dr. Lawrence Oliver.*)

VENOUS CALCIFICATION

Phleboliths are by far the most commonly encountered calcification in the pelvis. By age 40, one or more phleboliths can be found in at least 35% of patients. Frequently they are multiple and bilateral. Although they generally have an easily recognizable shape, they can be confused with ureteral stones or calcifications in a pelvic mass. Because they are asymptomatic and have not been conclusively shown to be associated with other diseases, they are usually regarded as innocuous and inconsequential and are often not mentioned on radiographic reports. At times, however, the location and movements of phleboliths may provide practical clinical information, and a knowledge of their radiological characteristics can be important in assessing the presence or growth of masses and in evaluating the nature of pelvic opacities.

In 1852, Von Rokitansky was the first to describe pelvic phleboliths in dissections of periprostatic veins in males. In 1881, Von Recklinghausen stated they were harmless entities. Nevertheless, in the early 1900s, because it was felt by some physicians that phleboliths were the cause of pelvic pain and were frequently associated with tumors, they were often surgically removed.[210] In 1908, Orton discussed their radiological appearance, and, in the following year, Clark proved that phleboliths were intravenous concretions by demonstrating, in autopsy studies, their disappearance on pelvic radiographs after the veins were dissected.[211,212]

Phleboliths are concretions of thrombi attached to the walls of veins. They consist of thickly packed laminae of platelets sandwiched between a reticulum of red blood cells and fibrin. Calcification usually takes place after the phleboliths have fully formed.[213] Culligan analyzed 20 venous stones and found they were remarkably similar in chemical constituents.[214] Approximately 50% by weight was calcium carbonate with lesser amounts of ammonium phosphate and magnesium ammonium phosphate. Between 12% and 20% of the stones' mass consisted of organic matter.[214]

Shenult has shown that, in the adult, pelvic veins are valveless and poorly supported in loose connective tissue.[210] Sudden intermittent increase in intra-abdominal pressure, such as with straining at defecation, may damage the venous wall and predispose to thrombosis. Burkitt et al offered epidemiologic data supporting the notion that episodic marked increases in intra-abdominal pressure lead to the formation of pelvic vein thrombi.[215] Phleboliths are most frequent in people residing in industrial countries and uncommon in rural people living in developing nations and eating a traditional diet.

For example, the incidence of phleboliths is 48% in adults in the United Kingdom but only 11.5% in Fiji.[215] Genetic factors do not seem significant; blacks and whites in the United States have a similar prevalence. Burkitt suggested that a diet low in fiber, the diet of many people in developed countries, leads to constipation and thus to straining at stools. Interestingly, phleboliths have not been described in veterinary radiology, possibly because the pelvic veins are not subjected to intermittent elevations of pressure in four-footed animals.[213]

That phleboliths may be the result of decreased consumption of cereals and fiber requires confirmation. There is strong evidence that colonic diverticulosis is a consequence of a long history of constipation.[216] We charted the number and position of phleboliths in 200 patients over age 40 undergoing barium enema examinations and demonstrated no difference in either the incidence or number of phleboliths in patients with diverticula and in those with normal colons.[217] In this sample, pelvic phleboliths also appeared unrelated to a history of appendicitis, being as common in normal patients as in those who have had an appendectomy. Contrary to past assumptions, there appears to be no relationship between phleboliths and a history of urinary tract disease.[218] Hence, although there are interesting clues to the cause of pelvic venous concretions, their pathogenesis is by no means fully understood.

Most studies have indicated that phleboliths increase in prevalence up to the fifth decade of life. We have not observed them in patients under age 16 but they are not a rare phenomenon by the third decade.[213] In some series, phleboliths continue to increase in prevalence to old age, but other investigations have noted a leveling off in the fifth and sixth decades, with no further increases in later years.[213–216] A study evaluating 1555 consecutive pelvic radiographs found phleboliths in 50% of men and in only 40% of women.[214] In 1934 Butzler,[219] and, in 1980, Mattson[220] observed a definite female prevalence. Others have shown an equal sex prevalence.[213,218] In the pelvic radiographs of patients over 40 that we have examined, concretions were present in 48% of 71 men and 54% of 131 women, a difference of 6%, which is not statistically significant.[217]

Phleboliths are dense, oval to round, and well defined. Usually there are no discontinuities in their outer margin, but often there is a concentric or slightly eccentric interior lucency. Sometimes the lucency may be large, with only a thin rim of calcification visible. Generally, they are 1.5 to 5 mm in diameter, but larger concretions occur occasionally. These ''giant'' stones may represent fused phleboliths and often contain multiple lucencies, suggesting the mottled appearance of solid masses (Fig 3–74). Uncom-

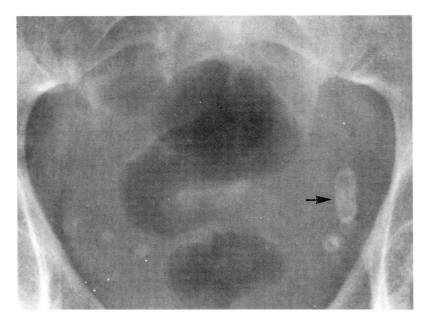

Figure 3–74. Fused phlebolith. Oblong density (*arrow*) with smooth margins and two areas of internal lucency located along the course of a pelvic vein.

monly, a fused phlebolith can even simulate the pattern of calcification seen in leiomyoma of the uterus. Usually between one and six phleboliths are present, but on occasion up to two to three dozen pelvic concretions may be noted. When there are numerous phleboliths in the pelvis they are almost always bilateral and tend to be arrayed in gently curing chains that follow the course of the distal ureters (Fig 3–75).

In men, phleboliths are found in perirectal and perivesical veins.[221] In women they occur also in veins in the broad ligament, where they are situated near the termination of the vein and hence are laterally placed. Occasionally, phleboliths are located in a more medial position but are still off the midline. The great preponderance of phleboliths lie at or just below a line drawn from the ischial spine to the fourth sacral segment. When there are many phleboliths, the majority are below that line and their course proceeding caudally will be from lateral to medial. Often phleboliths may be noted slightly below the superior margin of the symphysis pubis. In men, phleboliths may occasionally be present in scrotal veins, sometimes in large numbers (Fig 3–76).

Occasionally, a pelvic radiograph will reveal

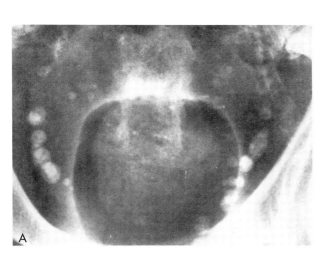

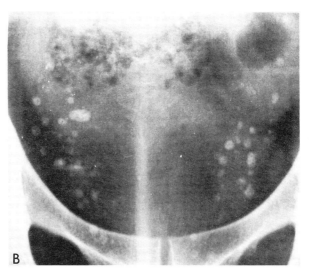

Figure 3–75. Numerous phleboliths. **A.** Bilateral, multiple phleboliths arranged in chains directed obliquely inferiorly. **B.** Multiple phleboliths in perivesical veins and veins of the broad ligament. More than one chain of phleboliths is present on each side.

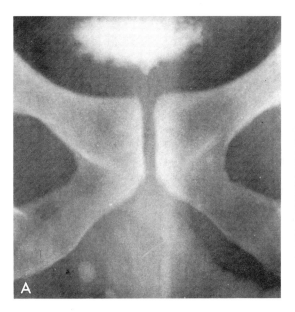
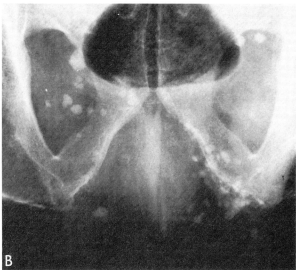

Figure 3–76. Phleboliths in scrotal veins. **A.** Two scrotal vein phleboliths below the right inferior pubic ramus. **B.** Many scrotal vein phleboliths on the left and one on the right.

one or several concretions in the superior pelvis, often without phleboliths present inferiorly. If the concretion is outside the genitourinary tract, it may be in a phlebolith located in a gonadal vein (Fig 3–77. These concretions tend to be multiple and are seen along the course of the vein as it ascends in the abdomen adjacent to the ureter (Fig 2–97). Gonadal phleboliths are almost exclusively seen in multiparous women, most of whom also have pelvic masses. Stasis in the gonadal veins during pregnancy has been suggested as a predisposing factor in the formation of these concretions.[222]

It is often difficult to distinguish between a ureteral calculus and a phlebolith in the pelvis or in gonadal veins.[223] Ureteral calculi are often angulated and usually lack a central lucency. However, their appearance may exactly mimic a phlebolith. One way of differentiating between the two is to obtain serial films a few hours or 1 day apart. Ureteral calculi may move in either an antegrade or retrograde fashion whereas phleboliths are usually fixed in position (Fig 3–78). If there is no movement of the ureteral stone, however, it may be impossible to distinguish the two types of concretions even on repeated plain films.

Careful attention to the position of phleboliths may be rewarding in determining the presence of pelvic masses or ascertaining the nature of previous surgery.[221,224] Normally, phleboliths situated in perivesical veins may be displaced slightly inferiorly and laterally if the bladder enlarges to a great degree

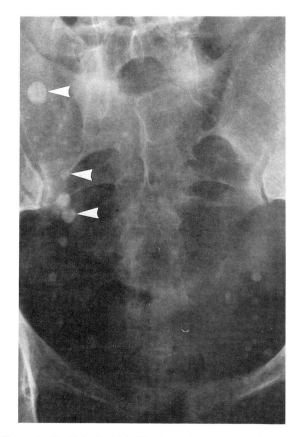

Figure 3–77. Multiple phleboliths in the right ovarian vein (*arrowheads*). They may simulate ureteral stones on a plain film.

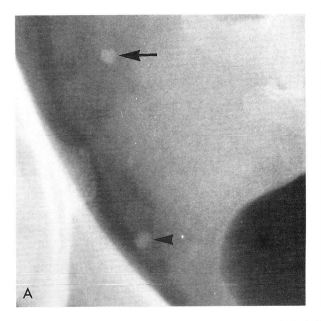
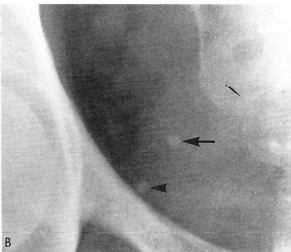

Figure 3–78. A phlebolith and a ureteral calculus may look similar on pelvic films. **A.** The initial films show a ureteral calculus (*arrow*) superior to a phlebolith (*arrowhead*). **B.** A film taken the next day demonstrates movement of the ureteral stone inferiorly (*arrow*), while the phlebolith is fixed (*arrowhead*).

(Fig 3–79). Occasionally, perirectal phleboliths are deviated laterally in the presence of rectal distention. These movements are usually minimal, however. Greater motion may be observed in the presence of masses. In fact, when a phlebolith is displaced, its migration may be all that is necessary to monitor the growth or shrinkage of tumefactions.[221,224–226]

Periurethral masses can elevate phleboliths as well as displace them to either side. Prolapse of the uterus move phleboliths inferiorly, sometimes dis-placing them below the superior margin of the pubic bone (Fig 3–80).

The veins of the pelvis are connected across the midline through the inferior vesical plexuses in both sexes, and the periprostatic plexus in men. However, crossing veins are usually small and are not the site of roentgenographically visible phleboliths. Hence, a phlebolith in the midline should always be regarded as abnormal. It may be deviated by a mass and, in women, medial migration is usually a con-

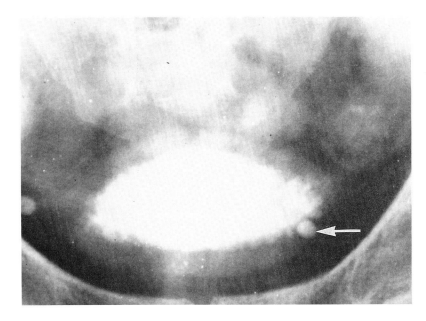

Figure 3–79. The intimate relationship of the bladder to a perivesical vein phlebolith (*arrow*). Distention of the bladder can push phleboliths inferiorly and laterally.

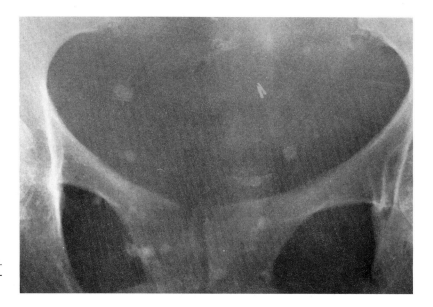

Figure 3–80. A woman with uterine prolapse. Phleboliths have moved below the superior margin of the pubic bone.

sequence of hysterectomy (Fig 3–81). Abnormally sited phleboliths are found in hemangiomas. Radiologically visible phleboliths have been noted in many abdominal locations in hemangiomas. Although an uncommon tumor in the pelvis, an hemangioma should be considered when phleboliths are seen at the midline in the absence of previous operation, or when multiple phleboliths are seen on only one side of the midline.[227] A spectacular appearance of phlebolith type calcification can be found in the Klippel–Trenaunay syndrome, which consists of bony abnormalities and large hemangiomas that may occur in the abdominal wall or within solid organs (Fig 3–82).[228]

Not all concretions with central lucencies in the pelvis are phleboliths. Many other densities simulating venous stones may be mistaken for them. In addition to ureteral calculi, concretions such as appendicoliths in low-lying appendices can be seen in the pelvis. Bladder stones, rectal stones, calcified appendices epiploicae, and calculi passing through the gastrointestinal tract may also be present in the pelvis. Ossification and tooth formation in ovarian dermoids can occasionally look like phleboliths (Fig 3–83). Bilateral clusters of discrete densities, suggestive of concretions, characterize calcification of ovarian corpora albicantia.[229]

From time to time foreign bodies may be mis-

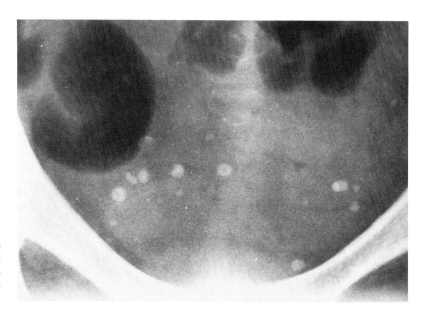

Figure 3–81. After a simple hysterectomy, phleboliths in broad ligament veins may be brought closer together. Observe the abnormal arrangement of the phleboliths. They are aligned horizontally and one is situated at the midline.

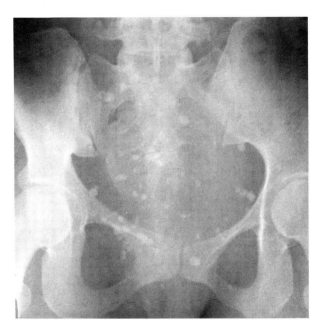

Figure 3–82. Klippel–Trenaunay syndrome. A large subcutaneous hemangioma with numerous phleboliths projects over the pelvis.

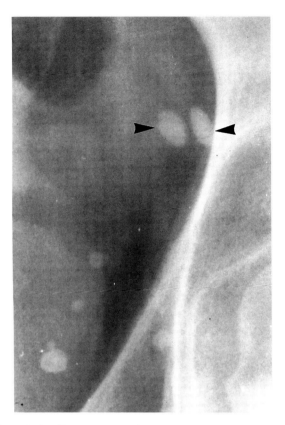

Figure 3–84. Two opaque pills (*arrowheads*) and phleboliths. Pills lack both a central lucency and a marginal rim of enhanced density.

taken for phleboliths. Radiopaque pills can resemble venous calculi but their homogeneous mass, absence of central lucency, and movement on sequential films are points of differentiation (Fig 3–84). Fallopian tube occlusion rings are implanted devices used in tubal ligations. They consist of siliconized synthetic rubber impregnated with barium sulfate, which makes them appear as annular opacities on plain radiographs. Often, they can closely simulate phleboliths (Fig 3–85).

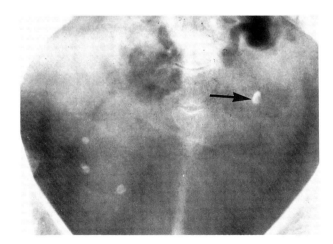

Figure 3–83. Three phleboliths on the right and calcification in an ovarian dermoid on the left (*arrow*). While simulating a phlebolith in configuration, the superior location of the dermoid calcification is atypical. An adjacent lucency represents fat in the dermoid.

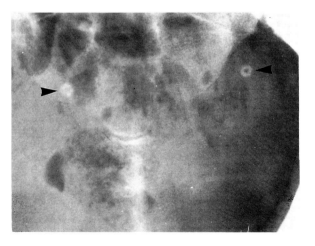

Figure 3–85. Bilateral fallopian tube occlusion rings (*arrowheads*) placed at the sites of tubal ligation. The central lucency and complete border of increased density in these devices give them the appearance of phleboliths.

CALCIFICATIONS IN THE ILIAC VEINS AND INFERIOR VENA CAVA

Aside from pelvic and gonadal vein pheboliths, calcification is seldom noted in abdominal veins on plain films. Veins are not subjected to either high pressure or large pulsatile flow and are therefore relatively protected from the risk of intimal injury. Consequently, venous walls, with the exception of the veins of the portal system, are rarely damaged sufficiently to be the site of intimal calcification. Mostly, calcification occurs in intraluminal clots in obstructed vessels.

Inferior vena cava calcification in adults is exceedingly rare.[230] Most examples have occurred in children who have a calcified thrombus in the intrahepatic portion of that great vessel, which is the narrowest region of the inferior vena cava.[231]

Like the inferior vena cava, the iliac veins are seldom the site of thrombus calcification, although thrombi are not unusual within the lumens of these vessels. Calcifications in the iliac veins appear as thick linear densities in the lateral portion of the pelvis converging toward the inferior vena cava (Fig 3–86).[232,233] They should be distinguished from calcifications in the sacrotuberous ligament, which have a similar appearance but a different location in the pelvis.

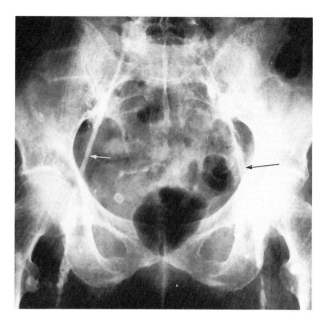

Figure 3–86. Iliac vein calcification. Thick linear calcification in the iliac veins (*arrows*) extending from the femoral veins to the inferior vena cava. The patient had chronic venous thrombosis. (*Courtesy of Dr. G.A. Goodman.*)

REFERENCES

1. Samuel E, Duncan JG, Philip T, et al. Radiology of the Post-operative abdomen. *Clin Radiol.* 1963;14:133–148.
2. Harrison I, Litwer H, Gerwig WH. Studies on the incidence and duration of post-operative pneumoperitoneum. *Ann Surg.* 1957;145:591–594.
3. Felson B, Wiot JF. Another look at pneumoperitoneum. *Semin Roentgenol.* 1973;8:437–444.
4. Bryant LR, Wolf JF, Kloecker RJ. A study of the factors affecting the incidence and duration of post-operative pneumoperitoneum. *Surg Obstet Gynecol.* 1963;117:145–150.
5. Miller, RE. The radiological evaluations of intraperitoneal air (pneumoperitoneum). *CRC Crit Rev Radiol Sci.* 1973;4:61–85.
6. Miller RE, Becker GJ, Slabaugh RD. Nonsurgical pneumoperitoneum. *Gastrointest Radiol.* 1981;6:73–74.
7. Gottfried EB, Plumser AB, Clair MR. Pneumoperitoneum following percutaneous endoscopic gastroscopy: A prospective study. *Gastrointest Endosc.* 1986; 32:397–399.
8. Thompson WM, Seigler HF, Rice RP. Ileocolonic perforation: A complication following renal transplantation. *Am J Roentgenol.* 1975;125:723–730.
9. Miller RE, Nelson SW. The roentgenological demonstration of tiny amounts of free intraperitoneal gas: Experimental and clinical studies. *Am J Roentgenol.* 1971;112:574–585.
10. Beneventano TC, Schein CJ, Jacobson HG. The roentgen appearance of some appendiceal abnormalities. *Am J Roentgenol.* 1966;961:344–360.
11. Keeffe EJ, Gagliardi RA. Significance of ileus in perforated viscus. *Am J Roentgenol.* 1973;117:275–280.
12. Cass LJ, Dow EC, Brooks JR. Pneumoperitoneum following pelvic examination. *Am J Gastroenterol* 1966; 45:209–211.
13. Lozman H, Newman AJ. Spontaneous pneumoperitoneum occurring during post-partum exercises in the knee-chest position. *Am J Obstet Gynecol.* 1956;72:903–905.
14. Ashai S, Lipton D, Cohen A, et al. Pneumoperitoneum secondary to cunnilingus. *N Engl J Med.* 1976; 295:117.
15. Freeman RK. Pneumoperitoneum from oral–genital insufflation. *Obstet Gynecol.* 1970;36:162–163.
16. Macklin MT, Macklin CC. Malignant interstitial emphysema of the lungs and mediastinum as an important occult complication in many respiratory diseases and other conditions: An interpretation of the clinical

literature in the light of laboratory experiment. *Medicine.* 1944;23:81–358.

17. Macklin CC. Transport of air along sheaths of pulmonic blood vessels from alveoli to mediastinum. Clinical implications. *Arch Intern Med.* 1939;64:913–926.

18. Rohlfing BM, Webb WR, Schlobohm RM. Ventilator-related extra-alveolar air in adults. *Radiology.* 1976;121:25–31.

19. Kleinman PK, Brill PW, Whalen JP. Anterior pathway for transdiaphragmatic extension of pneumoperitoneum. *Am J Roentgenol.* 1978;131:271–275.

20. Fataar S, Schulman A. Recurrent non-surgical pneumoperitoenum due to spontaneous pneumothorax. *Br J Radiol.* 1981;54:1100–1102.

21. Campbell, RE, Boggs TR Jr, Kirkpatrick JA Jr. Early neonatal pneumoperitoneum from progressive massive tension pneumomediastinum. *Radiology.* 1975;114:121–126.

22. Glanz S, Ravin CE, Deren MM. Benign pneumoperitoneum following median sternotomy incision. *Am J Roentgenol.* 1976;131:257–269.

23. Rohrmann CA Jr, Ricci MT, Krishnamurthy S, et al. Radiologic and histologic differentiation of neuromuscular disorders of the gastrointestinal tract: visceral myopathies, visceral neuropathies and progressive systemic sclerosis. *Am J Roentgenol.* 1984;143:933–941.

24. Dunn V, Nelson JA. Jejunal diverticulosis and chronic pneumoperitoneum. *Gastrointest Radiol.* 1979;4:165–168.

25. Wright, FW, Lumsden K. Recurrent pneumoperitoneum due to jejunal diverticulosis with a review of the causes of spontaneous pneumoperitoneum. *Clin Radiol.* 1975;26:327–331.

26. Papp JP, Sullivan BH Jr. Spontaneous peritoneum without peritonitis. Report of case. *Cleve Cin. Q.* 1965;32:149–155.

27. Allison DJ, Fletcher DR, Gordon-Smith EC. Therapeutic arterial embolisation of the spleen. A new cause of free intraperitoneal gas. *Clin Radiol.* 1981;32:617–621.

28. Miller RE. The technical approach to the acute abdomen. *Semin Roentgenol.* 1973;8:267–279.

29. Paster S, Brogdon BG. Roentgenographic diagnosis of pneumoperitoneum. *JAMA.* 1976;235:1264–1267.

30. Miller RE, Becker GJ, Slabaugh RA. Detection of pneumoperitoneum: Optimum body position and respiratory phase. *Am J Roentgenol.* 1980;138:487–490.

31. Rigler LG. Spontaneous pneumoperitoneum: A roentgenologic sign found in supine position. *Radiology.* 1941;37:604–607.

32. Schultz EH Jr. An aid to the diagnosis of pneumoperitoneum from supine abdominal films. *Radiology.* 1958;70:728–731.

33. deLacey G, Bloomberg T, Wignall BK. Pneumoperitoneum: The misleading double wall sign. *Clin Radiol.* 1977;28:445–448.

34. Miller RE. Perforated viscus in infants: A new roentgen sign. *Radiology.* 1960;74:65–67.

35. Jelaso DV, Schultz EH Jr. The urachus—An aid to the diagnosis of pneumoperitoneum. *Radiology.* 1969;92:295–296.

36. Weiner CI, Diaconis JN, Dennis JM. The "Inverted V": A new sign of pneumoperitoneum. *Radiology.* 1973;107:47–48.

37. MacGillivray PC, Stewart AM, MacFarlane A. Rupture of the stomach in the newborn due to congenital defects in the gastric musculature. *Arch Dis Child.* 1956;31:56–58.

38. Bray JF. Pneumoscrotum with testicular delineation—A new sign of pneumoperitoneum. *Br J. Radiol.* 1982;55:867–868.

39. Han SY, Shin MS, Tishler JM. Plain film findings of hydropneumoperitoneum. *Am J Roentgenol.* 1981;136:1195–1197.

40. Han, SY. Variations in falciform ligament with pneumoperitoneum. *J Can Assoc Radiol.* 1980;31:171–173.

41. Hoswell DM, Berne AS, Schneider B. Plain film recognition of the ligamentum teres hepatis. *Radiology.* 1975;114:263–267.

42. Menuck L, Siemers PT. Pneumoperitoneum: Importance of right upper quadrant features. *Am J Roentgenol.* 1976;127:753–756.

43. Pyle R. The liver edge silhouette. A specific sign of perforated duodenal ulcer. *Br J. Radiol.* 1963;36:503–504.

44. Hajdu N, deLacey G. The Rutherford Morison Pouch: a characteristic appearance on abdominal radiographs. *Br J. Radiol.* 1970;43:706–709.

45. Jackson DM. Letter re the liver edge silhouette. A specific sign of perforated ulcer. *Br J. Radiol.* 1963;36:783.

46. Movsas I. Gas in the hepato-renal space. An unusual radiologic sign of perforated appendicitis. *S Afr J Radiol.* 1965;3:35–37.

47. Rubenstein WA, Yong HA, Whalen JP. The perihepatic spaces: Computed tomographic and ultrasound imaging. *Radiology.* 1983;149:231–239.

48. Walker LA, Weens HS. Radiological observations on the lesser peritoneal sac. *Radiology.* 1963;80:727–737.

49. Goodwin CA, Lewicki AM. Sigmoid colon perforation into the lesser sac. *Am J Roentgenol.* 1977;128:491–492.

50. Mellins HZ. The radiological signs of disease in the lesser peritoneal sac. *Radiol Clin N Am.* 1964;2:107–120.

51. Cimmino CV, Sholes DM. Gas in the lesser sac in perforated ulcer. *Am J Roentgenol.* 1952;68:19–21.

52. Joffe N. Some uncommon roentgenologic findings associated with acute perforative appendicitis. *Radiology.* 1974;110:301–305.

53. Han SY, Tishler JM. Perforation of the abdominal segment of the esophagus. *Am J Roentgenol.* 1984;143:751–754.

54. Healy ME, Mindelzun RE. Lesser sac pneumoperitoneum secondary to perforation of the intraabdominal esophagus. *Am J Roentgenol.* 1984;142:325–326.

55. Stankey RM. Intestinal herniation through the foramen of Winslow. *Radiology.* 1967;89:929–930.

56. McKail RA. Hernia through the foramen of Winslow, hernia traversing the lesser sac, and allied conditions. *Br J. Radiol.* 1961;34:611–618.

57. Henisz A, Matesanz J, Westcott JL. Cecal herniation

through the foramen of Winslow. *Radiology.* 1974; 112:575–578.

58. Cimmino CV. Lesser sac hernia via the foramen of Winslow. A case report. *Radiology.* 1953;60:57–59.

59. Elliott KA, Elliott GB, Pow RE. Gas-containing abscess of the lesser sac. *Br J. Radiol.* 1961;34:622–624.

60. Grillo IA, Bohrer SP. Pseudopneumoperitoneum. Linear atelectasis simulating pneumoperitoneum. *Am Surg.* 1973;39:60–62.

61. Fisher MS. The simulation of pneumoperitoneum by basal atelectasis. *Br J. Radiol.* 1968;41:701.

62. Vessal K. Borhanmanesh F. Hepatodiaphragmatic interposition of the intestine (Chilaiditi's syndrome). *Clin Radiol.* 1976;27:113–116.

63. Melester T. Burt ME, Chilaiditi's syndrome. Report of three cases. *JAMA.* 1985;254:944–945.

64. Mokrohisky JF. Pseudopneumoperitoneum. Simulated free air in the peritoneal cavity. *Am J Roentgenol.* 1958;79:293–300.

65. Martinez LO, Raskin MM. Fat under diaphragm simulating pneumoperitoneum. *Br J. Radiol.* 1974;47:308–309.

66. Rao KG, Woodlief RM. Excessive right subdiaphragmatic fat: A potential diagnostic pitfall. *Radiology.* 1981;138:15–19.

67. Connell TR, Stephens DH, Carlson AC, et al. Upper abdominal abscess: A continuing and deadly problem. *Am J Roentgenol.* 1980;134:759–765.

68. Halber MD, Daffner RH, Morgan CL, et al. Intraabdominal abscess: Current concepts in radiologic evaluation. *Am J Roentgenol.* 1979;133:9–13.

69. Lundstedt T, Hederstrom E, Holmin T, et al. Radiological diagnosis in proven intraabdominal abscess formation: A comparison between plain film of the abdomen, ultrasonography and computerized tomography. *Gastrointest Radiol.* 1983;8:261–266.

70. Miller WT, Talman EA. Subphrenic abscess. *Am J Roentgenol.* 1967;101:961–969.

71. Masters SJ, Rice RP. The homogeneous density of gas in the diagnosis of intraabdominal abscess. *Surg Gynecol Obstet.* 1974;139:370–375.

72. Sands WW. Extraluminal localized gas vesicles: An aid in the diagnosis of abdominal abscesses from plain roentgenograms. *Am J Roentgenol.* 1955;74:195–203.

73. Rice RP, Masters SJ. Intraabdominal abscess. *Semin Roentgenol.* 1973;8:365–374.

74. Calenoff L, Poticha SM. Combined occurrence of retropneumoperitoneum and pneumoperitoneum. *Am J Roentgenol.* 1973;117:366–372.

75. Schulman A, Fataar S, Vander Spuy JW, et al. Air in unusual places: Some causes and ramifications of pneumomediastinum. *Clin Radiol.* 1982;33:301–306.

76. Toxopeus MD, Lucas CE, Krabbenhoft KL. Roentgenographic diagnosis in blunt retroperitoneal duodenal rupture. *Am J Roentgenol.* 1972;115:281–288.

77. Older RA, Rice RP, Kelvin FM, et al. Extraperitoneal gas following nephrectomy. Pattern and duration. *J Urol.* 1978;120:24–27.

78. Fataar S, Schulman A. Pseudo-subphrenic abscess. *Clin Radiol.* 1981;32:157–161.

79. Meyers MA. Radiological features of the spread and localization of extraperitoneal gas and their relationship to its source. An anatomical approach. *Radiology.* 1974;111:17–26.

80. Christensen EE, Landay MT. Visible muscle of the diaphragm: Sign of extraperitoneal air. *Am J Roentgenol.* 1980;135:521–523.

81. Gould RJ, Thorwarth WT. Retroperitoneal rupture of the duodenum due to blunt non-penetrating abdominal trauma. *Radiology.* 1963;80:743–747.

82. Karnaze GC, Sheedy PF II, Stephens DH. Computed tomography in duodenal rupture due to blunt abdominal trauma. *J Comput Assist Tomogr.* 1981;5:267–269.

83. Peterson N, Rohrmann CA, Lennard ES. Diagnosis and treatment of retroperitoneal perforation complicating the double contrast barium enema examination. *Radiology.* 1982;144:249–252.

84. Pickels RF, Karmody AM, Tsapogas MJ, et al. Subcutaneous emphysema of the lower extremity of gastrointestinal origin. Report of a case. *Dis Colon Rectum.* 1974;17:82–86.

85. Ainsworth J. Emphysema of the leg following perforation of the pelvic colon or rectum. *Br J. Radiol.* 1959; 32:54–55.

86. Fiss TW Jr, Cigtay OS, Miele AT, et al. Perforated viscus presenting with gas in the soft tissues (subcutaneous emphysema). *Am J Roentgenol.* 1975;125:226–233.

87. Korsten J, Mattey WE, Bastida J, et al. Subcutaneous emphysema of the thigh secondary to ruptured diverticulum of the ascending colon. *Radiology.* 1973; 106:555–556.

88. Nichols GB, Schilling PJ. Pseudo-retroperitoneal gas in a rupture of aneurysm of abdominal aorta. *Am J Roentgenol.* 1975;125:134–137.

89. Bryk D, Young RS, Morris N. Retroperitoneal lipomatosis report of two cases with an unusual distribution. *Gastrointest Radiol.* 1979;4:309–312.

90. Weissman B, Van Houten FX, Smith EH. Factitious retroperitoneal emphysema due to attempted epidural anesthesia. *Radiology.* 1973;107:345–347.

91. Margulies M, Stoane L. Hepatic angle in roentgen evaluations of peritoneal fluid. *Radiology.* 1967;88:51–56.

92. Jorulf H. Roentgen diagnosis of intraperitoneal fluid. *Acta Radiol.* 1975;343 (suppl):7–126.

93. McCort JJ. Intraperitoneal and retroperitoneal hemorrhage. *Radiol Clin N Am.* 1976;14:391–405.

94. Meyers MA, Whalen JP, Peelle K, et al. Radiologic features of extraperitoneal effusions. An anatomic approach. *Radiology.* 1972;104:249–257.

95. Keeffe EJ, Gagliardi RA, Pfister RC. The roentgenographic evaluation of ascites. *Am J Roentgenol.* 1967; 101:388–396.

96. Budin E, Jacobson G. Roentgenographic diagnosis of small amounts of intraperitoneal fluid. *Am J Roentgenol.* 1967;99:62–70.

97. Cimmino CV. More on the roentgenology of the paracolonic gutter. *Radiology.* 1969;92:638–639.

98. Cimmino CV. Further experience with the roentgen-

ology of the paracolonic gutter: Differentiation between free fluid and localization within the serosa. *Radiology.* 1968;90:761–764.

99. Frimann-Dahl J. *Roentgen Examinations in Acute Abdominal Diseases.* (3rd ed). Springfield, Ill: Charles C Thomas Publishers; 1974:40–87.

100. Meyers MF. Distribution of intra-abdominal malignant seeding: Depending on dynamics of flow of ascitic fluid. *Am J Roentgenol.* 1973;119:198–206.

101. Harris JH Jr, Loh CK, Perlman HC, et al. The roentgen diagnosis of pelvic extraperitoneal effusions. *Radiology.* 1977;125:343–350.

102. Hellmer H. Die Konturen des rechten leberlappens beim ascites. *Acta Radiol.* 1942;23:533–540.

103. Love L, Demos TC, Reynes CJ, et al. Visualization of the lateral edge of the liver in ascites. *Radiology.* 1977;122:619–622.

104. Proto AV, Lane EJ. Visualization of differences in soft-tissue densities: the liver in ascites. *Radiology.* 1976;121:19–23.

105. Wixson D, Kazam E, Whalen JP. Displaced lateral surface of the liver (Hellmer's sign) secondary to an extraperitoneal fluid collection. *Am J Roentgenol.* 1976;127:679–682.

106. Hoffman RB, Wankmiller R, Rigler LG. Pseudoseparation of bowel loops: A fallacious sign of intraperitoneal fluid. *Radiology.* 1966;87:845–847.

107. Morales O. Calcified appendices epiploicae as freely mobile bodies in the abdominal cavity. *Acta Radiol.* 1944;25:653–661.

108. Harrigan AH. Torsion and inflammation of the appendices epiploicae. *Ann Surg.* 1971;66:467–478.

109. Klingenstein P. Some phases of the pathology of the appendices epiploicae. *Surg Gynecol Obstet.* 1924;38:376–382.

110. Borg SE, Whitehouse GH, Griffiths GJ. A mobile calcified amputated appendix epiploica. *Am J Roentgenol.* 1976;127:349–350.

111. Morson BC. The large intestine. In: *Systemic Pathology by Thirty-Eight Authors,* 2nd ed. Edinburgh: Churchill Livingstone; 178:1099–1152.

112. Patterson DC. Appendices epiploicae. *N Engl J Med.* 1933;209:1255–1259.

113. Barder RP. Calcified epiploic appendages: A radiological curiosity. *Radiology.* 1939;33:768–769.

114. Pear BL, Boyden FM. Intraperitoneal lipid granuloma. *Radiology.* 1967;89:47–51.

115. Cohen WN, Safaie-Shirazi S. Starch granulomatous peritoneals. *Am J Roentgenol.* 1973;117:334–339.

116. Whitaker WG Jr, Walker ET, Canipelli J. Lipogranuloma of the peritoneum. *JAMA.* 1948;138:363–365.

117. Bennett HS, Collins EN. Oil granuloma of the peritoneum. *Gastroenterology.* 1952;20:485–491.

118. Pugh DG. A roentgenologic aspect of pseudomyxoma peritoneii. *Radiology.* 1942;39:320–322.

119. Weig CG, Koenig EC, Culver GH. Pseudomyxoma peritoneii report of a case with unusual roentgen findings. *Am J Roentgenol.* 1944;52:505–509.

120. Elliott CE. Two cases of pseudomyxoma peritonaeii from myxoma of the appendix. *Br J. Surg.* 1957;45:15.

121. Morson BC. The peritoneum. In: *Systemic Pathology by Thirty-Eight Authors,* 2nd ed. Edinburgh: Churchill Livingstone; 1978:1179–1190.

122. Dodds HW, Pitt MJ. Calcified rims: Characteristic but uncommon radiologic findings of pseudomyxoma peritoneii. *Gastrointest Radiol.* 1980;5:263–266.

123. Fernandez RN, Daly JM. Pseudomyxoma peritonaeii. *Arch Surg.* 1980;115:409–414.

124. Weig, CG, Koenig EC, Culver GJ. Pseudomyxoma peritonaeii: Report of a case with unusual roentgen findings. *Am J Roentgenol.* 1944;52:505–509.

125. Mittelstaedt C. Ultrasonic diagnosis of omental cysts. *Radiology.* 1975;117:673–676.

126. Teplick SG, Haskin ME. *Surgical Radiology.* Philadelphia: WB Saunders Co; 1981:267.

127. Morson BC. The peritoneum. In: *Systemic Pathology by Thirty-Eight Authors,* 2nd ed. Edinburgh: Churchill Livingstone; 1978:1191–1198.

128. Frank LW. Tuberculous peritonitis. *Am Rev Tuberc.* 1937;36:279–282.

129. Burack WR, Hollister RM. Tuberculous peritonitis. *Am J Med.* 1960;28:510–523.

130. Stassa G. Tuberculous peritonitis. *Am J Roentgenol.* 1967;101:409–413.

131. McCort JJ. Roentgen features of chronic tuberculous peritonitis. *Arch Surg.* 1944;49:91–99.

132. Auerbach O. Pleural, peritoneal and pericardial tuberculosis. *Am Rev Tuberc.* 1950;61:845–861.

133. Webster AJ, Semple T. Calcification of the peritoneum. *Br Med J.* 1951;2:1069–1070.

134. Steinberg B. Infections of the peritoneum. New York: Paul B. Hoeber Inc; 1944:253–260.

135. Stambaugh JE Jr, Burrows S, Jacoby J, et al. Peritoneal mesothelioma associated with diffuse abdominal ossification and unusual presentation. *J Med Soc NJ.* 1977;74:689–693.

136. Miller DLG, Pirani M. Calcified intraperitoneal and mediastinal implants in malignant ovarian teratoma. *J Can Assoc Radiol.* 1984;35:217–219.

137. Berliner L, Redmond P. Calcified papillary tumor of the peritoneum. *Br J. Radiol.* 1980;53:1200–1203.

138. Corner EM. The surgical treatment of tuberculous glands in the mesentery. *Lancet.* 1905;2:1825–1827.

139. Schechter S. Calcified mesenteric lymph nodes: Their incidence and significance in routine roentgen examination of the gastrointestinal tract. *Radiology.* 1936;27:485–493.

140. Pauson M (ed). *Gastroenterologic Medicine.* Philadelphia: Lee & Febiger; 1969.

141. Morson BC, Dawson IMP. *Gastrointestinal Pathology.* Oxford: Blackwell Scientific Publications; 1979:276.

142. Pfuetze KH, Radner DB (eds). *Clinical Tuberculosis.* Springfield, Ill: Charles C. Thomas; 1966:317.

143. Wilson GS. *The Hazards of Immunization.* London: Athlone Press; 1967:67–68.

144. Branson WPS. The surgical treatment of tuberculous glands in the mesentery. *Lancet.* 1905;2:1825–1827.

145. Dobroklonski V. The significance of calcified abdominal lymph nodes. *Am J Roentgenol.* 1929;22:305–317.

146. Barrowman JA. *Physiology of the Gastrointestinal Lym-*

phatic System. Cambridge: Cambridge University Press;178:54–56.

147. Symmers W. The Lymphoreticular System. In: *Systemic Pathology by Thirty-eight Authors.* Edinburgh: Churchill Livingstone; 1978.

148. Rich AR. *The Pathogenesis of Tuberculosis.* Springfield, Ill: Charles C Thomas Publishers; 1951.

149. Dunham EC, Smythe AM. Tuberculosis of abdominal lymph nodes, diagnosis by means of the roentgen ray. *Am J Dis Child.* 1926;31:815–831.

150. Nolan DJ, Norman WJ, Airth GR. Traction diverticula of the colon. *Clin Radiol.* 1971;22:458–461.

151. Phillips S. *Current Problems in Tuberculosis.* Springfield, Ill: Charles C Thomas Publishers; 1966:88.

152. Opie EL. Active and latent tuberculosis in the Negro race. *Am Rev Tuberc* 1924;10:265–274.

153. Fred HL, Eiband JM, Collins LC. Calcifications in intra-abdominal and retroperitoneal metastases. *Am J Roentgenol.* 1964;91:138–148.

154. Lingley JR. The significance of psammoma calcification in roentgen diagnosis of papillary tumors of the ovary. *Am J Roentgenol.* 1964;91:138–148.

155. Moncada R, Cooper RA, Garces M. Calcified metastases from malignant ovarian neoplasm. *Radiology.* 1974;133:31–35.

156. Stiedl RA. Extensive calcified retroperitoneal lymph node metastases from a primary carcinoma of the cecum. *Radiology.* 1967;89:263–264.

157. Ghahremani GG, Straus FH II. Calcification of distant lymph node metastases from carcinoma of the colon. *Radiology.* 1971;99:65–66.

158. Zboralske FF, Amberg JR, Subby WL. Calcified mucinous adenocarcinoma of the colon. *Am J Gastroenterol.* 1962;38:675–681.

159. Hermann G, Rozin R. Calcification in gastrointestinal carcinomata. *Clin Radiol.* 1964;15:139–141.

160. McNair M, Trapnell DH. Calcification in lymph node mestastases from adenocarcinoma of the colon. *Br J. Radiol.* 1971;44:468–470.

161. Hutcheson J, Page DL, Oldham RR. Calcified lymph nodes. *Br J. Radiol.* 1975;48:396–400.

162. Dolan PA. Tumor calcification following therapy. *Am J Roentgenol.* 1963;89:166–174.

163. Batlan LE. Calcification within the stomach wall in gastric malignancy. *Am J Roentgenol.* 1954;72:788–794.

164. Butler RL, Cotran R. Petrified stomach. *N Engl J Med.* 1969;261:84–86.

165. Case 42242, Case Records of the Massachusetts General Hospital. *N Engl J Med.* 1956;254:1139–1141.

166. Fisher AMH, Kendall B, Van Leuven BD. Hodgkin's disease: A radiological survey. *Clin Radiol.* 1962; 13:115–127.

167. Le Treut A, Dilhuydy MH, Denepoux R. Ossified lymph nodes metastatic from osteosarcoma. *J Radiol Electrol Med Nucl.* 1974;55:317–320.

168. Senturia HR, Schechter SE, Hulbert B. Heterotopic ossification in an area of metastasis from rectal carcinoma. *Am J Roentgenol.* 1948;60:507–510.

169. Valentin E. In: Dunham EC, Smythe AM eds. Tuberculosis of abdominal lymph nodes, diagnosis by

means of the roentgen ray. *Am J Dis Child.* 1926; 31:815–831.

170. Calmette A. Channels of tuberculous infection. *Br J. Tuberc.* 1909;3:199–201.

171. DeGiuli E. Lymph node calcification after radiotherapy in 2 cases of seminoma testis. *Tumori.* 1977; 63:543–548.

172. Oh KS. Mottled areas of intra-abdominal calcification. *JAMA.* 1969;208:521–523.

173. Syman SM, Weber AL. Calcification in intrathoracic nodes in Hodgkin's disease. *Radiology.* 1969;93:1021–1024.

174. McLennan TW, Castellino RA. Calcification in pelvic lymph nodes containing Hodgkin's disease following radiotherapy. *Radiology.* 1975;115:87–89.

175. Bertrand M, Chen JTT, Libshitz HI. Lymph node calcification in Hodgkin's disease after chemotherapy. *Am J Roentgenol.* 1977;129:1108–1110.

176. Korek-Amorosa J, Scheinman HZ, Clemett AR. Hypercalcemia and extensive lymph node calcification in a patient with Hodgkin's disease prior to therapy. *Br J. Radiol.* 1974;47:905–907.

177. Wright C, Payling, Heard BE. The lungs. In: *Systemic Pathology by Thirty-eight Authors.* Edinburgh: Churchill Livingstone; 1976;1:269–428.

178. Winchester PH, Cerwin R, Dische R. Hemosiderin laden lymph nodes. *Am J Roentgenol.* 1973;118:222–226.

179. Halbrecht I. Diagnosis, pathogenetic role and treatment of the sequels of female genital tuberculosis. In: Rippmann ET, Wenner R, eds. *Latent Female Genital Tuberculosis.* Basel: S Karger; 1966:232–238.

180. Eggen DA, Strong JP, McGill HC. Calcification in the abdominal aorta. *Arch Pathol.* 1964;78:575–583.

181. Hyman JB, Epstein FH. A study of the correlation between roentgenographic and post-mortem calcification of the aorta. *Am Heart J.* 1954;48:540–543.

182. Reid MM, Fannin TF. Extensive vascular calcification in association with juvenile rheumatoid arthritis and amyloidosis. *Arch Dis Child.* 1969;43:607–610.

183. Choube BS. Extensive aortic calcification in a case of primary arteritis. *Angiology.* 1972;23:618–634.

184. Ibels LS, Alfrey AC, Heffer WEK, et al. Arterial calcification and pathology in uremic patients undergoing dialysis. *Am J Med.* 1979;66:790–796.

185. Meema HE, Oreopoulos DB, de Veber GA. Arterial calcifications in severe chronic renal disease and their relationship to dialysis treatment, renal transplant, and parathyroidectomy. *Radiology.* 1971;121:315–321.

186. Boukhris R, Becker KL. Calcification of the aorta and osteoporosis. *JAMA.* 1972;219:1307–1311.

187. Epstein FH, Boas EP, Simpson R. The epidemiology of atherosclerosis among a random sample of clothing workers of different ethnic origins in New York City. *J Chron Dis.* 1957;5:300–325.

188. Peterson FG. Atherosclerosis of the abdominal aorta, a roentgenologic study. *Acta Radiol.* 1952;37:356–363.

189. Elkeles A. A comparative radiological study of calcified atheroma in males and females over 50 years of age. *Lancet* 1957;2:714.

190. Anderson JB, Barnett E, Nordin BEC. The relation between osteoporosis and aortic calcification. *Br J. Radiol.* 1964;37:910–912.

191. Burhenne HJ, Strasser E. A simple radiographic method and epidemiological study of atherosclerosis. *Radiology.* 1970;97:180–182.

192. Tejada C, Strong JP, Montenegro MR, et al. Distribution of coronary and aortic atherosclerosis by geographic location, race and sex. In: McGill HC, ed. *The Geographic Pathology of Atherosclerosis.* Baltimore: Williams & Wilkins Co; 1968:49–66.

193. Auerbach O, Garfinkel L. Atherosclerosis and aneurysm of aorta in relation to smoking habits and age. *Chest.* 1980;78:805–809.

194. Lawton G. Cigarette consumption and atherosclerosis. Their relationship in the aorta and iliac and femoral arteries. *Br J. Surg.* 1973;60:873–876.

195. Sackett DL, Winkelstein W Jr. The relationship between cigarette usage and aortic atherosclerosis. *Am J Epidemiol.* 1967;86:264–270.

196. Elkeles A. Calcified atherosclerosis and cancer. *Br J. Cancer.* 1959;13:403–407.

197. Elkeles A. Gastric ulcer in the aged and calcified atherosclerosis. *Am J Roentgenol.* 1964;91:744–750.

198. Fotopoulos JP, Crampton AR, Burkhead HC. Calcification of the abdominal aorta as an aid in diagnosis of gastric carcinoma vs benign ulcer. *Radiology.* 1962;79:637–643.

199. Winkelstein W Jr, Lilienfeld R, Pickren JW, et al. The relationship between aortic atherosclerosis and cancer. *Br J. Cancer.* 1959;13:606–613.

200. Charnsangavej C. Intraluminal calcification and occlusion of the abdominal aorta above the renal arteries. *Cardiovasc Intervent Radiol.* 1981;4:242–244.

201. Lipchik EO, Rob CG, Schwartzberg S. Obstruction of the abdominal aorta above the level of the renal arteries. *Radiology.* 1964;82:433–445.

202. Estes, JE Jr. Abdominal aorta aneurysm: A study of one hundred and two cases. *Circulation.* 1950;2:258–264.

203. Steinberg I, Stein HL. Visualization of abdominal aortic aneurysm. *Am J Roentgenol.* 1965;95:684–695.

204. Loughran CF. A review of the plain abdominal radiograph in acute rupture of abdominal aortic aneurysms. *Clin Radiol.* 1986;37:383–387.

205. Janower ML. Ruptured arteriosclerotic aneurysm of abdominal aorta: Roentgenographic findings on plain films. *N Engl J Med.* 1961;265:12–16.

206. Prystein S, Cavoto FV, Gerritsen RW. Spontaneous mycotic aneurysm of the abdominal aorta. *J Comput Assist Tomogr.* 1979;3:681–683.

207. Wilson JL, Marks JH. Calcification of the vas deferens: Its relation to diabetes mellitus and arteriosclerosis. *N Engl J Med.* 1951;245:321–325.

208. Hafiz A, Melnick JC. Calcification of the vas deferens. *J Can Assoc Radiol.* 1968;19:56–60.

209. King JC Jr, Rosenbaum HD. Calcification of the vasa deferentia in non diabetes. *Radiology.* 1971;100:603–606.

210. Shenult P. The origin of phleboliths. *Br J. Surg.* 1972;59:695–700.

211. Orton GH. Some fallacies in the x-ray diagnosis of renal and ureteral calculi. *Br Med J.* 1908;2:716–719.

212. Clark GD. Peri-ureteric pelvic phleboliths. *J Urol.* 1909;80:913–921.

213. Dovey P. Pelvic phleboliths. *Clin Radiol.* 1966;17:121–125.

214. Culligan JM. Phleboliths. *J Urol.* 1926;15:175–188.

215. Burkitt DP, Latto C, Janvrin SB et al. Pelvic phleboliths: Epidemiology and postulated etiology. *N Engl J Med.* 1977;296:1387–1391.

216. Burkitt DP. Hemorrhoids, varicose veins, and deep vein thrombosis: Epidemiologic features and suggested causative factors. *Can J Surg.* 1975;18:483–488.

217. Baker SR, Shapiro M. Unpublished data.

218. Green M, Thomas ML. The prevalence of pelvic phleboliths in relation to age, sex, and urinary tract infections. *Clin Radiol.* 1972;23:492–494.

219. Butzler O. Zur differential Diagnose der Phlebolithen und Ureterokonkremente im Rontgenbild des kleinen Becken. *Fortschr Roentgenstr.* 1934;49:253–262.

220. Mattson T. Frequency and location of pelvic phleboliths. *Clin Radiol.* 1980;31:115–118.

221. Steinbach HL. Identification of pelvic masses by phlebolith displacement. *Am J Roentgenol.* 1960;83:1063–1066.

222. Curry NS, Han FC, Schabel SI. Suprapubic phleboliths: Prevalence, distribution and clinical association. *Clin Radiol.* 1983;34:701–705.

223. Berlow ME, Azimi F, Carsky EW. Gonadol vein phlebolith simulating a mid-ureteral stone. *Am J Roentgenol.* 1979;133:919–920.

224. Dodd GD, Rutledge F, Wallace S. Postoperative pelvic lymphocysts. *Am J Roentgenol.* 1970;108:312–323.

225. Fenlon JW, Augustin C. The significance of pelvic phlebolith displacement. *J Urol.* 1971;106:595–598.

226. Kolman MA. Radiologic soft tissues in the pelvis: Another look. *Am J Roentgenol.* 1977;130:493–498.

227. Grieco RV, Bartone NF. Roentgen visualization of phleboliths in hemangioma of the gastrointestinal tract. *Am J Roentgenol.* 1967;101:406–408.

228. Taybi H. *Radiology of Syndromes.* Chicago, Ill: Year Book Medical Publishers; 1975:137.

229. Buhrow CJ, Gary TM, Clark WED. Ovarian corpora albicentia calcification. *Radiology.* 1966;87:746–747.

230. Gammill SL, Nice CM Jr. Calcification in the inferior vena cava. *Radiology.* 1969;92:1288–1290.

231. Singleton EB, Rosenberg HS. Intraluminal calcification of the inferior vena cava. *Am J Roentgenol.* 1961;86:556–560.

232. Banker VP. Calcified external iliac vein thrombosis. *Radiology.* 1975;117:311–314.

233. Goodman, GA. Intraluminal iliac venous calcification. *Br J. Radiol.* 1975;48:457–459.

CHAPTER FOUR

The Plain Film Assessment of the Stomach and Duodenum

STOMACH

Gastric Dilatation

The stomach and the large intestine are the two organs most amenable to plain film evaluation, as both of these hollow viscera usually contain at least a few milliliters of gas. Each has expected points of fixation that help determine its position in the upper abdomen. The stomach begins just beyond the esophageal hiatus, and movement of its distal end is limited by the retroperitoneal attachments of the descending duodenum. The transverse colon is confined by the anchorings of the anatomic hepatic and splenic flexures to the posterior peritoneal wall. Nevertheless, both organs are distensible structures capable of wide variability in caliber and volume. Even more than the colon, the stomach is subject to rapid changes in size because intraluminal contents may enter promptly by ingestion or leave as rapidly through peristalsis, vomiting, or iatrogenic manipulations.

The large intestine and the stomach share an intimate spatial relationship, tied to each other by the gastrocolic ligament. Recognition of the transverse colon on supine films helps to locate the stomach whereas observation of the gastric air bubble permits prompt identification of adjacent large intestinal segments. Hence, the two organs should be assessed in tandem. In general, the finding of gas in the transverse colon is more predictable than the presence of air in the stomach and therefore should be looked for first.

Downward depression of the transverse colon accompanies marked gastric enlargement. In massive distension, the transverse colon may overlie the true pelvis. A low-lying transverse colon in elderly patients need not necessarily indicate gastric dilatation because ptosis of the stomach and large intestine as well as stretching of the gastrocolic ligament are common occurrences in this age group. An elongated J-shaped stomach, a normal variation seen most often in ectomorphic individuals, may cause the distal transverse colon to be displaced downward. It is important not to assume that every inferiorly positioned transverse colon indicates a fluid-filled dilated stomach above it. Such a radiographic diagnosis should only be made in the presence of corroborating clinical signs and symptoms.

Depression of the transverse colon by an enlarged stomach can involve the entire length of this bowel segment or only its proximal, central, or distal portions. A localized impression on the mid or distal transverse colon is characteristic of the dilatation of vertically elongated stomachs (Figs 2–21, 4–1). Distension of a horizontally positioned gastric lumen often affects the proximal transverse colon preferentially. If the stomach is gasless and consequently similar in density to adjacent solid organs, its enlargement can simulate the appearance of massive hepatomegaly (Fig 4–2). A smooth extrinsic impression on the superior colonic wall is a helpful, but not an essential feature of gastric dilatation, as considerable displacement of the colon can occur without any accompanying deformation of its contour.

At times, the transverse colon is free of feces and gas and cannot be discerned on plain films. Without delineation of the contour of the transverse colon a markedly dilated stomach can resemble ascites, appearing on plain films as a homogenously dense abdomen. Nevertheless, there are points of differentiation between excessive intraperitoneal and intragastric fluid. A dilated stomach displaces small bowel loops laterally, not towards the midline, as in a large peritoneal effusion. With ascites, a diffuse accentuation of radiodensity is distributed evenly throughout the peritoneal cavity. Even in a stomach that seems to be completely liquid filled, however, a small amount of air is almost always present, collecting anteriorly and medially when the patient is placed in the supine position. Such gastric air, although not always a sharply outlined lucency,

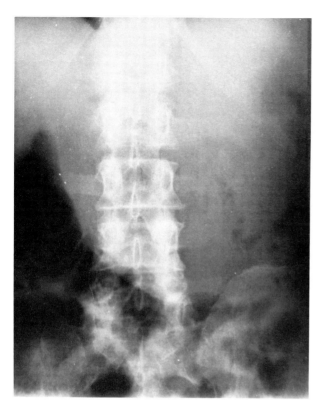

Figure 4–1. Gastric dilatation. The transverse colon has been impressed upon by the fluid-filled stomach. Downward depression is more marked at the mid and distal segments of the transverse colon.

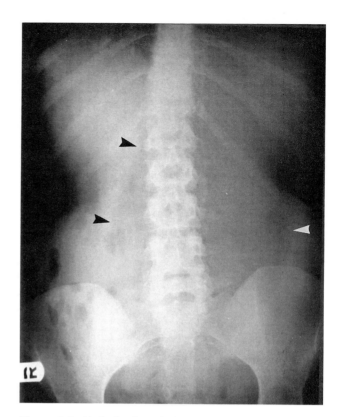

Figure 4–3. Markedly distended stomach in a patient with the superior mesenteric artery compression syndrome. The central abdomen contains no air-filled intestinal loops. Evidence of the location of the stomach is the faint but large gastric air collection outlined by arrowheads.

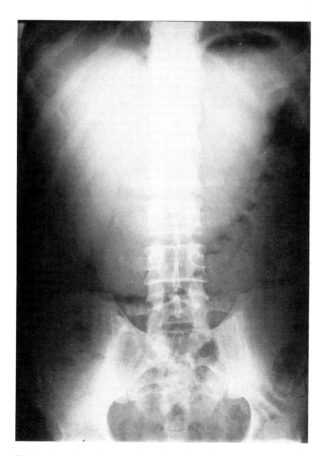

Figure 4–2. Gastric dilatation. The fluid-filled stomach has displaced the proximal transverse colon. This plain film appearance simulates hepatomegaly.

evenly throughout the peritoneal cavity. Even in a stomach that seems to be completely liquid filled, however, a small amount of air is almost always present, collecting anteriorly and medially when the patient is placed in the supine position. Such gastric air, although not always a sharply outlined lucency, can still be detected because the paramedian region of the abdomen appears slightly less opaque than the periphery when the stomach is massively distended (Fig 4–3). Confirmation of the presence of an enlarged gastric lumen can be accomplished by upright or decubitus projections that reveal an air–fluid level extending across the width of the stomach. If these maneuvers are not diagnostic, a repeat film taken soon after partial evacuation of the stomach contents should demonstrate a significant change in overall density of the abdomen and in the location of gas-filled large- and small-bowel intestinal segments.

If swallowed air is the major intraluminal constituent, distension of the stomach is easily recognized in most cases (Figs 4–4, 4–5). Not every large lucency extending from the left upper quadrant across the abdomen to the pelvis or right lower quadrant is a distended stomach, however. In cecal volvulus, the distended caput cecum and even much of the right colon may lie below the left hemidiaphragm. It can usually be identified by the presence

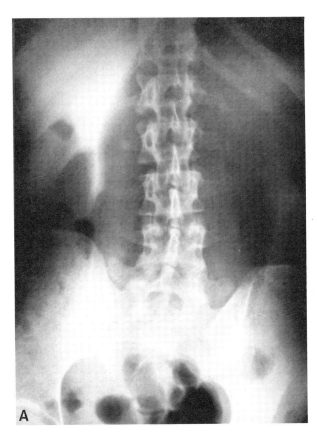
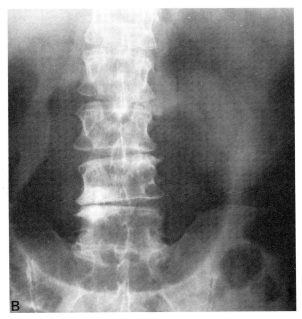

Figure 4–4. Air-filled dilated stomachs. Vertical configuration. **A.** The distended gastric air shadow descends to the pelvis. **B.** An air-filled stomach has displaced the transverse colon below it. The gray shadow within the proximal gastric body is liquid intraluminal contents.

gastric distension, in which the transverse colon must be caudal to the stomach (Fig 4–6). Occasionally, a redundant colon distended by retained feces may simulate the mottled shadows of food particles within a distended stomach. Differentiation of the two conditions can be achieved by tracing the large intestine between the hepatic and splenic flexures and from there to the ascending and descending colon. Almost always, a huge, feces-filled transverse colon is accompanied by a likewise dilated right colon (Fig 4–7).

Gastric distension may have a functional, metabolic, neurogenic, surgical, pharmaceutical, inflammatory, or obstructive etiology (Table 4–1). By far the most frequent cause is aerophagia, which although sometimes painful and often recurrent, is usually self-limited. Most of the time, the physician or the patient recognizes air swallowing, but, occasionally, ingestion of large quantities of air may not be apparent by history or observation of the patient. Dilatation is a common finding in diabetic gastropathy. Stomach distension need not correlate well with the control of blood glucose or the other man-

ifestation of this multisystem disease. In gravely-ill patients burdened by hypokalemia or uremia, gastric distension can be seen out of proportion to dilatation of other bowel segments. A similar preference for the stomach is a feature of porphyria and lead poisoning.

Truncal vagotomy and any other interruption of vagal impulses produces dilatation and delayed stomach emptying, necessitating simultaneous pyloroplasty to facilitate drainage of gastric contents. Transient, reversible distension of the stomach can be caused by morphine and atropine-like drugs. The short-acting paralysis and dilatation of the stomach after intravenous or intramuscular injection of glucagon can be put to good use in the evaluation of the areae gastricae during double-contrast upper GI roentgenographic series.

Inflammation of the stomach produces atony, which leads to gastric distension as swallowed air accumulates more quickly than it can be removed or resorbed. Pancreatitis and other inflammations adjacent to the stomach also result in a decrease in gastric peristalsis. Postoperative atony is a well-

130

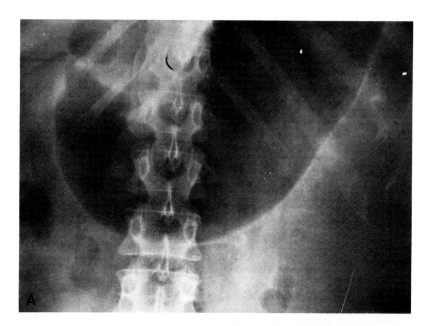

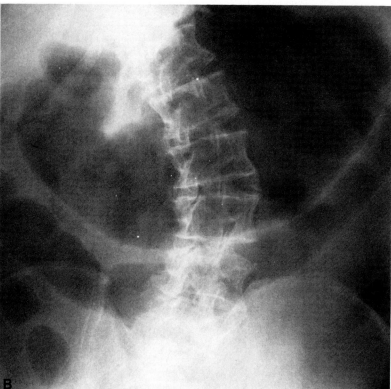

Figure 4–5. Air-filled dilated stomachs. Horizontal configuration. In both **(A)** and **(B)** the direction of gastric enlargement is primarily lateral rather than caudal. Note how the distal antrum in each case extends peripheral to the airfilled duodenal bulb.

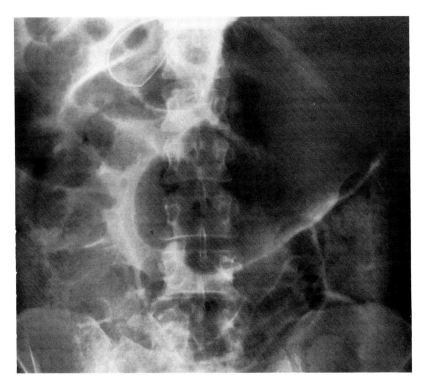

Figure 4–6. Cecal volvulus. The dilated cecum, twisted on a long mesentery, has come to lie in the left upper quadrant. The linear septation arising from its medial border identifies this large gas shadow as a colonic segment. An opaque nasogastric tube lies in the nondilated stomach.

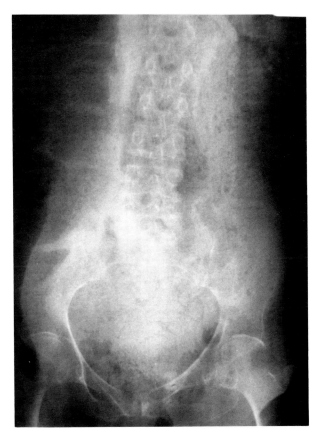

Figure 4–7. A markedly dilated colon simulates a distended stomach filled with particulate matter. The ascending colon, U-shaped transverse colon, sigmoid colon, and rectum are distended with gas and feces. The vertically oriented stomach contains gas and liquid and overlies the lumbar spine.

TABLE 4–1. CAUSES OF GASTRIC DISTENTION

Functional—aerophagia
Metabolic
  Diabetes
  Hypokalemia
  Uremia
  Lead poisoning
  Porphyria
Neurogenic
Surgical
  Postoperative Atony
  Post truncal Vagotomy
Pharmaceutical
  Morphine
  Atropine-like drugs
  Glucagon
Inflammation
  Gastritis
  Pancreatitis
  Other inflammations adjacent to the stomach
Obstructive
  Gastric obstruction
    Pyloric obstruction
    Gastric mass
    Bezoar
    Gastric volvulus
  Duodenal obstruction
    Ulcer
    SMA syndrome
    Other duodenal obstruction
  Jejunal and ileal obstruction

recognized concomitant of general anesthesia and is particularly frequent after abdominal surgery.

Duodenal and jejunal obstructions dilate small bowel proximal to the point of blockage. Sometimes the stomach expands as well, but the frequent vomiting characteristic of mechanical obstruction usually prevents marked gastric enlargement. The body cast syndrome,[1] the superior mesenteric artery syndrome,[2-4] and other causes of duodenal obstruction of the second and third portion of the duodenum have marked gastric distension as their hallmark. A typical presentation of pyloric channel ulcers is persistent dilatation of the stomach. Bezoars, which may themselves be a consequence of gastric surgery, can be responsible for intraluminal obstruction and distension (Fig 4–8).

In most cases of volvulus of the stomach, at least a part of the gastric lumen is situated in the thorax. Occasionally, the twisted stomach lies entirely below the diaphragm and appears on plain films much like a typical distended stomach. However, if the patient complains of unremitting pain

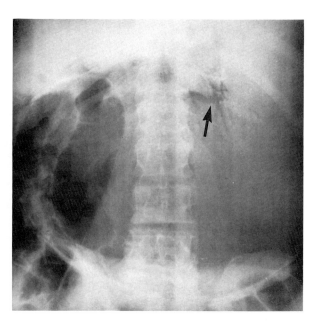

Figure 4–9. Volvulus of the stomach below the diaphragm. The large featureless lucency is the stomach, which has undergone a 360-degree twist. The arrow points to retroperitoneal air, which has resulted from the dissection of air through a posterior perforation of the infarcted gastric wall.

and dysphagia, volvulus must still be considered and confirmation by a contrast study should be done before the dire consequences of gastric ischemia or perforation ensue (Fig 4–9). In addition to air, liquid, and food particles, the ingestion of metallic or other radiodense objects by deranged patients may help outline the stomach. Also, retained radiopaque iron pills and multivitamin preparations containing iron that are designed to resist dissolution by gastric juices can provide a clue about the dimensions of an enlarged stomach (Fig 4–10).

Gastric Displacement

Despite its points of fixation at the esophagogastric junction and at the adjacent proximal duodenum, the stomach in part or in whole may change its position even without distending. The most common direction of migration is upwards through the esophageal hiatus. The plain film radiology of hiatus hernia is complicated and fascinating, fully deserving of a separate chapter. However, because most of its manifestations are in the thorax and often not observable on plain films of the abdomen, it is not discussed further here.

Within the abdomen, the stomach may be pushed backwards by masses in the left lobe of the liver or forwards by retroperitoneal tumefactions.

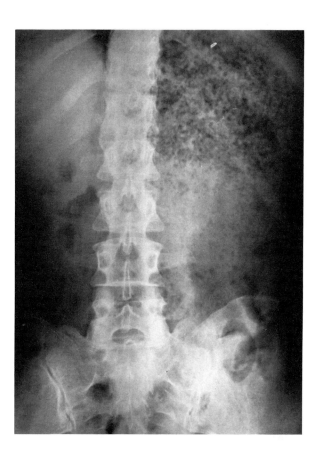

Figure 4–8. Bezoar. Post gastric surgery. A dilated stomach filled with air and undigested vegetable matter, producing a mottled pattern in the left abdomen.

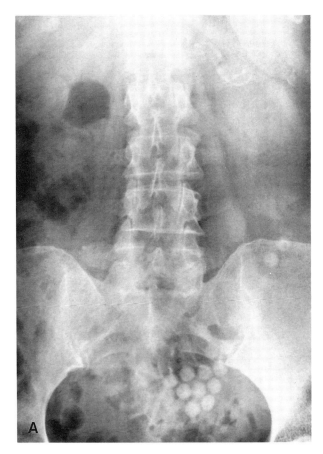
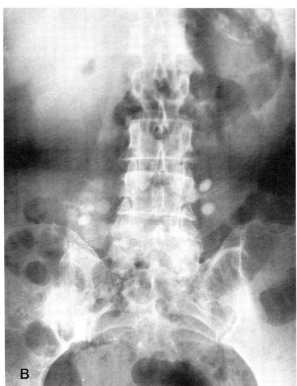

Figure 4–10. A. The only clue to a distended stomach is the collection of undissolved radiopaque iron tables in the expanded gastric lumen. **B.** Decompression of the stomach after placement of a nasogastric tube. The radiodense medications have migrated superiorly as the gastric lumen has decreased in size. The transverse colon is also seen clearly just below the stomach. (*Courtesy of Dr. James Naidich.*)

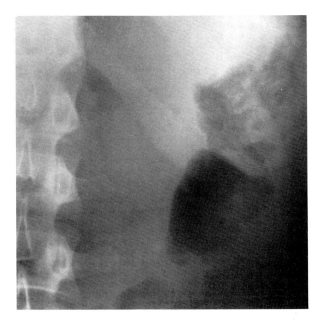

Figure 4–11. The spleen has been removed. The partially filled gastric air shadow is now positioned laterally.

Displacement along a purely anterior–posterior axis is difficult to detect on supine views. Medial repositioning is accomplished most frequently by an enlarging spleen (Fig 2–82) but may also be due to an expanding abscess in the lesser sac. Lateral displacement can be achieved by an adjacent liver mass (Fig 2–80) or by splenectomy, which provides an empty space for the stomach to enter (Fig 4–11). Often, slight lateral displacements are surgically induced, created during partial gastrectomy as the gastric pouch is affixed to a laterally positioned efferent loop of proximal jejunum (Fig 4–12).

ABNORMALITIES OF CONTOUR

Irregular Indentations

The presence of intraluminal swallowed air provides an opportunity to evaluate the shape of the stomach. However, plain film analysis of the configura-

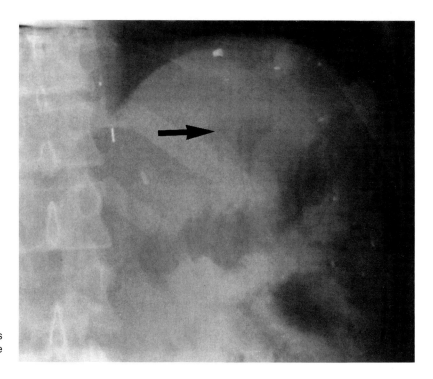

Figure 4–12. The small gastric remnant has been pushed laterally (*arrow*) to accommodate an anastomosis with the proximal jejunum.

tion of the gastric wall has considerable limitations that tend to restrict diagnostic confidence. Most importantly, the air shadow may not depict the dimensions of the lumen when admixed with gastric juices or ingested food particles. Instead, its lucent pattern reflects the distribution of gas, liquid and solid densities, rather than the wall of the stomach itself (Fig 2–5). Thus, the gastric bubble only supplies reliable contour information when air is the predominant constituent of the lumen.

Inexperienced interpreters of plain films of the abdomen sometimes incorrectly regard the thin lucency of air in an empty stomach as evidence of a constricting carcinoma. The nearly empty stomach preserves its rugal topography even if only one or two of these submucosal ridges are seen (Fig 2–1). The normal gas shadow generally has smooth, gently curving margins, with the greater and lesser curvatures describing roughly parallel courses. On successive films, there are almost always changes in the configuration of the stomach bubble, reflecting gastric distensibility and peristaltic activity.

In contrast, infiltrating gastric lesions tend to obliterate or deform the rugae of a nondistended stomach (Fig 2–3). Irregular contours with areas of narrowing between more distended regions characterize diffuse involvement of the wall by neoplasm,

granulomatous inflammation, or fibrosis (Fig 4–13). An unvarying gas pattern with a persistently similar contour on all films in a series of radiographs also strongly suggests a constricting gastric tumor.

A discrete mass can be seen on plain films as a focal interruption of an otherwise normal gas shadow. In such cases, the lumen at the site of the tumor often appears fixed and angulated (Fig 4–14). Normally, the entire stomach is not air-filled even though air may enter the duodenal bulb. Typically, in nondilated lumens, the air shadow fades imperceptibly near the midline. A sharp termination of the distal gastric bubble at its medial edge, often in association with apparent lateral displacement of the proximal stomach, indicates an extensive lesion of the stomach. In the body and antrum, the only manifestation of a deforming tumor may be an abrupt interruption of the gastric air shadow (Fig 4–15). Equally revealing is the double-lucency sign, the superimposition of two irregularly shaped air containing spaces demarcating the eccentric growth of a mass within the lumen (Figs 4–16, 2–34).

A fixed, narrowed stomach has been considered strongly suggestive of scirrhous carcinoma. For the past several decades, carcinoma of the stomach has been declining in frequency while the incidence of gastric lymphoma has been relatively stable. In

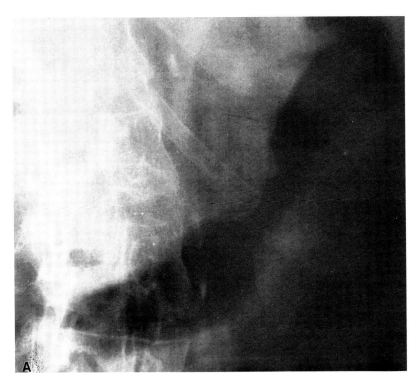

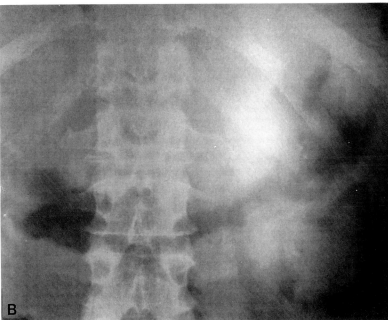

Figure 4–13. Lymphomas of the stomach narrowing the lumen. **A.** A segment of the body of the stomach is constricted by tumor infiltrating the gastric wall. **B.** The narrowing involves nearly the complete extent of the body. The distal antrum is still distensible.

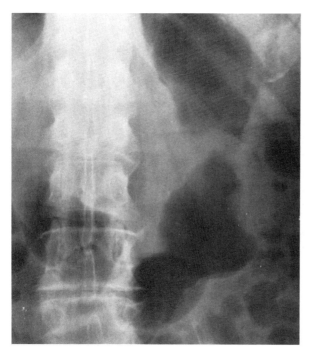

Figure 4–14. Carcinoma of the stomach. A focal interruption in the gastric air shadow delimits an endophytic tumor.

our experience, the plain film findings of a persistently narrowed lumen have been seen more often in lymphoma than in carcinoma. Other tumors that mimic gastric adenocarcinoma and lymphoma on plain films are metastatic deposits to the stomach,

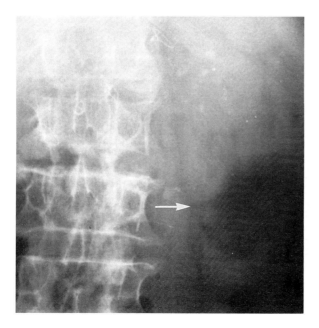

Figure 4–15. A constricting carcinoma has caused an abrupt termination of luminal air far from the midline (*arrow*).

especially from primary sites in the lung and breast and local extension of pancreatic carcinoma. Lye ingestion, radiation fibrosis, and granulomatous diseases, including sarcoidosis, actinomycosis, Crohn's disease, and syphilis, can have a similar appearance. A constricted lumen may also be a plain film manifestation of scarring from an extensive but benign gastric ulcer (Fig 4–17).

Not every markedly abnormal stomach is a result of inflammation or neoplasm. Patients may not be knowledgeable or forthright about previous abdominal operations. Because gastrectomy is a relatively common procedure with obvious deforming effects on the contour of the stomach bubble, postsurgical changes should also be considered in the differential diagnosis in all individuals with an upper abdominal scar, even when patient recollection is not edifying or old records are not available. In most instances, the air-filled efferent loop is located lateral to the stomach (Fig 2–29). Sometimes, the anastomosis itself can be seen with the gastric remnant and its small-bowel attachment both filled with air (Fig 4–18). Occasionally, air is apparent only in the gastric fundus and the configuration and location of the lucency mimics an obstructing mass (Fig 4–19).

Smooth Contour Defects

Gastric polyps are the most common neoplasms of the stomach. Usually, they are small lesions, rarely more than 2 cm in diameter. Their low malignant potential, small size, and infrequent bleeding make them clinically silent and innocuous in most patients. Rarely, they can be multiple, with each polyp having sufficient mass to project into the lumen, where they can be seen on plain films as a grouping of smooth filling defects (Fig 4–20).

Leiomyomas are the most frequently encountered smooth-walled benign gastric neoplasms. Exogastric leiomyomas, which arise from the stomach but grow away from it, are detected by the deviation of the gastric air shadow, not by focal indentation of it. On the other hand, mural leiomyomas may enlarge into the lumen, where they can be observed on plain films as a nonlobulated filling defect that rarely obstructs the lumen even when it becomes very large. The distinctive plain film findings of gastric leiomyomas are often the first evidence of their presence, as they are frequently asymptomatic at the time of their incidental discovery during imaging assessment for other clinical problems (Fig 4–21). Leiomyomas have a tendency to ulcerate and bleed. Almost always, the ulcer is near the center of the mass and is a sufficiently deep excavation to permit radiographic visualization during barium studies.

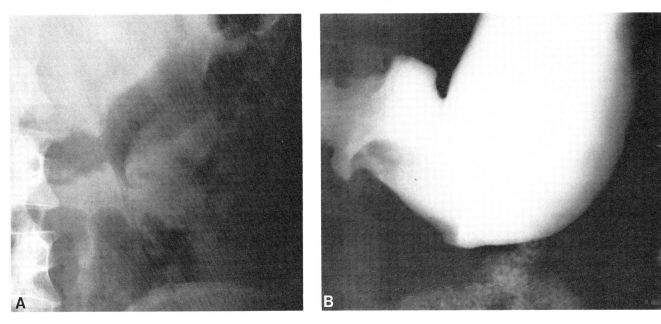

Figure 4–16. Double-lucency sign. **A.** A large carcinoma protruding into the lumen from the inferior wall is superimposed over an uninvolved segment of the air filled stomach. **B.** Barium contrast confirms the presence of a mass.

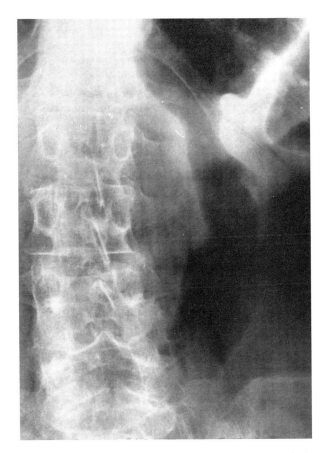

Figure 4–17. Extensive narrowing of the body of the stomach due to scarring from a healed benign gastric ulcer.

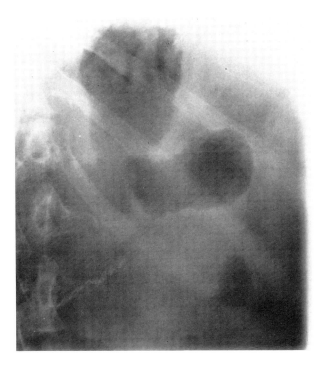

Figure 4–18. Billioth II anastomosis. The gastric pouch and the proximal jejunum are both air-filled and the point of connection between them is clearly seen.

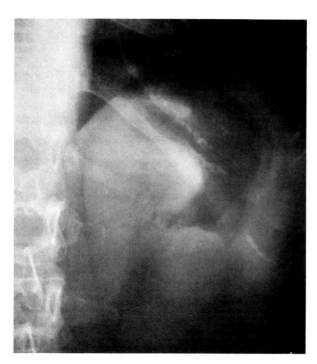

Figure 4–19. Abrupt termination of air in the gastric pouch and lateral position of the stomach. The stomach is air-filled but the small bowel is fluid-filled in this patient who had a partial gastrectomy with gastroenterostomy.

On occasion, the air-filled ulcer crater may be seen on plain films standing out in sharp contrast to the homogeneous density of the tumor (Fig 4–22).

In recent years, direct access to the stomach has been achieved through the percutaneous placement of gastrostomy tubes that permit intestinal feeding of patients with obstructive carcinoma of the esophagus and other debilitating conditions. Gastrostomy tubes are secured to the gastric wall by an inflatable balloon that prevents migration of the tube out of the lumen of the stomach. The balloon produces a filling defect unmistakable when seen en face (Fig 4–23). Viewed in profile, it can closely resemble, both in size and configuration, the plain film appearance of a gastric leiomyoma (Fig 4–24).

Gastric Ulcerations

Small ulcers of the stomach and duodenal bulb are difficult to appreciate by barium examination and are impossible to discern on plain films. Large ulcers, which extend beyond the expected borders of the gastric wall, can be observed if the radiographic beam views them in profile. Most often, they are giant, benign ulcers arrayed along the lesser curvature. Their ample craters, when filled with air, are recognizable as rounded lucent projections in contiguity with the gastric lumen (Fig 4–25). In most cases, the communication with the lumen is clear but in some ulcers, edema of its mucosal collar casts a grey shadow that falsely suggests a separation of the ulcer sac from the remainder of the stomach bubble. Also, cellular debris accumulating in the base of the crater can deform the ulcer shadow (Fig 4–26).

An air-filled ulcer should never be confused with a gastric diverticulum, which is always found in the fundus of the stomach far from the lesser curvature location of giant ulcers. Moreover, the

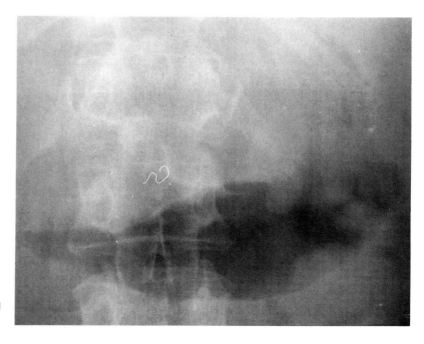

Figure 4–20. Gastric polyps. Several rounded densities indent the stomach bubble.

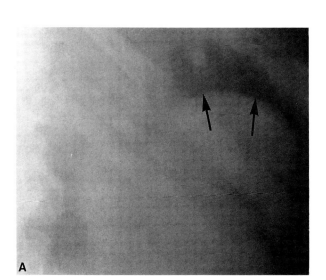
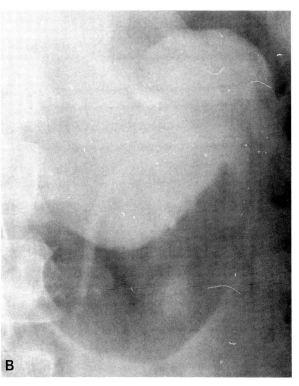

Figure 4–21. A. Gastric leiomyomas. The arrows point to a large, smooth, convex upward indentation of the gastric air shadow. **B.** A large leiomyoma growing into the lumen divides the gastric air shadow into separate segments for the body and the fundus. It was discovered incidentally at intravenous venography.

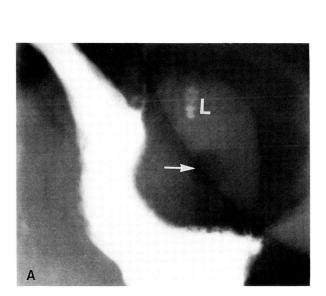
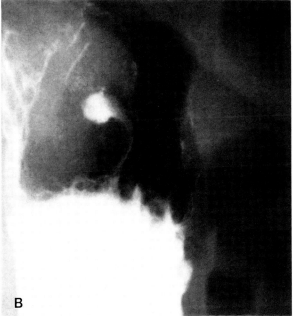

Figure 4–22. Ulcerated gastric leiomyoma. **A.** Initial film after the first swallow of barium during an upper GI series. A large smooth mass (L) protrudes into the fundus. Within the tumor is a rounded lucency (*arrow*) demarcating a central ulceration. **B.** A later film demonstrates barium entering the ulcer crater.

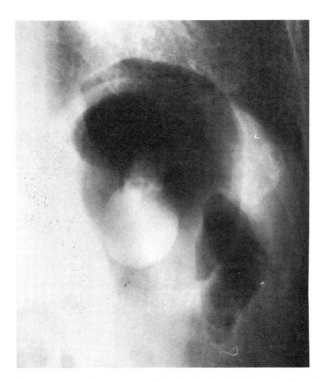

Figure 4–23. Gastrostomy. The intraluminal balloon is almost completely surrounded by air.

predictable posterior location of gastric diverticula inhibits plain film obstruction because they are almost always fluid filled when the patient is supine. A gas-filled, small-intestinal segment superimposed on the lesser curvature is usually easily distinguish-

able from an ulcer crater by its identifying signature of valvulae conniventes. However, the homogeneous lucency of a diverticulum of the fourth portion of the duodenum or proximal jejunum may very closely resemble the appearance of a giant ulcer of the stomach (Fig 4–27).

Air in the Stomach Wall

Air in the wall of the stomach is an unusual radiographic finding, encountered much less often than intestinal intramural gas. Despite its rarity, it can be a consequence of a diverse list of conditions ranging from acute asthma[5] to fulminant gastric inflammation (Table 4–2).[6] Moreover, gastric wall gas has several distinctive X-ray appearances. To bring order to this confusing array of causes and radiographic manifestations, it is best to consider intramural gas in the stomach as belonging to one of two categories, namely emphysematous gastritis or gastric emphysema.[7]

Emphysematous gastritis is seen most often after massive ingestion of alkaline corrosives.[8] It has also been reported in severe gastroenteritis,[6] acute alcohol abuse,[9] ischemic infarction of the stomach[10] and as a complication of gastroduodenal surgery.[11] Abrupt denudation of the epithelium leads to infiltration of the submucosa and muscular layers by gas-forming bacteria. Streaks of lucency may be noted, but the predominant pattern is small bubbles interspersed between large bullae.[12] Such a collection of rounded lucencies can be simulated by food particles and liquid in the gastric lumen as well as by

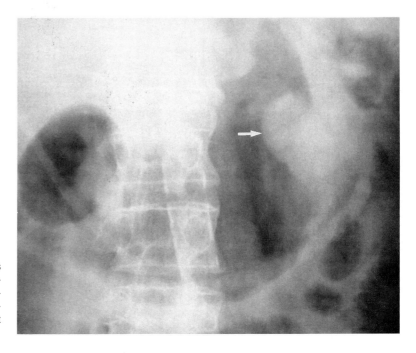

Figure 4–24. Gastrostomy. The balloon lies against the wall of the stomach. Its smooth contour suggests the plain film appearance of a leiomyoma (*arrow*). Note the drainage tube overlying the greater curvature of the stomach as it approaches the balloon tip.

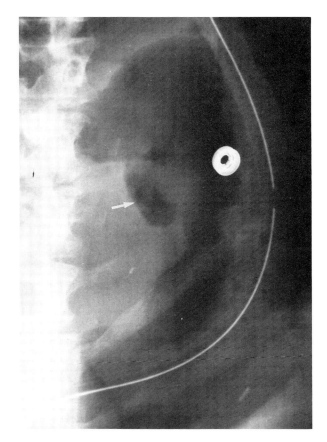

Figure 4–25. An air-filled large ulcer (*arrow*) extending beyond the expected contour of the lesser curvature of the stomach.

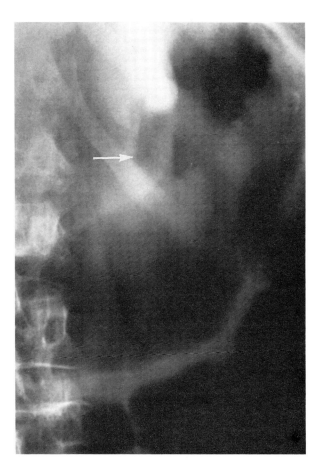

Figure 4–26. Giant air-filled gas ulcer (*arrow*). Cellular debris at the ulcer base has deformed the outline of this large excavation. (*Courtesy of Dr. Murray Rosenberg.*)

abscesses in the lesser sac, pancreas, spleen, left kidney, and left subphrenic space. The presence of streaks along the expected outline of the stomach helps to distinguish emphysematous gastritis from other gas-containing infections in the left upper abdomen.

Usually, the stomach is not markedly distended and its contents are meager.[13] The weakened gastric wall is liable to perforation, and pneumoperitoneum is a well-recognized complication.[9] Passage of gas into veins draining the stomach can lead to the presence of portal venous gas.[13]

The majority of patients with mural air have gastric emphysema, which appears as a streak of variable width outlining much of the stomach contour. Although small bubbles may be seen, a continuous linear lucency is the hallmark of gastric emphysema. Unlike with emphysematous gastritis, affected individuals are often asymptomatic and seldom have complaints directly referable to the stomach.[5] The stomach remains distensible and is usually moderately dilated, often containing considerable fluid (Fig 4–28). Not all streaks in the stomach represent mural air, however. A lucency of limited extent can result from the almost complete narrowing of the lumen by an expanding endophytic mass (Fig 4–29).

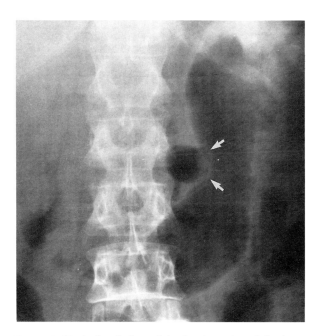

Figure 4–27. A diverticulum of the fourth portion of duodenum superimposed on the lesser curvature of the stomach mimicking a gastric ulcer. The thin line of the lateral margin of the diverticulum (*arrows*) is a helpful sign that this lucency overlies rather than projects from the stomach bubble.

141

TABLE 4–2. CAUSES OF AIR IN THE STOMACH WALL

Emphysematous gastritis
    Ingestion of corrosives
    Severe gastroenteritis
    Acute alcohol abuse
    Ischemic infarction
    Gastroduodenal surgery
Gastric emphysema
    Postendoscopy
    Severe vomiting
    Pyloric obstruction
    Small-bowel obstruction
    Asthma
    Chronic obstructive lung disease

Today, with the increasing popularity of endoscopic evaluation of the upper GI tract, gastroscopy is probably the most frequent cause of emphysema of the stomach wall.[14] It is a benign complication, producing little discomfort and usually resolving within 2 or 3 days.[15] Severe vomiting in the absence of obstruction is another cause.[16] In both conditions, inspection of the lumen does not often reveal a mucosal rent. Perhaps in most of these cases, microscopic tears through the epithelial lining allow air to enter the stomach wall.[17]

Gastric emphysema can be seen with mechan-

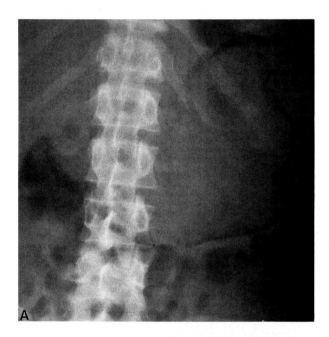

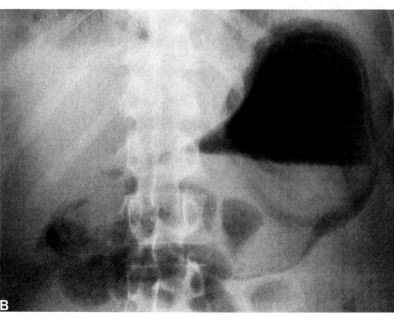

Figure 4–28. Supine (A) and upright **(B)** films in a patient with gastric emphysema after an episode of vomiting. A streak of varying width involves the wall of much of the dilated stomach.

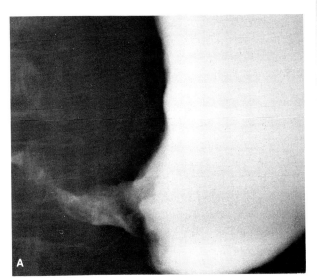
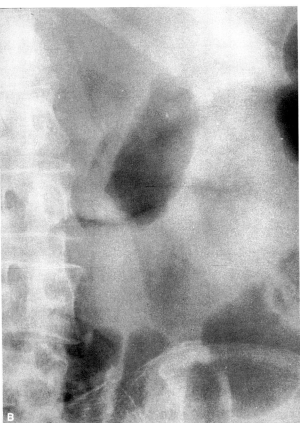

Figure 4–29. Stimulation of mural air by a carcinoma growing into the gastric lumen. **A.** Plain film reveals a short streak of gas. **B.** Barium study demonstrates a constricting tumor nearly occluding the lumen.

ical obstruction of the duodenum, jejunum, or ileum.[18,19] The frequency of blockage of the small intestine and the uncommonness of mural air suggests that a point of mucosal weakness such as the site of an active or healed ulcer may also be necessary before air can penetrate the gastric wall. Surprisingly, mural lucencies have been reported only twice in the duodenal bulb,[5,20] notwithstanding the fact that the bulb mucosa is often permanently scarred by peptic ulceration. The mechanism of formation of gastric emphysema as a concomitant of small bowel obstruction remains obscure.

Similarly mysterious is air in the stomach wall in patients with chronic or acute obstructive lung disease. It has been proposed that gas can dissect through the pulmonary interstitium, the mediastinum, the retroperitoneal space, and, finally, the muscular layers of the stomach.[21] Nevertheless, mediastinal air is often absent on X-ray, and gas bubbles elsewhere in the wall of the gut in association with gastric wall gas are not seen in most cases. It is not clear if a pathophysiological relationship exists between pulmonary and gastric abnormalities or if

there is merely an incidental association between the two, as both lung and stomach emphysema are found most often in the elderly.

Previous classification schemes mention a third source of gastric wall air—idiopathic cystic pneumatosis of the stomach. Just as the colon may spontaneously form innumerable gas cysts so, too, can the stomach have rounded mural lucencies that appear without an evident cause. Convincing examples of this phenomenon have yet to be demonstrated in the radiological literature, however, and cystic pneumatosis of the stomach may not be a real entity.[7,13,18,22]

RADIODENSITIES IN THE STOMACH

Mural Lesions

Opacification of all or a part of the wall of the stomach is rare, with the most frequent cause being calcification in adenocarcinoma of the stomach (Table 4–3). In recent years, there has been a growing list of small series and single case reports of calcified

TABLE 4–3. CALCIFICATIONS AND OTHER DENSITIES IN THE STOMACH

Mural calcification
  Carcinoma of the stomach
  Gastric leiomyoma
  Hemangioma
  Calcified duplication cyst
Intraluminal densities
  Foreign bodies
  Undissolved pills
  Gallstone migration
  Oral bismuth preparations

gastric malignancy. It is striking how similar all the cases appear. On plain films, the gastric air shadow is narrowed and a large infiltrating mass is suggested by numerous homogeneously punctate or granular calcifications that are most often faintly opaque (Fig 4–30). Sometimes, the calcifications may be so closely spaced that they give a hazy, poorly defined pattern of opacity, but individual densities can usually be recognized.[23] Calcification in adenocarcinoma of the stomach is seldom flocculent or streaky, a diagnostic point that serves to differentiate it from the less commonly observed calcified gastric leiomyoma.

Calcified gastric carcinoma, also known as petrified stomach, is almost always a large lesion when discovered on X-ray.[24,25] Behaving no differently from other bulky stomach carcinomas, it often metastasizes to the liver, but calcification in hepatic de-

posits is extremely rare. Although initial reports suggested that calcified tumors appear in younger individuals, later series have indicated that the age of onset is roughly the same as that of gastric adenocarcinomas in general.[26,29] The cause of calcification is still a matter of conjecture. On microscopic section, calcium salts are extracellular and are usually found in necrotic sections of the tumor. According to Gemmell, areas of ischemia are associated with a diminution of cellular respiration and an increase in carbon dioxide concentration and alkalinity.[30] Dystrophic calcification occurs in the petrified stomach supposedly because the tumor has outgrown its blood supply.[31] Hence, in the well-vascularized stomach, calcification does not occur until the tumor becomes large. This theory fails, however, to account for the fact that most large gastric carcinomas may grow rapidly and contain areas of necrosis and yet fail to calcify.

Batlan[32] and Khilnani,[33] noting that calcification occurs only in mucin-producing tumors, offer a different explanation. They claim that mucin, a glycoprotein with a special avidity for calcium, has a chemical composition similar to the cartilage in the provisional zone of calcification at the epiphysis of a growing bone. This is an intriguing but still unsubstantiated theory that fails to explain why only some tumors concentrate calcium in sufficient amounts to be seen on a plain film of the abdomen.

Leiomyoma of the stomach is a common neo-

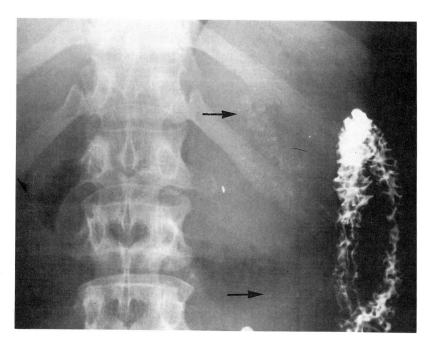

Figure 4–30. Calcified adenocarcinoma of the stomach. The arrows point to two areas with mottled calcification within the tumor. Almost the whole stomach is infiltrated with carcinoma. (*Courtesy of Dr. D. Randall Radin.*)

plasm that can vary in size from an insignificant wall lesion to a huge, mostly exophytic mass, larger than the stomach itself. Although microscopic calcification is often found in gastric leiomyomata, roentgenographically visible opacities are exceedingly uncommon. In fact, only a few cases have been reported. There is usually insufficient calcium in these tumors for plain film detection, but more sensitive imaging techniques such as computed tomography may reveal a closer correlation between pathological and radiological findings. Unlike carcinoma of the stomach, leiomyoma calcification tends to be mottled, coarse, and dense, with irregular streaks and clumps. The calcifications can project away from the gastric lumen (Fig 4–31) or appear within the gastric margin as a smooth, bulky tumor (Fig 4–32).

It is not always possible to distinguish carcinoma from leiomyoma by the pattern of calcification. Calcification in leiomyoma can be simulated by radiodense solid lesions in the left adrenal or left kidney or spleen. In some cases, the calcification

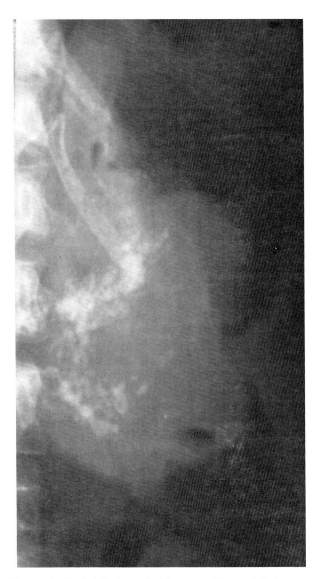

Figure 4–32. Calcified gastric leiomyoma. This calcified tumor stretches, indents, and nearly obstructs the stomach.

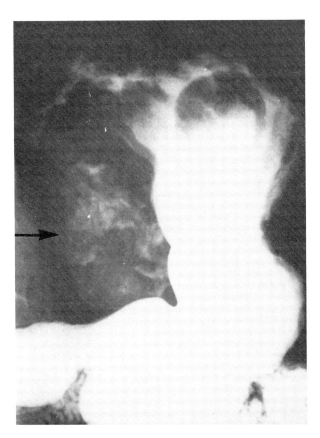

Figure 4–31. Exogastric calcified leiomyoma of the stomach. A film from an upper gastrointestinal series show a large exophytic mass with dense clumps of calcification (*arrow*).

extends far from the stomach.[34–37] For example, a gastric leiomyoma presenting as a calcified mediastinal mass has been reported.[38]

Other calcifying gastric tumors arising from the stomach are rare. Milk of calcium in a duplication cyst arising from the upper lesser curvature of the stomach has been observed (Fig 4–33). Phlebolithic calcification has been noted in hemangiomas of the stomach, although the presence of radiopaque phleboliths in this tumor is very infrequent.[39] In a series of 26 cases of hemangioma of the stomach, only one example of a mass with calcified phleboliths was recognized on plain films.[40]

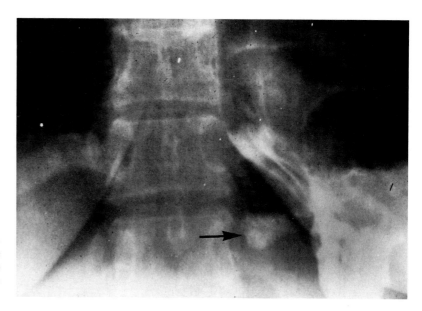

Figure 4–33. Upright film during an upper gastrointestinal series. Milk of calcium in a gastric duplication cyst (*arrow*). A level demarcating the boundary between the calcified contents in the cyst and radiolucent fluid is seen.

Intraluminal Opacities

Calcified concretions are formed and remain opaque in an alkaline environment. Hence, the acid contents of the lumen of the stomach do not favor calcium deposition. Thus, opaque gastric calculi forming de novo do not occur here. Bezoars are not radiodense and will be seen on plain films only if they are coated by an opaque material or outlined by air.[41]

Although calcified gallstones may pass in a retrograde fashion through the pyloric sphincter, almost all discrete intraluminal opacities in the stomach represent ingested substances.[42] Pills are the most frequently observed radiopaque objects in the stomach. To be recognized in the stomach, a pill must be both radiodense and remain undissolved. Most medications opaque enough to be seen on plain films either pass through the stomach quickly or break apart and enter into solution in the gastric lumen. In general, for an intragastric density to be visualized, an abdominal film must be taken soon after the ingestion of the substance (Fig 4–34). Occasionally, however, some pills resist dissolution and remain intact in the stomach. In particular, iron-containing medications can be seen as well-defined densities within the stomach lumen (Fig 4–10).[43] Often other iron pills that have passed beyond the stomach into the small intestine will also be observed on the same radiograph (Fig 4–35).

If ingested in large quantities, bismuth preparations in the stomach may be detected on plain films. They coat particulate material in the lumen and appear as numerous amorphous opacities within the contents of the gastric margins. At times,

bismuth preparations simulate the pattern of opacity of a calcified carcinoma of the stomach (Fig. 4–36). Bismuth disappears with peristalsis or gastric drainage, however, and it usually changes its configuration on upright, decubitis, or prone views or on successive supine radiographs. Hence, a repeat abdominal film may be the most informative study in the differentiation of intraluminal from intramural gastric opacities.

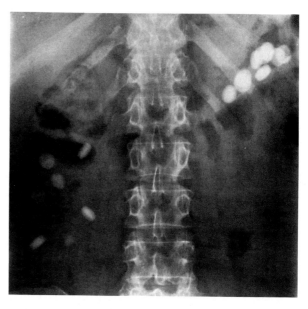

Figure 4–34. Dense pills in the stomach and colon. This patient was known to be a frequent consumer of iron-containing vitamin tablets.

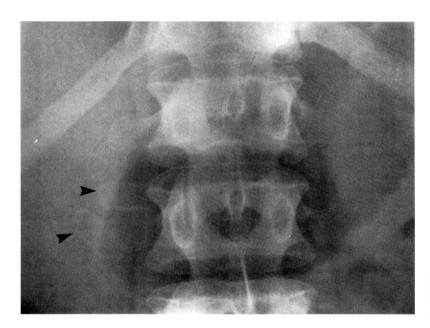

Figure 4–35. Capsules with radiopaque margins in the distal antrum (*arrowheads*). This film was obtained moments after the capsules were swallowed.

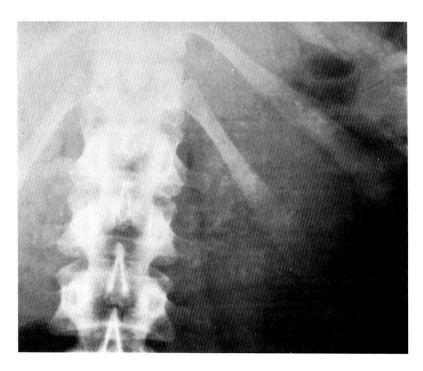

Figure 4–36. Scattered densities of recently ingested Bismuth subsalicylate in the stomach resemble diffuse calcification in a tumor.

PROXIMAL DUODENUM

Air in the duodenum bulb has many appearances, almost all of which are variants of normal. A small, rounded lucency to the right of the midline in the upper abdomen is the usual appearance of air in a nearly empty bulb. As the first portion of the duodenum fills with air, its margins become more angulated, typically assuming a triangular shape. Most often, a three-sided bulb is seen in individuals with an air-filled J-shaped stomach. In more horizontally oriented stomachs, the classical geometric configuration is less common. The bulb is apt to be situated dorsal rather than superior to the antrum, and on supine views its long axis is oblique to the radiographic beam. In such individuals, the acute angulation of both the pylorus and the immediately distal descending duodenum further modifies its contours, even causing apparent filling defects to appear within its lucent shadow.

Prolapse of gastric mucosa is a well-recognized phenomenon of little clinical significance. Occasionally, it can be recognized on plain films if the bulb distends with air. At times, transient intrusion of the pylorus becomes very marked and resembles a nodular mass surrounded by duodenal air (Fig 4–37). The pylorus itself may be outlined within the bulb in patients with transversely oriented stomachs. Less frequently, the proximal portion of the second part of the duodenum can project upwards in a capacious air-filled bulb (Fig 4–38).

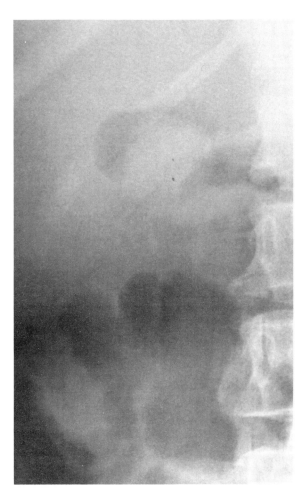

Figure 4–38. The proximal descending duodenum projects as a filling defect within a large but otherwise normal duodenal bulb.

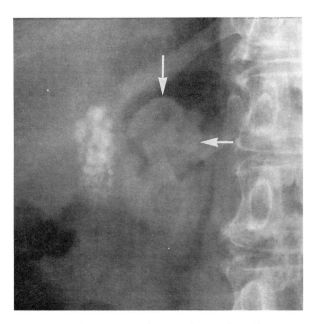

Figure 4–37. The arrows point to prolapse of gastric mucosa within a large duodenal bulb. Numerous opaque calculi are present in the gallbladder.

The plain film recognition of an active ulcer crater of the proximal duodenum is distinctly uncommon but secondary effects of ulcer disease may be seen. Nodularity of the bulb wall can represent scarring of the mucosa or hyperplasia of Brunner's glands, both of which are sequelae of peptic disease (Fig 4–39). Almost always, "bumps" in the bulb are either these postulcer changes or merely evanescent indentations consequent to peristalsis. Rarely, a persistent defect may indicate intraluminal extension of a neoplasm of the duodenum or adjacent structures (Fig 4–40). Unlike gastric ulcers, in which giant craters filled with gas or barium are well-recognized findings, benign postbulbar ulcers are identified on barium studies by their cicatrizing effect rather than by their excavation beyond the lumen. The plain film observation of a rounded lucency closely associated and medial to the bulb accompanied by deformity and narrowing of the duodenal lumen should suggest infiltration of the bowel wall by a

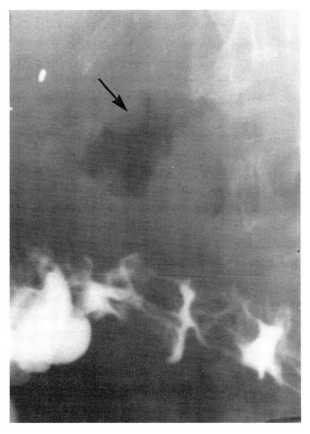

Figure 4–39. Brunner gland hyperplasia, confirmed at biopsy (*arrow*), producing nodular indentations on the air-filled bulb.

biliary, pancreatic, or other retroperitoneal malignancy (Fig 4–41).

The upper limit of the duodenal bulb is approximately 3.5 cm across its base and 4 cm from base to apex. The bulb may distend in paralytic and obstructive conditions that dilate other segments of the small intestine as well. More often, megabulbus is related to focal conditions that narrow the immediate postbulbar area.[44,45] The differential diagnosis of a large bulb in infants and young children is extensive, including all congenital obstructions that distend the proximal duodenum and the stomach, producing the "double-bubble" sign. In adults, megabulbus is limited to relatively few acquired diseases, the most common being benign postbulbar ulceration. Much less frequently, benign or malignant tumors can present with this finding.

The location of the bulb also has considerable variation. In most cases, it is positioned just to the right of the spine, but in a patient with repeated gastric dilatation, the bulb may be displaced from its initial location, migrating far laterally, sometimes even peripheral to the right kidney. The pseudotumor phenomenon of the stomach seen in the left upper quadrant in individuals with a horizontal gastric orientation has a duodenal bulb analogue in the right upper quadrant.[46] A fluid-filled laterally positioned bulb outlined by retroperitoneal fat can mimic a distended gallbladder projecting from the liver edge (Fig 4–42).

Duodenal Diverticula

Duodenal diverticula are very common, demonstrated in 20% of the population at autopsy and in

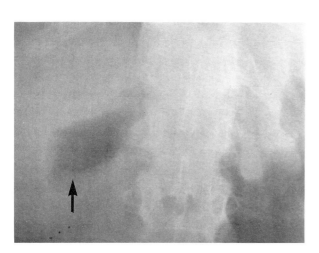

Figure 4–40. Metastatic leiomyosarcoma to the duodenal bulb. The small nodular density projecting into the inferior aspect of the bulb (*arrow*) was one of several tumor deposits in the duodenum and the pancreas.

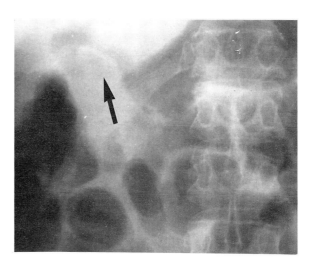

Figure 4–41. Post–bulbar ulcer due to malignancy. The duodenal bulb is narrowed and stretched around a large but faint lucency (*arrow*) that proved to be a post–bulbar ulcer within a lymphomatous mass extending to the wall of the bulb.

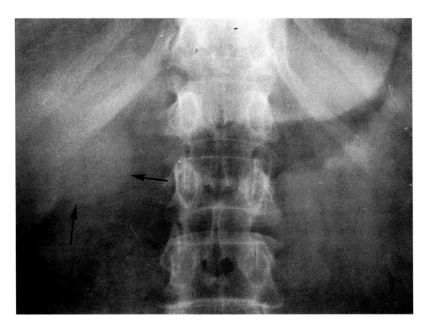

Figure 4–42. The arrows outline a fluid-filled duodenal bulb. Its superior margin overlies the lower margins of the liver.

1% to 5% of patients undergoing upper GI roentgenographic series. They are found in the second and third portion of the duodenum in 80% of cases, but they may occur anywhere from the bulb to the ligament of Treitz.[47] Although the overwhelming majority of duodenal diverticula are less than 2 cm in diameter and clinically insignificant, a small percentage may bleed, become infected, or even block the common bile duct and the main pancreatic duct. Most are unseen on plain films, but lateral and posterior duodenal diverticula have a tendency to attain a large size.[48] When filled with air, they appear on supine films as a homogeneous lucency lacking internal markings. Duodenal diverticula can simulate a distended bulb, but their typically rounded or oval configuration is an unusual shape for a megabulbus (Fig 4–43). Gas-containing abscesses in the liver, pancreas, or right kidney are filled with fluid as well as gas and, therefore, are not as lucent as an almost purely air-containing duodenal diverticulum. Gas in Morison's pouch is limited superiolaterally by the 11th rib and often has a triangular contour (Fig 4–44). A duodenal diverticulum may be mistaken for air in the gallbladder on plain radiographs. As infection in the gallbladder proceeds, however, luminal air is often accompanied by a thin lucent stripe in the gallbladder wall (Fig 2–47). Duodenal diverticula, on the other hand, have a relatively constant appearance on a successive films (Fig 4–45). In elderly and emaciated patients, lucent pockets between skin folds can be confused with the large, featureless gas shadow of a duodenal diverticulum. Skin folds often have bizarre configurations without sharp demarcations in all sections of their perimeter. Also mimicking a duodenal diverticulum is a giant diverticulum of the transverse colon and the lucent blind pouches occasionally seen after side-to-side intestinal anastomoses.[49] A very large diverticulum situated at the juncture of the second and third portions of the duodenum can even resemble a dilated cecum.

Duodenal diverticula can perforate and become infected. Lucent streaks adjacent to the diverticular cavity indicate penetration into the retroperitoneal space[50] and numerous small bubbles close to the diverticular cavity suggest a gas-containing abscess (Fig 4–46).[51,52]

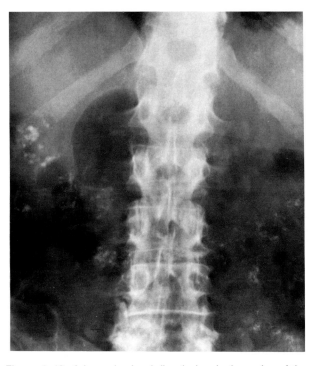

Figure 4–43. A large duodenal diverticulum in the region of the duodenal bulb. Its rounded configuration and unchanging size on successive film help differentiate it from a megabulbus.

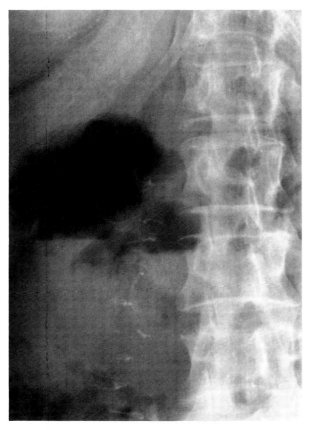

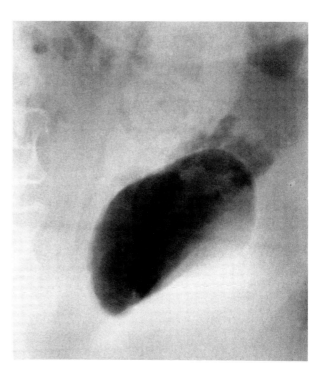

Figure 4–45. A huge duodenal diverticulum mimics emphysematous cholecystitis.

Figure 4–44. Upright film shows air and fluid in a duodenal diverticulum superiorlateral to the bulb. It simulates gas in Morison's pouch.

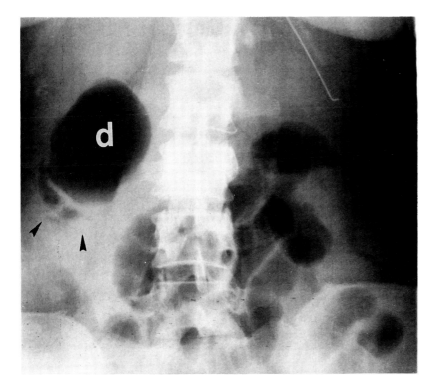

Figure 4–46. Infected, perforated duodenal diverticulum: The diverticulum (d) is filled with air. The smaller gas pockets (*arrowheads*) represent air in abscesses adjacent to the diverticulum. (*Courtesy of Dr. Stanford Goldman. Reprinted with the permission of the* American Journal of Roentgenology.)

REFERENCES

1. Berk RN, Coulson DB. The body cast syndrome. *Radiology.* 1970;94:303–305.
2. Wallace RG, Howard WB. Acute superior mesenteric artery syndrome in the severely burned patient. *Radiology.* 1970;94:307–310.
3. Gondos B. Duodenal compression defect and the "superior mesenteric artery syndrome." *Radiology.* 1977; 123:575–580.
4. Mindell HJ, Holm JL. Acute superior mesenteric artery syndrome. *Radiology.* 1970;94:299–302.
5. Chin WS. Interstitial gastric and duodenal emphysema. *J Can Assoc Radiol.* 1978;29:136–137.
6. Meyers HI, Parker JJ. Emphysematous gastritis. *Radiology.* 1967;89:426–431.
7. Martin DF, Hartley G. Gastric emphysema demonstrated by computed tomography. *Br J Radiol.* 1986; 59:505–507.
8. Bernardino ME, Lawson TL. Emphysematous gastritis and gastric perforation: An unusual manifestation of alkaline corrosive ingestion. *Gastrointest Radiol.* 1977;2:107–108.
9. Kinkhabwala MN, Conradi H, Farman J, et al. Acute emphysematous gastritis. The significance of the angiographic findings. *Radiology.* 1973;109:553–554.
10. Dassel PM. Roentgen demonstration of gangrene of the stomach and intestine. A late finding in infarction of the gastrointestinal tract. *Am J Roentgenol.* 1964; 91:819–825.
11. Isdale JM. Interstitial emphysema of the stomach. *Br J Radiol.* 1970;43:141–148.
12. Levitt R, Stanley RJ, Wise L. Gastric bullae. *Radiology.* 1975;115:597–598.
13. Berens SV, Moskowitz H, Mellins HZ. Air within the wall of the stomach. Roentgen manifestations and a new roentgenographic sign. *Am J Roentgenol.* 1968; 103:310–313.
14. Seaman WB, Fleming RJ. Intramural gastric emphysema. *Am J Roentgenol.* 1967;101:431–435.
15. Schorr S, Marcus M. Intramural gastric emphysema. *Br J Radiol.* 1962;35:641–644.
16. Cancelmo JJ. Interstitial gastric emphysema with report of a case. *Radiology.* 1954;63:81–83.
17. Fierst SM, Robinson HM, Lasagna L. Interstitial gastric emphysema following gastroscopy; its relation to the syndrome of generalized emphysema with no evident perforation. *Ann Intern Med.* 1951;34:1202–1212.
18. Ward PR. Interstitial gastric emphysema. *Br J Radiol.* 1961;33:458–459.
19. Lumsden D. Radiologic demonstration of gas in stomach wall. *Br J Radiol.* 1956;29:596–600.
20. Kay-Butler JJ. Case of interstitial gastric emphysema. *Br J Surg.* 1962;50:99–101.
21. Plachta A, Speer FD. Nonbacterial gastric emphysema: Review of literature and report of a case. *Gastroenterology.* 1961;40:248–252.
22. Colguhom J. Intramural gas in hollow viscera. *Clin. Radiol.* 1965;16:71–86.
23. Bloch C, Peck HM. Calcification in gastrointestinal malignancy: An important clue in radiologic diagnosis. Mt Sinai J Med. 1971;38:405–416.
24. Myo Lwin TO, Soodeen TH. A case report on calcified mucinous adenocarcinoma of the stomach. *J Can Assoc Radiol.* 1973;24:370–373.
25. Ghahremani GG, Meyers MA, Port, R.B. et al. Calcified primary tumors of the gastrointestinal tract. *Gastrointest Radiol.* 1978;2:331–339.
26. Kendig TA, Gaspar MD, Secrest PG. Calcification in gastric carcinoma: Case report. *Radiology.* 1957;68;80–82.
27. Hermann G, Rozin R. Calcification in gastro-intestinal carcinomata. *Clin Radiol.* 1964;15:139–141.
28. Balthazar E, Rosenthal M. Calcifying mucin producing adenocarcinoma of the stomach. *NY State J Med.* 1973;73:2704–2706.
29. Thomas RL, Rice RP. Calcifying mucinous adenocarcinoma of the stomach. *Radiology.* 1967;88:1002–1003.
30. Gemmell NI. Calcification within a gastric carcinoma. *Am J Roentgenol.* 1964;91:779–783.
31. Robertson JW, Osterhout S. Calcification in scirrhous carcinoma of the stomach. *Am J Surg.* 1952;83:830–832.
32. Batlan LE. Calcifications within the stomach wall in gastric malignancy. *Am J Roentgenol.* 1954;72:788–794.
33. Khilnani MT. Calcifying mucous-cell carcinoma of the stomach. *Am J Dig Dis.* 1960;5:479–483.
34. Leigh TF. Calcified gastric leiomyoma: Report of case. *Radiology.* 1950;55:419–422.
35. Garbarini J, Price HP. Calcified leiomyoma of the stomach. *N Engl J Med.* 1950;243:405–407.
36. Crummy AB Jr, Juhl JH. Calcified gastric leiomyoma. *Am J Roentgenol.* 1962;87:727–728.
37. Koloski EL, Shallenberger PL, Hawk AW. Large partially calcified gastric leiomyoma. *Am J Surg.* 1950; 80:245–248.
38. Graham JC Jr, Blanchard IT, Scatliff JH. Calcified gastric leiomyoma presenting as a mediastinal mass. *Am J Roentgenol.* 1972; 114:529–531.
39. Kerekes ES. Gastric hemangioma: A case report. *Radiology.* 1964;82:468–469.
40. Flannery MG, Caster MP. Hemangioma of the stomach with a roentgenologic diagnostic point. *Am J Roentgenol.* 1957;77:38–40.
41. Canlas EM, Fildes CE. Radiopaque phytobezoar: A case report. *Radiology.* 1953;60:261–264.
42. Afflerbaugh JK, Cole HA. Intragastric gallstone. *Radiology.* 1955;64:581–583.
43. Staple TW, McAlister WH. Roentgenographic visualization of iron preparations in the gastrointestinal tract. *Radiology.* 1964;83:1051–1056.
44. Evison G. Unusual presentation of a megabulbus. *Br J Radiol.* 1969;42:64–65.
45. Fischer HW. The big duodenum. *Am J Roentgenol.* 1960;83;861–873.
46. Balthazar E. Right Upper quadrant pseudotumor, a fluid filled viscus. *Radiology.* 1974;112;11–12.
47. Lukes PJ, Rolny P, Nilson AE. Clinical significance of

duodenal diverticula and value of hypotomic duode-nography. *Acta Radiol* (Diagn). 1979;20:93–99.

48. Millard JR, Ziter FMH Jr, Slover WP. Giant duodenal diverticula. *Am J Roentgenol.* 1974;121:334–337.
49. LeVine M, Katz I, Lampros PJ. Blind pouch formation secondary to side-to-side intestinal anastomosis. *Am J Roentgenol* 1963;89:706–719.
50. Wolfe RD, Peral MJ. Acute perforation of duodenal diverticulum with roentgenographic demonstration of localized retroperitoneal emphysema. *Radiology.* 1972; 104:301–302.
51. Beachley MC, Lankau CA Jr. Inflamed duodenal diverticulum, preoperative radiographic diagnosis. *Am J Dig Dis.* 1977;22:149–154.
52. Glasser CM, Goldman, SM, Pio Roda CL, et al. Preoperative Diagnosis of a Perforated Duodenal Diverticulum. *Am J Roentgenol.* 1978;130:563–564.

CHAPTER FIVE

Plain Film Radiology of the Intestines and Appendix

SMALL BOWEL OBSTRUCTION

The normal small intestine may be entirely gas free, but scattered lucent collections are often seen within the duodenum, jejunum, and ileum, resulting from the swallowing of air or, to a lesser degree, from the liberation of carbon dioxide in the stomach by the neutralization of hydrochloric acid.[1-3] The absorptive capacity of the bowel is so great that even massive ingestions fail to distend an unobstructed lumen persistently.[4] These gaseous agglomerations are generally nondescript, appearing as rounded or amorphous foci of decreased density. A quite different roentgenographic pattern characterizes small intestinal obstruction. Luminal blockage eventuates in the proximal accumulation of succus entericus and gas as the obstructed bowel is less able to resorb fluid. The intestine dilates and peristalsis becomes more strenuous in a heightened effort to propel bowel contents distally. Hypertonic contractions of the muscularis mucosa within the valvulae conniventes thickens these encircling indentations.[5] The hallmark of small-bowel obstruction is the demonstration of adjacent or continuous loops, each of which are distended and contain prominent valvulae that stand out in contrast to the air-filled lumen (Fig 5–1).

The arrangement of these tubular lucencies depends upon the site, duration, and completeness of obstruction and the relative proportions of liquid and gas within each segment of occluded bowel. The more proximal the blockage, the fewer the number of loops available for distension. Hence, obstruction within the first few feet of the jejunum may go unnoticed on plain films whereas ileal obstruction usually is recognized on the basis of extensive small bowel dilatation (Fig 5–2). Since gas does not accumulate instantaneously, the longer the period of obstruction, the greater the likelihood of observing proximal dilatation. Even this rule requires modifi-

cation, however, if the obstruction is incomplete or intermittent, allowing for partial decompression of the bowel.[6] Swallowing of air is not inevitable in obstruction. Stoic individuals tend to ingest little air and abdominal radiographs may reveal a gasless abdomen even if their obstruction is complete and prolonged. In others, pain, crying, a sense of apprehension, and even a lack of teeth promote the swallowing of air that then occupies and distends numerous small intestinal loops.[2,5] Poor posture plays a role, too, as excessive gas in the stomach lumen may not be expelled through the esophagus as easily as it can pass distally into the small intestine. The volume of small bowel air is constantly changing. Ingested oxygen and carbon dioxide are rapidly resorbed, requiring continuous replenishment by swallowing. At the same time, gas can be withdrawn through nasogastric suction and by vomiting. Such a complex interplay of competing influences on jejunal and ileal gas accumulation is an inherent limitation of the plain film, reducing its efficacy for the detection of obstruction of the small bowel.

Another factor that confounds plain film assessment of small bowel obstruction is the variable quantity of flatus in the large intestine. A moderate volume of colonic gas, identified by haustral outpouchings and intervening septa, is a normal finding. It may occupy much of the lumen but in the supine position tends to collect in the transverse and sigmoid colons, the least dependent large intestinal segments. Obstruction of the small intestine does not necessarily mean the total and immediate disappearance of distal gas, as it usually takes 1 to 2 days for the colon to empty after the onset of small-intestinal occlusion. Hence, the persistence of large-bowel gas is an expected observation early in the course of a more proximal obstruction. Incomplete blockage also permits ingested air to pass distally (Figs 5–2B, 5–3). Even after total occlusion, the fer-

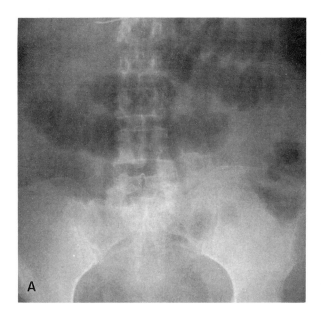
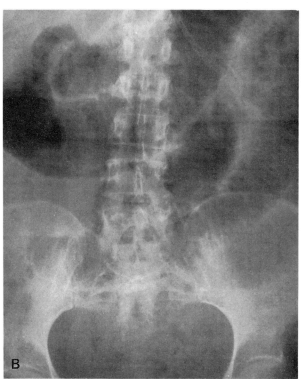

Figure 5–1. Two examples of uncomplicated small bowel obstruction. **A.** Ileal obstruction due to a congenital band. Dilated small bowel loops in the mid abdomen are identified by the vertically oriented valvulae conniventes. Little gas remains in the colon. **B.** Distal jejunal obstruction caused by a postoperative adhesion. Even the most dilated loops reveal the regular impressions of valvulae.

mentation of residual fecal matter may continue for a while, resulting in the sustained production of colonic gas. In the course of the clinical evaluation of obstruction, gas may be introduced into the colon in a retrograde fashion via a sigmoidoscope, colonoscope, or enema tip.

In approximately one fourth of patients with large bowel obstruction, an incompetent ileocecal valve decompresses the colon and an inflow of flatus distends the distal small bowel. Hence, what appears to be an ileal blockage may, in fact, be a colonic occlusion (Fig 5–4).[7,8] Furthermore, mechanical occlusion can be mimicked by a diverse group of conditions—including adjacent inflammation[9] and mesenteric ischemia[10]—in which no luminal blockage occurs but functional obstruction exists because of a focal paralysis of bowel.

Faced with the limitations imposed by the lack of sensitivity and specificity of the patterns of small bowel obstruction, it is understandable why the diagnosis cannot be made with certainty in every case. The probability of a correct diagnosis by plain films alone varies from 55%[11] to 80%, with a roughly equal likelihood of false-positive and false-negative interpretations.[12] Accuracy can be increased by at-

tention to subtle signs of gas accumulation and distribution and by close coordination between the radiologist and referring physician. Nonetheless, there will always be a significant minority of cases in which the plain film is misleading or unhelpful.

Proximal Small Bowel Obstruction

The principles of interpretation of small bowel obstruction can be applied to luminal blockage at any level. The appearances of proximal and distal occlusion are often so dissimilar, however, that they must be considered separately. Obstruction of the proximal jejunum frequently goes undetected on plain films, as the diagnosis rests exclusively on the visualization of one or two air-filled loops. Evacuation of gas by vomiting or by placement of a tube into the stomach or duodenum often removes such telltale lucencies. Moreover, even if gas-filled jejunal loops are observed, they are usually not markedly dilated.[5] In almost every case, the valvulae are evident but this sign is not specific as it can be present with air swallowing (Figs 2–6, 5–5) and in the atonic sentinel loop of proximal bowel sometimes seen in acute pancreatitis (Figs 5–6, 7–4A) and other upper abdominal inflammations. Although the plain film

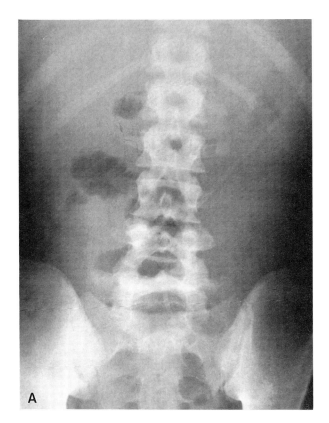
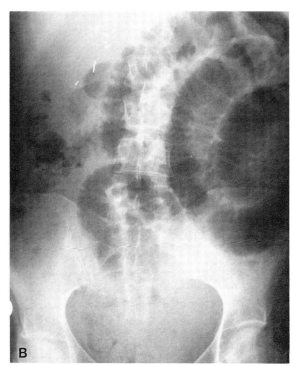

Figure 5–2. A. Proximal jejunal obstruction. Only a single slightly dilated air-filled loop suggests the diagnosis. **B.** Distal ileal obstruction. Many dilated small bowel loops are seen, each with prominent valvulae conniventes.

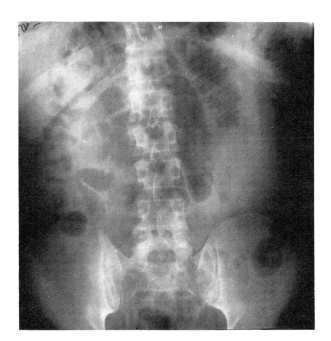

Figure 5–3. Small bowel obstruction. Central dilated small bowel loops proximal to the obstruction. Gas is also present in the non-dilated ascending, transverse, and sigmoid colon.

signs of proximal obstruction are meager and not pathognomonic, in the appropriate clinical context even one dilated small-bowel loop should be regarded with suspicion (Fig 5–7).

Distal Small Bowel Obstruction

As more loops become air-filled the radiographic distinctiveness of mechanical obstruction, air swallowing, and adynamic ileus become more obvious. Meteorism, the rapid ingestion of air, deposits a large volume of gas within non-obstructed bowel. The prompt resorption of gas prevents dilatation, and the valvulae in the distal jejunum and ileum do not thicken as the intestinal wall is not placed under increased pressure. The bowel lumen appears as continuous rounded or polyhedral-shaped lucencies and the pattern of gas distribution can change rapidly, even on two films taken several minutes apart (Figs 2–6B,5–8).[2,5] In the upper abdomen a focal ileus, evidenced by the appearance of a sentinel loop, seldom affects more than one or two small intestinal segments. Yet, a focal ileus in the lower small bowel may be radiologically akin to a mechanical obstruction in the same location, as air swallowing and bowel dilatation can involve many proximal loops.

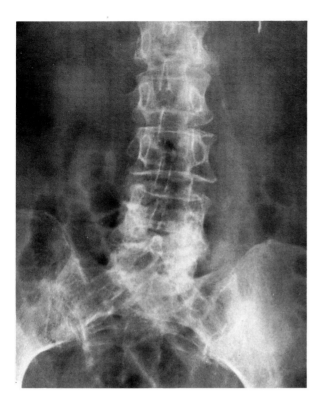

Figure 5–4. Cecal tumor. The only plain film manifestation is dilated ileal loops. The cecum was decompressed because the ileocecal valve was incompetent, allowing retrograde flow of gas into the distal small intestine.

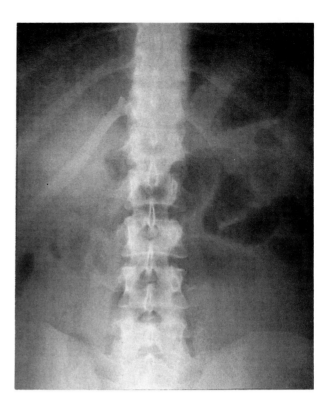

Figure 5–6. Jejunal obstruction. The roentgenographic pattern is also suggestive of a sentinel loop secondary to pancreatic inflammation.

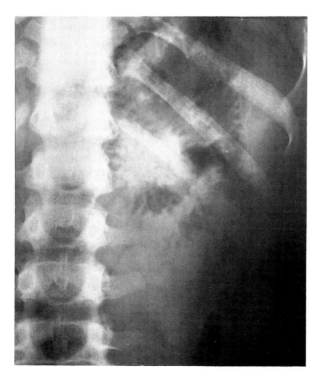

Figure 5–5. Air swallowing. A preliminary film before a barium enema examination. The proximal jejunal loops are air-filled but not dilated. The valvulae conniventes stand out clearly.

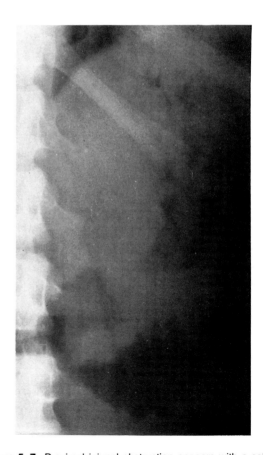

Figure 5–7. Proximal jejunal obstruction appears with a solitary dilated air-filled loop.

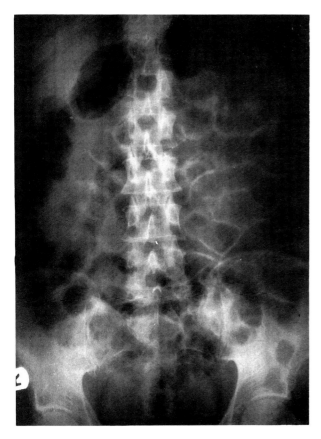

Figure 5–8. Air swallowing in an anxious patient. Numerous segments of small bowel contain air, but the lumen is not widened and valvular indentations are not evident.

Moreover, in obese patients in whom the obstruction is caused by adhesions or herniation at the ventral abdominal wall, several intestinal loops can relocate far anteriorly. The displaced bowel may appear to have a widened caliber on supine views solely because of the magnification effect of structures located relatively close to the source of the roentgenographic beam (Fig 5–10).

The majority of ileal and distal jejunal obstructions occur in the pelvis, and the site of blockage, whether caused by tumor or an adhesive band, is seldom observed on plain films. Occasionally, however, an elongated stenotic segment contains enough gas to be seen amidst adjacent dilated loops (Fig 5–11). In the absence of a conspicuous deformity or narrowed bowel, it is hazardous to suggest the exact point of obstruction based upon the distribution of gas-filled bowel loops, as many feet of completely fluid-filled intestine are often interposed proximal to the site of blockage but distal to the visualized gas-filled segments.[13]

It is customary for some radiologists to comment on the temporal course of a small intestinal occlusion as defined by information discerned on the plain film. The designation of "early obstruction" is proffered at times when gas and feces are still present in a nondistended large bowel. In fact, the duration of a small bowel obstruction cannot be

A generalized adynamic ileus usually affects the small and large intestines together, with both distending and often filling with air as flaccidity becomes the muscular response of the bowel wall. In the jejunum and ileum, the atonic valvulae efface and each retracts toward the bowel wall, making a relatively short impression on luminal contour.

The archetypical appearance of distal small bowel obstruction consists of multiple dilated loops of bowel, all bearing the "signature" of small bowel, unaccompanied by colonic lucencies (Fig 2–7).[13] In actuality, some large intestinal gas usually remains but there is a discrepancy in the degree of intestinal distension proximal and distal to the point of obstruction (Fig 5–9). Valvulae conniventes can be seen in all dilated air-filled segments, although they are less prominent in the distal ileum where these mucosal protuberances are more widely spaced. Obstructed small bowel segments rarely exceed 5 cm in diameter, but, in long-standing blockage, muscular fatigue or superimposed adynamic ileus may develop, allowing small bowel to distend to such a degree that it may be mistaken for colonic dilatation.

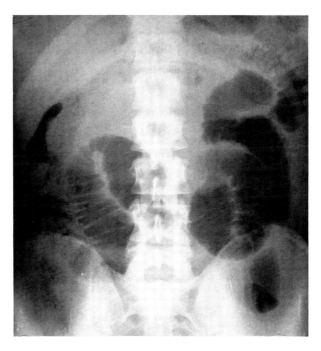

Figure 5–9. Distal ileal obstruction in a patient with colonic obstipation. Best seen in the right colon and splenic flexure, the large intestine is feces-filled, but not occluded. The ileum is blocked by an adhesion and proximal loops are air-filled and distended.

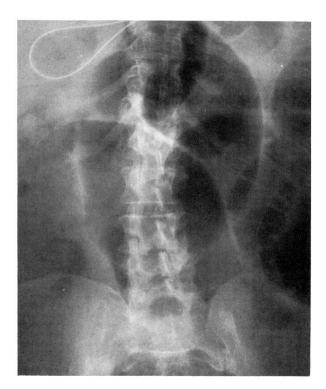

Figure 5–10. Markedly dilated and obstructed small bowel loops. The widening of the central loops reflects the magnification effect caused by fixation of the ileum at the anterior abdominal wall.

determined on a single abdominal film without corroborating clinical data. For example, an incomplete luminal occlusion is often associated with the accumulation of colonic gas and may look exactly like a so-called early obstruction. The notion of partial blockage has also gained wide currency. Yet, what may be considered an unremitting but incomplete narrowing may just as well be an intermittent obstruction distinguished by alternating intervals of total blockage and luminal patency. The essential fact to report is that an obstruction exists. Further information about the degree of bowel narrowing and its persistence over time requires additional radiological studies, including follow-up plain films or barium contrast studies as well as continual monitoring of the patient's signs and symptoms.

Reliance on the demonstration of fluid levels on upright or decubitus projections is also a part of radiology lore. The clinical value of these additional views has been questioned by several investigators, however. Intestinal fluid levels per se do not indicate disease.[2,5,13] Donahue et al observed gas–liquid interfaces in bowel on erect films of normal, postpartum women, at the moment they experienced abdominal pain after having taken a cathartic medication several hours earlier in the day.[14] Gammill and Nice noted fluid levels in healthy individuals

who had no intestinal abnormalities or recent bowel preparation.[15] In most instances, fluid and gas were confined to the colon. They regarded the presence of two or more small bowel fluid levels as a sign of luminal stasis but were unable to use this finding to differentiate between adynamic ileus and mechanical obstruction (Fig 5–12).[15] In both conditions, fluid is retained and the bowel distends because of failure of transport across the intestinal wall.

The seminal work of Frimann-Dahl popularized the clinical pertinence of fluid levels.[16] He maintained that in obstruction the tense loops proximal to the point of blockage become arrayed as a series of inverted "U"s, with many containing short fluid levels that could be seen on upright films. Often, a single loop could have differing fluid heights in its two limbs, a reflection of the enhanced peristalsis secondary to obstruction. On the other hand, in adynamic ileus, whatever its cause, motor activity is diminished, individual loops are longer, and the fluid interface is wider. Also, Frimann-Dahl suggested that the differential level sign should not be seen in ileus because passive mixing of liquid and gas in a hypotonic intestine results in an equilibration of fluid heights.

These observations were made during continuous fluoroscopic evaluation of bowel patterns. They have not been borne out in careful studies using

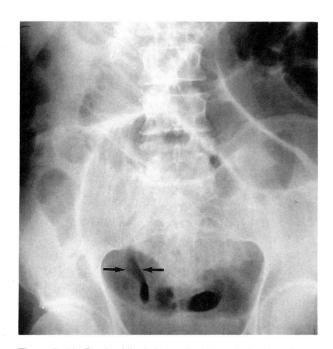

Figure 5–11. Proximal ileal obstruction due to ischemic stricture. Fortuitously, the narrowed intestinal segment is partially air-filled and can be seen on this plain film (*arrow*).

In cases in which the gas pattern is inconclusive, a valuable, supplementary view is a repeat radiograph taken minutes to several hours after the initial film. Bryk has demonstrated that successive supine films obtained in conjunction with close monitoring of physical findings can help clarify the presence and evolution of an intestinal blockage with minimal discomfort to the patient.[17]

In some patients, gas is not the predominant intraluminal fluid and succus entericus and ingested liquids occupy much of the dilated segments. The remaining scant gas appears as black slits sandwiched between hypertrophied valvulae. The "stretch sign" consisting of parallel straight radiolucencies perpendicular to the long axis of bowel is pathognomonic of fluid-filled small intestine with prominent valvulae (Figs 2–10,5–13). When even less gas is present the "stretch sign" is not seen, as the residual lucencies may be reduced to small bubbles, each trapped beneath a single valvula. Often hidden from view on supine films, they may be observed on horizontal beam projections as a chain of black circles oriented along the course of the bowel. The "string of pearls" sign has been noted in adynamic ileus, gastroenteritis, and after the ingestion of cathartic medications.[5,13] It is, however, almost always indicative of intestinal obstruction and is one of the few situations in which an upright or decubitus film of the abdomen contributes crucial information about small bowel obstruction (Figs 1–12, 5–14).

Strangulated Obstruction

A gasless abdomen may be a normal finding in an individual habituated to avoid swallowing gas. It can be seen in mesenteric ischemia, obstruction of the stomach or esophagus, and in any condition associated with severe persistent vomiting, including pancreatitis and gastroenteritis.[5] In small bowel obstruction, a gasless abdomen is an uncommon presentation. Williams found such a pattern in only 18 of 300 patients with mechanical blockage of the small bowel. One third of these had gas demonstrated on erect or decubitus views. Of the 18 with gasless abdomens, 12 had an uncomplicated bowel occlusion and the other six had a strangulated intestinal obstruction.[18] The urgent need for treatment of vascular compromise makes strangulated bowel occlusion a disease that mandates identification without delay. Frequently the lack of specific findings hinders plain film recognition, however. Rarely, a closed loop obstruction may remain distended, with air appearing as featureless lucencies that can mimic a dilated sigmoid colon, a cecal or sigmoid volvulus

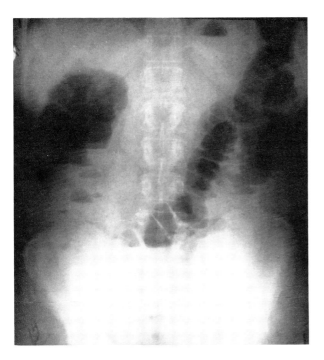

Figure 5–12. Adynamic ileus. The upright views reveals gas in the colon and small intestine. Note the differential heights in the hepatic flexure and in small bowel loops overlying L5. The patient had no intestinal blockage.

plain films alone. Fluid-filled loops are usually broader than gas-filled loops regardless of etiology. Contrary to Frimann-Dahl, Levin observed longer fluid levels in obstruction than in adynamic ileus, but there was such variation for each that this feature of gas accumulation was not reliable.[13] Differential levels can occur in ileus as in obstruction. In any circumstance in which a bowel loop contains liquid or gas, there may be flow from one limb to another in much the same way as water and air course through the arms of a siphon as the siphon's position and orientation are disturbed. Before equilibrium can be restored, fluid heights need not be in the same horizontal plane.[2] Equally important on erect or decubitus films is the difficulty of assigning nearly fluid levels to one continuous section of intestine. Two noncontiguous but adjacent gas-containing segments can often be mistaken for the separate ends of one loop.

The inherent ambiguities in the interpretation of small-bowel fluid levels limits the effectiveness of films taken with a horizontal beam. As long as there is sufficient gas in the bowel, the supine projection is usually adequate for the determination of intestinal obstruction. Eliminating the upright film can hasten the radiographic examination and frees a sick patient from the unnecessary rigor of assuming the erect position as a matter of routine.

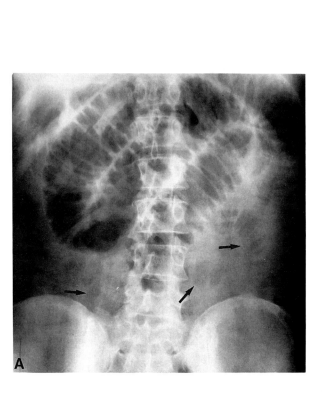

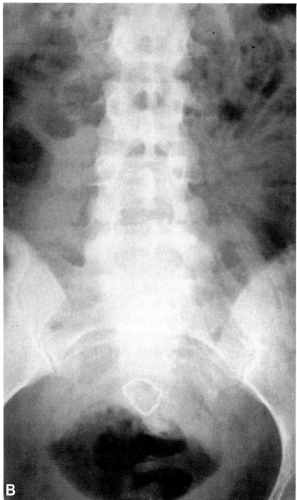

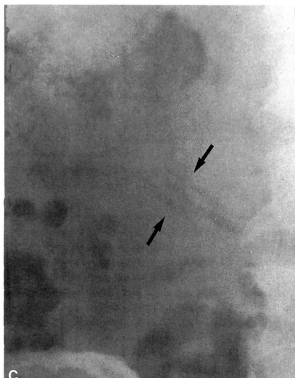

Figure 5–13. Varying appearance of fluid in small bowel obstruction. **A.** The proximal loops are predominantly air-filled. Several more distal loops contain more liquid than air and appear grayer, with the gas shadow demarcated by valvulae conniventes (*arrows*). **B.** Adhesions secondary to colon resection. A large segment of dilated jejunum and ileum contains much liquid. The intraluminal gas appears as parallel separated bands. **C.** Small bowel obstruction. The only indication of intestinal obstruction are faint slits of gas in one small area in the right mid abdomen. The lumen was filled with liquid contents and little air (*arrows*).

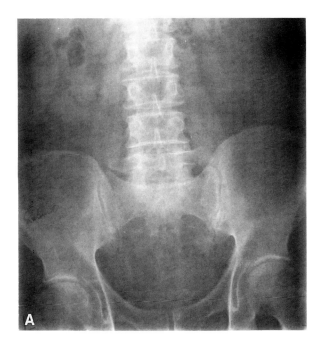 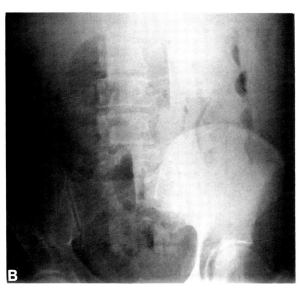

Figure 5–14. String of pearls sign, distal ileal obstruction. **A.** Supine film reveals a gasless abdomen. **B.** Left decubitus view. Several rows of bubbles are arrayed as a "string of pearls" (*arrow*) indicative of intestinal obstruction.

(Fig 5–15), a gas-containing abscess, or a gas-filled giant duodenal or sigmoid diverticulum. Its typical ovoid appearance prompted the term the "coffee bean sign." The valvulae that identify simple mechanical small-bowel obstruction become effaced in the strangulated segment. More often, the distended intestinal segment is fluid-filled and undetected on plain films. When outlined by serosal or mesenteric fat, however, it can resemble a solid mass—hence the term "pseudotumor sign."[19] Successive films may show fixation of the pseudotumor, a feature that distinguishes it from normal fluid-filled bowel, which should change in configuration on follow-up radiographs. To demonstrate fluid-filled loops or the pseudotumor sign, a high-contrast, low-voltage technique is required to contrast these intestinal segments with adjacent fat.[20] In many cases, the strangulated segment is obscured by gas accumulation proximally, and the plain film appearance is identical to simple mechanical obstruction (Fig 5–16). Persistence of discomfort, a decrease in bowel sounds, and a change from crampy to continual pain are indications of the development of strangulation.

Large Bowel Distension and Small Bowel Obstruction

The diagnosis of small intestinal obstruction depends upon differences in the width of segments of air-filled bowel with proximal loops distended and

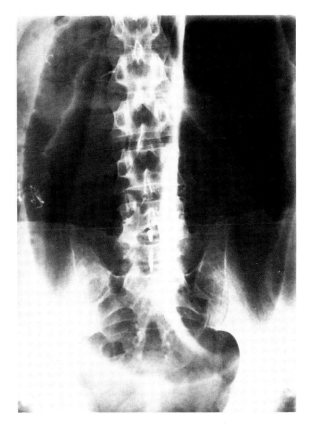

Figure 5–15. Small bowel volvulus. Massively dilated closed loop obstruction of the small bowel. Gas could not exit and the bowel distended to such an extent that it simulated the appearance of sigmoid volvulus.

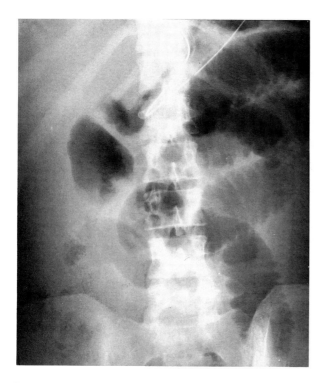

Figure 5–16. Strangulated obstruction in an internal hernia through a mesenteric defect. The fluid-filled closed loop cannot be seen on plain film. Only the air-filled loops proximal to the closed loop are identified. The configuration of small bowel is identical to the pattern of a simple mechanical obstruction.

distal segments of normal caliber. There are occasions, however, in which the colon is also abnormally dilated even though the obstruction is in the jejunum or ileum. In such circumstances, plain film diagnosis becomes more problematical and even greater reliance should be placed on correlation with clinical information and on comparison with previous and successive roentgenograms.

After an abdominal operation, dilatation of all intestinal segments is a normal occurrence, often lasting up to 10 days. In this interval, abdominal radiographs can be very misleading. There are no plain film criteria to differentiate postsurgical ileus from mechanical obstruction, although it is tempting to request this examination in an attempt to seek the reason for pain or vomiting in the immediate postoperative period, the plain film is only definitive for the recognition of gastric dilatation.[21] To avoid a misdiagnosis of acute intestinal obstruction it may be more prudent to wait until bowel tone returns to normal. Not only surgery but any type of insult to the peritoneal membranes, including trauma, perforated viscus, and infection, can be occasioned by a reflex ileus involving colon and small bowel.

Intestinal obstruction need not be confined to one focus in the bowel. Adhesions, tumors, and inflammatory masses can all produce simultaneous obstructions in the small and large bowel (Fig 5–17). Multiple sites of bowel occlusion are seen in peritoneal carcinomatosis and in the diffuse fibrosis of radiation therapy.[22] Moreover, a single mass may trap adjacent loops. For example, a large diverticular abscess can occlude the sigmoid colon and nearby ileal segments at the same time. If the colon is fluid-filled, small bowel findings may predominate on abdominal films.[23] In another manifestation of combined obstruction by one lesion, evidence of colon occlusion can be obvious, but signs of jejunal or ileal blockage are subtle, partially masked by dilatation of gas-filled large intestine (Fig 5–18).

Causes of Small Bowel Obstruction

In most populations in industrialized countries, postoperative adhesions are the commonest cause of adult-onset small bowel obstruction (Fig 5–19, Ta-

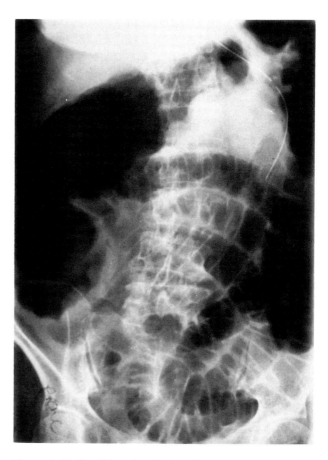

Figure 5–17. Small bowel and colon dilatation due to metastatic carcinoma, etiology unknown. Simultaneously, pelvic metastases have obstructed the sigmoid colon and the ileum. A single nonobstructing mass indents the inferior wall of the transverse colon.

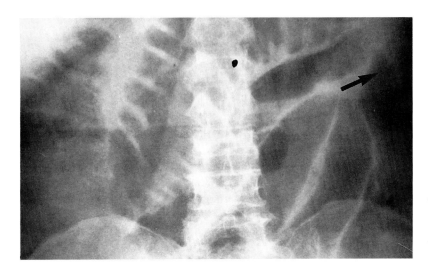

Figure 5–18. Obstructing sigmoid colon carcinoma with separate small-bowel obstruction. The dilated large intestine is feces-filled and the right colon is clearly seen. The only clue to co-incidental small bowel occlusion from tumor extension is a few valvulae conniventes in a dilated jejunal loop at the edge of the film (*arrow*).

ble 5–1). Congenital bands may occlude the intestines but they usually come to attention in childhood. The probability of an adhesive band etiology is especially great in patients who suffer recurrent episodes of obstruction over several years. Adhesions can be found anywhere in the peritoneal cavity. For example, the fashioning of abdominal wall stomas can also lead to a fibrous reaction, with the small bowel becoming trapped at the ventral peritoneal surface (Fig 5–20).

External hernias are the second most common cause of small intestinal occlusion, with inguinal and femoral protrusions the most frequent. The finding of gas-containing bowel in these herniations may be missed on plain films if the radiograph is centered too high with its lower edge above the level of the obturator foramen (Fig 1–10). Small bowel occlusion

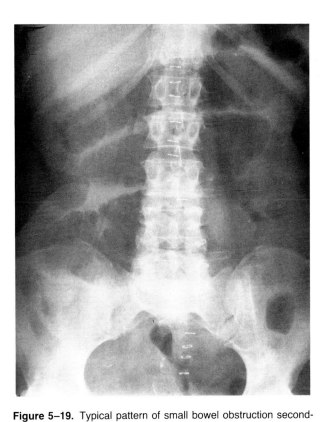

Figure 5–19. Typical pattern of small bowel obstruction secondary to adhesion occluding the mid-ileum. Midline clips indicate previous abdominal surgery.

TABLE 5–1. CAUSES OF SMALL BOWEL OBSTRUCTION

1. Adhesions
   Postoperative
   Congenital
   Inflammatory
   Radiation
   Peritoneal malignancy
2. External hernias
   Inguinal
   Femoral
   Ventral
   Umbilical
   Spigelian
   Rarer external hernias of the lateral abdominal wall
3. Internal hernias
   Paraduodenal fossae
   Lesser sac
   Lower abdominal mesentery
4. Masses
   Intrinsic obstructions
   Extrinsic obstructions
   Inflammatory masses
   Metastatic masses
5. Volvulus of the small bowel
6. Ileosigmoid knot
7. Meckel's diverticulum
8. Obturation obstruction
   Parasite
   Foreign body
   Gallstone

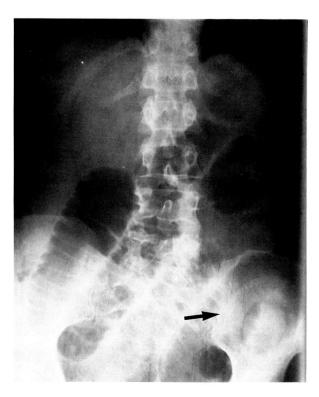

Figure 5–20. Small bowel obstruction at a colostomy site (*arrow*). The dilated air-filled loops extend to the point of blockage.

due to an umbilical hernia resembles adhesive obstruction. A subtle plain film clue is the clustering of dilated bowel around the midline at the L3–L4 level rather than in the pelvis or in the lower abdominal quadrants (Fig 5–21). For all anterior protrusions a helpful projection is a cross-table lateral film with the patient supine. This view can demonstrate fixation of bowel at or within the hernial sac (Fig 1–15). In ventral hernias, the abdominal defects can be extensive, allowing much of the small bowel to enter the sac. As a result, the dilated bowel may be seen on supine films well beyond the expected margin of the peritoneal cavity, sometimes even overlying pelvic soft tissues below the ischial tuberosity or lateral to the greater trochanter (Fig 5–22). The presence of so much bowel in a large ventral hernia raises the risk of torsion and fixation of both small intestine and proximal large bowel. The twisting of ileal loops tends to orient them vertically rather than horizontally on supine films—an important sign of acquired mid-gut volvulus. The cecum may be displaced as well, sometimes coming to rest in the left upper quadrant (Fig 5–23). Therefore, the plain film appearance of torsion of bowel within a ventral protrusion can be confused with cecal volvulus unaccompanied by hernia.

A distinctive, albeit rare (less than 2% of anterior wall hernias) lesion is the Spigelian hernia.[24] The posterior sheath of the rectus abdominus muscle is formed by the fused medial aponeuroses of the transversalis and internal oblique muscles. A separate internal oblique aponeurosis becomes the anterior sheath. Below the fold of Douglas, a semicircular fibrous band that marks the halfway point between the umbilicus and the symphysis pubis, the posterior sheath is often thin or incomplete. Thus, at the lateral margin of the lower rectus, there are many potential points of weakness through which hernial sacs can protrude. Since the much stronger external oblique muscle prohibits passage of the hernia through the abdominal wall, Spigelian hernias are apt to extend laterally within the space between the internal and external oblique muscles.[25,26] For this reason, they are also known as interstitial or interparietal hernias. Most are small, contain only fat, and are easily reducible.[27] However, some trap, obstruct, and deviate small-bowel loops far laterally. Spigelian hernias can be recognized as peripheral air- or fluid-filled structures that sometimes displace the peritoneal margin medially. They resemble an extraperitoneal abscess but until strangulation supervenes, affected individuals are not febrile, and the properitoneal and lateral intermuscular fat planes are usually preserved (Fig 5–24).[28,29] The radiographic findings are not pathognomonic, being closely simulated on occasion by laterally positioned incisional hernias (Fig 5–25).

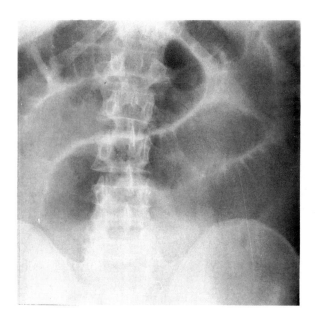

Figure 5–21. Small bowel obstruction within an umbilical hernia. The dilated loops do not extend below the level of the iliac wings.

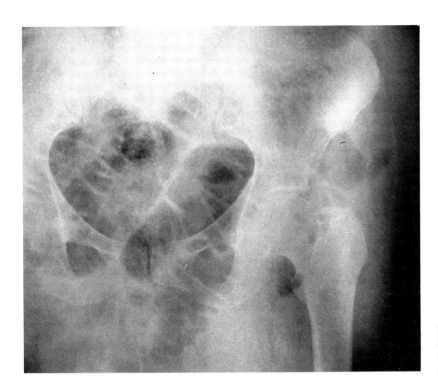

Figure 5–22. Obstructed ventral hernia. Dilated small bowel loops are seen beyond the pelvis laterally and inferiorly, well outside the expected peritoneal contours.

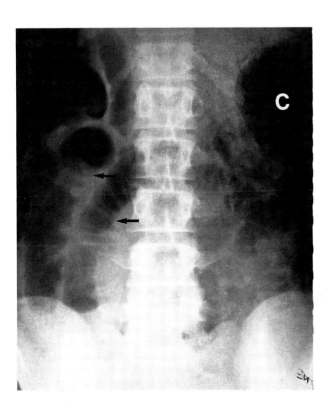

Figure 5–23. Ventral hernia with mid-gut volvulus. The cecum (C) has migrated to the left upper quadrant and ileal loops (*arrows*) have moved to the right, within the hernial sac.

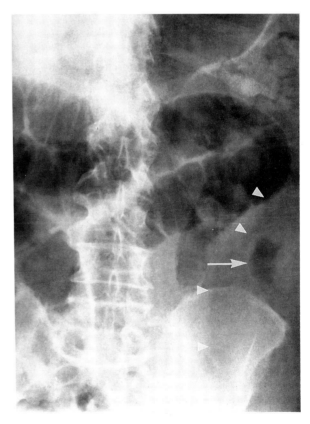

Figure 5–24. Spigelian hernia. Bowel in the hernial sac (*arrow*) with evidence of small intestinal obstruction. The properitoneal fat line is displaced medially (*arrowheads*). (*Courtesy of Dr. Murray Rosenberg.*)

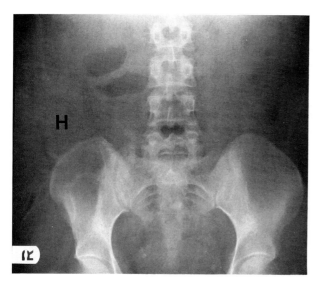

Figure 5–25. Nonobstructing incisional hernia. The laterally situated hernial sac (H) contains scattered air collections within displaced bowel.

In industrialized countries, internal hernias are much less common than abdominal wall defects, comprising only 1% of small bowel obstructions. In less developed regions of the world, however, they are several times more frequent.[30] Internal hernias are seldom diagnosed definitively on plain films, because even when they totally occlude bowel they usually appear as simple mechanical obstruction. Also, the obstruction is usually intermittent, rather than persistent, with the bowel appearing normal between painful episodes. The most common sites are the right and left paraduodenal fossae, each of which possesses several points of potential weakness through which small-intestinal segments can protrude.[31,32] A well-defined collection of closely packed bowel loops, often situated between the transverse colon and stomach, either all to one side or astride the midline, should raise suspicion of these posterior paramedian protrusions (Fig 5–26). Herniation into the lesser sac also occurs in the upper abdomen, with bowel entering through the foramen of Winslow or across a mesenteric defect in the gastrocolic ligament. Most often, a cecum on a long mesentery passes into the lesser sac: ileal or jejunal involvement is very rare. In the lower abdomen, a frequent site for internal hernia is the mesentery adjacent to the cecum. The most common defect is found in the field of Treves, the right lower quadrant area between the most distal ileal artery and the ileocolic artery. This relatively avascular space may contain congenital or acquired defects through which ileal loops can become trapped and

twisted, appearing on plain films as a distal small bowel bowel obstruction.[33]

Intraperitoneal tumors block small bowel by one of several mechanisms. Local extension of a mass often associated with bowel perforation and abscess formation can constrict adjacent bowel. Both inflammatory cicatrization and fibrous reaction to an encroaching neoplasm can contribute to intestinal obstruction (Fig 5–27). The shear bulk of intraperitoneal carcinomatosis and its attendant fibrosis can stiffen, straighten, and narrow trap bowel loops, an appearance often distinctive on plain films (Fig 5–28). Occasionally, occlusion of vessels by expanding malignancies causes ischemic strictures of bowel. The most common primary tumors with intraperitoneal extension are carcinomas of the colon, ovary, stomach, and pancreas, but metastases from more remote primary lesions, especially lung and breast carcinoma and melanoma, also cause small-bowel obstruction.

Volvulus of the small bowel, appearing for the first time after childhood, is much less common than either sigmoid or cecal volvulus. It can be a primary lesion or a complication of a preexisting intestinal deformity. Idiopathic small bowel volvulus is rare in the United States but surprisingly frequent in Africa, where, in one series, it was the cause of 15% of

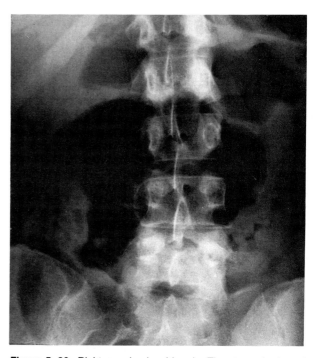

Figure 5–26. Right paraduodenal hernia. The stomach above is horizontally oriented. The transverse colon below contains feces. Between the two is a hernial sac containing proximal small bowel. The sac extended across the midline. The patient was not obstructed clinically when this film was obtained.

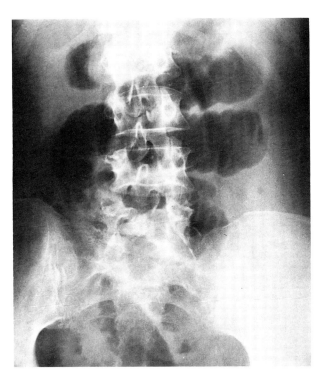

Figure 5–27. Perforated sigmoid carcinoma with abscess. The tumor and associated inflammatory mass have occluded the ileum with plain film evidence of small bowel obstruction.

factors include multiple adhesions and mesenteric defects into which bowel can become fixed.[38] The radiographic appearance is similar to other forms of strangulated obstruction.

Inflammatory lesions in and near the gut are sometimes neglected in the differential diagnosis of intestinal blockage. Such an oversight does not reflect the rarity of inflammatory occlusion but rather the subsidiary role obstructive signs and symptoms play in the typical clinical presentation of an intra-abdominal abscess. Moreover, even though clear-cut evidence of a focus of inflammation may be lacking at times, it must still be considered when plain films reveal small bowel obstruction because intestinal occlusion may be its first roentgenographic manifestation.

In the large bowel, diverticulitis almost always affects the sigmoid colon. It is primarily an extraluminal disease and the close approximation of ileal loops to the sigmoid can help explain the relatively frequent involvement of the small bowel. Usually, plain film findings of small bowel obstruction do not reveal a specific etiology, but one feature of diverticular abscess merits special consideration. In the

all intestinal obstructions.[30] Occurring predominantly in males, it is a disease of young adults who are usually healthy until they present with the abrupt onset of severe pain. At risk are patients with an abnormally mobile small intestine that is attached to a long mesentery. An adhesive band, usually a congenital fiber strand, causes twisting of the intestine, leading to a closed loop obstruction. Plain films may be unremarkable if all intestinal segments are fluid-filled, but widely separated gas-containing bowel loops, often accompanied by a persistent pseudotumor sign, are suggestive plain film findings.[34]

A complication of primary small bowel volvulus is the ileosigmoid knot. If there is also an elongated sigmoid colon, the small bowel loops can twist right to left around the large bowel mesentery, forming a knot with two closed loops. The dilated sigmoid colon is seen in the right abdomen and the dilated small intestine occupies the left. The ileosigmoid knot has a grave prognosis and requires prompt recognition so that decompression of both the small and large bowel can be accomplished expeditiously.[35–37]

Secondary volvulus usually occurs at or near the point of a preexisting obstruction, where it is induced by strong contractions that convert a simple blockage into an irreducible torsion. Predisposing

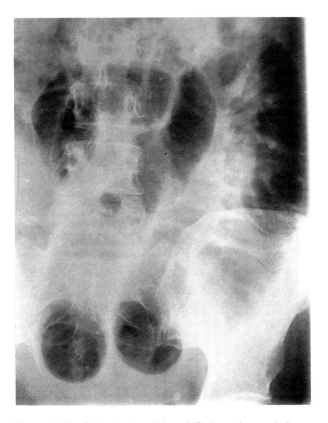

Figure 5–28. Obstructed small bowel. Peritoneal spread of ovarian carcinoma. The dilated loops are fixed in place, appearing stiff and oriented vertically.

elderly, or inebriated, diverticulitis can be initiated by the swallowing of a pointed foreign body that passes through most of the bowel uneventfully only to become held up in the narrowed lumen of a sigmoid colon containing many diverticula. The sharp object can then perforate one of these abnormal outpouchings, eventuating in a diverticular abscess. The plain film observation of a pelvic opaque foreign body, often an ingested bone, along with characteristic features of small bowel obstruction, should raise the suspicion of diverticulitis (Fig 5–29).

Appendiceal abscess is often accompanied by focal ileus, a result of the atonic effects of adjacent inflammation on bowel tone. In a minority of cases, the abscess itself may occlude the ileum and mechanical obstruction can complicate the clinical course. Generally, however, the distinction between luminal occlusion and localized ileus cannot be established definitively on plain films, as both may appear with findings of small bowel dilatation involving much of the small bowel (Fig 5–30). A Meckel's diverticular abscess can have a similar configuration of bowel loops (Fig 5–31).[39] Small bowel obstruction is an infrequent complication of Crohn's disease. Usually the diagnosis rests on barium ex-

amination of the intestine, but, at times, a segment of involved bowel can be discerned on plain films if it remains air-filled (Fig 5–32).

Obturation obstruction of the small intestine can be caused by a heterogeneous group of conditions associated with blockage of the lumen by particulate substances. A common etiology in elderly women is gallstone ileus, discussed in detail in Chapter 6. Hydroscopic bulk laxatives, cholestyramine, Amphogel (a nonabsorbable antacid), vitamin C tablets, and Isocal tube feedings can all occlude the small intestinal lumen.[40,41] The typical sufferer is a bedridden, inactive patient subjected accidentally to an excessive dose of one of these medications. After gastric surgery, phytobezoars are more apt to occur in the proximal small intestine.[42] An obtunded, dentureless, inebriated, or careless individual may ingest a fibrous food without chewing it well, thereby delivering a large bolus to the gastric remnant, through which it passes quickly, remaining intact and undigested. Orange sections are frequently found at the site of obstruction.[43] In parts of the United States, the unripe persimmon is sometimes implicated. Its skin contains shiboul, which becomes a cementlike substance in the acid medium of the stomach. Passing into the small bowel the coagulum of seeds and persimmon fibers forms a hard unyielding mass that snugly fills the intestinal lumen. Even in the presence of an intact stomach, fiber-laden vegetable matter such as fruit pits, cherry stones, and even uncooked cauliflower and eggplant fragments can resist decomposition to become an obstacle to bowel transit.[44]

The smuggling of drugs has become a profitable activity for an increasing number of people willing to take great risks. One means of crossing international borders with the contraband intact and undiscovered is to ingest the drug wrapped in a condom or other smooth, soft covering. The medical dangers of such a deception are twofold. The package can break, delivering a fatal dose to the carrier, or may become obstructed in the small or large bowel. In the air-filled intestine the condom covering stands out as a smooth, rounded density,[45,46] sometimes having irregular margins at its tied end (Fig 5–33).[47] If two or more condoms are used for additional protection, air may be trapped between the folded surfaces, with the overall appearance being a well-defined circular or ovoid lucency.[48] Drug-filled condoms are readily observed in the small bowel when there is sufficient gas in the bowel surrounding them. In the large intestine they can be distinguished from feces by their sharp margins and lack of mottling.

Ascaris lumbricoides is the most common helm-

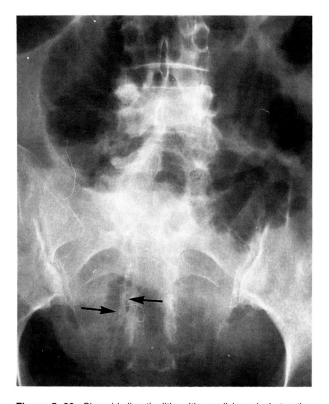

Figure 5–29. Sigmoid diverticulitis with small bowel obstruction due to penetrating chicken bone (*arrows*).

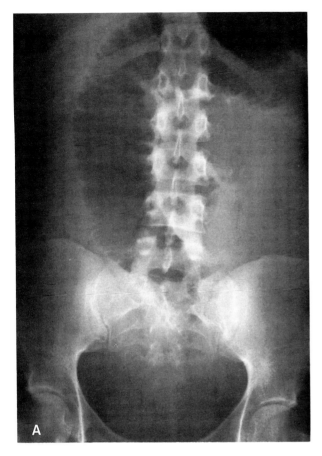
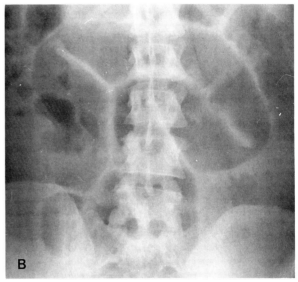

Figure 5–30. Appendiceal abscess. Mechanical obstruction vs. ileus. **A.** Appendiceal abscess with complete obstruction of the distal ileum. The small bowel proximal to the occlusion is dilated, with prominent valvulae conniventes. **B.** Periappendicitis with dilated small bowel loops. Ileus led to the dilatation of intestine proximal to the inflammation. There was no mechanical obstruction.

inth infestation in the world, affecting approximately one billion persons. The worm resides in the small bowel for long periods and only traverses the large intestine as it is excreted from the body. In children, especially, masses of worms may obstruct the small intestine.[49] The duodenum, jejunum, and ileum normally contain no particulate material so a careful search of air-filled intestinal loops can reveal ascaris on plain films. En face, a worm appears as a smoothly marginated, rounded density.[50] In profile, it is seen as a slightly undulated band extending for several centimeters within the lumen of gas-filled small intestine (Fig 5–34). Masses of worms distend the bowel, and the overall pattern of parasite and luminal gas suggests a medusa-like or swirly array of black and gray strips (Fig 5–35).[51,52] Another worm that may be seen in the small bowel outlined by gas is *Taenia saginata*, the beef tapeworm. It rarely obstructs because it is thinner and less numerous than *A lumbricoides*.[53,54]

Simulators of Mechanical Small Bowel Obstruction

Gas-filled small bowel, dilated to a greater extent than more distal intestinal segments, is a distinctive radiographic pattern, but it is not exclusive for mechanical occlusion. A variety of conditions are included in the category of small intestinal pseudo-obstruction, all of which may be confused on plain films with jejunal or ileal blockage (Table 5–2). They range in severity from the innocuous to the life-threatening, encompassing both transient and irreversible abnormalities. Urinary retention can cause adynamic distension. Often, in obtunded patients, the clinical picture is not specific for bladder dilatation, and an incidental plain film may reveal numerous gas-filled small bowel loops. A repeat radiograph taken after bladder drainage often shows a markedly altered configuration of the intestinal gas as the distension of small bowel resolves promptly.[13] Frequently, the oral administration of

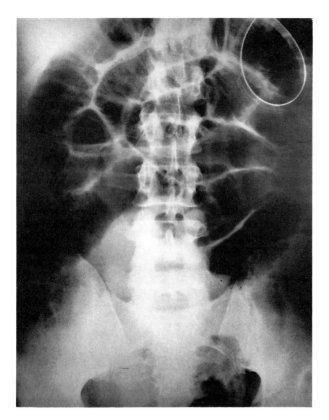

Figure 5–31. A large soft tissue mass overlying L4, L5, and the sacrum is a Meckel's diverticular abscess. The dilated bowel loops are evidence of a small bowel obstruction caused by extrinsic compression on the ileal lumen by the abscess.

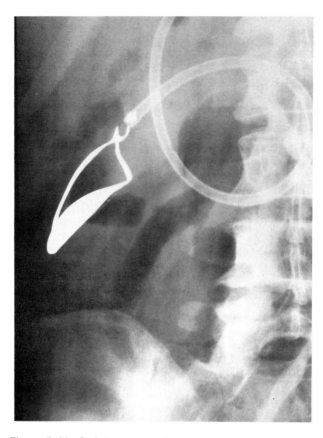

Figure 5–32. Crohn's disease. Obstruction of the small bowel. Gas in dilated jejunal and ileal loops has been removed by drainage through the intestinal tube. The narrowed featureless ileal loop is involved by Crohn's enteritis. (*Courtesy of Dr. Jutta Greweldinger.*)

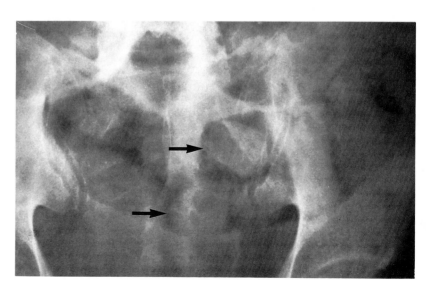

Figure 5–33. "Cocaine balls" (*arrows*) in the sigmoid colon. The rounded densities are condoms enclosing the powdered drug.

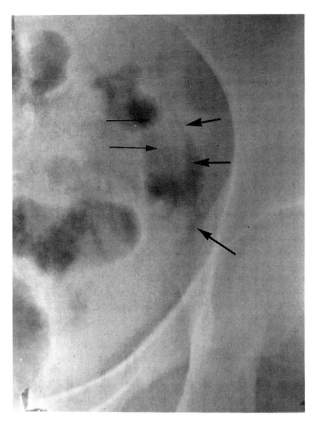

Figure 5–34. Two *Ascaris* worms in a small bowel segment (*arrows*).

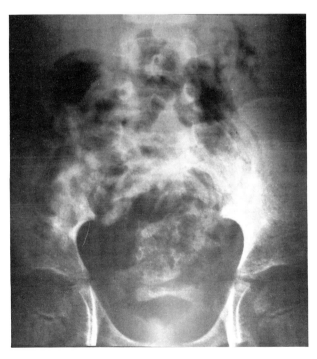

Figure 5–35. Masses of *Ascaris lumbricoides* occupying much of the small bowel in a child. The swirly pattern suggests a heavy intestinal worm burden.

TABLE 5–2. SIMULATORS OF MECHANICAL SMALL BOWEL OBSTRUCTION

1. Inflammatory masses
2. Mesenteric ischemia
3. Urinary retention
4. Air swallowing
5. Small bowel pseudo-obstruction
    Distant disease (acute)
        Pneumonia
        Congestive heart failure
    Distant disease (subacute)
        Myxedema
        Uremia
    Acute abdominal disease
        Blunt trauma
        Pancreatitis
        Mesenteritis
        Enterocolitis
        Peritoneal irritation
    Collagen defect diseases
        Ehler's–Danlos syndrome
        Scleroderma
    Sprue
    Idiopathic pseudo-obstruction

saline cathartics is accompanied by air swallowing. If the colon is dilated and contains much feces before evacuation, fluid and air can remain in the small bowel in a configuration that resembles mechanical obstruction.[13]

Small bowel pseudo-obstruction is a frequent concomitant of blunt trauma, pneumonia, congestive failure, myxedema, and uremia. In each of these entities temporary neuromuscular dysfunction of the small bowel initiated by a poorly understood mechanism can be manifested as adynamic distension.[11,55] Pancreatitis, diffuse mesenteritis, gastroenteritis, and enterocolitis are all occasioned by marked abdominal discomfort.[9] Air swallowing is increased and resorption of oxygen and carbon dioxide is retarded in an inflamed bowel segment. The result is retention of gas in dilated small bowel loops. In some cases of intestinal inflammation, the valvulae may appear edematous, but in most instances there are no roentgenographic findings that distinguish inflammation from obstruction. Once again, an appreciation of the clinical context is crucial in reaching a correct diagnosis.

Occasionally, persistent small bowel distension is seen in scleroderma[11] and in Ehlers–Danlos syndrome.[56] In both diseases, bowel dilatation is probably due to deficiencies in collagen formation in the intestinal wall. In some patients with nontropical sprue, intermittent small bowel distension may be a consequence of transient intussusceptions.[57] There is also a poorly delineated entity of idiopathic small bowel pseudo-obstruction. The typical patient is a young adult who complains of recurrent episodes of abdominal pain. The diagnosis is one of exclusion entertained only after additional examinations, including barium contrast studies, fail to demonstrate luminal occlusion in the small bowel.[58]

Mesenteric ischemia is a common and often fatal disease associated with pseudo-obstruction of the small bowel. It cannot be overemphasized that a bowel pattern identical to distal ileal obstruction may be the only plain film presentation of acute small intestinal vascular insufficiency. Although this appearance is not specific for mesenteric ischemia, it is quite common, occurring in up to 50% of cases.[59] Occasionally, helpful ancillary findings of ischemia are seen such as air in the bowel wall and a dilated lumen without indenting valvulae but, in many cases, the radiographic appearance is identical to distal small bowel obstruction (Fig 5–36).

Large Bowel Obstruction

The plain film recognition of large bowel obstruction is no less challenging than the interpretation of small intestinal occlusion. The colon has a wide range of normal configurations. In addition, the pattern of large bowel obstruction is influenced by the site and duration of blockage, the composition of luminal contents, competence of the ileocecal valve, and the coincident dilatation of small bowel loops. Moreover, adynamic distension is also common in the large bowel and often resembles obstruction. At times, the arrangement of bowel loops can make the diagnosis obvious, but, more often, correct evaluation rests on the observation of subtle roentgenologic signs with an awareness of clinical findings.

In a typical configuration of mechanical obstruction, all colonic segments proximal to the point of luminal narrowing are dilated (Fig 5–37). Unlike the small intestine, which can only receive gas introduced into it through the pylorus or ileocecal valve, the colon has an endogenous source of flatus produced by the bacterial decomposition of feces. The constituents of colonic or gas include methane and hydrogen and lesser amounts of other volatile products of fermentation, but the major component is poorly absorbable nitrogen derived from the ingestion of air. Thus, in large bowel obstruction, it is aerophagy that contributes most prominently to gaseous accumulation.[1,3]

When the large bowel distends with gas and the ileocecal valve prohibits retrograde flow into the ileum, the diagnosis of large bowel obstruction is often readily apparent on plain films. The colonic segments up to the site of luminal blockage stand out clearly and the septa indenting the lumen are sharply demarcated. However, such an appearance is found in only a minority of cases. In most pa-

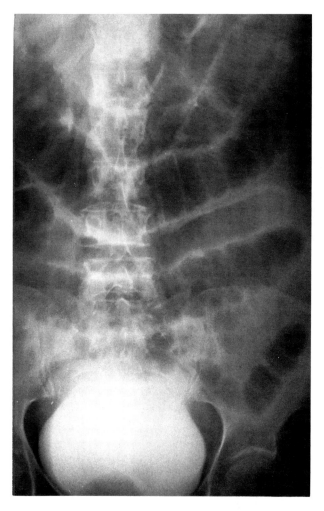

Figure 5–36. Mesenteric ischemia. A film from an intravenous urography. Several horizontally oriented small bowel loops are more dilated from the gas-filled sigmoid colon, which overlies the left iliac fossa. The appearance resembles distal small bowel obstruction. Note the infarcted small bowel lacking valvulae covering the abdomen at the level of the L4–L5 disc space.

tients, intestinal secretions and particulate fecal matter also occupy the distended lumen, and the relative proportion of solid, liquid and gaseous constituents determine the extent of lucency in the obstructed colon. Completely fluid-filled large intestine may go undetected on plain films, as the dilated bowel cannot be distinguished from adjacent abdominal soft tissues. Usually, the combination of gas and feces imparts a mottled character to the large intestine. On supine views less dependent segments, such as the transverse and sigmoid colon, may contain much gas and appear black whereas other sections of the large bowel are more gray, reflecting the admixture of feces and fluid. Typically, the septa are thickened, due in part to muscular hypertonicity engendered by obstruction and also

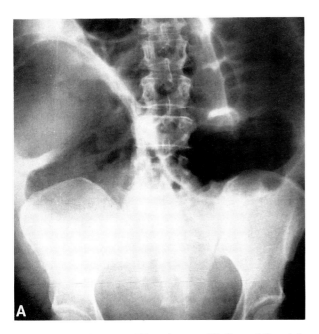 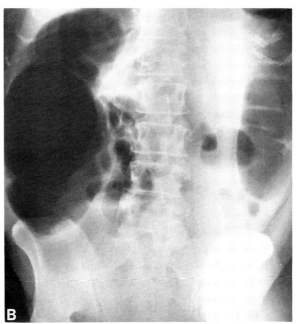

Figure 5–37. Supine **(A)** and prone **(B)** films of the abdomen in a patient with distal descending colon obstruction by a carcinoma. Gas fills the entire large bowel proximal to the occlusion, with minimal gas in the small intestine.

because retained secretions displace remaining gas away from the luminal surfaces. Copious adherent fecal material can give the bowel wall a shaggy margin (Fig 5–38). Eventually, in long-standing obstruction, muscular exhaustion can ensue, resulting in the effacement of intraluminal septa and haustra.[60]

The confinement of gas entirely within the colon without small bowel dilatation has been termed type IA obstruction according to a classification scheme devised by Love in 1960.[61] Despite its classic appearance on plain films type IA obstruction is relatively uncommon, having been observed in only 8% of Love's cases. Much more frequent is type IB obstruction, in which the large bowel is distended but there is also superimposed small-bowel obstruction with antegrade luminal transit restricted by the ileocecal valve (Fig 5–39). Types 1A and 1B are, in effect, closed looped obstructions with the stenotic segment of large bowel at the distal end and a competent ileocecal valve defining the proximal point of colonic occlusion. Cecal distension is common, and with marked dilatation there is an increased risk of rupture.

Type 2 obstruction comprises approximately 33% of cases. It results from an open ileocecal valve allowing gas to escape proximally into the small bowel. Incompetence of the ileocecal valve is independent of the location of the large intestinal blockage and is equally likely in ascending colon and sigmoid obstructions. The colon is not dilated and

usually free of gas, but the ileal and jejunal loops may become quite distended (Fig 5–40).[8] The pattern of gas accumulation in type 2 obstruction mimics ileal occlusion.

The exact point of a large bowel obstruction is difficult to detect on supine views. Occasionally, a persistent difference in the caliber of gas-filled colonic segments immediately proximal and distal to an obstructing lesion identifies the site of stricture (Fig 5–41). In most cases, the location of the terminus of the colonic gas shadow does not necessarily correspond with the site of bowel occlusion.[62] A typical pattern is continuous dilatation of the cecum, right colon, and transverse colon up to the splenic flexure caused by an obstructing tumor in the sigmoid colon. The intervening descending colon lacks gas, as it is distended by fluid and solid feces only (Fig 1–14). An abrupt interruption of colonic gas in either the midtransverse or middescending colon more often closely approximates the point of obstruction. The cross-table view with the patient in the right decubitus position can be helpful in confirming the presence of a luminal mass in the left colon because with this projection liquid intraluminal contents move away and the remaining gas outlines the tumefaction (Fig 5–42).

In the supine position the rectum is the most dependent large bowel segment and need not fill with gas. Consequently, the standard recumbent projection cannot differentiate distal sigmoid block-

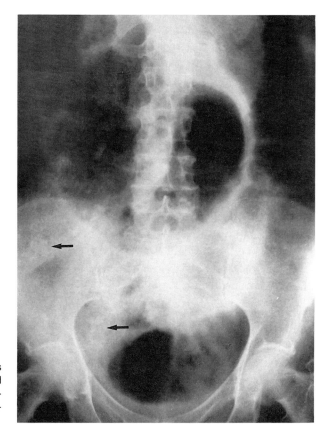

Figure 5–38. Obstruction by a sigmoid carcinoma. The colon is dilated and filled with gas and feces, giving the lumen a mottled appearance. Stasis has led to formation of coproliths (calcified feces). The absence of small bowel gas makes this a type 1A obstruction.

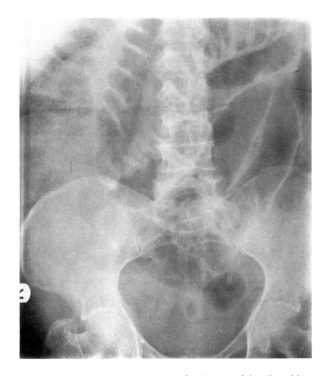

Figure 5–39. Type 1B obstruction. Carcinoma of the sigmoid colon. The transverse colon is gas-filled and the dilated right colon contains feces. There are also dilated distal small bowel loops situated in the pelvis and to the right of the lower lumbar spine.

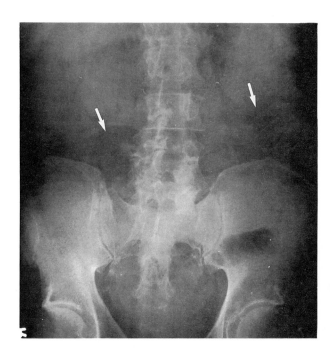

Figure 5–40. Splenic flexure carcinoma. Type 2 obstruction. No gas is seen in the colon, but numerous small bowel loops are dilated (*arrows*), an appearance also suggestive of ileal obstruction.

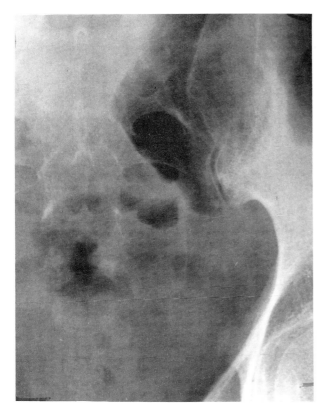

Figure 5–41. Obstructing sigmoid carcinoma. Dilated bowel proximal to the occlusion and normal caliber colon immediately distal identify the site of the lesion on this plain film.

age from colonic ileus. The prone view places the rectum superiorly, allowing flatus to flow into it from the sigmoid colon. If gas is seen to fill the rectum a distal sigmoid obstruction can be ruled out with assurance (Fig 5–43).

Colonic Pseudo-obstruction

Diffuse dilatation of the large bowel unrelated to mechanical blockage of the lumen is a relatively common condition in hospitalized patients. Also known as colonic ileus or pseudo-obstruction of the large intestine, it is associated with a wide array of diseases and may be an acute, chronic, or an intermittent disturbance (Table 5–3). In most cases, the plain film appearance is sufficiently characteristic to differentiate it from large bowel occlusion.

On supine views, flatus-filled, dilated colon extends as a continuous lucency from cecum to left colon. In some cases, the gas shadow may end abruptly at the splenic flexure, descending colon, or rectosigmoid, but decubitus and frontal views usually reveal luminal patency throughout the bowel. Occasionally, the dilatation may spare the rectum or distal left colon, but there is no persistent narrowing to retard the flow of gas or feces.

In large intestinal pseudo-obstruction the haustra are regularly spaced and the septa are thin, smooth and sharply marginated. Inasmuch as gas is the predominant intraluminal constituent, bowel wall contour is clearly demarcated, a pattern markedly different from the shaggy interfaces often seen in colonic obstruction.[60,63] Plain film recognition of pseudo-obstruction is important because in the absence of a focal occlusion barium enema is not only unnecessary but may be painful and excessively demanding for debilitated individuals. In a small percentage of patients with either obstruction or adynamic ileus of the colon, the radiographical appearance is indeterminate, but in most cases, the two types of colonic dilatation are distinguishable on plain films.

Transient pseudo-obstruction is most often seen as a complication of acute abdominal disorders. Cholecystitis, pancreatitis, and pelvic abscess frequently present with large-bowel dilatation.[64] In a study of 50 patients with ileus treated successfully by colonoscopy, 35% developed persistent distension after abdominal surgery.[65] Spinal disease, including disc herniation, osteomyelitis, and painful spondylolisthesis, is another group of conditions in which non-obstructive distension of the colon is seen. Imbalances in sympathetic and parasympathetic neurological influences may be responsible for the bowel distension, although the exact mechanism still remains largely undeciphered.[66]

Metabolic derangements accompanied by pseudo-obstruction include hypokalemia[67] and hypercalcemia.[64] Low serum potassium may explain the appearance of megacolon in diabetes. It is a relatively infrequent occurrence and the dilatation is almost always confined to the sigmoid colon.[68] Severe abnormalities whose major manifestations are remote from the colon also appear to induce pseudo-obstruction. It has been reported in such diverse conditions as pneumonia, congestive heart disease, and acute renal failure.[63,64] Ogilvie's syndrome is an eponym for acute colonic pseudo-obstruction without a specific etiology.[69] Perhaps Ogilvie's syndrome is a separate entity; more likely, however, all cases of unexplained pseudo-obstruction have a specific cause, although other manifestations of the predisposing disease are not clinically evident.[70–72]

A particularly severe form of colonic ileus is found in severely retarded or psychotic individuals who may have few other physical abnormalities. Rapidly progressive dilatation of the colon, uncontrolled by rectal tube or colonoscopic decompression, is a recurring danger in these patients. Unless promptly treated, dilatation may continue un-

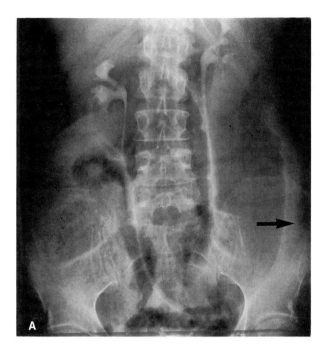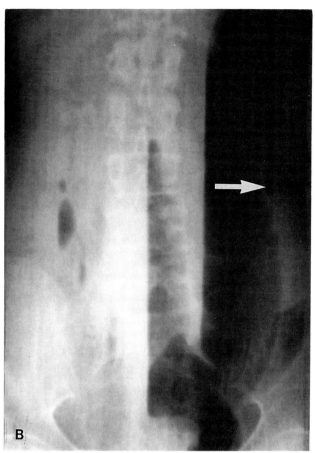

Figure 5–42. Descending colon obstruction by carcinoma. **A.** Supine view shows a dilated colon with an abrupt end of the gas shadow in the descending colon (*arrow*). **B.** Right decubitus view also defines the point of blockage (*arrow*).

abated, leading to cecal perforation and death (Fig 5–44).[73,74]

Two syndromes of intermittent dilatation in young adults are familial and idiopathic pseudo-obstruction. Both entities typically present with repeated episodes of pain and bloating. Affected individuals may eventually undergo several unrewarding laparotomies. Inasmuch as no characteristic pathological changes are seen on biopsy, the diagnosis is usually one of exclusion.[75,76]

Recurrent or persistent pseudo-obstruction accompanies the administration of phenothiazine and related medications.[77] Antiparkinsonian drugs are particularly apt to lead to colonic ileus. Usually massive dilatation does not appear unless the drug has been administered continually for at least 1½ years.[78] Lactulose, effective in the treatment of cirrhosis, is metabolized by colonic bacteria, with the release of hydrogen and other gases. Persistent ingestion of lactulose may result in the development of marked gaseous dilatation of the large bowel (Fig

5–45). Colonic ileus is a side effect of vincristine, a chemotherapeutic agent most often employed in combination drug therapy for lymphoma. Vincristine ileus is no different roentgenographically from other causes of pseudo-obstruction, most often developing 10 to 15 days after an intravenous bolus administration of the drug (Fig 5–46).[79]

Chronic dilatation of the colon occurs in myxedema[80,81] and in a range of intrinsic bowel wall disorders, including sprue,[82,83] amyloidosis,[64] plexiform neurofibromatosis,[84,85] and familial dysautonomia.[86] In scleroderma,[87] myotonic dystrophy,[88,89] and Chagas' disease,[90] large bowel dilatation is seen, along with distension and hypomotility of the small bowel and esophagus.

Etiology of Large Bowel Obstruction

Mechanical obstruction of the large intestine is most often due to primary carcinoma of the colon, which occludes the bowel either by direct intraluminal growth or by encroachment of an enlarging exo-

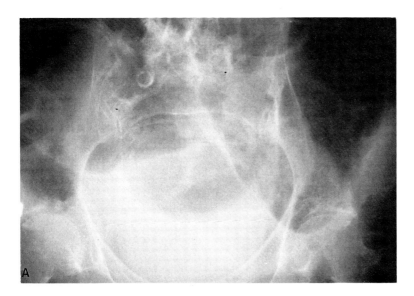

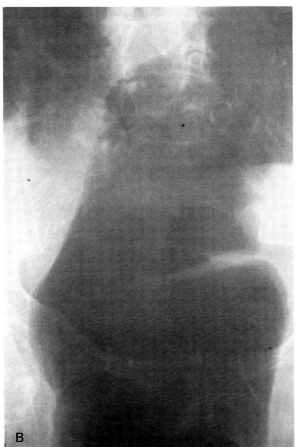

Figure 5–43. The value of the prone film. The supine view **(A)** shows dilatation of the large bowel proximal to the rectum. The prone projection **(B)** clearly demonstrates gas filling a nonobstructed prolapsed rectum.

TABLE 5–3. COLONIC PSEUDO-OBSTRUCTION

1. Transient pseudo-obstruction
   - Acute peritoneal insult
     - Post-operative
     - Peritonitis
     - Cholecystitis
     - Pancreatitis
     - Pelvic abscess
   - Spinal disease
     - Spondylitis
     - Spondylolisthesis
     - Metabolic derangements
     - Hypokalemia
     - Diabetes
     - Hypercalcemia
   - Acute extraintestinal disease
     - Pneumonia
     - Congestive heart failure
     - Renal failure
   - Idiopathic colonic pseudo-obstruction (Ogilvie's Syndrome)
   - Familial pseudo-obstruction
   - Pseudo-obstruction of the psychotic or retarded
   - Drug-induced pseudo-obstruction
     - Phenothiazines
     - Antiparkinsonian medications
     - Lactulose
     - Vincristine
   - Postprocedure colon dilatation
     - Colonoscopy
     - Barium enema
2. Chronic dilatation
   - Myxedema
   - Amyloidosis
   - Plexiform neurofibromatosis
   - Familial dysautonomia
   - Myotonic dystrophy
   - Chagas' disease

phytic lesion on an adjacent large intestinal loops. In one series, obstruction by colonic tumor was exceeded only by small intestinal postoperative adhesions as a cause of bowel blockage.[91] Inflammatory adhesions, a frequent complication of diverticulitis, has a predilection for the small intestine and yet is not rare in the colon. On the other hand, postsurgical adhesive bands rarely block the large intestinal lumen (Fig 5–47).[92] Both external and internal hernias are ten times more likely to obstruct small intestine than the colon;[91] the one exception to this rule is herniation into the lesser sac, which involves the cecum more than any other bowel segment.

In developed countries where the prevalence of *Ascaris* infestation is low, obturation obstruction is predominantly a large bowel affliction. The prime cause is fecal impaction, a frequent occurrence in the elderly and neurologically impaired. It is also seen in younger patients who are chronic abusers of narcotic medications (Figs 2–12,5–48). The serious

consequences of intractable constipation in the aged or infirm is sometimes underestimated. Marked dilatation of the colon or rectum may restrict blood flow to the bowel wall, especially in patients with preexisting aortic or splanchnic arteriosclerosis. The abrasive effect of solid feces on the mucosa of large bowel can lead to stercoral ulcers of varying sizes. The combination of ischemia and mucosal rents increases the risk of perforation, a catastrophic and often fatal event. Gallstone ileus is another cause of colonic obturation, but in only 3% to 5% of patients with luminal blockage by gallstones is the colon occluded.[93,94] Strangulation obstruction is also more often a small-bowel problem. On the other hand, perforation, although rare in both small and large intestinal occlusions, is slightly more common in the colon.

If there is free flow of gas and fluid along a segment of bowel, intraluminal pressure must be constant throughout. Laplace's law states that the pressure needed to distend a hollow viscus varies inversely with its radius. Thus, the cecum, often the widest part of the colon, expands to the greatest extent as the large bowel dilates.[95] The propensity for cecal disruption in obstruction was studied by Lowman and Davis, who observed that perforation becomes a clinical consideration if cecal diameter exceeds 9 cm.[96] Most cases of rupture involve a diastasis of the weaker outer wall of muscle at the anterior surface of the caput cecum. The mucosa first protrudes through a linear gap in muscle before it, too, splits. Kottler and Lee reported that marginal rupture could be recognized on plain films by the presence of intraluminal gas along the lateral aspect of the cecum.[97] Nevertheless, this is a rare and transient finding that can be closely simulated by normal properitoneal fat adjacent to the bowel wall. After perforation, the cecum does not return to normal size despite the formation of an egress for intestinal gas. Apparently, the ileus induced by peritoneal irritation keeps the cecum distended.

Cecal width is not the only factor that influences perforation. The duration of distension is also important, with a rapid accumulation of gas more poorly tolerated than a slower progression of dilatation. Moreover, preexisting disease in the proximal colon can hasten the process of diastatic rupture independent of cecal size. The validity of the 9 cm standard is limited by the geometric uncertainty implicit in all radiographic measurements of abdominal structures. Such a consideration must always be taken into account in obese patients because the cecum is usually significantly magnified on supine films. Furthermore, the position of the cecum in the abdomen varies. In some patients, it is located just

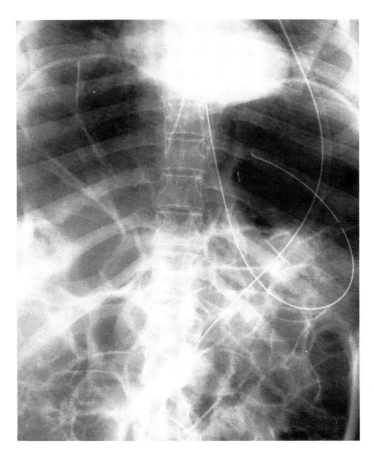

Figure 5–44. Colonic ileus in a retarded young adult with phenylketonuria. The dilated colon retains septa and is free of feces. The patient had repeated episodes of pseudo-obstruction. The last attack was precipitous leading, quickly to colonic perforation, pneumoperitoneum and death.

beneath the anterior abdominal wall, and measurements of the gas shadow may overestimate cecal size whereas in others it is more posteriorly situated and its radiographic dimensions more closely approximate actual bowel width.

Cecal rupture is more common in colon pseudo-obstruction than in bowel occlusion by tumor, as rapid distension of gas in colonic ileus puts the cecum at risk for perforation. Hence, with slowly obstructing carcinomas of the left and transverse colon, cecal rents are uncommon. Desai and Rodko observed perforation in only 10 in 860 cases of colonic malignancy.[98] None were in the cecum and all cases were caused by the infiltration of the bowel wall by the advancing tumor.

Cecal Volvulus

Volvulus of the cecum is an uncommon abnormality, accounting for only 1% to 2% of intestinal obstruction in adults. Its share of colonic occlusion is, of course, higher, and in one series, 10% of large-bowel obstructions were due to cecal volvulus,[99] although most other reports place its relative incidence between 2% and 3%.[99,100] Unlike volvulus of the small bowel, which usually appears with a roentgenographic pattern similar to simple mechanical obstruction, most cases of cecal volvulus can be definitively identified in plain films. Moreover, because the clinical presentation of cecal volvulus is rarely specific, supine noncontrast films are crucial in the ascertainment of a correct preoperative diagnosis.

A mobile cecum is a necessary prerequisite for the later development of cecal volvulus. Between 11% and 22% of individuals have congenital defects in the fixation of the right colon to the lateral abdominal wall.[99,101] The nonobstructed cecum, attached to an elongated mesentery, is likely to wander from its expected position in the right lower quadrant. Often, a gas-filled mobile right colon can be seen on plain films in a median location, sometimes with small bowel loops interposed between it and the ipsilateral properitoneal fat stripe (Fig 5–49). Typically, a mobile cecum is repositioned near the midline, with the caput cecum oriented horizontally.

It is not possible to determine from plain films which patients who have a poorly fixated cecum will develop a volvulus. In the pre–World War II era, volvulus was thought to be more frequent among Scandinavians than among other Europeans, especially among those eating a high-fiber diet.[102] There

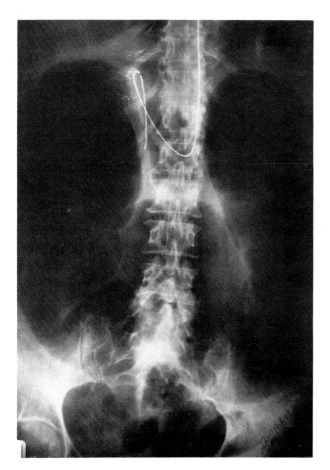

Figure 5–45. Lactulose ileus. Severe colonic dilatation without mechanical obstruction. The distension eased with cessation of therapy.

has been little recent epidemiologic investigation of this matter, however. Cecal volvulus can be precipitated by any procedure that causes large bowel dilatation, including colonoscopy and barium enema. Distal colonic obstruction from any cause is another risk factor. Patients with a mobile right cecum are particularly vulnerable to cecal volvulus in the recuperative period after laparotomy. The combined effects of postoperative ileus and a lax abdominal wall permit unrestricted dilatation of the cecum, which may then go on to twist upon itself. Intraperitoneal adhesive bands are sometimes the focal point of a cecal volvulus. Among the many complications of radiotherapy to the abdomen should be added cecal volvulus precipitated by the entanglement of a mobile cecum in one or more intraperitoneal adhesions caused by this form of therapy.[101]

In a recent study of 55 cases of cecal volvulus, the radiological report of abdominal plain films indicated the diagnosis in 53% of cases.[101] In retrospect, diagnostic roentgenographic findings of cecal volvulus were present in an additional 36%. Thus,

the value of survey radiographs is undebatable. The presence of a dilated cecal gas shadow is seen in at least 75% of cases.[101] Characteristically, the haustra are preserved and the bowel walls are smooth. Most often the cecum is relocated to the mid-abdomen or to the left upper quadrant as it twists on an oblique axis (Fig 2–26), sometimes even overlying or displacing the stomach (Figs 4–6,5–50). A mobile, markedly distended cecum and ascending colon can migrate to the mid or lower left side of the abdomen and the pelvis, but the right lower quadrant is an unusual site of dilated bowel in cecal volvulus.

If the ileocecal valve is competent, a closed loop obstruction is created in cecal volvulus. Coexistent small bowel distension is not a hallmark of the disease, however. In fact, in more than 50% of patients in a recent study, little gas was seen in the ileum and jejunum, and marked small bowel dilatation occurred in only 10% of cases (Fig 5–51).[99] Even less common is dilated gas-filled small bowel with a completely fluid-filled cecum—a pattern indistinguish-

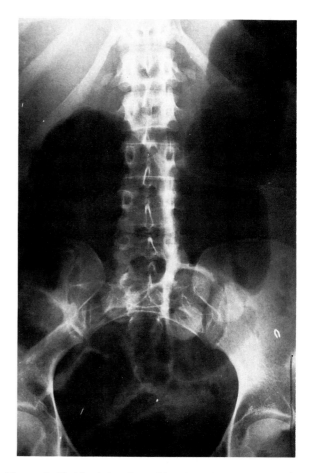

Figure 5–46. Vincristine ileus. Dilatation of the colon resulting from administration of vincristine for the treatment of Hodgkin's disease.

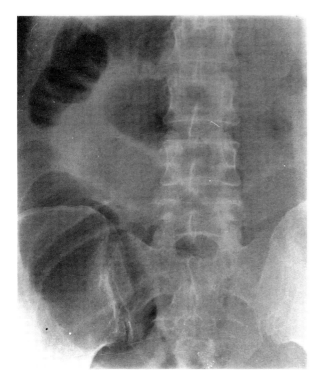

Figure 5–47. Obstruction of the large bowel at the mid-transverse colon by a postoperative adhesion. The proximal transverse colon, right colon, and several distal small bowel loops are dilated.

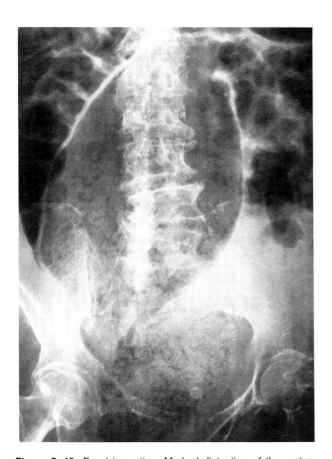

Figure 5–48. Fecal impaction. Marked distention of the rectum and the sigmoid, which rises out of the pelvis filled with gas and feces. The patient had rectal bleeding from a stercoral ulcer at the rectosigmoid junction.

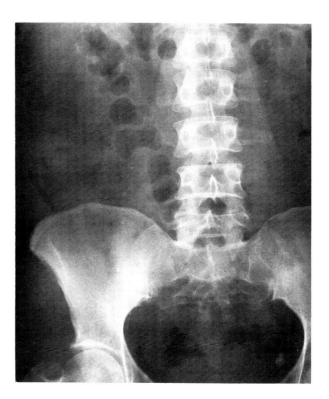

Figure 5–49. Mobile cecum. The right colon, including the cecum, has relocated medially, with faintly lucent, nondistended small bowel more lateral. The poorly fixated proximal large bowel on a long mesentery can wander in the lower abdomen and is perfectly set up to twist on itself.

able from distal ileal obstruction. Persistent dilatation of the colon distal to the volvulus is seldom noted unless perforation and peritonitis ensue, causing a diffuse paralytic ileus. Marked distension of a displaced cecum, along with gas-filled loops oriented vertically, suggests the possibility of cecal volvulus within an extrinsic hernia sac.

In 1938, Weinstein called attention to an abnormality in the anchoring of the wall of the proximal right colon to the posterior peritoneal surface.[102] A defect in mesenteric attachment causes an obstructive angulation of the cecum. The pattern of abrupt folding of the right colon resembles a pan balance, with the posterior kink as the fulcrum—hence, the term cecal bascule (from the Latin "bascula," or scale). It can be suggested on plain films if a dilated cecum is directed medially from the right lower quadrant.[103,104]

Recently, the concept of cecal bascule was challenged by Johnson et al, who showed that most examples of a cecum dilated out of proportion to the rest of the large intestine resulted from adynamic distension rather than mechanical obstruction at a crease in the ascending colon.[105] They termed the abnormality cecal ileus because they observed gas filling of the more distal colon but no luminal occlusion. The key to the diagnosis is the predominance of cecal distension and its anteriomedial rotation

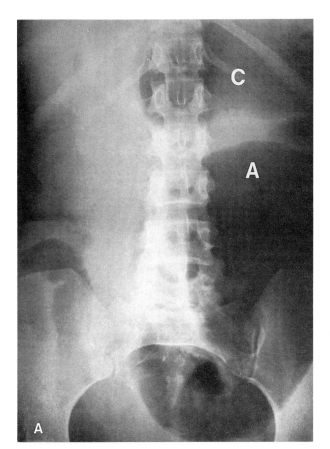

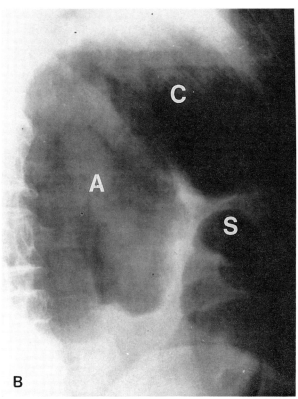

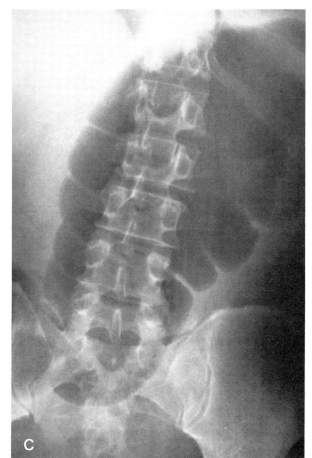

Figure 5–50. Three examples of cecal volvulus. **A.** The entire right colon has twisted and lies in the left abdomen. The ascending colon (A) occupies part of the pelvis and much of the left lower quadrant. The cecum (C) is a featureless lucency in the left upper quadrant. **B.** The cecum (C) and the ascending colon (A) have rotated upwards into the left upper quadrant. (S) denotes the sigmoid colon. **C.** The dilated proximal colon rises from the right lower quadrant to the left upper abdomen. Haustra and septa denote its colonic signature.

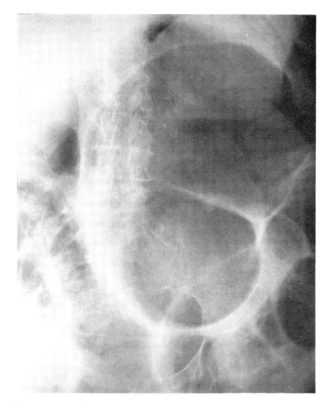

Figure 5–51. Cecal volvulus with small bowel dilatation. The markedly distended cecum occupies the left side of the abdomen. Air-filled dilated ileal loops are seen in the right abdomen.

(Fig 5–52). As in generalized colonic ileus, in cecal ileus the bowel contains much gas but little feces. Prompt recognition of this abnormality is important because prolonged distension brings with it an increased risk of perforation. Cecal volvulus can respond to treatment by colonoscopy, however, and, unlike cecal bascule, does not need eventual surgery if decompression can be accomplished endoscopically.[105]

Sigmoid Volvulus

Sigmoid volvulus, although similar in incidence to cecal volvulus, differs from it in etiology. Congenital abnormalities of the sigmoid mesocolon are rare; the susceptibility to torsion depends almost exclusively on environmental, dietary, and behavioral factors. The length and configuration of the large intestine is greatly influenced by the fiber content of ingested foods. Several studies have shown that a lifelong diet high in bran tends to elongate the distal large intestine. Undigestible fiber increases the bulk of the stool, which gradually widens and lengthens the bowel. In countries and regions where unrefined cereals remain the staple food, dolichocolon is expected in the majority of adults.[106] It can be rec-

ognized on plain films and barium enema by redundancy of the sigmoid colon. Instead of appearing as a gentle S-bend in the left lower quadrant, the convoluted sigmoid loop and its accompanying mesentery may be located in the right lower quadrant (Fig 2–25,5–49) and even in the mid-abdomen just below the transverse colon (Figs 2–24,5–53).

Increasing affluence and urbanization are global factors that have tended to decrease the percentage of people subsisting on unprocessed grain. Nevertheless, dolichocolon should be considered a normative bowel configuration for much of the world's population, especially in the less developed areas of Asia, Africa, and Latin America.

Although all individuals with redundancy of the large bowel are at risk for sigmoid volvulus, it appears to be more prevalent in those who eat a traditional diet and reside at high altitudes. By far the most common abdominal surgical emergency in the high Andes among the Quechua Indians in Cuzco, Peru, is sigmoid volvulus. It is seen less often in mestizo city dwellers in Cuzco, who participate in the money economy and are thus more likely to consume processed bread. In Lima, on the seacoast, sigmoid volvulus is relatively less frequent, even among Indian residents.[107] Bolivian tin miners who live and work above 10,000 feet also have a high prevalence of sigmoid volvulus.[108] It is commonplace as well in elevated areas of East Africa. In fact, sigmoid volvulus is the most important cause of large bowel obstruction at Black Lion Hospital in Addis Ababa, Ethiopia.[107] It is endemic on the north shore of Lake Victoria, in Uganda, primarily in those locales where the major source of calories is the bulky, high-residue green banana.[109] In miners in Zimbabwe, sigmoid volvulus was more prevalent when the staple was coarsely ground maize. The substitution of finely ground maize was associated with a decline in the incidence of this form of volvulus.[109] The added risk of altitude has not been fully explained. Perhaps an elongated sigmoid is more distended in its resting state and thus more apt to twist in individuals living in high plateaus and mountains who subsist on fiber-laden carbohydrates.

In Western countries, the effect of altitude is insignificant because the habitual consumption of low-residue grain retards colonic elongation. Most often, dolichocolon is seen in the senile, the retarded, and in long-time sufferers of Parkinson's disease. Unlike the thick-walled bowel found in sigmoid volvulus in otherwise normal people in the Third World, the twisted colon of impaired individuals in industrialized countries typically has thin walls reflecting muscular atrophy. In these patients,

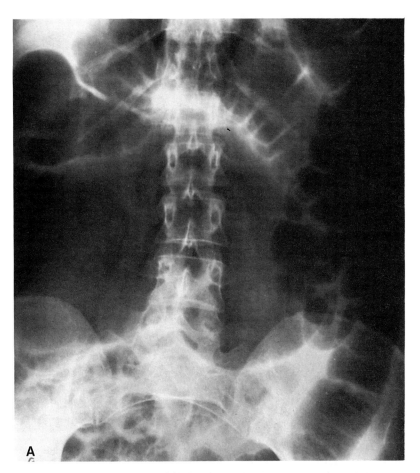

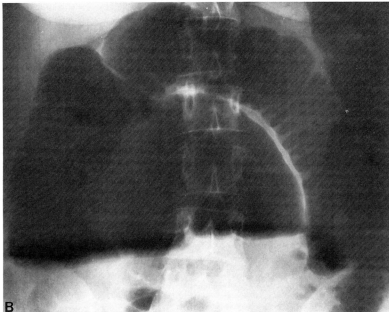

Figure 5–52. Cecal ileus. **A.** Supine view. There is diffuse dilatation of the colon, which is gas-filled but contains little feces. The cecum is especially dilated and extends from the periphery of the right abdomen across the midline. **B.** Upright projection confirms the preponderance of gas in both the dilated distal colon and the large cecum.

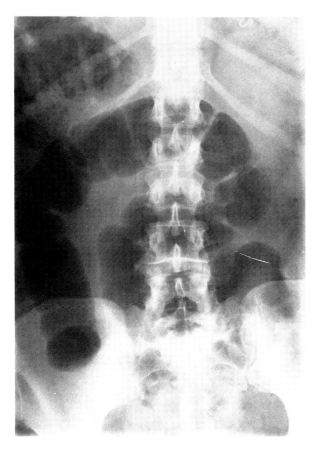

Figure 5–53. Elongated sigmoid colon rises first across the midline and then turns to the right before descending into the pelvis. Such a configuration predisposes to sigmoid volvulus.

chronic fecal impaction gradually leads to an increase in the dimensions of the sigmoid lumen, thereby favoring the development of volvulus.

Sigmoid volvulus involves torsion along both the mesenteric axis and the long axis of the bowel. It is the axial rotation that is responsible for the beak-like obstruction best seen on barium enema.[110] The occluded sigmoid loop may twist between 180 and 540 degrees. Hence, there is a heightened possibility of vascular insufficiency if the obstruction is not relieved. The sigmoid loop fills with gas, rapidly ballooning superiorly from its point of fixation, which usually overlies the sacrum or upper pelvis. Although intraluminal secretions also occupy the distending segment, it is gas that predominates (Fig 5–54). A characteristic finding, seen in nearly every case, is the upward migration of the sigmoid loop crossing above the transverse colon, almost always ascending superior D10. The loop may be situated in the midline but more often it rises either to the right or left upper quadrants where it can elevate a hemidiaphragm. Superimposed over the hepatic shadow, the gas-filled sigmoid colon may simulate

the appearance of a pneumoperitoneum (Fig 5–55).[111]

Other features that identify a sigmoid volvulus are the lack of haustra and septa in the gas-filled loop and its inverted "U" configuration. The dilated sigmoid lacks the undulating course of normal bowel, appearing as a continuous single curve reminiscent of a bent inner tube (Fig 5–56).[112] A frequently sought plain film finding is the pelvic convergence of three vertical lines, lines representing the two lateral walls of the loop as it abuts other bowel segments and the middle line is the shadow of the coapted medial walls. Such a configuration requires that the two arms of a sigmoid volvulus lie side by side with respect to the X-ray beam. The "three-line" sign is uncommon because in the majority of cases on supine films the two limbs of the volvulus are not aligned astride each other but rather overlap to some extent.

Inasmuch as sigmoid volvulus is a closed-loop obstruction, the more proximal colon is also blocked. Hence, dilatation of the right, transverse, and left colon complicates the radiographic appearance. The

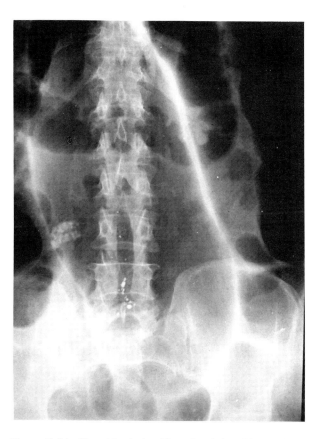

Figure 5–54. Sigmoid volvulus. The twisted sigmoid extends superiorly from the pelvis. It contains mostly gas and lacks haustra or septa.

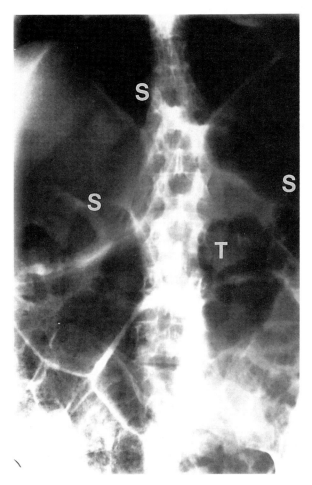

Figure 5–55. The upward extent of a sigmoid volvulus is clearly seen in this case. The twisted sigmoid loop (S) fills the upper abdomen well above the transverse colon (T).

moid torsion. In colonic ileus, distension of the sigmoid can be seen as a large lucency emanating from the pelvis but regardless how dilated the unobstructed sigmoid becomes, it does not reach above the transverse colon. Additionally, prone films show a continuous intraluminal expanse of gas extending to the rectum. Simple blockage of the rectosigmoid can resemble a sigmoid volvulus. Usually, differentiation between the two forms of obstruction rests on the demonstration of the characteristic upward migration of the twisted sigmoid colon to just beneath the diaphragm. In some cases, however, uncomplicated mechanical obstruction and volvulus appear remarkably similar on plain films, especially if the large intestine is elongated. Finally, ileosigmoid knot, also common in Africans eating a traditional diet, is recognized by the rightward position of the sigmoid colon and the presence of dilated ileal loops in the left abdomen. Rarely is colonic dilatation as marked in ileosigmoid knot as it is in the usual case of sigmoid volvulus.

Transverse Colon Volvulus

The third most common large bowel twisting obstruction is transverse colon volvulus. Although it is

distended proximal loops maintain their septa and haustra and usually remain in their expected location (Fig 5–57). Despite the dilatation of the proximal colon, in most cases of sigmoid volvulus, small bowel distension is absent.

Several conditions, both normal and abnormal, can mimic sigmoid volvulus. A redundant but gas-filled transverse colon can descend into the pelvis. An elongated transverse colon, however, retains septa and haustra and still maintains its position as the most superior large-bowel segment in the mid-abdomen (Fig 5–58).[113] Typically, small-bowel volvulus or other closed-loop obstructions are fluid-filled, but in rare cases, air distends the occluded segment. The convex margin of the U-shaped lucent loop in small-bowel volvulus is oriented inferiorly, distinctly different from the inverted U of a sigmoid volvulus (Fig 5–15). The absence of proximal colonic dilatation, an origin outside the pelvis, and retention of septa distinguish cecal volvulus from sig-

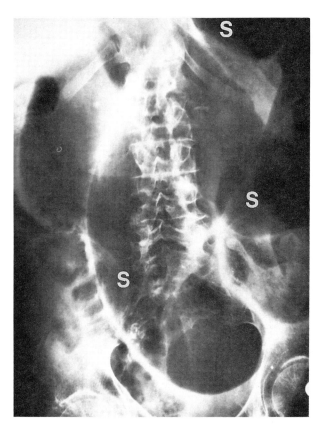

Figure 5–56. Torsion of the sigmoid loop (S) appears as a stiff curvilinear segment of dilated bowel.

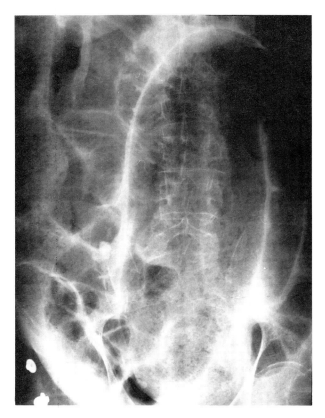

Figure 5–57. Sigmoid volvulus. The markedly distended sigmoid is superimposed on the lumbar spine. The more proximal colon is also obstructed by the volvulus. It is distended and contains feces but is not displaced from its expected location. (*Courtesy of Dr. Jutta Greweldinger.*)

responsible for only 4% to 11% of colonic torsions, its mortality rate is three times that of cecal volvulus and more than 50% greater than sigmoid volvulus. The configuration of the bowel and its mesenteric attachments are the important predisposing factors. A lax mesentery and a mobile redundant transverse colon are essential, but there must also be a relatively narrow base of fixation of the transverse mesocolon, which enables the bowel to twist on itself. Precipitating factors include adhesions, which limit the unimpeded movement of the transverse colon, and distal occlusion, which causes proximal bowel distension. Decreased abdominal wall muscular tone during pregnancy or after surgery also provides space for the torsion to develop.[114,115]

The radiographic appearance is variable on supine views. Typically, the proximal colon is dilated and is situated near its expected position. The small bowel is also distended and air-filled (Fig 5–59). This is sometimes a plain film pattern of simple transverse colon obstruction, however, and often a barium enema is needed to demonstrate the characteristic beak at the point of occlusion of the volvulus.

Splenic Flexure Volvulus

Splenic flexure volvulus is very rare, with only 15 cases reported by 1979.[116] Because the anatomic splenic flexure is almost always fixed to the posterior peritoneal wall, there is little opportunity for a normally attached bowel to undergo torsion. Mobility of the splenic flexure, often a result of disruption of anchoring ligaments at previous surgery, allows for mobility of the splenic flexure. A helpful plain film finding is a large featureless left upper quadrant lucency that can be mistaken for a distended stomach. It is usually seen in association with a separate stomach bubble and with proximal dilatation of the colon.[116,117]

Cecosigmoid Volvulus

Cecosigmoid volvulus is a twisting together of the cecum and sigmoid colons (Fig 5–60). It should be distinguished from ileosigmoid knot, which occurs without cecal involvement. Despite the frequency of mobility at the cecum and sigmoid this is a very rare lesion. On plain films it resembles a cecal volvulus, with the involvement of the sigmoid colon initially revealed at surgery unless a preoperative barium enema has been performed.[118]

Intussusception

Unlike childhood intussusception, which is painful and has an abrupt onset, adult intussusception is a more insidious form of intestinal obstruction. Bowel occlusion may wax and wane over several months, often experienced by the patient as intermittent bouts of bloating, pain, and constipation. More than 90% of affected individuals have underlying lesions.[119] In 50% to 70% of cases, there is an intestinal tumor at the site of the occlusion.[120] Most of these lesions are malignant, but benign neoplasms may also lead to intussusception. Other causes include inflammatory strictures and Meckel's diverticulum.[121] The intermittent nature of the obstruction may prompt repeated plain films. If the intussusception is of the ileocolic or colicolic type the pathognomonic crescent sign may be seen on occasion. As the intussuscipiens invaginates into the intussusceptum it stretches the outer bowel wall. Intraluminal gas trapped between the two intestinal surfaces can appear as a semilunar lucency lacking septa and valvulae conniventes. The crescent is wider than the normal bowel diameter and is often superimposed on a rounded soft tissue density representing the mass created by the telescoping of the bowel.[122,123] Within this lucent arc may be seen trapped gas situated in the lumen of the intussuscipiens. It has a less distinctive configuration than the more peripheral crescent sign. A helpful ancil-

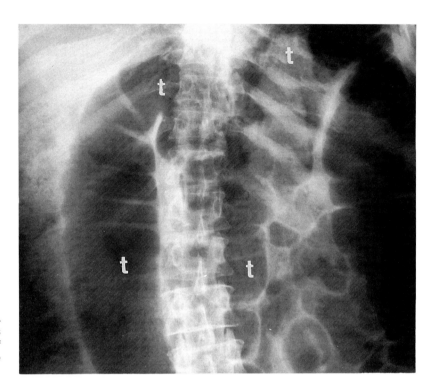

Figure 5–58. Pseudosigmoid volvulus. A widely undulating transverse colon (t) simulates a twisted sigmoid loop. Note the maintenance of septa. There is no loop above the transverse colon.

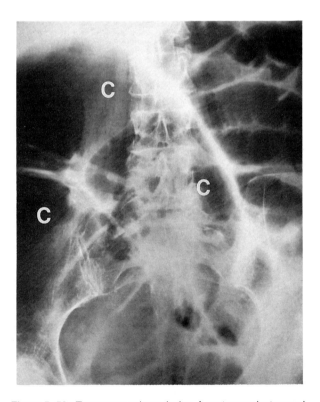

Figure 5–59. Transverse colon volvulus. A postappendectomy adhesion at the proximal transverse colon was the focus of the twist. The right colon (C) is markedly dilated. There is also a secondary small bowel obstruction evidenced by dilated paramedian and left sided ileal and jejunal loops. A normal transverse colon gas shadow is not seen.

lary finding of intussusception on supine views is absence of the transverse colon gas shadow because this bowel segment is usually displaced distally (Fig 5–61).[124]

Diverticulosis of the Left Colon

There is an interesting epidemiologic relationship between volvulus and diverticulosis of the sigmoid colon. In regions in which volvulus is endemic, diverticulosis is almost unknown. On the other hand, diverticular disease is common and increasing in incidence in industrialized countries even as volvulus remains an infrequently encountered abnormality. In the United States diverticulosis is seldom present in persons under age 40 but with advancing age the prevalence of the disease rises,[125,126] so that by age 80, more than 70% of women and 50% of men have at least one or more diverticula.[127] It can occur in any colonic segment (although it is exceedingly rare in the rectum), but the sigmoid is involved in 90% of cases.[128] Indeed, most commonly, diverticula are distributed exclusively in the sigmoid segment. Approximately one third of patients with sigmoid diverticulosis have fewer than five outpouchings, another third have 6 to 15, and the remaining third have many protrusions through the bowel wall.[129] Occasionally, diverticula retain colonic gas, and massed diverticulosis can be identified on plain films as a collection of small, sharply margined round lucencies in the pelvis or left lower quadrant. They

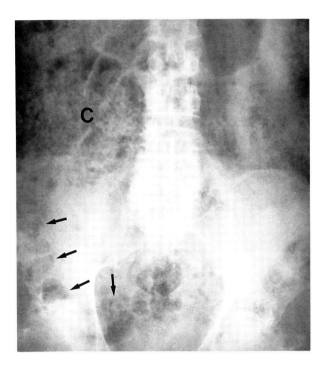

Figure 5–60. Sigmoid on a long mesentery (*arrows*) in the right lower quadrant. Cecum on a long mesentery (C) directed medially. This patient is at risk for a cecosigmoid volvulus.

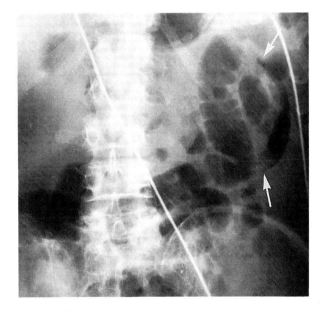

Figure 5–61. Intussusception of the colon. Gas between the intussuscipiens and the stretched intussusceptum appears as a crescent (*arrows*). Within the arc of the crescent are nondescript collections of gas that are in the lumen of the intussuscipiens. A dilated small bowel loop indicates obstruction more distally. Transverse colon gas is absent because that colonic segment is participating in the intussusception.

often have a range of sizes reflecting the varying diameters of colonic diverticula. In 1955, Massik and Wheatley identified gas in diverticula on scout films of the abdomen in approximately 3% of patients undergoing barium enema examination.[130] Most likely plain film recognition is even more frequent today as diverticulosis has become more prevalent.

As seen on supine films, the convoluted course of the sigmoid colon in the pelvis may group the diverticula in a roughly circular (Fig 5–62) or ovoid conformation (Fig 5–63). Pelvic gas-containing abscesses from whatever cause (including diverticular abscesses) can resemble gas-filled diverticula. Pus collections tend to be roughly spherical and contain an admixture of gas and liquid. Therefore, each separate bubble is usually smaller and less black than the lucent shadows that identify gas-filled diverticula (Fig 5–64). Another mimic is an ulcerating rectal tumor with the extraluminal penetration of flatus similar in shape but less numerous than those seen in massed sigmoid diverticulosis (Fig 5–65).

Rising out of the pelvis the colon can be seen in profile along the left lower edge of the peritoneal cavity. Gas-containing diverticula situated at the colonic margin sometimes stand out in a row along the medial aspect of the bowel (Fig 5–66). Other diverticula attached to the anterior or posterior colonic surface project within the outline of the lumen (Fig 5–67). If small rounded lucencies are seen along the lateral aspect of the left colon, they are usually not diverticula but discrete, intraluminal collections of flatus in a normal large intestine separated from the rest of the colonic gas shadow by solid feces and liquid secretions (Fig 5–68).

Giant Colonic Diverticulum

A rare complication of diverticulosis is the giant colonic diverticulum (GCD). Also known as a giant gas cyst,[131] giant solitary gas cyst,[132], giant diverticulum of the sigmoid colon,[133] and giant sigmoid diverticulum,[134] GCD appears to form within an extramural abscess after an episode of diverticulitis.[135,136] Evidence for the inflammatory etiology of a GCD is the histology of its wall, which is composed of fibrous and vascular granulation material surrounding isolated strands of mucosal epithelium. Varying amounts of other colonic layers, including muscularis mucosa and muscularis propria may be scattered in its cystic lining, raising the question as to whether this is a pseudodiverticulum or a true diverticulum containing all bowel wall constituents.[137] One explanation for the genesis of a GCD is that it results from an asymptomatic gas-forming infection occurring in a preexisting normal sized diverticulum with an occluded neck. Bacterial

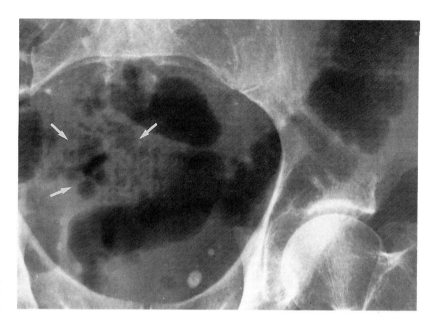

Figure 5–62. Gas in sigmoid diverticula (*arrows*). They have varying diameters and are situated along the convoluted course of the bowel.

excavation widens and weakens the diverticular walls, expanding the dimensions of the outpouching. Rarely, however, is diverticulitis clinically silent. More likely, the partial resolution of a diverticular abscess narrows the neck of a single diverticulum, allowing ingress of gas but restricting egress. Such a ball valve type process can lead to the slow but steady enlargement of a gas-filled sac.[137] Often the aperture is very small, preventing the entry of barium (Fig 5–69). In some cases, however, the opening is wide, allowing free flow of gas and barium in and out of the diverticulum (Fig 5–70).[138]

GCD is found in middle-aged and elderly individuals—the youngest patient reported was 38 years old.[139] More than 90% of cases of GCD involve the sigmoid, with the remainder found in the transverse[140,141] or descending[142] colon. Most patients complain of a protracted history of poorly defined pain, others note an expanding but otherwise asymptomatic mass, and a few present with a rapid onset of signs and symptoms of acute diverticulitis.[139,143] On occasion, the lesion is discovered incidentally on plain films or at barium enema. Reported complications of GCD include perforation with and without pneumoperitoneum,[142,144] volvulus,[145] and carcinoma.[142]

The diverticulum is always located on the antemesenteric border of the colon. It may attain a large size, sometimes exceeding 20 cm in diameter.[134] Most are between 5 and 15 cm in width, appearing as a round or oval unilocular gas collection.[141] The radiological hallmarks of a GCD are its marked lucency, because it contains mostly flatus and little fluid, its smooth walls, and its featureless interior.

Since it is attached to the sigmoid colon it may change position on successive radiographs obtained minutes to hours apart.[139] After initial recognition, it can enlarge steadily over weeks to months. Usually, a GCD is situated over the sacrum or left iliac fossa but it may appear anywhere in the lower peritoneal cavity.

Simulators of a Giant Colonic Diverticulum

The roentgenographic appearance of a giant colonic diverticulum (GCD) is striking but not pathognomonic. Several other conditions also appear on plain films as a well-marginated single lucency (Table 5–4). Generally, they can be distinguished from GCD on the basis of age of onset and clinical presentation.

Meckel's diverticulum is the persistent remnant of the embryonic omphalomesenteric duct and is found in approximately 2% of the population.[146] In most cases, it is small and innocuous. In less than 5%, it is clinically apparent—usually in children or young adults—when it ulcerates, becomes infected, or causes obstruction. Bowel occlusion can result from diverticulitis, volvulus, intussusception, incarceration within an internal hernia, or compression of adjacent bowel loops. It is very rare for a large Meckel's diverticulum to accumulate gas. When it does, it usually has an elongated configuration, but it can resemble a GCD if it appears as a homogeneous ovoid lucency in the lower abdomen.[147]

Duplication of the colon can be either total or partial. An incomplete duplication may have a spherical or a tubular configuration and almost always contains fluid. Rarely, a duplication is seen

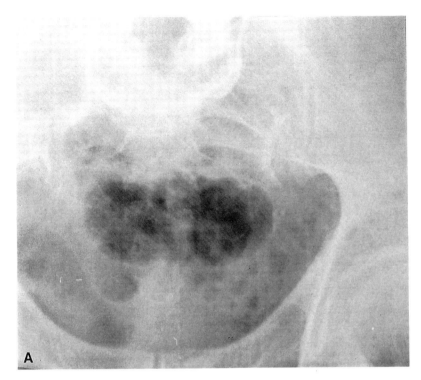

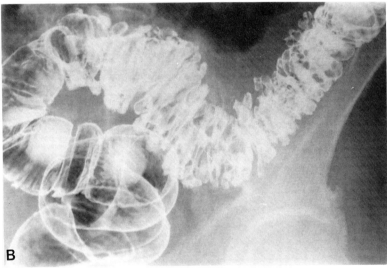

Figure 5–63. A. Diverticula appear as a group of black circles in the left pelvis. **B.** Barium enema confirms the presence of extensive diverticulosis in the same location.

on plain films as a featureless lucency if it communicates with adjacent bowel.[148] Large bowel duplications are less common than those arising from the small intestine, and in most cases they are situated near the ileocecal valve.[149] Confined to the mesenteric margin of the bowel, they are located lateral to the ascending and descending colon and superior to the transverse colon.[150] Duplications are almost always recognized in infancy or in the first two decades of life. The incidental appearance of colonic duplication on plain films in an adult patient is distinctly uncommon.

Giant duodenal diverticula resembles GCDs in appearance, although they sometimes have a more angulated margin. They are seen in the upper or mid-abdomen because of their connection to the duodenal sweep. On plain films a giant diverticulum of the descending or transverse colon may be indistinguishable from a large duodenal diverticula (Fig 2–38).

A homogeneously lucent blind pouch of small bowel may develop 5 to 15 years after a side-to-side intestinal anastomosis (Fig 5–71). It forms more often on the afferent side. To avoid this complication, the distal remnant of the afferent loop should be made as small as possible, as even a three-quarter

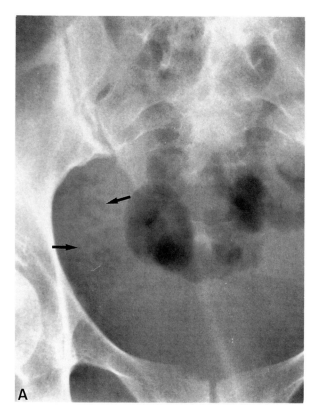
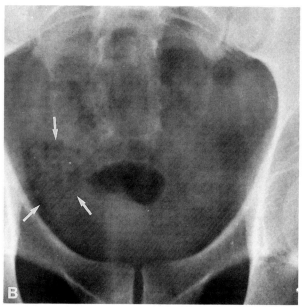

Figure 5–64. Two examples of pelvic abscesses both due to diverticulitis. **A.** The bubbles are faint and of similar size (*black arrows*). **B.** The abscess is more discrete (*white arrows*) but each bubble lacks the sharp margination of gas in a noninflamed diverticulum.

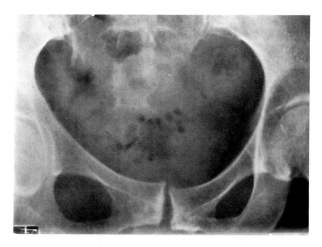

Figure 5–65. Several rounded lucencies adjacent to a larger but fainter and more amorphous lucency are plain film findings of an ulcerating rectal leiomyosarcoma.

inch excluded segment may dilate into a large balloon-like cul-de-sac after several years.[151] Like the more familiar blind loop created by intestinal surgery, a blind pouch can cause bloating, failure to thrive, anemia, and hemorrhage. Generally, blind pouches are fluid-filled and asymptomatic. On occasion, they can be seen as a homogeneous saccular lucency that lacks the signature of large or small bowel.[152] Although seldom located in the pelvis, they can be seen anywhere in the mid-abdomen, either centrally or peripherally, dependent, of course, on the location of the anastomosis.

Gas in the normal cecum may lack the identifying marker of a colonic septum (Fig 5–72). A repeat film usually reveals a change in configuration of the cecal gas bubble that distinguishes it from the fixed dimensions of a blind pouch or a GCD.

Emphysematous cystitis typically appears as a large, round pelvic lucency. The inevitable location of its lower border across the midline just above the symphysis pubis is a distinctive finding (Fig 2–48). Gas-containing abscesses and ulcerating intestinal neoplasms may both be noted on plain films as a single area of decreased density. Generally, they are

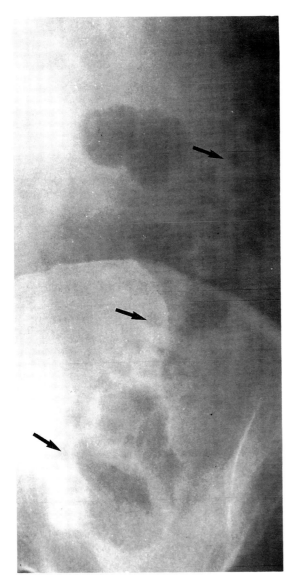

Figure 5–66. A chain of lucencies primarily along the medial aspect of the descending colon (*arrows*) represent gas in diverticula.

gray, not black, reflecting the presence of fluid in the cavity. Pus collections often contain small bubbles adjacent to a larger unilocular lucency (Fig 2–50).[153] Typically, ulcerating tumors have irregular margins (Fig 2–53). In almost every case large abscesses and excavating neoplasms can be distinguished from a GCD.

Bowel Neoplasms—Deformity of the Intestinal Gas Pattern

Usually, plain film evidence for a neoplasm of the small and large bowel is based on a recognition of its complications. Intestinal obstruction is the most common adverse consequence of bowel tumors that can be discerned on survey radiographs. However,

the location and extent of the tumor is rarely seen in association with obstructive changes. Bowel masses can also perforate, becoming manifest on noncontrast abdominal X-rays with signs of a localized abscess (Fig 5–73), a pneumoperitoneum (Fig 3–19), a pneumoretroperitoneum (Fig 2–44), or gas in the soft tissues in the abdominal wall (Fig 2–45). With these complications too, the presence and the site of the bowel lesion are deduced but rarely displayed.

Direct signs of an intestinal mass require either calcification within the tumor (see below), displacement of adjacent structures by the growing lesion, or deformity of the bowel wall. The latter is often an inconstant finding, dependent entirely on intraluminal gas to outline the margins of the tumor.

There are four ways in which an intestinal mass alters the bowel gas pattern. The most frequent appearance is a narrowing of the lumen. Typically, the strictured segment is seen as a thin band of lucency that persists on successive studies (Figs 2–33, 5–74). Usually, it has a straightened or rigidly curving contour, markedly different from the gentle arcs described by normal bowel. There can be great variation in the contour of the stricture. In some tumors,

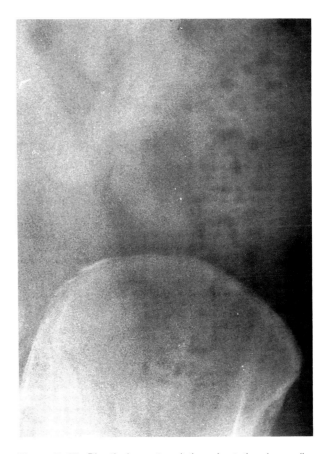

Figure 5–67. Diverticula scattered throughout the descending colon.

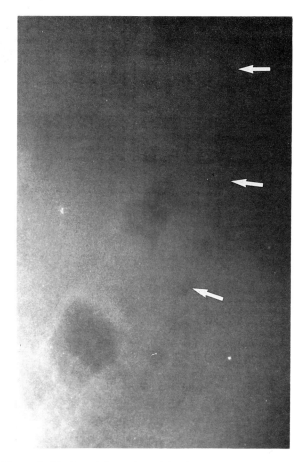

Figure 5–68. Coned-down view of the descending colon. The lateral, round lucencies (*arrows*) are not within diverticula. They are isolated intraluminal gas in normal, nondistended bowel.

the walls are smooth and roughly parallel whereas in others nodularity and irregular widths characterize the mucosal margin. Long, narrowed segments may contain only scattered gas, appearing as separated areas of slit-like lucencies (Fig 5–75). Occasionally, both the bulkiness and cicatrizing tendencies of a carcinoid tumor can be appreciated on plain films as a large mass that has trapped and constricted several loops of bowel (Fig 5–76).

Luminal stenosis is by no means an exclusive feature of indigenous malignancy of the bowel. Ischemic fibrosis, intramural hemorrhage, radiation change, metastatic deposits, and inflammatory bowel disease can also narrow the lumen. Generally, long strictures are not due to primary cancer, but there are too many exceptions to this rule to rely on it unreservedly.

Ulceration within an intestinal mass allows intraluminal gas to enter the excavation. Such an occurrence is rare in carcinoma but can be seen occasionally in small bowel leiomyosarcomas and leiomyomas (Fig 2–53). Infrequently, a polypoid le-

sion can be seen as a rounded intraluminal density if it is surrounded by gas in a dilated bowel. Nevertheless, the presence of adjacent feces usually makes it very difficult to recognize most endophytic, nonobstructing colon carcinomas. Large, smooth benign lesions in both intestines may be recognized if they project within gas-filled distended bowel. Lipoma is the most readily visible because its intermediate density provides a contrast with both intraluminal gas and the bowel wall (Fig 2–31).

Aneurysmal dilatation, the fourth deforming pattern, is an uncommon but distinctive characteristic of non-Hodgkin's lymphoma of the intestine.[154] Infiltration of the bowel wall by this nonfibrosing tumor weakens intestinal muscle and obliterates colonic septa and valvulae conniventes. The plain film findings are often spectacular (Fig 5–77). One or several long segments can appear as rigid, sausage-shaped lucencies. The adjacent bowel may be normal or narrowed. Such elongated and featureless black shadows are not pathognomonic for non-Hodgkin's lymphoma, however. Dilated distorted gas-filled bowel can be seen in Crohn's disease, mesenteric ischemia, and closed loop obstruction. Rarer causes include Meckel's diverticulum, which is more often tubular than round or oval, and partial duplication of the terminal ileum or right colon (Table 5–5).

Ulcerative Colitis

The plain film is rarely helpful if ulcerative colitis is confined to the rectum alone or if only superficial

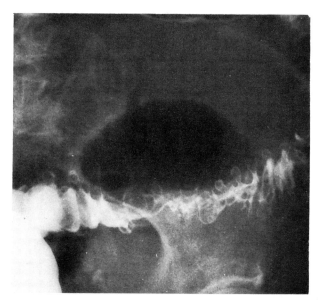

Figure 5–69. A giant colonic diverticulum that does not fill with barium.

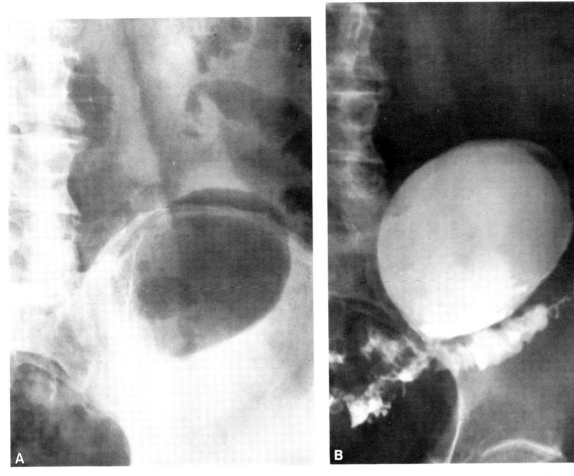

Figure 5–70. Giant colonic diverticulum. **A.** Plain film reveals a large lucency overlapping the left iliac bone. **B.** At barium enema, the diverticulum fills with contrast material. (*Courtesy of Dr. John Adler*).

layers of the colon are involved, even if all of the large intestine is affected. Nonetheless, noncontrast abdominal radiographs can be diagnostic in both the subacute and chronic phases of ulcerative colitis if the inflammation penetrates deep into the bowel wall. Previous reports have emphasized observation

TABLE 5–4. LOWER ABDOMEN—ROUNDED FEATURELESS LUCENCY

1. Giant colonic diverticulum
2. Normal cecum
3. Cecal distension
   Ileus
   Volvulus
   Bascule
4. Meckel's diverticulum
5. Communicating partial duplication
6. Blind pouch
7. Emphysematous cystitis
8. Gas-containing abscess
9. Ulcerating intestinal tumor

of mural thickening as a good radiographic sign of extensive involvement in ulcerative colitis. Normally, the wall should not exceed 2 mm in width, but in severe cases, a 1-cm thickness is not uncommon.[155] The determination of bowel width requires gas in the lumen and a clearly defined interface between the serosa and pericolic fat. Incomplete distension of the bowel and the failure to discern bordering adipose tissue limit the applicability of this sign.

More rewarding is the assessment of the mucosal margin of the large bowel. Approximately 50% of patients with extensive, nonfulminant ulcerative colitis have sufficient intraluminal gas in at least one segment of large bowel to evaluate the mucosal interface.[156] On supine views, gas tends to collect in the least dependent segment, usually the sigmoid or transverse colon. When seen in profile, the pseudopolyps of active ulcerative colitis can be recognized by their lumpy impressions on the bowel gas shadow. En face, they appear as well-defined nodular densities within the lumen.[155] These nodular

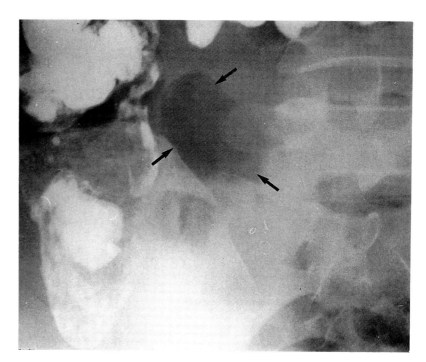

Figure 5–71. A blind pouch (*arrows*) appearing as a featureless lucency that came to attention several years after a side-to-side intestinal anastomosis.

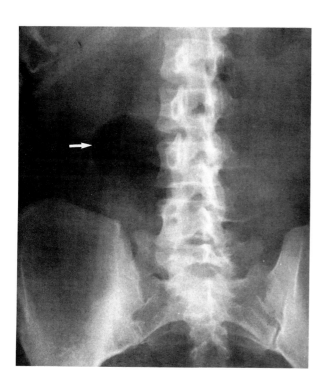

Figure 5–72. A cecum filled with gas (*arrow*) in an otherwise gasless abdomen. It can be mistaken for other causes of a simple featureless lucency.

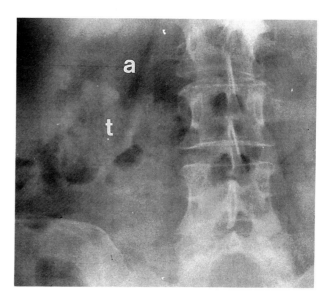

Figure 5–73. Perforated carcinoma of the transverse colon. Feces in the bowel lumen (t) is situated inferior to a contiguous gas-filled abscess cavity (a).

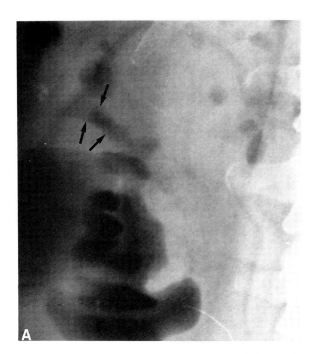
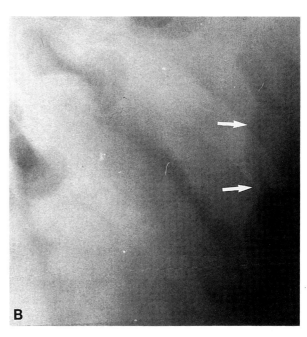

Figure 5–74. Narrowed lumen due to constricting carcinoma. **A.** Malignant stricture of the ascending colon (*arrows*). **B.** Descending colon carcinoma. The stenotic bowel has smooth walls.

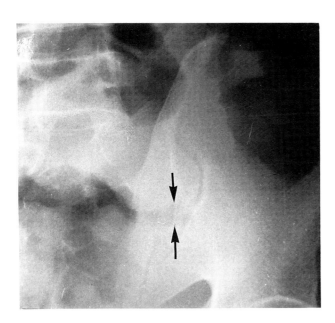

Figure 5–75. Sigmoid carcinoma. The arrows indicate the distal end of a long malignant stricture. The proximal end does not contain gas. The normal distal descending colon is dilated.

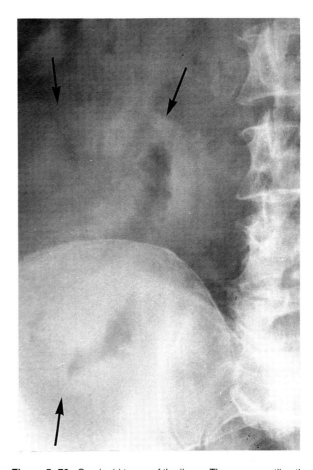

Figure 5–76. Carcinoid tumor of the ileum. The arrows outline the extent of the mass. Within it are fixed loops of distal small bowel.

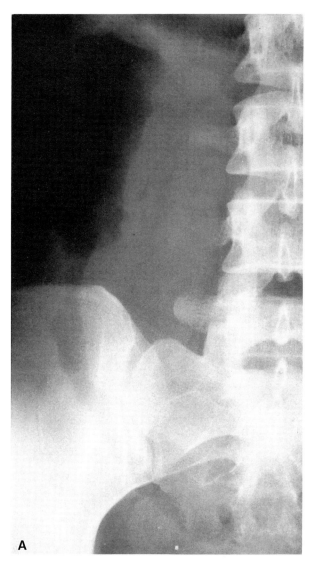
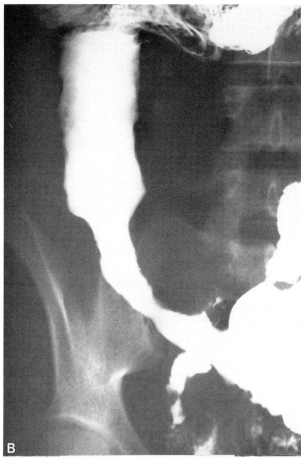

Figure 5–77. Non-Hodgkin's tumor of the distal small bowel. **A.** The plain film demonstrates a long narrowed segment of bowel with irregular walls. Immediately proximal is an aneurysmally dilated segment also infiltrated with tumor. **B.** The barium-filled small bowel study confirms the plain film findings.

impressions are usually numerous and closely grouped, and although many of the pseudopolyps have similar diameters it is distinctly unusual for them all to be of uniform size.

As the disease becomes quiescent, pseudopolyps resolve, leaving a scarred, narrowed, and short-

TABLE 5–5. LOWER ABDOMEN—ELONGATED FEATURELESS LUCENCY

1. Infarcted small bowel
2. Infarcted large bowel
3. Bowel tumor—aneurysmal dilatation
4. Inflammatory bowel disease
5. Meckel's diverticulum
6. Partial duplication

ened bowel whose walls lack the arcuate convexity of haustra and the intervening indentations of plica semilunaris.[157] The pattern of normal bowel has been altered by the intramural fibrosis induced by the disease. Moreover, the absence of feces is a peculiar feature of both active and quiescent ulcerative colitis. The typical gas-filled bowel in chronic ulcerative colitis resembles a stiff, hollow pipe with parallel walls having smooth or slightly irregular margins (Fig 5–78).

A dreaded complication of long-standing ulcerative colitis is the malignant degeneration of a segment of chronically inflamed mucosa. In most cases, such carcinomas are not polypoid, endophytic lesions but constricting tumors that sometimes come

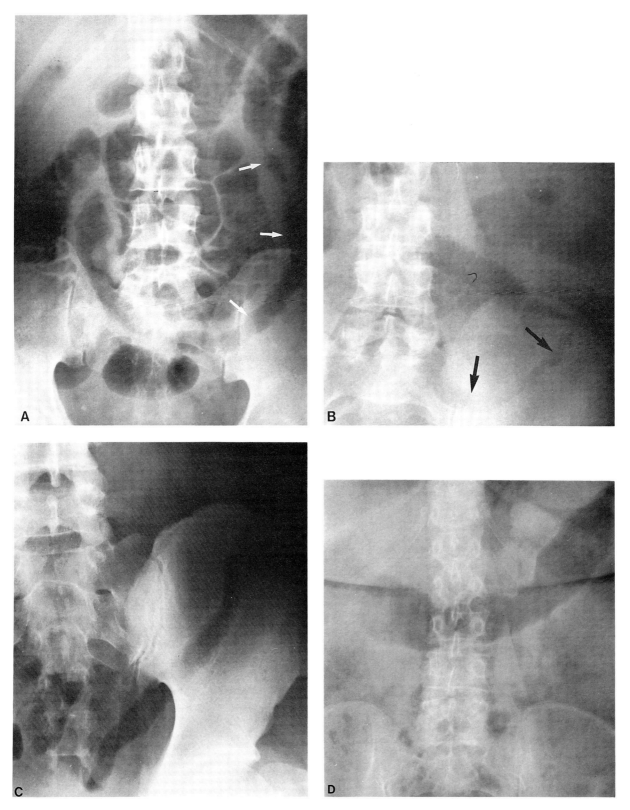

Figure 5–78. Four examples of chronic ulcerative colitis. **A.** Narrowed slightly irregular gas-filled descending and sigmoid colon (*arrows*). **B.** Long strictured area of sigmoid colon (*arrows*). **C.** Stiff pipelike sigmoid colon. **D.** An ahaustral gas-filled transverse colon.

to notice as a result of colonic obstruction. Marked accumulations of feces proximal to the lesion and an ahaustral but nondilated colon distally characterize the plain film appearance (Fig 5–79).

An interesting drug interaction can be responsible for some episodes of recurrence of active disease after long asymptomatic intervals. Azulfidine, which consists of equal parts of a 5-aminosalicylic acid and sulfapyridine, is an oral preparation effective in many patients with diffuse disease. The aspirin-like compound is the anti-inflammatory component, which becomes effective as it enters the colonic mucosa. Sulfapyridine is merely a carrier, preventing small bowel absorption of 5-aminosalicylic acid so that it can be delivered to the large bowel surface. Simultaneous administration of an opiate medication to prevent or treat diarrhea results in constipation, which inhibits the intraluminal transit of azulfidine. The drug cannot reach its destination and a recrudescence of acute inflammation is apt to occur. Affected patients are, in a sense, "constipated colitics," as the left colon is deprived of the benefit of azulfidine by the accumulation of

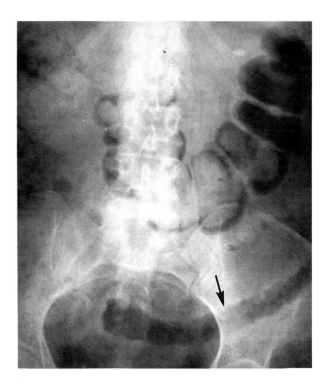

Figure 5–80. The "constipated colitic." This patient, well maintained on azulfidine, took Paregoric for several days in preparation for a trip abroad. The constipating effect of the medication resulted in the deposition of feces throughout the right and transverse colon. Azulfidine could not reach the left colon and a recurrence of acute ulcerative colitis is seen in the sigmoid colon. The arrow points to one of many pseudopolyps indenting the bowel wall.

feces more proximally. Withholding the constipating drug and continued treatment with azulfidine often can reverse the inflammation, restoring the patient to his or her previous asymptomatic state (Fig 5–80).

Not all instances of diffuse ulceration and pseudopolyp formation are due to idiopathic ulcerative colitis. Stenosis of the colon from carcinoma or any other chronic constriction can lead to proximal changes indistinguishable from ulcerative colitis.[158,159] It has been observed in diverticulitis, volvulus, Hirschsprung's disease, fecal impactions, radiation changes, and postoperative stricture. All these conditions can lead to proximal dilatation, with a decrease in mesenteric blood flow. Of all the bowel layers the mucosa is least able to withstand persistent or repeated periods of vascular insufficiency and is, therefore, most apt to develop ulcerations and edema.[160]

Rarely, the stenotic lesion may be seen on plain films but more often its consequences in the aboral colon are noted. A differentiating point between ulcerating colitis secondary to obstruction and idiopathic ulcerative colitis is the appearance of the large bowel distal to the site of narrowing. In obstructive

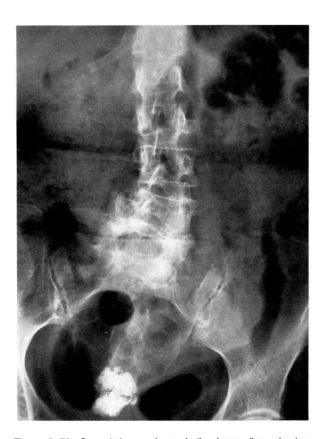

Figure 5–79. Constricting carcinoma in the descending colon in a patient with chronic ulcerative colitis. No haustra or plica are seen in the gas-filled descending and sigmoid colon. Obstruction by the tumor has resulted in massive fecal accumulation in the more proximal colon.

proximal colitis due to carcinoma, stricure, or abscess, the distal bowel is normal whereas in most cases of ulcerative colitis there is inflammatory involvement all the way to the rectum.

Toxic Megacolon

There are but very few life-threatening conditions in which the abdominal roentgenogram still remains the sole imaging study required to render an unequivocal diagnosis. Along with pneumoperitoneum, mesenteric ischemia, small bowel obstruction, colonic volvulus, and emphysematous cholecystitis, toxic megacolon must be included on this short list. In most instances, the plain film appearance is so distinctive that no other diagnosis need be considered. Furthermore, because the barium enema is a dangerous examination in fulminant colitis, exposing the patient to a heightened risk of large bowel perforation, the crucial role of noncontrast abdominal radiographs cannot be overemphasized.

Toxic megacolon is an acute dilatation of a segment of the large intestine. A typical clinical presentation is the rapid onset of abdominal pain and diarrhea, accompanied by high fever and severe debilitation. In untreated cases the mortality approaches 20% to 30%. The characteristic pathological features are diffuse transmural inflammation accompanied by focal to confluent areas of necrosis. Pseudopolyps, either singly or in clusters, are commonplace and are often present in juxtaposition with mucosal ulcerations. In areas of marked inflammation the colon is thickened but in adjacent bowel sloughing of mucosa results in a thin, fragile wall.[161] Usually, the rectum is spared but the more proximal large intestinal segments are involved, sometimes in isolation but also as a continuous lesion damaging much of the colon. In the past, the transverse colon has been thought to be particularly susceptible to toxic megacolon. The focus on transverse colon involvement may merely reflect the usual distribution of bowel gas in the supine position, however. Gas rises to the transverse colon because it is the least dependent section of the large intestine. Almost always, decubitus films can reveal similar changes in the ascending and descending colon.[162] Nevertheless, these additional projections are usually unnecessary because the extent of toxic megacolon is less important than the observation of its presence in at least one segment of the large bowel.

Dilatation is moderate in toxic megacolon, never as marked as the massive distension seen in cecal volvulus. Inasmuch as it is observed most often in the transverse colon, which can be far from the film in obese patients, the magnification effect makes the lumen appear even wider. Almost always, there is little feces within the dilated bowel. In areas of severest inflammation the haustra are effaced and the plica semilunaris are either absent or thickened. Pseudopolyps intrude into the lumen as homogeneous, rounded densities, and ulcerations can be appreciated as small protrusions of gas within the mucosal margin (Figs 2–37,5–81). The proximal accumulation of gas distends even noninvolved bowel, which maintains its normal landmarks of haustra and plica. In fact, pseudopolyps and a thickened, irregular wall need not be seen on every abdominal radiograph. McConnell et al studied the plain abdominal films of 27 patients with the fulminant form of ulcerating colitis.[163] Sixteen had nodular impressions on the colonic gas shadow but only 11 had large bowel dilatation. Thus, there can be a resemblance between the radiographic appearance of some cases of toxic megacolon and adynamic ileus. The characteristic clinical presentation of toxic megacolon helps to differentiate it from other causes of large intestinal distension, however.

Although ulcerative colitis is the most common cause of toxic megacolon, an identical roentgenographic and clinical picture has been reported in granulomatous[164] amebic,[165,166] and pseudomembranous colitis.[167]

Crohn's Disease

Crohn's disease, also known as granulomatous colitis when confined to the large bowel, may look ex-

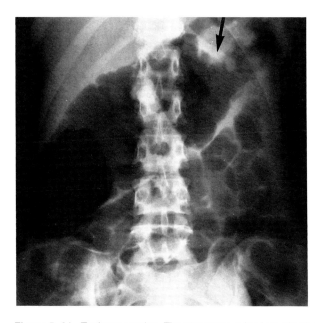

Figure 5–81. Toxic megacolon. The transverse colon is markedly dilated. The arrow points to a confluent area of pseudopolyps. Other pseudopolyps are also seen in this feces-free segment. The bowel wall is thin in the proximal transverse colon but thick near the splenic flexure.

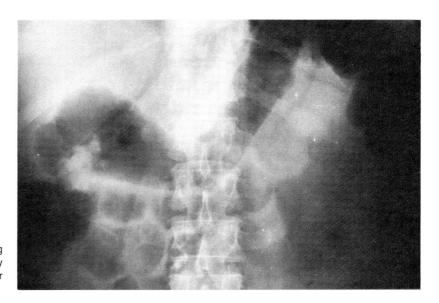

Figure 5–82. Granulomatous colitis involving the transverse colon. The bowel has a slightly bumpy contour superiorly and lacks haustra or plica semilunares.

actly like ulcerative colitis on plain films. The similarities can be seen in both the chronic form of the disease (Fig 5–82) and in its more fulminant manifestations. The tendency for stricture formation is a feature of granulomatous colitis that can be detected on noncontrast roentgenographs. An extended gas-filled stricture following the course of the colon is consistent with Crohn's disease (Fig 5–83) but can also be seen in ulcerative colitis, carcinoma, and in the healing phase of ischemic colitis.

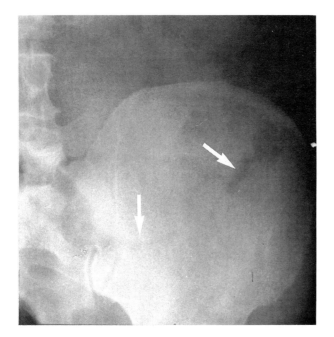

Figure 5–83. Granulomatous colitis. The arrows point toward a long stricture of the sigmoid colon.

Narrowing of the small bowel lumen is a feature of Crohn's disease not shared by ulcerative colitis. Nevertheless, it is uncommon to observe a stenotic small bowel segment on plain films because the gas is present less frequently in the jejunum and ileum than in the colon. In the right lower quadrant, Crohn's stricture can mimic air in the lumen of the appendix (Fig 5–84). After surgery, strictures may appear near the site of anastomosis (Fig 5–85). On occasion, marked stenosis results in the mechanical occlusion of the bowel lumen. Hence, a plain film manifestation of Crohn's disease is the pattern of simple small bowel obstruction (Fig 5–32). Less often, the intervening bowel between two stenoses can dilate markedly. If this segment contains air, it can be seen on plain films as an oblong lucency reminiscent of the dilated loop of small bowel volvulus, the configuration of a communicating partial duplication or even an elongated gas-filled Meckel's diverticulum (Fig 5–86).

Amebiasis

Amebiasis is endemic in many parts of the world. In most individuals, the parasite *Entamoeba histolytica* lives in a cyst form within the lumen of the large bowel, where it causes no symptoms. Invasive amebiasis with penetration of the colonic mucosa by the trophozoite form of the parasite is found in approximately 6% of cases. By far the most frequent manifestation of invasive amebiasis is ulcerative rectocolitis (greater than 90% of cases), which is usually undetected on plain films of the abdomen. In 3% of patients the infestation is confined to the cecum and appendix. Here, too, there is a paucity of plain film findings. Occasionally, the cecum may be gas-filled

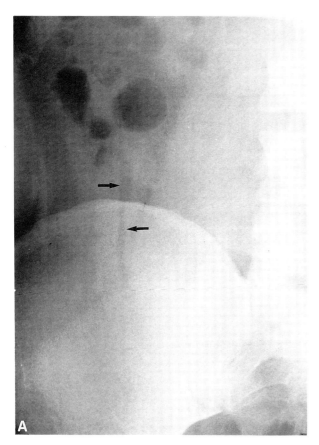 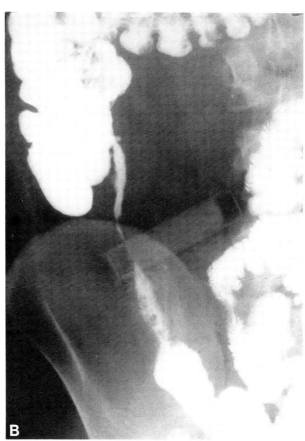

Figure 5–84. Crohn's disease. **A.** Long tubular stricture in the right lower colon contains gas (*arrows*). It resembles air in the appendix but its straightened configuration and the varying width of the lumen are unusual features of an appendiceal air pattern. The lucency is within a strictured segment of terminal ileum. **B.** A barium contrast small bowel series confirms the plain film findings.

and dilated, but this is a nonspecific indication of inflammation. In 1% to 2% of patients with invasive amebiasis, a discrete mass attached to the colonic wall develops. Amebomas may be single or multiple and are most frequent in the right colon but are rarely seen on plain films.[168]

In about 1% of patients with invasive amebiasis, the disease is fulminant.[168] Again, noncontrast films are usually unrewarding but two patterns of diffuse amebic colitis recognizable on plain films are toxic megacolon[168] and thumbprinting.[169] Amebiasis should always be considered in the differential diagnosis of fulminant colitis, especially in endemic areas or in travelers recently returning from places of high prevalence of the disease.

Pseudomembranous Colitis

Most bacterial infections of the large intestine are readily diagnosed without imaging tests. Moreover, the rapid course of these acute colitides usually obviates the need for roentgenographic studies.

Pseudomembranous colitis is an exception to the rule, as it often runs a protracted course. In almost every case, formation of the pseudomembranes is due to toxins elaborated by *Clostridium dificile*. Normally a minor component of the intestinal flora, *C dificile* is most apt to proliferate in patients receiving antibiotic therapy. Clindamycin was first implicated, but almost every other antimicrobial agent has been associated with the development of pseudomembranous colitis.

Endoscopic inspection of the large intestine reveals whitish deposits consisting of fibrin, mucus, inflammatory cells, and necrotic debris that appear either in patches or as extensive sheets on the mucosal surface. In severe cases, the entire epithelial lining of the colon may slough, but more often there are focal ulcerations placing the submucosa in contact with the pseudomembrane.[170] The lumen contains liquid feces often mixed with considerable amounts of bowel gas.

Stanley et al reported that plain films can be

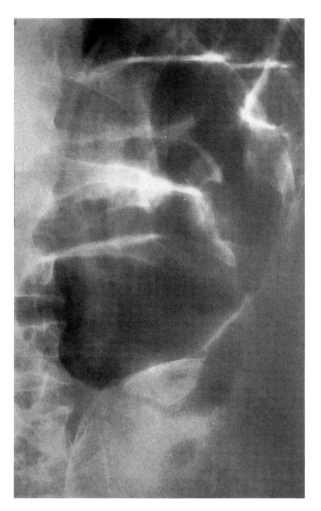

Figure 5–85. Recurrence of Crohn's disease after ileosigmostomy. Overlying the iliac crest is a stricture of the small bowel near the anastomotic site. The proximal small bowel is dilated.

diagnostic in severe forms of this entity. They observed distinctive wide transverse bands with shaggy edges, much thicker and more irregular than the normal plica semilunares.[171] Occasionally, thumbprinting also distorts the colonic contour.[172] Usually, the large bowel is moderately distended, but in some patients there is marked dilatation and the radiological and clinical features can be characterized as a toxic megacolon.[173] Small bowel dilatation is variable, but plain film changes in the jejunum and ileum are never as distinctive as those seen in the colon.[170,171]

Intestinal Hemorrhage

Bleeding into the bowel wall has many causes. A blow to the abdomen may induce an intestinal hematoma. Although most common in the duodenum, which is fixed in place and anchored to its retroperitoneal attachments, any segment of the more mobile small bowel or colon may be affected by blunt trauma. The intestinal mucosa is the mural layer most susceptible to anoxia. In both mesenteric ischemia and ischemic colitis, blood may escape into the lumen and into the submucosa, where it thickens folds and distorts the bowel contour. In the late stages of diffuse leukemia, tumor infiltrating the bowel wall causes intestinal hemorrhage. Anticoagulants must be carefully monitored so that their therapeutic effects are realized without inducing intraparenchymal bleeding. The widespread use of blood thinning agents has made intramural bowel hemorrhage a well-recognized complication, however. Any disorder of hemostasis, whether congenital or acquired, may present with intestinal wall accumulation of blood. Thus, it can be seen in such diseases as idiopathic thrombocytopenic purpura (ITP), hemophilia, and Henoch–Schonlein purpura.

None of the plain film findings of intestinal hemorrhage are specific, and a definitive diagnosis can only be made by correlating radiological evidence with the clinical story. Moreover, the plain film is also relatively insensitive, as the diagnosis rests on a deformation of the configuration of intraluminal air. In the absence of significant quantities of bowel gas the plain film is often an unrewarding examination for the recognition of intestinal hemorrhage.

Very large hematomas can appear as mass lesions that displace adjacent structures, especially nearby bowel loops. Intestinal segments may be moved toward the periphery of the hematoma if the blood is deposited eccentrically, but in circumferential mural accumulations the lumen is narrowed and usually confined within the center of the mass.[174] Large carcinoid tumors that trap bowel within them as they expand resemble giant hematomas of the bowel wall (Fig 5–76).

Smaller collections of blood within the intestinal wall narrow and straighten the bowel. Air-filled jejunum and ileum loops may appear as thin, rigid lucencies with irregular walls. In the right lower quadrant, a pencillike lumen surrounded by a swollen blood-filled bowel wall can be mistaken for a long ileal structure or even a gas-filled appendix (Fig 5–87).[175] A similar configuration of small intestine occurs in hereditary angioneurotic edema as the bowel is thickened by transudated fluid alone.[174,176.]

Another pattern of hemorrhage of the small bowel is the thickened fold sign. The submucosal penetration of blood into the valvulae conniventes widens these encircling indentations. The junction of each fold with the mural surface is no longer homogeneously perpendicular and sharply defined but assumes a more irregular and arcuate configu-

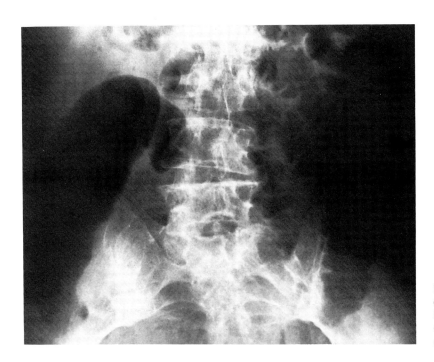

Figure 5–86. An elongated loop of dilated ileum in the right side of the abdomen is located between proximal and distal stricture due to Crohn's disease. The air-filled jejunum has an obstructive pattern.

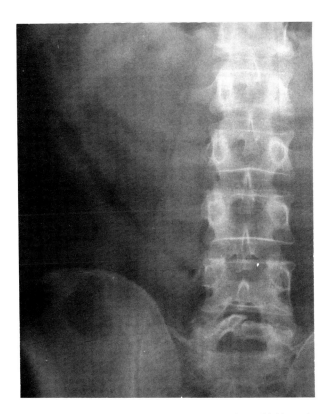

Figure 5–87. A long rigid loop of ileum in a patient with Henoch–Schonlein purpura. Blood in the wall narrows the lumen and straightens the bowel.

ration, reflecting the simultaneous infiltration of valvulae and bowel wall (Fig 5–88). In some cases, the appearance of the air-filled bowel segment suggests a stack of coins, each lucent band separated from the next by a broadened valvula.[174] The thick fold sign is usually observed in the jejunum because of the greater prominence of valvulae in the proximal bowel, but it may be evident in any portion of the small intestine.

The classic finding of thumbprinting helps identify segments of small bowel and colon infiltrated with blood. These smooth indentations of the luminal contour are not specific for hemorrhage, however, and can be found in any condition which widens the bowel. Thumbprinting may be seen in subacute and chronic inflammations of the large intestine, including ulcerative colitis (Fig 5–89),[155] Crohn's disease, amebiasis,[169] and pseudomembranous colitis.[172] Lymphoma, leukemia, and metastatic malignancy can produce numerous focal enlargements of the submucosa and subserosa. In ischemia of the large or small intestine, thumbprinting occurs in an adynamic bowel that is often air-filled, distended, and unchanging on successive views.[177] In the colon, however, thumbprinting need not be a harbinger of pathology but merely an evanescent finding reflecting spasm in an otherwise normal bowel (Fig 5–90).[178,179] As is true of other plain film signs the clinical significance of thumbprinting must be interpreted within a specific clinical context (Table 5–6).

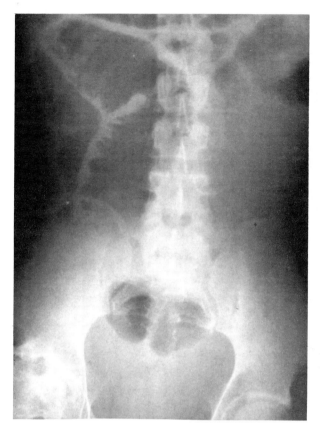

Figure 5–88. Thick wall sign due to intramural hemorrhage. Several small-intestinal loops are dilated and in one the valvular folds are thick and the bowel wall is bumpy. The patient has Christmas disease (clotting factor IX deficiency). Note also degenerative change in the right hip and evidence of aseptic necrosis of the femoral head, another feature of the disease due to chronic bleeding.

Acute Mesenteric Ischemia

Acute mesenteric ischemia, with its predilection for progressing rapidly to infarction, is almost always a dire emergency requiring expeditious treatment. Sometimes the clinical picture is characteristic and unequivocal; in the majority of cases, however, presenting signs and symptoms do not point directly to vascular insufficiency, and a search for other diagnoses is undertaken. Probably the greatest impediment to increased survival in these patients is the lack of clinical suspicion of acute mesenteric ischemia at the time of initial evaluation.

Many sufferers complain of the rapid onset of acute abdominal pain so that a supine radiograph is often obtained early in the workup. Except for the demonstration of gas in the bowel wall, mesenteric veins, and the portal veins—all of which are uncommon findings—there are no definitive plain film signs of intestinal ischemia. Nevertheless, morphological changes in the bowel wall and a particular distribution of intraluminal gas that frequently accompanies the progression from ischemia to infarction can be detected on noncontrast abdominal films.

Anoxia results in the loss of intestinal muscular tone. In the small bowel, mild dilatation ensues and the valvulae conniventes become effaced. At the same time, impending infarction causes a weakening of membrane integrity in the mucosal epithelial cells and in the endothelium of its capillaries. Hemorrhage into the submucosa produces bumpy protrusions of the bowel wall into the luminal gas shadow. The remaining valvulae may also widen as they swell with blood and edema fluid. Occasionally, focal indentations in the wall have the configuration of thumbprints. More diffuse mural infiltration narrows the lumen, and the boggy wall may appear rigid and straightened (Fig 5–91). The increased hydrostatic pressure attending mesenteric venous occlusion helps account for the pronounced changes in intestinal contour often seen in this form of ischemia.[180–182] Bowel wall thickening can also be seen when two gas-filled loops lie next to one another. Infarction need not always thicken the bowel, however, and dilated paper-thin segments of gangrenous intestine may be contiguous to edematous ischemic segments (Fig 5–36). Successive films taken over several hours can reveal a continuum of contour deformities in one loop—first nodular and then, as the ischemia becomes irreversible, smoother and more featureless margins.[183] Even if the territory of vascular insufficiency includes the large bowel, mural changes predominate in the small intestine (Fig 5–92).[59,180]

This constellation of abnormalities has been categorized in the literature as part of the complex of "specific" signs of mesenteric infarction. The term is a misnomer because none of the signs are specific. Nonischemic bleeding, inflammatory bowel disease, and infiltration by tumor can each distort the bowel wall in a similar way.

In a study of 68 patients with acute mesenteric infarction, Scott et al evaluated the frequency of these signs on plain films.[59] Most often seen was an edematous mucosa in a loop of air-containing bowel, which was noted in 43% of cases. A smooth bowel wall indicating effaced mucosa was found in 16% and in only 4% was thumbprinting observed. The yield of mural signs on plain films was only 16% in an investigation by Tomchik et al.[180] All the signs were uncommon when the etiology of the vascular insufficiency was nonocclusive disease (low-flow state) or arterial thrombosis, but in arterial embolus and venous thrombosis the frequency was 46% and 30%, respectively.

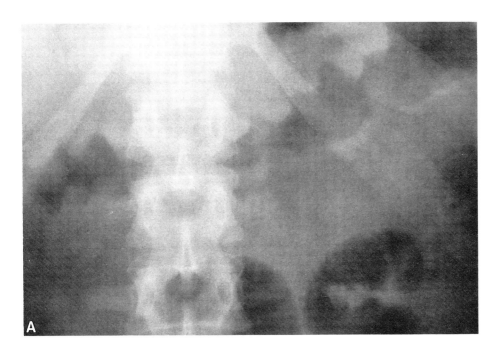

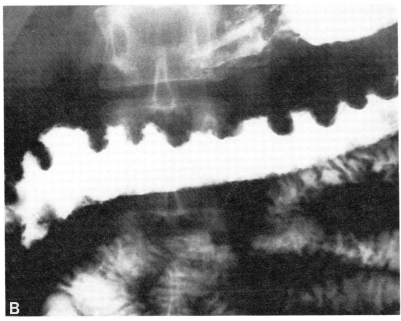

Figure 5–89. Thumbprinting in the transverse colon in a patient with ulcerative colitis. **A.** Plain film. **B.** Barium in the colon. Follow-up film from a small bowel series.

A distinctive distribution of gas in the small and large bowel is also a feature of acute mesenteric ischemia. In fact, the most common plain film finding is small bowel pseudo-obstruction (Fig 5–36) evidenced by minimal gas in the colon and air-filled distension of numerous jejunal and ileal loops. It was present in 50% of the patients studied by Scott et al[59] and in 36% of those reviewed by Tomchik et al.[180] Although no mechanical occlusion exists, atony in the distal small bowel induces a functional blockage to flow made visible on plain films by anxious patients who continue to swallow copious amounts of air. Sometimes, fluid predominates in one segment and the air appears as slits or streaks, a configuration identical to the stretch sign seen in fluid-filled intestinal segments proximal to a mechanical obstruction (Fig 5–93). A completely gasless abdomen is an unusual appearance in acute intestinal ischemia. Once a patient is placed on nasogastric suction, however, ingested air may be removed before it reaches the small bowel, and after residual intestinal gas is absorbed (a much slower process across the mucosa of ischemic bowel) the abdomen may become gasless.

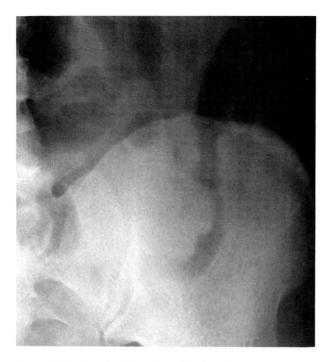

Figure 5–90. Thumbprinting. No wall lesion. A barium enema examination immediately afterwards revealed a normal sigmoid and descending colon.

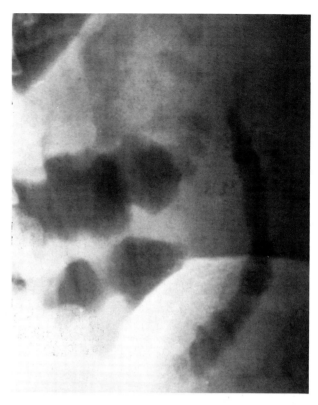

Figure 5–91. An infarcted gangrenous segment of jejunum appears as a stiff gas-filled loop situated over the left iliac crest. The wall is edematous, giving it a bumpy configuration.

The splenic flexure cutoff pattern in mesenteric ischemia was first described by Rendich and Harrington.[184] It consists of dilatation of the small bowel, the right colon, and the transverse colon to the splenic flexure with little gas beyond, a distribution of gas that matches the area of bowel sup-

TABLE 5–6. THUMBPRINTING

1. Nonischemic hemorrhage
   Trauma
   Anticoagulants
   Bleeding diatheses
     ITP
     Hemophilia
     Christmas disease
     Henoch–Schonlein purpura
     Acquired defects in hemostasis
2. Ischemia
   Arterial insufficiency
   Venous insufficiency
3. Inflammatory disease
   Ulcerative colitis
   Ulcerating colitis secondary to partial obstruction
   Crohn's disease
   Amebiasis
   Pseudomembranous colitis
4. Tumor
   Leukemic infiltrate
   Lymphoma
   Metastatic tumor
5. Functional
   Spasm

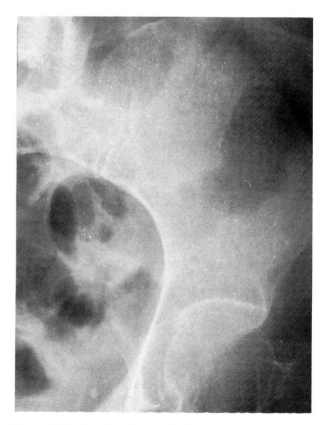

Figure 5–92. An ischemic sigmoid colon overlies the left iliac fossa. It lacks plica and smooth haustral margins. The bumpy appearance indicates mural edema.

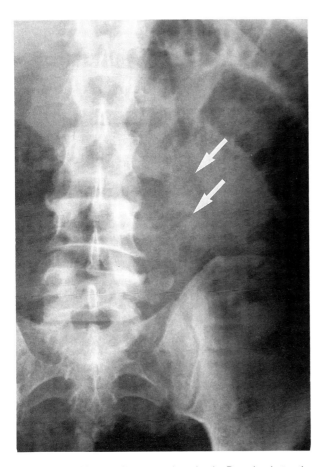

Figure 5–93. Mesenteric venous thrombosis. Pseudo-obstruction in mesenteric ischemia. The proximal jejunum is dilated and gas-filled. Two more distal loops (*arrows*) reveal the stretch sign—parallel streaks of intraluminal gas trapped surrounded by fluid. The gas lines up parallel to and between valvulae conniventes.

plied by the superior mesenteric artery. This sign's diagnostic value is limited by its rarity and its lack of specificity. Many other conditions, including pancreatic inflammation, mechanical obstruction, and even prolonged lack of mobility, can be associated with gas in the transverse colon and right colon. Moreover, even in intestinal infarction it is rarely noted on plain films.[185]

In adults, gas in the bowel wall extending throughout one or several loops and arrayed as tiny bubbles, crescents, or elongated streaks almost always indicates intestinal necrosis. In children, especially, similar lucencies can be seen in bowel infarction by a gas-forming organism, but the clinical presentation is usually distinctly different.[186,187] Intramural air can occur in both mesenteric ischemia and ischemic colitis, but it is seen in the large intestine in less than 10% of cases.[59,180] Typically, the gas within the wall appears as a continuous streak (Fig

5–94). In the large bowel it may project over the lumen as it extends within a plica semilunares (Figs 2–41,5–95). Small bowel gas can involve many valvulae conniventes and, thus, may appear as a chain of ringlike lucencies whose width conforms to the diameter of the bowel.[188] In nearly half the cases of intramural air, gas is seen in the branches of the portal vein within the liver shadow (Fig 1–5). Such a finding implies extensive infarction. An interesting, albeit exceedingly rare pattern, is gas within mesenteric veins without portal vein lucencies. This peculiar distribution of gas suggests obstruction of the portal circulation proximal to the liver. It has been observed in bowel infarction secondary to venous occlusion in small bowel volvulus[189] and in an obstructed, strangulated intestine entrapped in a transmesenteric hernia.[190]

There is no single roentgenographic sign or combination of signs that indicates a specific cause of mesenteric ischemia. Venous occlusion is apt to produce the most marked bowel changes per area of involvement, and embolus to the superior mesenteric artery and its branches has the highest frequency of plain film findings, but such tendencies are not predictive in an individual case.[59] The extent of disease seems to correlate with the likelihood of plain film evidence, but there are too many exceptions to this rule to rely upon it clinically. For example, infarction of most of the small bowel can be present even when the plain film appears completely unremarkable (Table 5–7).

Pneumatosis Cystoides Intestinalis

Pneumatosis cystoides intestinalis is an interesting condition in which the bowel wall contains innumerable lucent cysts. Its pathognomonic appearance in both the small intestine and colon is easily distinguishable from the mural streaks and tiny bubbles that are the hallmarks of mesenteric ischemia and necrotizing enterocolitis. The cysts vary in diameter from 0.5 to 3.0 cm, and in general the average cyst width is greater in the large bowel than in the jejunum or ileum.[191] Duodenal involvement is rare regardless of etiology.[192] The cysts may cluster in the intestinal wall only or extend into the adjacent mesentery.[193]

On pathological inspection air cysts are seen to lie either in the submucosa or subserosa. The lining contains scattered endothelial cells and the intervening stroma consists of bands of connective tissue. Apparently, the cysts do not communicate with each other, and in most cases the overlying mucosal margins are intact.[194]

The pathophysiological mechanisms for both the formation and persistence of these cystic spaces

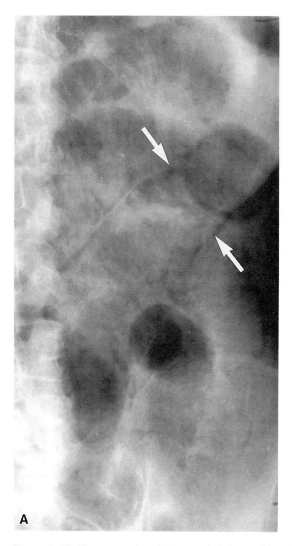
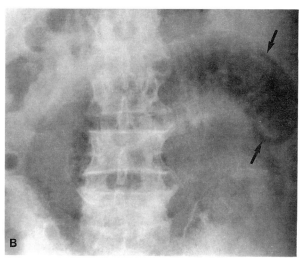

Figure 5–94. Four examples of intramural air in small bowel infarction. **A.** Gas in the wall appears as continuous streaks (*arrows*). **B.** A crescent of gas (*arrows*) in a small bowel loop folded on itself laterally.

remain a mystery. The vast literature on the subject is replete with theories, none of which are fully substantiated by physical evidence and all of which fail to explain the association of pneumatosis with a diversity of predisposing conditions.

The mechanical theory attempts to account for the relationship between jejunal and (especially) ileal pneumatosis with peptic ulcer disease and pyloric stenosis. It is presumed that increased pressure forces air through gastric mucosal rents, from which it then enters lymphatics that drain towards the intestines. The absence of duodenal pneumatosis and the rarity of gastric air cysts are puzzling.[195] Apparently, an undernourished state in peptic ulcer disease predisposes to cyst formation for still unclear reasons.[196]

Keyting et al proposed that some cases of colonic gas cysts are caused by the tracking of air from

the lung interstitium through the mediastinum and retroperitoneum, with further passage downward along the mesenteric vessels to the bowel wall.[197] That such a pathway of dissection exists was proved in 1944 by Macklin and Macklin.[198] The association of asthma and pulmonary fibrosis with colonic pneumatosis suggests that coughing and bronchospasm are responsible for the egress of air from the pulmonary alveoli.[199] Nevertheless, no case has yet provided a roentgenographic demonstration of the coexistence of pneumomediastinum or with pneumatosis.

Trauma to the colonic mucosa may result in definite but occult mucosal disruptions that allow gas to enter the bowel wall, but the failure to show actual gaps in the epithelial lining is bedeviling. Although pneumatosis has been reported in Crohn's disease,[200] colonic volvulus,[201] and after sigmoid-

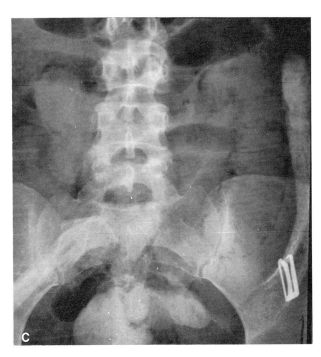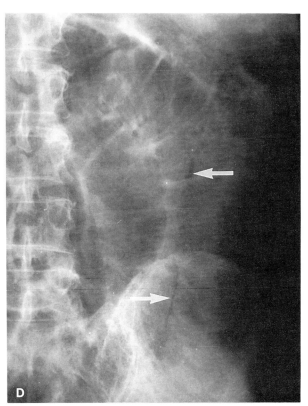

Figure 5–94. (cont.) C. Mural air stands out in a dilated fluid-filled loop. The transverse lucencies are gas streaks within the valvulae conniventes. The contrast-filled descending colon is lateral to the dilated small bowel. **D.** Mural gas appears as a streak (*lower arrow*) and as a chain of short interrupted lucencies (*upper arrow*).

oscopy,[192] it is hard to explain its extreme rarity in ulcerative colitis, a disease whose characteristic finding is a disturbed mucosa.

Pneumatosis cystoides intestinalis has been described in many small bowel diseases. Rounded lucencies and more streaky collections of wall gas have been noted in the small intestine, and, in both types of accumulations, the clinical course is typically benign and self-limited. In a study of 32 patients who underwent intracatheter feeding after percutaneous placement of a jejunostomy tube, 5 developed intestinal air cysts. Apparently air irrigation of the tube was responsible for the development of mural gas.[202] Jejunoileal bypass predisposes to pneumatosis, which appears primarily in the unbypassed intestinal segment.[203,204] Jejunal diverticulosis[206] and celiac disease[206,207] may also be complicated by bowel wall air cysts. Pneumatosis has even been reported in appendicitis.[208]

An important relationship exists between some collagen diseases and pneumatosis cystoides intestinalis. In scleroderma, wall cysts and lucent streaks develop in patients who are severely malnourished. The presence of cysts is a grave sign, signaling further clinical deterioration.[209] A poor prognosis is

suggested by the appearance of pneumatosis in systemic lupus erythematosus.[210,211] In dermatomyositis, however, air cysts in the colonic wall are typically transient and innocuous.[212]

Decreased immunologic competence is related to pneumatosis, probably through the complex mediation of several factors. In recent years, there have been reports of intestinal gas cysts in acute leukemia,[213] non-Hodgkin's lymphoma,[214] bone marrow transplantation,[215] and graft-versus-host disease.[216] Steroid therapy appears to play a role in these patients. It leads to atrophy of Peyer's patch, which may create minute openings in the covering ileal mucosa, permitting gas to enter the wall.[217] Chemotherapy and radiation therapy can directly damage the mucosa as well.[218] In addition, opportunistic infection by gas-forming bacteria may penetrate the mucosa of the sterilized bowel.[219]

Pneumatosis cystoides intestinalis is most often an incidental finding but on occasion bleeding can occur into the bowel lumen.[192] Other complications are simple obstruction and volvulus. Rarely, pneumoperitoneum occurs, resulting from rupture of a cyst. Almost always, it resolves spontaneously.[220]

The plain film diagnosis is easy if the cysts are

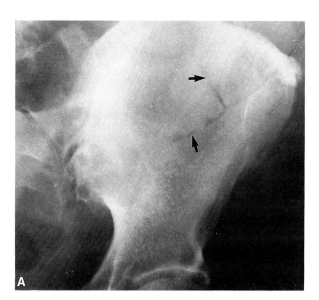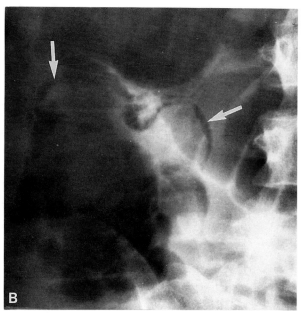

Figure 5–95. Mural gas in the colon. **A.** Sigmoid colon. The vertical arrow points to gas in the wall. The horizontal arrow highlights gas in a plica semilunares. **B.** Gas in the wall of the ascending colon (*arrows*).

diffusely distributed throughout the colon (Fig 5–96). Each lucency is larger and more sharply defined than abscess bubbles. Often, the thin wall of individual cysts can be seen when two of these rounded lucencies lie adjacent to each other. Localized pneumatosis can be identified as it follows the course of the colon. Unlike the more widely spread discrete gaseous deposits residing within colonic diverticula, mural air cysts are closely clustered, packed together like a bunch of grapes (Figs 2–39,5–97). Occasionally, intraperitoneal air may insinuate itself between colonic folds, thereby simulating mural gas. The

TABLE 5–7. PLAIN FILM SIGNS OF MESENTERIC ISCHEMIA

1. Mural contour abnormalities
   Effaced valvulae conniventes
   Thickened valvulae conniventes
   Bumpy bowel wall
   Thumbprinting
   Featureless bowel
   Thickened bowel wall
   Rigid bowel loop
2. Extraluminal gas
   Gas in wall
   Gas in mesenteric veins
   Gas in portal vein branches
3. Intraluminal gas distribution changes
   Pseudo-obstruction pattern
   Gasless abdomen
   Stretch sign—fluid and gas in bowel
   Splenic flexure cutoff pattern

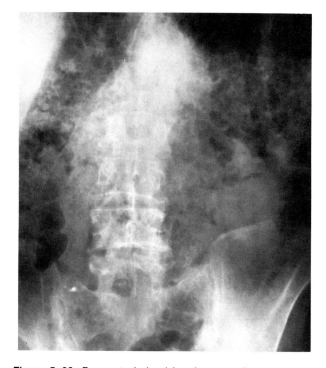

Figure 5–96. Pneumatosis involving the ascending, transverse and descending colon. There are innumerable cysts all confined to the bowel wall.

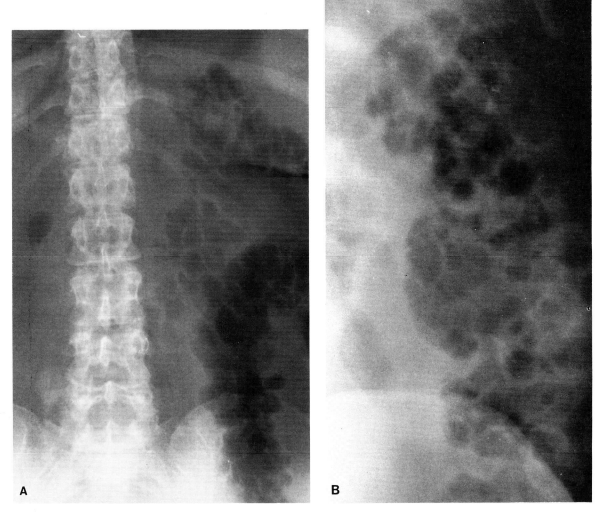

Figure 5–97. Two examples of pneumatosis coli. **A.** The cysts are confined to the distal transverse colon and descending colon in grapelike clusters. Some even extend slightly beyond the expected contours of the bowel. **B.** Cysts in the descending colon. The superimposed lucencies all have rounded contours.

presence of free air elsewhere in the abdomen separate from the bowel allows it to be distinguished from pneumatosis cystoides intestinalis.[221]

INTESTINAL CALCIFICATION AND OTHER OPACITIES

Many widely varying conditions in the gastrointestinal tract may be recognized on plain films by the presence of single or multiple opacities. The lumina of the stomach, small intestine, appendix, and large intestine should, in a sense, be considered extracorporeal, and these organs can contain pills, bones, and other ingested foreign bodies. Calculi may form

in the intestines and appendix or enter the gastrointestinal tract through a fistula. An awareness of the appearance of the various types of gastrointestinal concretions and other radiodensities is sometimes crucial for the diagnosis and management of serious abdominal disorders. Moreover, the walls of these hollow organs can be the site of calcification in both benign and malignant masses, some of which have a characteristic radiographic appearance on plain films.

In the discussion that follows, a distinction is made between intraluminal and extraluminal densities. Attention is given to densities that are not so clearly discerned rather than to readily recognizable foreign bodies. Emphasis is placed on pattern recognition and the clinical implications of the various densities both endogenously produced and introduced from outside.

OPACITIES IN THE SMALL INTESTINE

Intramural Lesions

Calcification in small bowel tumors is very uncommon (Table 5–8). Carcinoid tumors calcify occasionally, and they represent the majority of lesions in the small bowel with detectable calcification on plain films. Most of the reported cases have revealed small, scattered, well-defined spherical densities, similar to but somewhat larger than phleboliths.[222] Less often, combinations of flecks and arcuate lines of radiodensity are seen with this tumor. All reported examples of calcified carcinoid tumors arise from the ileum, and the opacities are usually located away from the lumen in the midst of an area of fibrosis in the adjacent mesentery.[223-225] The calcifications are fixed and do not change position on successive films.

Approximately 5% of small-bowel hemangiomas contain radiographically demonstrable phleboliths.[226] Hemangiomas are soft, often bulky masses that do not restrict movement of the small bowel during peristalsis. These tumors and their calcific phleboliths may change position on sequential films. Occasionally, hemangiomas cause intussusception, forcing the tumor to traverse a long distance. Hemangiomas may occur anywhere in the small bowel but are most frequent in the distal jejunum and ileum.[226]

Leiomyomas and leiomyosarcomas are rela-

tively common small-bowel tumors, but radiographically detectable calcium deposition within them is exceedingly rare. Like smooth muscle tumor elsewhere, calcification usually has a mottled configuration. Surprisingly, metastases to pelvic and retroperitoneal nodes may become radiodense even if a primary small-bowel leiomyosarcoma remains uncalcified.[227]

Intraluminal Opacities

Ingested Substances. The ingested substances most often visible in the small bowel are medications. Liquid preparations containing calcium or other high-atomic-number elements such as bismuth are infrequently recognized because they are diluted by gastric juices and rapidly disperse through the intestines with peristalsis. On the other hand, intact solid medications are often seen in the small bowel. Pills may be observed if they are sufficiently radiopaque and if they have withstood disintegration in the stomach and small intestine.[228]

Medications containing iron are the most commonly observed foreign bodies in the small bowel. These pills often resist dissolution and can appear intact anywhere in the small or large intestine. The sizes and shapes of iron-containing medications vary because ferrous sulfate and ferrous gluconate may be incorporated into a number of preparations, including vitamin complexes.[229]

Enteric coating is often applied to iron medications to render the active ingredient of a pharmaceutical resistant to decomposition. The purpose of enteric coating is to protect the integrity of the pill from breakdown in the stomach, thereby sparing the patient the irritative effect of iron on the gastric mucosa. Occasionally, however, the coating may be so impregnable that the drug cannot be released into the lumen and absorbed. Most often this occurs in elderly patients and in pills with a hardened shell after a long shelf life. Some enteric-coated medications such as potassium chloride can be faintly radiopaque, owing to the chemical composition of the coating material.[230] Unfortunately, information about the constituents of the protective coating are generally unavailable to consumers and physicians because the ingredients are often trade secrets.

Iodine-containing pills are radiodense but are usually not seen on plain radiographs because they dissolve rapidly in the stomach or proximal small bowel. At times, nonabsorbed Telepaque, an iodine compound, will appear as clumps of density in the distal small bowel and colon (Fig 5–98). This is to be distinguished from the amorphous appearance of

TABLE 5–8. CALCIFICATIONS AND OTHER DENSITIES IN THE SMALL BOWEL

Intramural lesions
  Carcinoid tumors
  Hemangiomas
  Leiomyoma
  Leiomyosarcoma
Intraluminal opacities
  Ingested materials
    Solid opaque medication
    Metallic objects
    Eggshells
    Bones
  Enteroliths
    Intraluminal stones
    Meckel's stones
  Stones entering through a fistula
    Gallstones

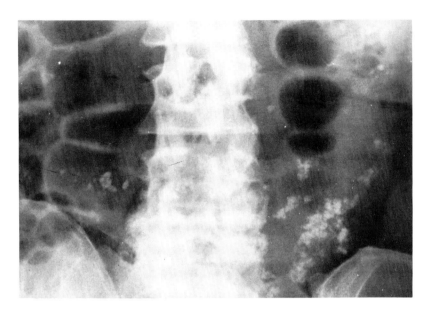

Figure 5–98. Unabsorbed nonconjugated Telepaque in the small bowel. Scattered clumps of mottled density resemble mesenteric lymph node calcification.

conjugated Telepaque, which, after having been absorbed in the small bowel and transported to the liver and biliary ductal system, reenters the gut through the enterohepatic circulation. Conjugated Telepaque is seen as a diffuse increase in density within small bowel loops.[231]

Radiographic Appearance. Most pills can be recognized easily on a scout radiograph, but if they are small they can be confused with concretions. Pills are sometimes disc-shaped, a conformation seldom seen with stones. Also, they are homogeneous, with their radiodensity varying in direct proportion to their thickness (Figs 3–84,4–34,5–99). Consequently, ovoid or round pills are less dense at the periphery. On the other hand, concretions may be laminated or at least have a band of increased density at their margins.

The recognition of pills in the gut can be significant in modifying patient management. If a medication is intact in the colon, then it is most probable that it is of no benefit to the patient because it will not be absorbed.[230] A switch to another agent may be necessary. Moreover, the presence of many pills, such as ferrous sulfate medications, in the intestine when none are prescribed may be an indication of overdose.[229]

Any radiopaque material passing through the stomach intact can be seen in the small bowel. Large objects like pins and coins rarely cause diagnostic difficulty because their appearance is readily discerned. Small objects, however, ingested in large quantities, may look like contrast material and with-

out historical information may be misinterpreted on plain films (Fig 5–100).

In edentulous patients, fragments of eggshells are sometimes swallowed inadvertently. As they pass through the small bowel, they can be recognized as smooth, slightly arcuate linear opacities. The thinness of eggshells enables them to be visualized only when they are aligned parallel to the X-ray beam. Since these fragments change in posi-

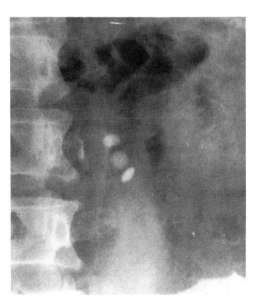

Figure 5–99. Three disc-shaped opaque pills in the small bowel. The radiographic beam passes through the long axis of the upper and lower pills. Hence, they appear more dense than the middle pill, which is aligned with its narrow axis to the beam.

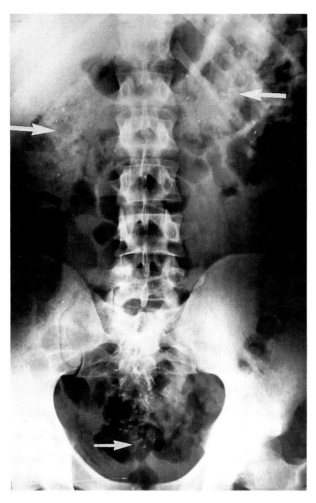

Figure 5–100. Numerous small fragments of metal are scattered throughout the colon (*arrows*). They represent fragments of razor blades ingested by a disturbed patient to induce gastrointestinal bleeding.

tion and orientation as they are transported distally by peristalsis, the number of discernible densities can vary from film to film even if two radiographs are obtained moments apart (Fig 5–101).

Enteroliths. Occasionally, concretions form in the small-bowel lumen. Sometimes undigested vegetable matter, such as plum or prune pits, serves as a nidus (Fig 5–102).[232] In most instances, however, there is no nucleus of insoluble material.[233] The formation of enteroliths requires retardation of flow of intestinal contents. Hence, they are found proximal to a stenosis or in a diverticulum with a narrowed neck.[234] Calcified intestinal stones form only if there is both stasis and a favorable pH for calcium deposition.[235] In the upper small bowel the intestinal contents are too acidic for the precipitation of calcium. Here nonopaque choleic acid stones may

be present, occurring almost exclusively in women and often located in duodenal diverticula.[232] Calcified enteroliths are encountered only in the distal small intestine where the bowel contents are more alkaline. In the ileum, the pH of intestinal secretions can reach 9.0.[236] Analysis of distal small bowel enteroliths usually reveals calcium oxalate or calcium carbonate as the main chemical constituent.[234] They have been reported in patients with Crohn's disease, intestinal tuberculosis, and other abnormalities causing bowel constriction, even carcinoma of the cecum.[237–239] Usually multiple calculi are present, and, although the shape of the stones may vary, they are typically all of similar size. Enteroliths are rarely laminated and usually have a thin complete rim of calcification and a lucent or faintly opaque center (Fig 5–103).[236]

Most small bowel diverticula have wide mouths that permit easy inflow and egress of intestinal contents. Therefore, they are not likely sites for stone formation. If they become inflamed, however, the neck may narrow, trapping the contents of the diverticulum. A prime example is an infected Meckel's diverticulum, where both stasis and an alkaline environment promote calcium precipitation. Only a few cases of opaque calculi in Meckel's diverticulum have been reported, and most of these were in men, even though the incidence of Meckel's diverticulum is equal in both sexes.[240] Typically, stones in a small bowel diverticulum are single and round, but multiple, faceted concretions have also been noted.[241,242] In a large diverticulum, movement of the stone on sequential films can be observed. In one report, a stone moved from the lower abdomen to the right upper quadrant within a single giant diverticulum.[243]

Differential Diagnosis of Enteroliths. Enteroliths, either in a diverticulum or proximal to an obstruction, can usually be distinguished from other calculi. Appendiceal stones are more densely calcified and fixed in position. Multiple gallstones are almost always confined to the gallbladder whereas enteroliths are apt to move within loops of bowel.[244] Calcified ectopic gallstones entering the gut through a cholecystoenteric fistula are usually faintly opaque, single, and larger than 2.5 cm in diameter, with nonangulated margins. In approximately one half of cases air can be seen in the biliary tree (Fig 6–57A). Ureteral calculi and phleboliths are generally smaller than intestinal stones. In most cases, enteroliths cause no symptoms in themselves, but their presence on plain films should alert one to the possibility of significant intestinal narrowing or diverticular inflammation.

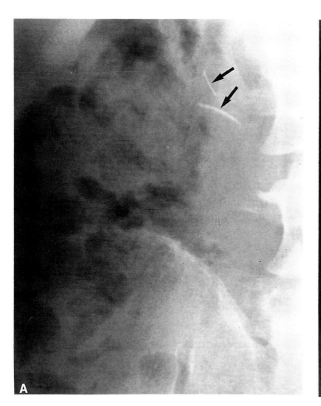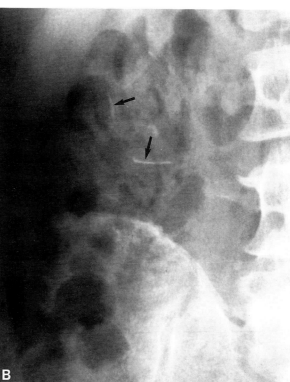

Figure 5–101. Eggshell calcifications due to eggshells. **A.** Two shell fragments (*arrows*) grouped closely together in the small bowel. **B.** A film obtained 10 minutes later. The two fragments (*arrows*) have moved considerably. Smaller fragments can now be seen as they have become aligned parallel to the radiographic beam.

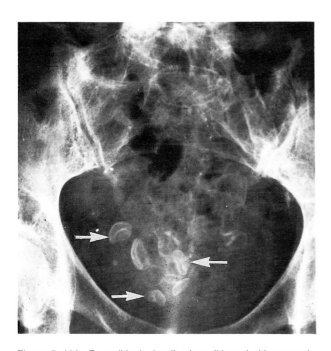

Figure 5–102. Enteroliths in the distal small bowel with prune pits as the nidi of the stones. The patient has intermittent obstruction owing to the descent of ileum into a femoral hernia. (*Courtesy of Dr. Harry Miller*).

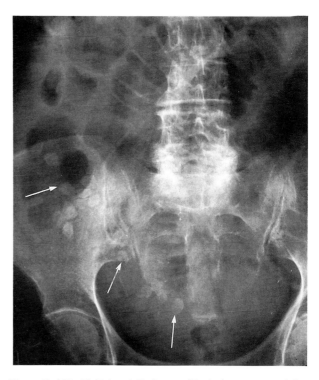

Figure 5–103. Multiple calcified enteroliths in the cecum and distal ileum (*arrows*). The patient has a constricting carcinoma in the proximal ascending colon. Note that the proximal colon is not distended but the small bowel is gas-filled and dilated, a pattern that conforms to a type 2 large bowel obstruction by Love's criteria.

219

RADIOPACITIES IN THE LARGE INTESTINE

Liquid Substances

The large bowel resorbs water and forms, stores, and expels feces. Nonabsorbable radiopaque substances suspended in luminal fluid may first become concentrated in the cecum as water is resorbed. Opaque liquid medications taken orally can concentrate in the right colon and may be observed in the large intestine on plain films (Fig 5–104).

Conjugated Telepaque is another substance that may become visible in the large bowel. Orally administered Telepaque enters the enterohepatic circulation, passing through liver cells and the biliary radicals and entering the duodenum through the common bile duct. Although usually not seen in the small bowel, Telepaque becomes visible in the right colon, where it coats feces (Fig 5–105).

Bones

Solid radiopacities may be found in the colon for a variety of reasons (Table 5–9). Ingested foreign bodies can pass through the large bowel and become fixed at some point. Most small and smooth objects will usually cause no problem, but larger angulated items can obstruct the colonic lumen or perforate the wall of the large bowel. The swallowing of radiopaque foreign bodies is more apt to occur in demented, inebriated, or neurologically impaired

individuals.[245] It has also been observed with heightened frequency in elderly denture wearers. In the aged, tactile sensation in the oral cavity is frequently diminished, and the wearing of a dental prosthesis further decreases awareness of unchewed material. The calcified foreign body most often recognized in the colon is a chicken breastbone. Often, it is inadvertently swallowed in soups, sandwiches, and salads, or other food where the patient does not expect to encounter a bone.[246] Chicken bones may be long and pointed and can penetrate the intestinal wall at any point.

Common sites for obstruction and penetration of chicken bones are the second portion of the duodenum, the duodeno-jejunal junction, Meckel's diverticulum, the ileocecal region, and the colonic flexures.[247,248] Moreover, in the aged, in whom there is a high incidence of diverticulosis, the sigmoid becomes a frequent site for obstruction, perforation, and abscess formation (Figs 1–9, 5–106). Even if a chicken bone is calcified, it may not be seen on plain films because it can overlie the pelvic bones. In a patient predisposed to accidental ingestion of a foreign body who presents with symptoms of obstruction and/or diverticulitis, the presence of an abnormal density should be carefully sought on plain films. After contrast material is introduced into the colon, it becomes more difficult to ascertain the presence of a bone or other opacity.

Other Foreign Substances

In West Africa primarily, but also in parts of the southern United States, geophagy is practiced. After the ingestion of calcareous clay, undissolved opacities can be seen throughout the gastrointestinal tract, from stomach to rectum. If much clay is consumed, the calcific densities may simulate the appearance of barium (Fig 5–107). After the inadvertent rupture of a mercury bag attached to a long intestinal tube, elemental mercury may move freely through the small intestine. Since mercury is very dense and is a liquid at body temperature it will assume the shape of small radiopaque globules in the small and large bowel (Fig 5–108).

Concretions

Concretions occur in the large bowel as well as in the small intestine. The colon is an occasional site of obstruction in gallstone ileus. Large-bowel obstruction promotes the formation of calculi in the same way that enteroliths are able to form in an occluded small-bowel lumen and in Meckel's diverticulum (Figs 5–38,5–109). Diverticula in the left colon are common, but calcific stones are unusual (Fig 2–125). This is surprising because of the prolonged transit

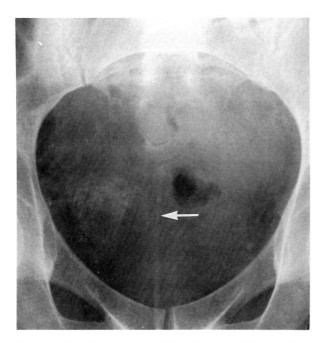

Figure 5–104. Concentration of bismuth in the right colon. Two days before, this patient took 4 oz. of bismuth subsalicylate by mouth. With resorption of water in the cecum, bismuth concentrates and becomes radiopaque as it coats feces (*arrow*).

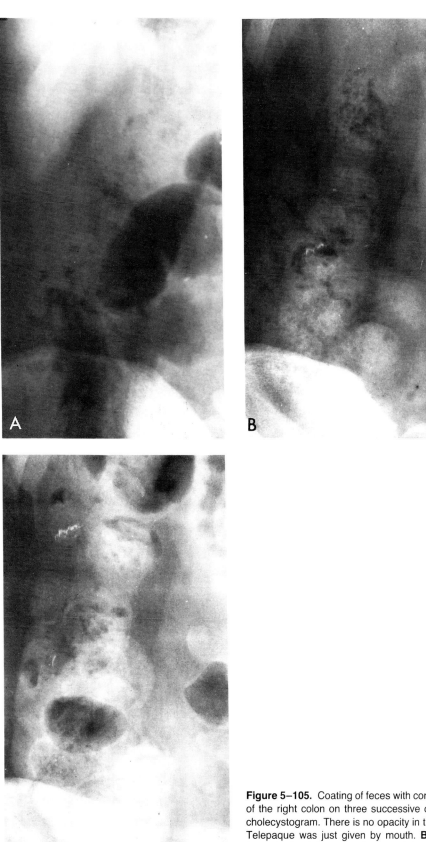

Figure 5–105. Coating of feces with conjugated Telepaque. Films of the right colon on three successive days. **A.** Day 1 of an oral cholecystogram. There is no opacity in the colon. A single dose of Telepaque was just given by mouth. **B.** Day 2—faint coating of feces in the right colon. A second dose of Telepaque was then given. **C.** Day 3—bright coating of feces in the colon caused by the accumulation of conjugated Telepaque.

TABLE 5-9. CALCIFICATIONS AND OTHER DENSITIES IN THE LARGE INTESTINES

1. Intraluminal densities
    Concentration of liquid substances
        Bismuth
        Conjugated Telepaque
    Ingested objects
        Pills
        Metallic densities
        Bones
        Calcareous clay
        Mercury globules
    Concretions
        Coproliths
        Gallstones
        Coating of feces in the distal colon
2. Intramural calcifications
    Tumors
        Adenocarcinoma
        Hemangioma
    Infections
        Schistosoma haematobium
        Schistosoma mansoni

time in patients with diverticulosis, the narrowed necks of colonic diverticula, and the alkaline pH of intraluminal contents. All these favor the formation of large bowel stones (Fig 5–110).[249–251]

Little has been written about concretions in the distal colon. In comparison to small bowel enteroliths, opaque calculi are uncommon in this area and their etiology may be different. We have observed a number of patients who had transient opacifications of feces in the absence of obstruction. In several

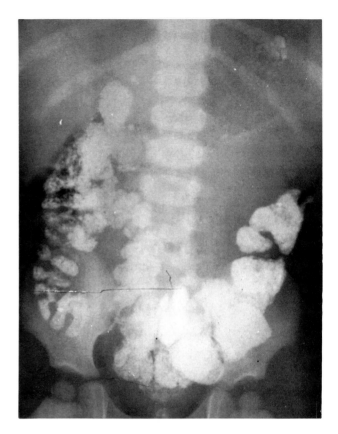

Figure 5–107. Undigested radiopaque material fills the colon and a smaller amount is present in the fundus of the stomach. The patient is a child who regularly ingested clay.

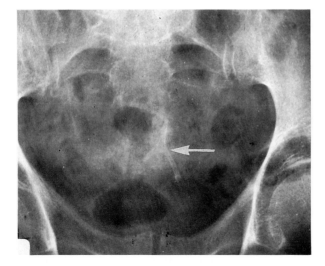

Figure 5–106. Chicken bone (*arrow*) in the sigmoid colon. An ingested chicken bone perforated a sigmoid diverticulum causing a diverticular abscess. Although diverticulitis may be diagnosed on a barium enema, a chicken bone or other density that precipitates acute inflammation can be missed if no preliminary film is obtained.

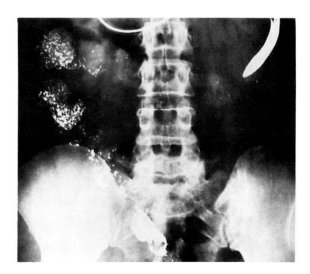

Figure 5–108. Globules of mercury in the colon after the rupture of a mercury bag attached to a long intestinal tube.

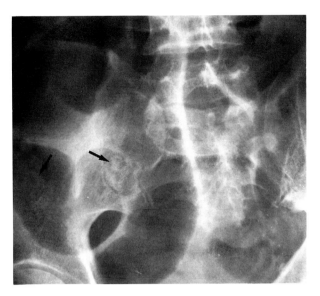

Figure 5–109. A patient with chronic obturation of the distal sigmoid colon. The sigmoid colon is elongated and projects to the right of the midline. Within the lumen are agglomerations of calcified coproliths (*arrows*).

patients, arcuate calcification coated fecal material on one day, and after a bowel movement both feces and their marginal opacities had been evacuated. In some instances transient opacification was extensive (Fig 5–111). Most of the patients in whom this finding was observed were elderly, but some were young and had no chronic colonic abnormalities. It is conceivable that transient elevations in pH could provide a favorable environment for calcium depo-

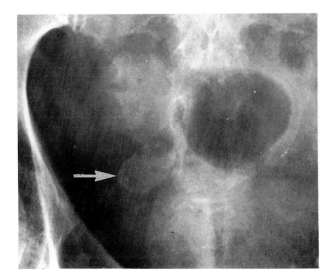

Figure 5–110. Single calculus in a sigmoid diverticulum. A large faintly calcified stone (*arrow*). On films following the barium enema, its position within a diverticulum was noted.

sition. Undoubtedly, in other patients, accumulations of radiopaque material such as bismuth at the margin of feces may be detectable on plain film.

Solid substances can enter the intestine per rectum. Usually the recognition of opaque objects in the rectum or distal colon poses no difficulty. Occasionally, dissolving suppositories may simulate masses or concretions. Most rectally administered medications are radiolucent, but hemorrhoid preparations containing bismuth and zinc can be seen on plain films.[252] Within minutes after insertion, opaque suppositories are rapidly fractured and dissolved. If a radiograph is taken soon after administration of such a suppository, the demonstrated radiodensities may resemble phleboliths (Fig 5–112), prostatic calculi, or calcification in solid masses.

Mural Lesions

Carcinoma of the Large Intestine. The most common cause of calcification in the wall of the large intestine is a mucin-producing adenocarcinoma. The cecum and rectum are the most frequent sites, but calcified malignancies have also been noted in other sections of the large bowel.[253] Typically, these tumors present with a mottled, speckled, or granular pattern of calcification, which may extend away from the intestinal lumen (Fig 5–113). At times, instead of numerous punctate opacities, only a few densities are seen. In other cases, just the metastatic deposits and not the primary colonic tumor contains calcium (Fig 3–55). By far the most common location of calcified metastases is the liver but, occasionally, calcified metastases appear exclusively in retroperitoneal lymph nodes. Isolated peritoneal calcific deposits are extremely unusual in colon cancer. This is an important point of differentiation from ovarian serous cystadenocarcinoma, in which psammomatous calcification can appear singly or in concert in the primary tumor, the liver, and in peritoneal metastases. Sometimes ossification occurs in rectal carcinomas. Generally, bone-forming carcinomas are small and slow-growing, but they can also spread rapidly into adjacent pelvic muscles (Fig 5–114).[254–256]

Many patients with calcified carcinoma are below age 40 at the time of initial recognition of the disease. Although there appears to be a predilection for younger age groups, only rarely has a calcified adenocarcinoma been reported in a patient with preexisting ulcerative colitis.[257]

Hemangioma. Another colonic tumor that presents with calcification on plain films is hemangioma. Colonic and rectal hemangiomas are uncommon le-

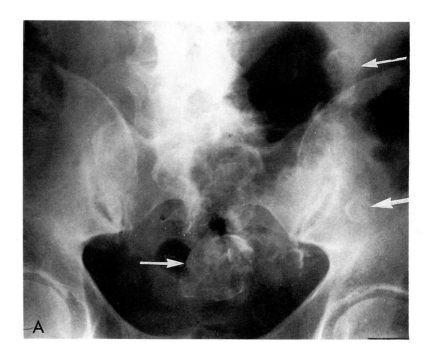

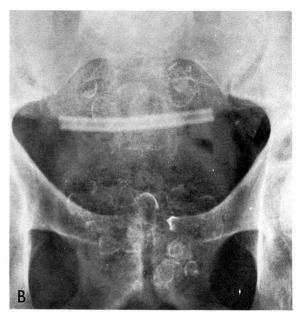

Figure 5–111. Two examples of transient intraluminal opacities in the colon. **A.** Multiple curvilinear densities in the rectum, sigmoid, and descending colon (*arrows*). They were not present on subsequent films obtained the next day. **B.** Many rounded opacities, which appear to coat feces. After an enema, they were evacuated from the colon.

sions but they often contain radiopaque phleboliths. In the rectum, a hemangioma is suggested by an abnormal position of phleboliths (Fig 5–115). In the more proximal colon, phleboliths and hemangiomas can move considerable distances with peristalsis.[258–260]

Schistosomiasis

Calcification in the wall of the large intestine has been reported in *Schistosoma haematobium* and *S mansoni* infestation. Most common in the rectum, calcium deposition occurs in the nonviable ova deposited within the submucosa of the bowel. In some cases, the densities appear as solid masses within polypoid excrescences.[261] In others, they have a distinctive circumferential distribution in a segment of large intestinal wall. A diagnostic feature of encircling schistosomal calcification is a change in configuration as the colon is emptied.[262] In the nonfilled bowel the calcification assumes a corrugated appearance analogous to the pattern of density seen in the vesical wall of an evacuated bladder infested by schistosomiasis (Figs 8–86,8–87). The variable appearance of colonic calcification is due to the fact that the muscle layers of the bowel are undisturbed by the calcified ova.

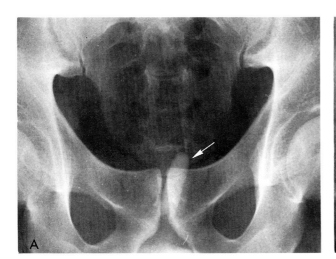 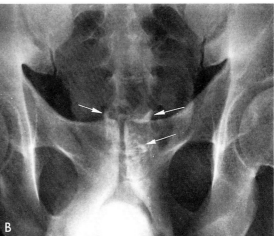

Figure 5–112. The appearance of radiopaque suppositories. A suppository containing bismuth and zinc was administered rectally. **A.** Immediately after placement, the opaque suppository is intact (*arrow*). **B.** Fifteen minutes later, the suppository had fragmented into multiple densities (*arrows*).

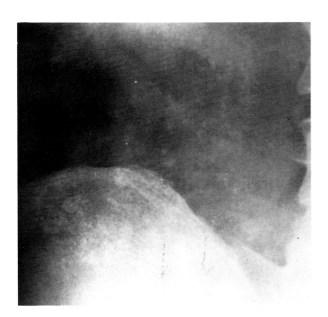 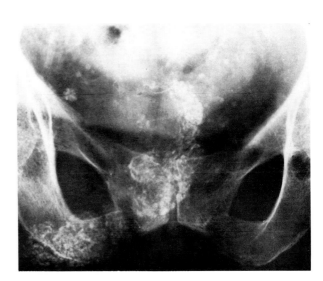

Figure 5–113. A large ascending colon adenocarcinoma. It contains innumerable speckled calcifications.

Figure 5–114. Calcified carcinoma of the rectum growing directly into the soft tissues of the right buttock. (*Courtesy of Dr. Paul Cohen.*)

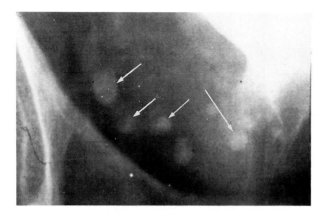

Figure 5–115. Hemangioma of the rectum. There are several phlebolith-type calcifications (*arrows*) in this large tumor.

APPENDIX

Acute Appendicitis

Appendicitis requires the occlusion of the appendiceal lumen by particulate material. Although an endogenously produced appendicolith is usually the offending agent, any solid, nonabsorbable substance can cause obstruction, either by blocking the orifice (Fig 5–116) or by forming a nidus upon which inspissated feces adhere and calcium salts are laid down.[263] For example, Indians in Northern Quebec derive much of their protein from the ingestion of game killed with shotguns. Appendicitis is surprisingly high in this population and shot is often found within the obstructed appendiceal lumen.[264] Elongated and pointed metallic objects such as straight pins may serve as the foci for stone formation (Fig 5–117). Barium can remain in the patent lumen of an appendix for months and even years. It appears to confer no added risk for the later development of inflammation despite the fact that it eventually becomes a hard, dry mass.[265] On occasion, however, flecks of barium may become trapped within the laminae of an appendiceal calculus (Fig 5–118).

Stones in the appendix are not rare. Among the many names that have been given to them, the most common are coproliths, fecaliths, stercoliths, and appendicoliths.[266] The best term is appendicolith because it signifies the origin of the stone and serves to distinguish it from other intraluminal calculi in the gastrointestinal tract. Stones in the appendix were first noted in 1813, and Weisflog in 1906 provided the initial description of the radiological appearance of calcified appendicoliths.[267] Since the turn of the century, appendiceal stones have been observed with increasing frequency. Initial reports stated they were very rare, but now they are not considered unusual.

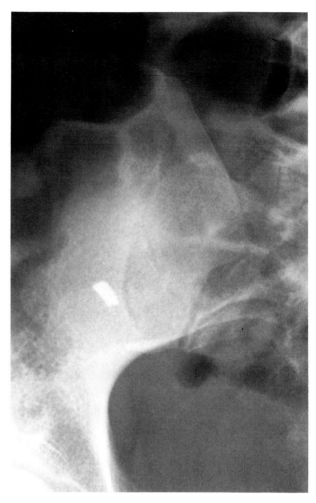

Figure 5–116. Appendiceal abscess. Ten days before, the patient inadvertently swallowed a piece of metal he was storing in his mouth as he changed a tire. The foreign body occluded the orifice of the appendix, leading to appendicitis and the formation of an abscess. The abscess deforms the cecal gas shadow. In its center is the ingested metal fragment.

Not all stones are calcified. In a study of 100 surgically removed, noninflamed appendices, four stones were found but only one was calcified. In 100 patients with acute appendicitis, 17 calculi were present and 12 were seen preoperatively on plain films (Figs 2–92,5–119).[268] Another study claimed that up to 60% of resected and diseased appendices contained stones but that calcification occurred in no more than 30% of them (Fig 5–120).[269] Opaque calculi are of clinical importance because they are frequently associated with perforation, especially in children with abdominal complaints. Brady found that 32 of 34 children with calcified appendicoliths had perforation at the time of operation.[270] Hence, it is generally agreed that in a symptomatic patient with a demonstrated appendiceal calculus, an appendectomy should not be delayed.

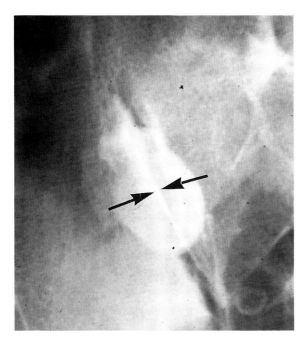

Figure 5–117. The nidus of this large appendicolith is a straight pin extending the length of the stone (*converging arrows*).

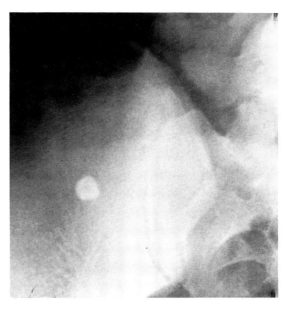

Figure 5–119. Typical appearance of an appendicolith. A dense, sharply outlined concretion is in the right lower quadrant.

Appendicoliths are found wherever the appendix is located. Usually, they are seen in the right lower quadrant. If the appendix is low-lying they occur in the pelvis (Fig 5–121) and if the appendix is retrocecal and posterior they can be seen in the right upper quadrant (Fig 5–122). In one case of a patient

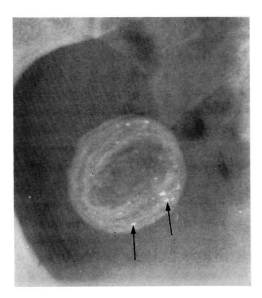

Figure 5–118. Laminated large appendiceal stone. The brighter punctate densities are flecks of barium within the laminae of the stone (*arrows*).

with malrotation of the colon, an appendiceal concretion was observed in the left upper quadrant.[270] Rarely, stones may be free in the peritoneal cavity (Fig 5–123). Like other calculi, appendicoliths are sharply marginated with curvilinear or faceted borders. Occasionally, smaller irregularities may appear on one surface (Fig 2–92), but generally they assume a regular, geometric shape. Appendicoliths often are densely calcified and approximately three fourths are clearly laminated (Fig 2–71). They can become very large and stones up to 4 cm in diameter have been noted (Fig 5–124).[271] Appendicoliths need not be solitary—in fact, multiple stones are not infrequent. A series of appendicoliths may have varying diameters, but almost always they are situated near to each other (Fig 5–125). Occasionally, if the appendiceal lumen is oriented in profile to the roentgenographic beam, the intraluminal stones may be linearly arrayed as an interrupted chain of radiodensities (Fig 5–126).

Appendicoliths are easily distinguished from mesenteric lymph nodes in the right lower quadrant because the latter have irregular margins and mottled interiors. Ureteral calculi are usually smaller and less prominently laminated, but, at times, differentiation between the two is difficult without oblique films or intravenous urography. Phleboliths are also smaller and have a central lucency, which is an uncommon finding in appendiceal stones. Moreover, phleboliths are generally restricted to pelvic locations whereas most appendiceal calculi are located

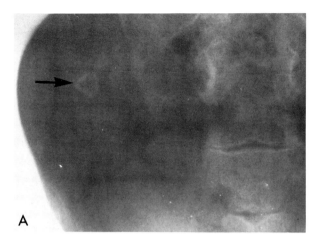
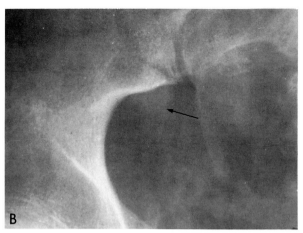

Figure 5–120. Sometimes appendicoliths may be faintly calcified. **A.** Only a marginal rim of calcification is seen (*arrow*). **B.** The appendicolith (*arrow*) is diffusely but minimally calcified, and if all of it were to overlie the iliac bone, it might be missed.

more superiorly. A rare entity that can be confused with an appendicolith is a calcified appendix epiploica (Fig 3–38). This concretion is often faintly calcified and freely movable in the peritoneal cavity. On occasion, stones form in an obstructed, inflamed Meckel's diverticulum and, if the pH of the diverticulumen is alkaline, the concretions can calcify. The appearance of these calculi is variable but typically they are rounded and homogeneously radiodense, simulating appendicoliths (Fig 5–127).[272,273]

A Meckel's stone is so infrequent, however, that an appendicolith must be considered the first diagnostic possibility in a patient with a right lower quadrant concretion that lies peripheral to the expected course of the ureter.

Other Signs of Acute Appendicitis

Acute occlusion of the appendix leads to the accumulation of mucus secretions and the growth of bacteria within the lumen. The ensuing infection extends to the wall of the appendix. Mural venules

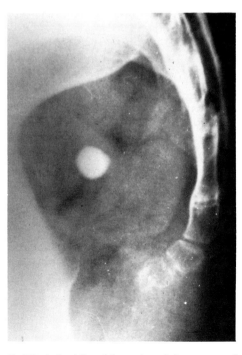

Figure 5–121. Lateral film of the rectum. A dense appendicolith in a retrocecal appendix occupies a low position in the pelvis.

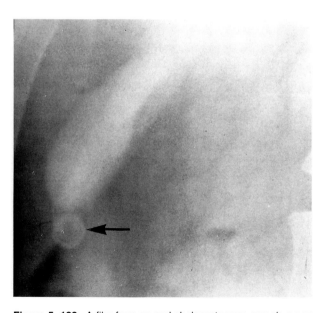

Figure 5–122. A film from an oral cholecystogram reveals a normal gallbladder and a calculus (*arrow*) adjacent to the fundus of the gallbladder. At operation a retrocecal appendix containing an appendicolith was found adherent to the gallbladder wall.

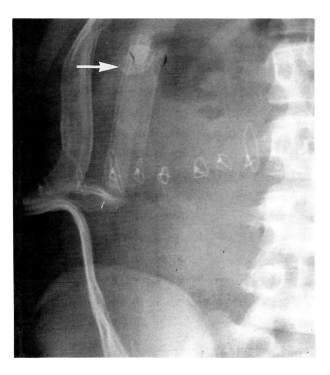

Figure 5–123. Calcified stone free in the peritoneal cavity (*arrow*). Drains in place from recent appendectomy. The freely moving stone was missed at the initial operation.

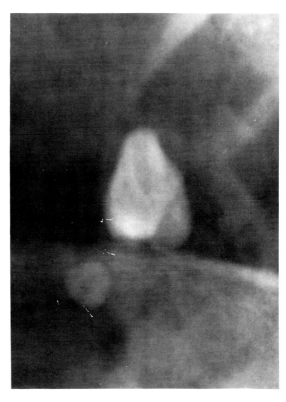

Figure 5–125. Two appendicoliths of dissimilar size and appearance. The upper stone is triangular and the lower stone resembles a phlebolith.

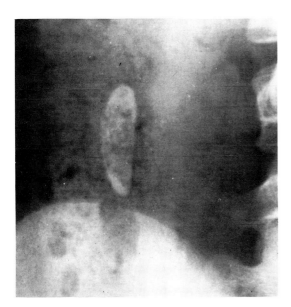

Figure 5–124. Very large appendicolith. It has the morphological characteristics of a concretion, ie, a complete perimeter of calcification and a regular if elongated shape.

become thrombosed by the spreading inflammation, and the resultant infarction of part of the damaged wall leads to perforation, local abscess formation, and peritonitis.[274] Often, the adjacent cecum becomes hypotonic and fills with gas. Although cecal ileus is a well-recognized feature of acute appendicitis (Fig 5–128), such an air-filled dilatation is not a specific sign because it may be seen in any other inflammation that abuts the cecal pouch. Cecal distension may even be an insignificant, transient plain film finding (Fig 5–129).[275,276]

Gas in the appendix has been regarded as an indicator of acute appendicitis.[277,278] In most patients, however, an air-filled appendix is normal, occurring when the lumen is situated anterior to its opening to the cecum.[279] An upward pointing appendix is particularly likely to contain gas when the patient assumes the supine position (Figs 2–14,5–130). Also, generalized ileus may involve the appendix as well as the intestines, and if its orifice is patent, it, too, can fill with gas.[280] An inflammatory process should be strongly suspected only when the appendiceal lumen is widened with irregular walls (Fig 2–16) or if a meniscus-type indentation abruptly and completely terminates the serpentine gas

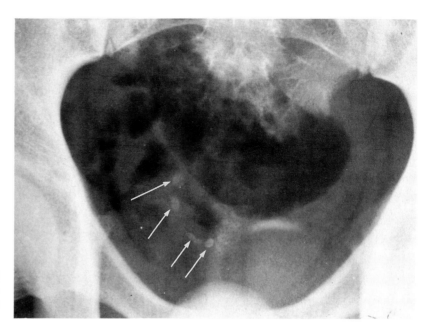

Figure 5–126. Four appendicoliths (*arrows*) occupying the lumen of a low-lying appendix. They should not be confused with phleboliths, which are usually positioned more laterally.

shadow. The meniscus represents the soft tissue density of a nonopaque appendicolith.[274]

Appendiceal abscesses are most easily discerned when they contain gas. Like pus collections elsewhere in the abdomen, the abscess may be identified by the presence of tiny bubbles (Fig 5–131), a large, irregularly shaped unilocular lucency (Fig 2–52), or a combination of the two (Fig 2–81). At times, only the soft tissue density of a non–gas-containing abscess is discernible, but this sign, in the absence of all other roentgenographic evidence, is nonspe-

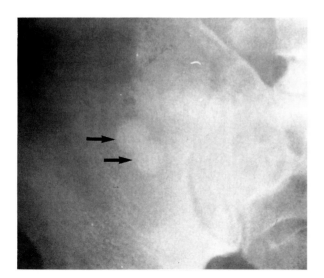

Figure 5–127. Two rounded opaque stones (*arrows*). Both reside within a Meckel's diverticulum.

cific, being simulated by fluid-filled bowel and by solid, noninfected right lower quadrant masses.

There is nothing pathognomonic about the plain film features of a gas-containing periappendiceal pus collection. Any localized inflammation of the right quadrant may have a similar appearance (Fig 5–132). Inasmuch as the appendix is frequently located below the level of the sacroiliac joint, appendiceal abscesses must be considered in the differential diagnosis of gas-containing pelvic inflammations. The demonstration of a calcified appendicolith in or near the abscess helps to confirm the diagnosis (Fig 5–133).

Large abscesses tend to ascend within the peritoneal cavity, especially in the right paracolonic gutter,[282] and evidence of a pus collection is often seen far from the appendiceal tip,[283] sometimes even reaching the subhepatic space anteriorly (Fig 3–50) and Morison's pouch posteriorly (Fig 5–134). Bubbles outside the bowel are the only clue to the presence of an expanding pus collection. A specific diagnosis becomes more secure if a calcified stone is also evident.

Other plain film findings of appendicitis include a generalized haziness in the right lower quadrant caused by the enlarging appendiceal mass[281] and separation of the bowel from the right flank stripe by the lateral accumulation of pus and ascites.[282] An abscess can be responsible for small bowel obstruction by extrinsic compression[284] or a generalized ileus[285]—both of which may be mistaken on plain films for an intrinsic mechanical occlusion of the dis-

Presumably the source of the lucency is a ruptured gas-containing abscess, not merely the residual contents of the lumen.[286–289]

Appendiceal Mucocele

Sometimes obstructed appendices do not form stones, even if luminal blockage is persistent. Especially when infection is absent, there is continuous production of mucus by appendiceal epithelial cells, so accumulation of fluid can distend the appendix. If the obstruction persists and mucus formation continues, a mucocele develops. It is a rare lesion found in less than 0.3% of all appendices removed at operation.[290,291] Occurring primarily in middle age, mucoceles are slightly more common in males. Some may be clinically silent, but often there is a history of multiple episodes of right lower quadrant pain,

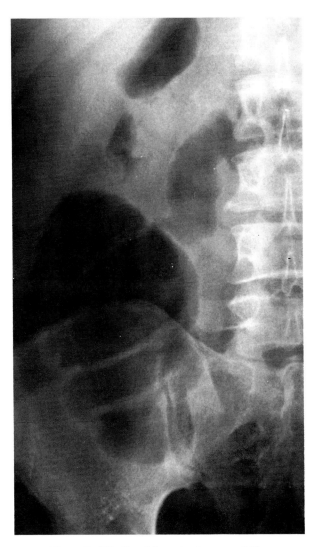

Figure 5–128. Cecal ileus due to appendicitis.

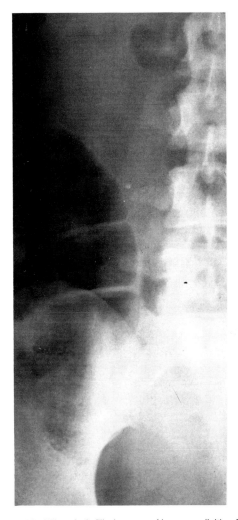

Figure 5–129. Dilated air-filled cecum. No appendicitis. An incidental finding in an asymptomatic patient. The film was obtained as a scout radiograph prior to a barium enema examination.

tal small bowel (Fig 5–30). Scoliosis of the lumbar spine, loss of the ipsilateral psoas shadow, and localized obscuration of the right flank stripe may be caused by appendicoliths, but, by themselves, they are not reliable signs of acute appendiceal inflammation.

Perforation of the appendix discharges gas into the peritoneal cavity. The volume of the lumen of the obstructed appendix is rarely more than a few cubic centimeters, however, and therefore the amount of released gas is insufficient to be noted on a supine roentgenograph even were it allowed to flow freely in an unrestricted fashion within the peritoneal space. Hence, roentgenographically detectable free air in appendicitis is quite rare. Nevertheless, there have been reports of massive pneumoperitoneum with appendiceal inflammation.

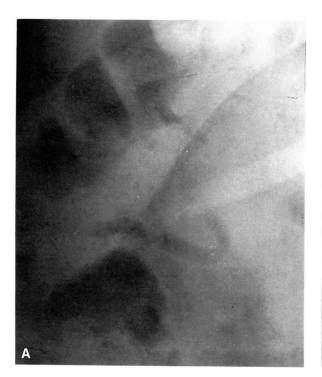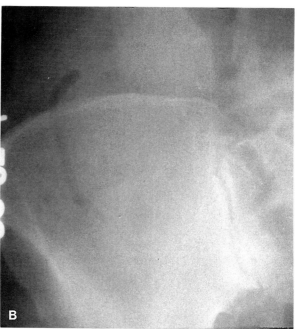

Figure 5–130. Two normal gas-filled appendices. **A.** Curvilinear appendix, horizontally directed proximally. The right 12th rib overlies a section of the lumen. **B.** Vertically oriented appendix overlying and projecting above the right iliac crest.

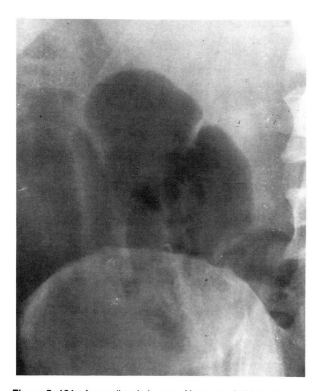

Figure 5–131. Appendiceal abscess. Numerous bubbles of gas in the abscess are superimposed on the shadow of a dilated, gas-filled cecum.

probably due to intermittent intussusception of the mass within the cecum.[292–294] Uncalcified mucoceles can be detected as smooth, filling defects indenting the medial wall of the cecum, and on plain films they closely resemble large lipomas or fibromas of the large bowel (Fig 5–135).

In a small percentage of patients, calcification of the wall of a cyst can be seen resembling that seen in cysts elsewhere. A thin, often continuous rim of calcification identifies the mucocele wall. Characteristically, there are no laminations or angulations in this annular opacity. Often, mucocele calcification is faint; because the appendix usually overlies the iliac bone, oblique films may be helpful in revealing the lesion. Cyst-type calcification in the right lower quadrant is not specific for mucocele. A mesenteric cyst may also be found here, and an echinococcal cyst can project from the inferior margin of the liver to overlie the right colon. Since appendiceal mucoceles are adjacent to the cecal pouch, they may be located in the pelvis. In women, leiomyoma of the uterus occasionally has a cystic appearance, causing confusion with mucocele calcification. A benign cystadenoma and a dermoid cyst of the ovary can also each have a similar appearance to a mucocele. One case of a hydrocele of the right spermatic cord in a

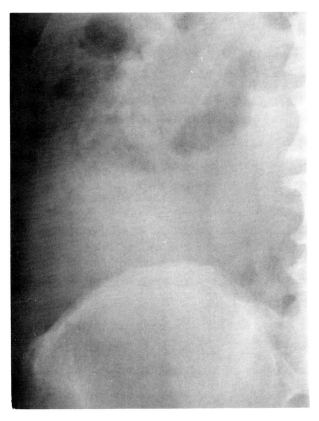

Figure 5–132. Right sided abscess due to perforated cecal diverticulitis. It resembles appendiceal abscess with a poorly defined mass just above the iliac crest and numerous bubbles more superiorly.

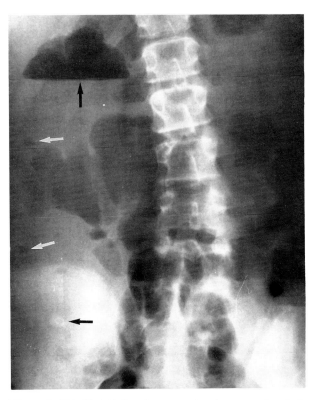

Figure 5–134. Upright film. Large gas-forming appendiceal abscess extending to Morison's pouch (*vertical black arrow*). Abscess bubbles (*white arrows*) are scattered in the right flank. A calcified appendicolith (*lower black arrow*) remains in the appendix. Note also the scoliosis, convex away from the abscess, a subsidiary sign of appendicitis.

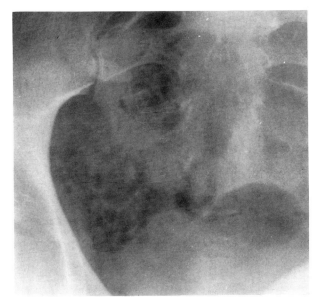

Figure 5–133. Pelvic appendiceal abscess. Bubbles in the right pelvis define the abscess. A bullet-shaped, horizontally oriented appendicolith overlies the lower right sacroiliac joint.

middle-aged man presented as rimlike calcification in the right pelvis and looked exactly like a radiodense mucocele.[295]

Myxoglobulosis

Approximately 5% of cystic lesions of the appendix contain free-floating intracystic bodies. Since the solid material contains mucin and assumes a globular shape, the term myxoglobulosis has been given to this uncommon variant of mucocele. The particulate densities within the cyst are termed globoid bodies. One explanation for their formation is that the lining cells of mucoceles slough and become nidi for the development of concretions containing mucin and cellular debris. Infrequently, globoid bodies calcify and appear as multiple concretions within the mucocele. In these cases, the wall of the cyst is not calcified. Since globoid bodies can move freely in the cyst, they change their location with respect to each other, a point of differentiation from multiple appendicoliths, which are usually fixed in a narrow lumen.[296–299]

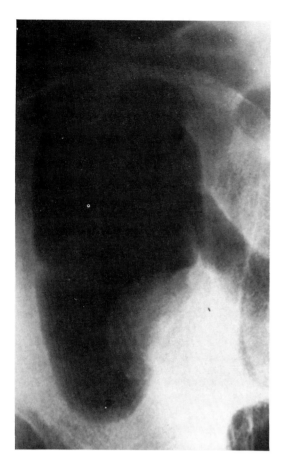

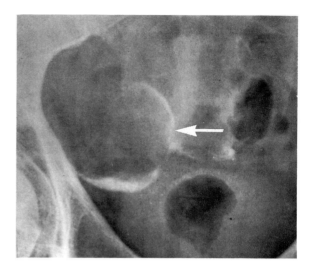

Figure 5–136. Large calcified mucocele (*arrow*) arising from an appendix situated in the right pelvis.

peritoneal cavity, implanting cells on the serosa of the bowel and solid organs. Like mucinous carcinoma of the ovary, pseudomyxoma peritoneii can develop; these can be identified on plain films by multiple foci of rimlike calcification representing the deposition of calcium salts at the margin of many of the intraperitoneal deposits.[300,301]

Figure 5–135. Noncalcified appendiceal mucocele creating a smooth indentation on the medial wall of the cecum.

Pseudomyxoma Peritonii

Mucoceles are usually confined to the right lower quadrant. They may, however, rupture into the

REFERENCES

1. Andersen K, Ringsted A. Clinical and experimental investigation on ileus with particular reference to the genesis of intestinal gas. *Acta Chir Scand.* 1943;88:475–502.
2. Schwartz SS. The differential diagnosis of intestinal obstruction. *Semin Roentgenol.* 1973;8:323–338.
3. Levitt MD, Bond JH Jr. Volume, composition and source of intestinal gas. *Gastroenterology.* 1970;59:921–929.
4. Williams JL. Obstruction of the small intestine. *Radiol Clin N Am.* 1964;2:21–31.
5. Bryk D, Wolf BS. A radiological evaluation of small bowel activity in the acute abdomen. *CRC Crit Rev Diagn Imag.* 1977;10:99–128.
6. Epstein BS. Simple distal ileal obstruction. *Radiology.* 1960;74:581–587.
7. Love L. Large bowel obstruction. *Semin Roentgenol.* 1973;8:299–322.
8. Kent KH, Raszkowski HJ. Colon lesions masquerading as small bowel obstruction on the plain roentgenogram of the abdomen. *Am J Roentgenol.* 1962;88:671–676.
9. Young BR. Significance of regional or reflex ileus in roentgen diagnosis of cholecystitis perforated ulcer, pancreatitis and appendiceal abscess: As determined by survey examination of the acute abdomen. *Am J Roentgenol.* 1957; 78:581–586.
10. Hodges P, Miller RE. Intestinal obstruction. *Am J Roentgenol.* 1955;74:1015–1025.
11. Seaman WB. Motor dysfunction of the gastrointestinal tract. *Am J Roentgenol.* 1972;116:235–248.
12. Tibblin S. Diagnosis of intestinal obstruction with spe-

cial regard to plain roentgen examination of the abdomen. *Acta Chir Scand.* 1969;146:249–252.

13. Levin B. Mechanical small bowel obstruction. *Semin Roentgenol.* 1973;8:281–297.

14. Donahue JK, Hunter C, Balch HH. Significance of fluid levels in x-ray films of the abdomen. *N Engl J Med.* 1958;259:13–15.

15. Gammill SL, Nice CM Jr. Air–fluid levels: Their occurrence in normal patients and their role in the analysis of ileus. *Surgery.* 1972;71:771–780.

16. Frimann-Dahl J. *Roentgen Examinations in Acute Abdominal Diseases,* 2nd ed. Springfield, Ill: Charles C Thomas Publishers; 1960.

17. Bryk D. Functional evaluation of small bowel obstruction by successive abdominal roentgenograms. *Am J Roentgenol.* 1972;116:262–275.

18. Williams JL. Fluid-filled loops in intestinal obstruction. *Am J Roentgenol.* 1962;88:677–686.

19. Mellins HZ, Rigler LG. The roentgen findings in strangulating obstructions of the small intestine. *Am J Roentgenol.* 1954;71:404–416.

20. Kelvin FM, Rice RP. Radiologic evaluation of acute abdominal pain arising from the alimentary tract. *Radiol Clin N Am.* 1978;16:25–36.

21. Samuel E, Duncan JG, Philp T, et al. Radiology of the post-operative abdomen. *Clin Radiol.* 1963;14:133–148.

22. Maruyama Y, Van Nagell JR Jr, Utley J, et al. Radiation and small bowel complications in cervical carcinoma therapy. *Radiology.* 1974;112:699–703.

23. Fataar S, Schulman A. Small bowel obstruction masking synchronous large bowel obstruction: A need for emergency barium enema. *Am J Roentgenol.* 1983;140:1159–1162.

24. Hunter TB, Freundlich IM, Zukoski CF. Pre-operative radiographic diagnosis of a spigelian hernia containing large and small bowel. *Gastrointest Radiol.* 1977;1:379–381.

25. Som PM, Khilnani MT, Wolf BS, et al. Spigelian hernia. *Acta Radiol (Diagn).* 1976;17:305–312.

26. Holder LE, Schneider HJ. Spigelian hernias: anatomy and roentgenographic manifestations. *Radiology.* 1974;112:309–313.

27. Bryk D. Spigelian hernia containing sigmoid colon. *Am J Roentgenol.* 1967;99:71–73.

28. Balthazar EJ, Subramanyam BR, Megibow A. Spigelian hernia. CT and ultrasonography diagnosis. *Gastrointest Radiol.* 1984;9:81–84.

29. Spiers TC, Rosenbloom MB, Palayew MJ. Spigelian hernia: plain film diagnosis. *J Can Assoc Radiol.* 1980; 31:147–148.

30. White A, Palmer PES. The radiology of intestinal obstruction in Rhodesia. *Clin Radiol.* 1963;14:211–218.

31. Meyers MA. Paraduodenal hernias. Radiologic and arteriographic diagnosis. *Radiology.* 1970;95:29–37.

32. Azouz EM, Doyon M. Waldeyer's hernia. *J Can Assoc Radiol.* 1976;27:108–110.

33. Harbin WP, Andres J, Kim SH, et al. Internal hernia into Treves' field pouch. *Radiology.* 1979;130:71–72.

34. Jules GL, Stemmer EA, Connolly JE. Pre-operative di-

agnosis of small bowel volvulus in adults. *Am J Gastroenterol.* 1971;56:235–247.

35. Young WS, White F, Grave GF. The radiology of ileosigmoid knot. *Clin Radiol.* 1978;29:211–216.

36. North LB, Weens HS. The intestinal knot syndrome. *Am J Roentgenol.* 1964;92:1042–1047.

37. Frimann-Dahl J. Roentgen findings in intestinal knots. *Acta Radiol.* 1942;23:22–33.

38. Lewis JL, Hoskins EO. Volvulus of the small bowel into a pouch in the field of Treves presenting with anaemia. *Br J Radiol.* 1985;58:1132–1134.

39. Dalinka MK, Wunder JF. Meckel's diverticulum and its complications with emphasis on roentgenologic demonstrations. *Radiology.* 1973;108:295–298.

40. Townsend CM Jr, Remmers AR Jr, Searles HE, et al. Intestinal obstruction from medication bezoars in patients with renal failure. *N Engl J Med.* 1973;208:1058–1059.

41. O'Malley JM, Ferrucci JT Jr, Goodgave JT. Medication bezoar: Intestinal obstruction by an Isocal bezoar. *Gastrointest Radiol.* 1981;6:141–144.

42. Moskowitz H. Phytobezoars of the small bowel following gastric surgery. *Radiology.* 1974;113:23–26.

43. Schlang HA, McHenry LE. Obstruction of the small bowel by orange in the postgastrectomy patient. *Ann Surg.* 1964;159:611–622.

44. Strauss S, Rubinstein ZJ, Shapiro Z. Food as a cause of small intestinal obstruction. A report of five cases without previous gastric surgery. *Gastrointest Radiol.* 1977;2:17–20.

45. Freed TA, Sweet LN, Gauder PJ. Balloon obturation bowel obstruction: a hazard of drug smuggling. *Am J Roentgenol.* 1976;127:1033–1034.

46. Balthazar EJ, Lefleur R. Abdominal complications of drug addiction: Radiologic features. *Semin Roentgenol.* 1983;18:213–220.

47. Sinner WN. The gastrointestinal tract as a vehicle for drug smuggling. *Gastrointest Radiol.* 1981;6:319–323.

48. Pinsky MF, Ducas J, Ruggere MD. Narcotic smuggling: The double condom sign. *J Can Assoc Radiol.* 1978;29:79–82.

49. Isaacs I. Roentgenographic demonstration of intestinal ascariasis in children without using barium. *Am J Roentgenol.* 1956;76:558–561.

50. Bean WJ. Recognition of ascariasis by routine chest or abdomen roentgenograms. *Am J Roentgenol.* 1965; 94:379–384.

51. Weissberg DL, Berk RN. Ascariasis of the gastrointestinal tract. *Gastrointest Radiol.* 1978;3:415–418.

52. Ellman BA, Wynee JM, Freeman A. Intestinal ascariasis: New plain film features. *Am J Roentgenol.* 1980; 135:37–42.

53. Gold BM, Meyers MA. Radiologic manifestations of *Taenia saginata* infestation. *Am J Roentgenol.* 1977; 128:493–494.

54. Fetterman L. Radiographic demonstrations of Taenia saginata—an unsuspected cause of abdominal pain. *N Engl J Med.* 1965;272:364–365.

55. Maldonado JE, Gregg JA, Green PA, et al. Chronic

idiopathic intestinal obstruction. *Am J Med.* 1970; 49:203–212.

56. Bughton PH, Murdoch JL, Vottela T. Gastrointestinal complications of the Ehlers–Danlos syndrome. *Gut.* 1969;10:1004–1008.

57. Cohen MD, Lintott DJ. Transient small bowel intussusception in adult coeliac disease. *Clin Radiol.* 1978; 29:529–534.

58. Naish JM, Capper WM, Brown NJ. Intestinal pseudo-obstruction with steatorrhea. *Gut.* 1960;1:62–65.

59. Scott JR, Miller WT, Urso M, et al. Acute mesenteric infarction. *Am J Roentgenol.* 1971;113:269–279.

60. Bryk D, Soong KY. Colonic ileus and its differential roentgen diagnosis. *Am J Roentgenol.* 1967;101:329–337.

61. Love L. The role of the ileocecal valve in large bowel obstruction. A preliminary report. *Radiology.* 1960; 75:391–398.

62. McIver JR, Don C. The fluid-filled bowel in acute large bowel obstruction. *Am J Roentgenol.* 1965;94:410–415.

63. Meyers MA. Colonic ileus. *Gastrointest Radiol.* 1977; 2:37–40.

64. Moss AA, Goldberg HI, Brotman M. Idiopathic intestinal pseudo-obstruction. *Am J Roentgenol.* 1972; 115:312–317.

65. Shirazi KK, Agha FP, Strodel WE. Non-obstructive colonic dilation: Radiographic findings in 50 patients following colonoscopic treatment. *J Can Assoc Radiol.* 1984;35:116–119.

66. Melamed M, Rabuschka SE, Malamet JL. Colon ileus associated with low spine disease. *Clin Radiol.* 1969; 20:47–51.

67. Lowman RM. The potassium depletion states and postoperative ileus. The role of the potassium ion. *Radiology.* 1971;98:691–694.

68. Berenyi MR, Schwarz GS. Megasigmoid syndrome in diabetes and neurologic disease. *Am J Gastroenterol.* 1967;47:311–319.

69. Ogilvie H. Large intestine colic due to sympathetic deprivation. *Br Med J.* 1948;II: 671–673.

70. Nanni GF, Garbini A, Luchetti P, et al. Ogilvie's syndrome (acute colon pseudoobstruction): Review of the literature (October 1948–March 1980) and report of four additional cases. *Dis Colon Rectum.* 1982;25:157–166.

71. Soreide O, Bjerkeset T, Fossdal JE. Pseudo-obstruction of the colon (Ogilvie's syndrome). A genuine clinical condition. Review of the literature and report of five cases. *Dis Colon Rectum.* 1977;20:487–491.

72. Gilchrist AM, Mills JOM, Russell CFJ. Acute large bowel pseudo-obstruction. *Clin Radiol.* 1985;36:401–404.

73. Watkins GL, Oliver GA. Giant megacolon in the insane: Further observations on patients treated by subtotal colectomy. *Gastroenterology.* 1965;48:718–727.

74. Ehrentheil DF, Wells EP. Megacolon in psychotic patients. A clinical entity. *Gastroenterology.* 1955;29:285–293.

75. Teixidor HS, Heneghan MA. Idiopathic intestinal pseudo-obstruction in a family. *Gastrointest Radiol.* 1978;3:91–95.

76. Schuffler MD, Rohrmann CA, Templeton FE. The radiologic manifestations of idiopathic intestinal pseudo-obstruction. *Am J Roentgenol.* 1976;127:729–736.

77. David JT, Nusbaum M. Chlorpromazine therapy and functional large bowel obstruction. *Am J Gastroenterol.* 1975;60:635–639.

78. Caplan LH, Jacobson HG, Rubinstein BM, et al. Megacolon and volvulus in Parkinson's disease. *Radiology.* 1965;85:73–79.

79. Rosenberg RF, Carichi JG. Vincristine-induced megacolon. *Gastrointest Radiol.* 1983;8:71–73.

80. Salerno N, Grey N. Myxedema pseudoobstruction. *Am J Roentgenol.* 1978;130:175–176.

81. Burrell M, Cronan J, Megna D, et al. Myxedema megacolon. *Gastrointest Radiol.* 1980;5:181–186.

82. Carlson DH, Ziter FMH Jr. Non-tropical sprue as a cause of megacolon. Report of a case. *J Can Assoc Radiol.* 1970;21:235–237.

83. Kappelman NB, Burrell M, Toffler R. Megacolon associated with celiac sprue. Report of four cases and review of the literature. *Am J Roentgenol.* 1977;128:65–68.

84. Staple TW, McAlister WH, Anderson MS. Plexiform neurofibromatosis simulating Hirschsprung's disease. *Am J Roentgenol.* 1965;91:840–845.

85. Anderson TE, Spackman TJ, Schwartz S. Roentgen findings in intestinal ganglioneuromatosis. Its association with medullary thyroid carcinoma and pheochromocytoma. *Radiology.* 1971;101:93–96.

86. Grossman HJ, Limiosani MA, Shore M. Megacolon as a manifestation of familial autonomic dysfunction. *J Pediatr.* 1956;49:289–296.

87. Rohrmann CA Jr, Ricci MT, Krishnamurthy S, et al. Radiologic and histologic differentiations of neuromuscular disorders of the gastrointestinal tract. Visceral myopathies, visceral neuropathies and progressive systemic sclerosis. *Am J Roentgenol.* 1984;143:933–941.

88. Simpson AJ, Khilnani MJ. Gastrointestinal manifestations of the muscular dystrophies. A review of roentgen findings. *Am J Roentgenol.* 1975;125:948–955.

89. Weiner MJ. Myotonic megacolon in myotonic dystrophy. *Am J Roentgenol.* 1978;130:177–179.

90. Gema AG, Raia A, Netto AC. Motility of the sigmoid colon and rectum. Contributions to the physiopathology of megacolon in Chagas disease. *Dis Colon Rectum.* 1971;14:291–304.

91. Smith GA, Perry JF Jr, Yonehiro EG. Mechanical intestinal obstruction: A study of 1,252 cases. *Surg Gynecol Obstet.* 1955;100:651–660.

92. Brodey RA, Schuldt DR, Magnuson A et al. Complete colonic obstruction secondary to adhesions. *Am J Roentgenol.* 1979;133:917–918.

93. Griffiths GC. Gallstone obstruction of the descending duodenum. *Br J Radiol.* 1962;38:869–870.

94. Fjermeros H. Gallstone ileus. Case reports and review of 178 cases from Scandinavia and Finland. *Acta Chir Scand.* 1964;128:188–192.

95. Novy S, Rogers LF, Kirkpatrick W. Diastatic rupture of the cecum in obstructing carcinoma of the left colon. Radiographic diagnosis and surgical implications. *Am J Roentgenol.* 1975;123:281–286.

96. Lowman RM, Davis C. Evaluation of cecal size in impending perforation of the cecum. *Surg Gynecol Obstet.* 1956;103:711–718.

97. Kottler RE, Lee GK. The threatened cecum in acute large-bowel obstruction. *Br J Radiol.* 1984;57:989–990.

98. Desai MG, Rodko EA. Perforation of colon in malignant tumors. *J Can Assoc Radiol.* 1973;24:344–349.

99. Young WS. Further radiological observations in caecal volvulus. *Clin Radiol.* 1980;31:479–483.

100. Hemingway AP. Caecal volvulus—a new twist to the barium enema. *Br J Radiol.* 1980;53:806–807.

101. Anderson JR, Mills JOM. Caecal volvulus: A frequently missed diagnosis? *Clin Radiol.* 1985;35:65–69.

102. Weinstein M. Volvulus of the cecum and ascending colon. *Ann Surg.* 1938;107:248–259.

103. Bobroff LM, Messinger NH, Subbarao K, et al. The cecal bascule. *Am J Roentgenol.* 1972;115:249–252.

104. Balthazar EJ. Congenital positional anomalies of the colon: Radiographic diagnosis and clinical implications of abnormalities of fixations. *Gastrointest Radiol.* 1977;2:49–56.

105. Johnson CD, Rice RP, Kelvin FP, et al. The radiological evaluation of gross cecal distensions: Emphasis on cecal ileus. *Am J Roentgenol.* 1985;145:1211–1217.

106. Painter MS. *Diverticular Disease of the Colon: A Deficiency Disease of Western Civilization.* London: Heinemann Medical Books; 1979.

107. Personal observation.

108. Figiel LS, Figiel SJ. Lesions of the large intestine producing acute symptoms. *Radiol Clin N Am.* 1964;2:33–54.

109. McAdam IWJ. Geographical pathology—East Africa. *Clin Radiol.* 1963;14:193–199.

110. Meyers MA, Ghahremani GG, Govoni AF. Ischemic colitis asociated with sigmoid volvulus: New observations. *Am J Roentgenol.* 1977;128:591–595.

111. Young WS, Englebrecht HF, Stoker A. Plain film analysis in sigmoid volvulus. *Clin Radiol.* 1978; 29:553–560.

112. Essenson L, Ginzburg L. Volvulus of the sigmoid. *Am J Surg.* 1949;77:24–249.

113. Evison G, Samuel E. Pseudo-volvulus of the colon. *Clin Radiol.* 1965;16:256–261.

114. Newton NA, Raines HD. Transverse colon volvulus: Case reports and review. *Am J Roentgenol.* 1977; 128:69–72.

115. Chalmers AG, Boddy JE, Franklyn PP. Transverse colon volvulus associated with a vascular and neuronal malformation. *Br J Radiol.* 1985;58:1134–1136.

116. Lantieri R, Teplick SK, Labell MJ. Splenic flexure volvulus: Two case reports and review. *Am J Roentgenol.* 1979;132:463–464.

117. Sachidananthan CK, Soehrer B. Volvulus of the splenic flexure of the colon: Report of a case and review of the literature. *Dis Colon Rectum.* 1972; 15:466–469.

118. Jones B. Ceco-sigmoid volvulus—a new entity? *Br J Radiol.* 1978;51:469–471.

119. Agha FP. Intussusception in adults. *Am J Roentgenol.* 1986;146:527–531.

120. Dean DL, Ellis FH Jr, Sauer WG. Intussusception in adults. *Arch Surg.* 1956;73:6–11.

121. Reymond RD. The mechanism of intussusception: A theoretical analysis of the problem. *Br J Radiol.* 1972; 45:1–7.

122. Jackson H. A sign of intussusception. *Br J Radiol.* 1953;26:323–325.

123. Schatzki R. The roentgenologic appearance of intussuscepted tumors of the colon with and without barium examination. *Am J Roentgenol.* 1939;41:549–563.

124. Dick A, Green CJ. Large bowel intussusception in adults. *Br J Radiol.* 1961;34:769–777.

125. Hughes LE. Post-mortem survey of diverticular disease of the colon—Part I: Diverticulosis and diverticulitis. *Gut.* 1969;10:336–344.

126. Parks TG. Natural history of diverticular disease of the colon. A review of 521 cases. *Br Med J.* 1969; 4:639–649.

127. Painter NS, Burkitt DP. Diverticular disease of the colon: A deficiency disease of western civilization. *Br Med J.* 1971;2:450–454.

128. Parks TG. Post-mortem studies on the colon with special reference to diverticular disease. *Proc R Soc Med.* 1968;61:932–934.

129. Baker SR, Alterman DD. False-negative barium enema in patients with sigmoid cancer and coexistent diverticulosis. *Gastrointest Radiol.* 1985;10:171–173.

130. Massik P, Wheatley FE Jr. The recognition of air in diverticula of the colon as a diagnostic aid. *Radiology.* 1955;64:417–419.

131. Vanapruks S, Fuhrman M. Giant solitary gas cyst of the sigmoid colon: A case report. *Radiology.* 1969; 92:1533–1534.

132. Frankenfeld RH, Waters CH, Schepeler TV. Giant air cyst of the abdomen: An unusual manifestation of diverticulitis of the sigmoid. *Gastroenterology.* 1959; 37:103–106.

133. Gallagher JJ, Welch JP. Giant diverticula of the sigmoid colon: A review of differential diagnosis and operative management. *Arch Surg.* 1979;114:1079–1083.

134. Foster DR, Ross B. Giant sigmoid diverticulum: Clinical and radiological features. *Gut.* 1977;18:1051–1053.

135. Johns ER, Hartley MG. Giant gas filled cysts of the sigmoid colon: a report of two cases. *Br J Radiol.* 1976; 49:930–931.

136. Rabinowitz JH, Farman J, Dallemand S, et al. Giant sigmoid diverticulum. *Am J Roentgenol.* 1974;121:338–342.

137. Muhletaler CA, Berger JL, Robinette CL Jr. Pathogenesis of giant colonic diverticula. *Gastrointest Radiol.* 1981;6:217–222.

138. Smulewicz JJ, Govoni AF. Giant air cysts of the colon. *J Can Assoc Radiol.* 1974;25:245–250.

139. Moss AA. Giant sigmoid diverticulum: Clinical and

radiological features. *Am J Dig Dis.* 1975;20:676–683.

140. Sager S. Giant sigmoid diverticulum of the transverse colon with diverticulosis. *Br J Clin Pract.* 1973; 27:145–146.

141. Wallers KJ. Giant diverticulum arising from the transverse colon of a patient with diverticulosis. *Br J Radiol.* 1981;54:683–684.

142. Kricun R, Stasik JJ, Reither RD, et al. Giant colonic diverticulum. *Am J Roentgenol.* 1980;135:507–512.

143. Swann JC, Giles, KW. Giant diverticulum of the sigmoid colon. *Br J Radiol.* 1971;44:551–553.

144. MacBeth WAAG, Riddle PR. Gas-filled abscess as a manifestation of diverticulitis of the colon. *Br J Radiol.* 1964;37:861–862.

145. Silberman ER, Thorner MC. Volvulus of giant sigmoidal diverticulum. *JAMA.* 1961;177:782–785.

146. White AF, Oh KS, Weber AL. Radiologic manifestations of Meckel's diverticulum. *Am J Roentgenol.* 1973; 118:86–94.

147. Dalinka MK, Wunder JF. Meckel's diverticulum and its complications with emphasis on roentgenologic demonstration. *Radiology.* 1973;106:295–298.

148. Govoni AF, Burdman D, Teicher I, et al. Enterogenous cyst of the colon presenting as a retroperitoneal tumor in an adult. *Am J Roentgenol.* 1975;123:320–329.

149. Kottra JJ, Dodds WJ. Duplication of the large bowel. *Am J Roentgenol.* 1971;113:310–315.

150. Bass EM. Duplication of the colon. *Clin Radiol.* 1978; 29:205–209.

151. LeVine M, Katz I, Lampros PJ. Blind pouch formation secondary to side-to-side intestinal anastomosis. *Am J Roentgenol.* 1963;89:706–719.

152. Maglintie DDT. "Blind pouch" syndrome: A cause of gastrointestinal bleeding. *Radiology.* 1979;132:314.

153. Telepak RJ, Huggins TJ, Bova JG. Tuboovarian abscess simulating giant colon diverticulum. *Gastrointest Radiol.* 1984;9:369–371.

154. Marshak RH, Lindner AE. *Radiology of the Small Intestine.* Philadelphia: WB Saunders; 1970.

155. Rice RP. Plain abdominal film roentgenographic diagnosis of ulcerative diseases of the colon. *Am J Roentgenol.* 1968;104:544–550.

156. Bartram CI, Preston DM, Lennard-Jones JE. The "air enema" in acute colitis. *Gastrointest Radiol.* 1983;8:61–65.

157. Simpson SA, Lewin JR. Plain roentgenography in diagnosis of chronic ulcerative colitis and terminal ileitis. *Am J Roentgenol.* 1960;84:306–315.

158. Bryk D. Ulcerative colitis proximal to an obstructing surgical colonic stricture. *Radiology.* 1968;91:786–787.

159. Senturia HR, Wald SM. Ulcerative disease of intestinal tract proximal to partially obstructing lesions: Roentgen appearance. *Am J Roentgenol.* 1967;99:45–51.

160. Schwartz SS, Boley SJ. Ischemic origin of ulcerative colitis associated with partially obstructing lesions of the colon. *Radiology.* 1972;102:249–252.

161. Wolf BS, Marshak RH. "Toxic" segmental dilatation in course of fulminating ulcerative colitis: Roentgen findings. *Am J Roentgenol.* 1969;82:985–995.

162. Kramer P, Wittenberg J. Colonic gas distribution in toxic megacolon. *Gastroenterology.* 1981;80:433–437.

163. McConnell F, Harelin J, Robbins LL. Plain film diagnosis of fulminating ulcerative colitis. *Radiology.* 1958;71:674–682.

164. Schaeter A, Goldstein MJ, Kirsner JB. Toxic dilatation complicating Crohn's disease of the colon. *Gastroenterology.* 1967;53:136–142.

165. Faegenburg D, Chiat H, Mandel PR, et al. Toxic megacolon in amebic colitis: Report of a case. *Am J Roentgenol.* 1967;99:74–76.

166. Wruble LD, Dachsworth JK, Duke DD, et al. Toxic dilatation of the colon in a case of amebiasis. *N Engl J Med.* 1966;275:926–928.

167. Tully TE, Feinberg SB. Those other types of enterocolitis. *Am J Roentgenol.* 1974;12:291–300.

168. Cardoso JM, Kimura K, Stoopen M, et al. Radiology of invasive amebiasis of the colon. *Am J Roentgenol.* 1977;128:935–941.

169. Hardy R, Scullin DR. Thumbprinting in a case of amebiasis. *Radiology.* 1971;98:147–148.

170. Tully TE, Feinberg SB. Those other types of entercolitis. *Am J Roentgenol.* 1974;121:291–300.

171. Stanley RJ, Nelson GL, Tedesco FJ, et al. Plain film findings in severe pseudomembranous colitis. *Radiology.* 1976;118:7–11.

172. Driscoll RH. "Thumb-printing" in pseudomembranous enterocolitis. *N Engl J Med.* 1978;299:1414–1415.

173. Brown CH, Ferrante WA, David WD Jr. Toxic dilatation of the colon complication pseudomembranous enterocolitis. *Am J Dig Dis.* 1968;13:813–821.

174. Khilnani MT, Marshak RH, Eliasoph J, et al. Intramural intestinal hemorrhage. *Am J Roentgenol.* 1964; 92:1061–1071.

175. Sears AD, Hawkins J, Kitgore BB, et al. Plain roentgenographic findings in drug induced intramural hematoma of the small bowel. *Am J Roentgenol.* 1964; 91:808–813.

176. Pearson KD, Buchignani JS, Shimkin PM, et al. Hereditary angioneurotic edema of the gastrointestinal tract. *Am J Roentgenol.* 1972;116:256–261.

177. Rosato EF, Rosato FE, Scott J, et al. Ischemic dilatation of the colon. *Am J Dig Dis.* 1969;14:922–928.

178. Damuth HD Jr, Greenbaum EI. Colonic spasm: A possible mechanism for thumbprinting. *J Can Assoc Radiol.* 1984;35:202–203.

179. Wittenberg J, Athanasoulis CA, Williams LF Jr, et al. Ischemic colitis radiology and pathophysiology. *Am J Roentgenol.* 1975;123:287–300.

180. Tomchik FS, Wittenberg J, Ottinger LW, et al. The roentgenographic spectrum of bowel infarction. *Radiology.* 1970;96:249–260.

181. Nelson SW, Eggleston W. Findings on plain roentgenograms of the abdomen associated with mesenteric vascular occlusion with a possible new sign of mesenteric venous thrombosis. *Am J Roentgenol.* 1960;83:886–894.

182. Wang CC, Reeves JD. Mesenteric vascular disease. *Am J Roentgenol.* 1960;83:895–908.

183. Frimann-Dahl J. Roentgen examination in mesenteric

thrombosis. *Am J Roentgenol.* 1950;64:610–616.

184. Rendich RA, Harrington LA. Roentgenologic observation in mesenteric thrombosis. *Am J Roentgenol.* 1944;52:317–322.

185. Schwartz S, Boley SJ, Robinson K, et al. Roentgenologic features of vascular disorders. *Radiol Clin N Am.* 1964;2:71–87.

186. Schorr S. Small intestinal intramural air. *Radiology.* 1963;81:285–287.

187. Rigler LG, Pogue WL. Roentgen signs of intestinal neurosis. *Am J Roentgenol.* 1965;94:402–409.

188. Rosenquist CJ. An unusual pattern of intramural gas in small bowel infarction. *Radiology.* 1971;99:337–338.

189. Cynn W-S, Hodes PT. A new sign of small bowel volvulus. Gas in mesenteric veins without gas in portal vein. *Radiology.* 1973;108:289–290.

190. Kessler RM, Levitz JC, Abdenour CE Jr. Mesenteric vascular gas secondary to ischemic bowel in transmesenteric hernia. *Radiology.* 1981;140:645–646.

191. O'Connell DJ, Dewbury KC, Green B, et al. The plain abdominal radiograph in pneumatosis coli. *Clin Radiol.* 1976;27:563–568.

192. Colquhon J. Intramural gas in hollow viscus. *Clin Radiol.* 1965;16:71–86.

193. Elliott GB, Elliott KA. The roentgenologic pathology of so-called pneumatosis cystoides intestinalis. *Am J Roentgenol.* 1963;89:720–729.

194. Koss L. Abdominal gas cysts (pneumatosis cystoides intestinorum hominis). *Arch Pathol.* 1952;53:523–549.

195. Kenney JL. Pneumatosis intestinalis. *Clin Radiol.* 1963;14:70–76.

196. Druckmann A, Schwartz A, Rabinovici N, et al. Pneumatosis of the intestines. *Am J Roentgenol.* 1961;86:911–919.

197. Keyting WS, McCarver RR, Kovacik JL, et al. Pneumatosis intestinalis: A new concept. *Radiology.* 1961;76:733–741.

198. Macklin MT, Macklin CC. Malignant interstitial emphysema of lungs and mediastinum as important occult complications in many respiratory diseases and other conditions: Interpretation of clinical literature in light of laboratory experiment. *Medicine.* 1944;23:281–358.

199. Doub HP, Shea JJ. Pneumatosis cystoides intestinalis. *JAMA.* 1960;172:1238–1242.

200. Ghahremani G, Post R, Beachley M. Pneumatosis coli in Crohn's disease. *Am J Dig Dis.* 1974;19:315–323.

201. Frimann-Dahl J. *Roentgen Examination in Acute Abdominal Diseases.* Springfield, Ill: Charles C Thomas Publishers; 1951.

202. Strain JD, Rudikoff J, Moore EE, et al. Pneumatosis intestinalis associated with intracatheter jejunostomy feeding. *Am J Roentgenol.* 1982;139:107–109.

203. Wandtke J, Skucas J, Spataro R, et al. Pneumatosis intestinalis as a complication of jejunoileal bypass. *Am J Roentgenol.* 1977;129:601–604.

204. Clements JL, Jr. Intestinal pneumatosis—A complication of the jejunoileal bypass procedure. *Gastrointest Radiol.* 1977;2:267–271.

205. Bryk D. Unusual causes of small bowel pneumatosis: Perforated duodenal ulcer and perforated jejunal diverticula. *Radiology.* 1973;106:299–302.

206. Frank PH, O'Connell DJ. Pneumatosis cystoides intestinalis and obstructing intussusception in celiac disease. *Gastrointest Radiol.* 1977;2:109–111.

207. Gefter WB, Evers KA, Malet PF, et al. Nontropical sprue with pneumatosis coli. *Am J Roentgenol.* 1981;137:624–625.

208. Didonato LR. Pneumatosis coli secondary to acute appendicitis. *Radiology.* 1976;120:90.

209. Miercourt RD, Merrill FG. Pneumatosis and pseudo-obstruction in scleroderma. *Radiology.* 1969;92:359–362.

210. Kleinman F, Meyers MA, Abbott G, et al. Necrotizing enterocolitis with pneumatosis intestinalis in systemic lupus erythematosus and polyarteritis. *Radiology.* 1976;121:595–598.

211. Freiman D, Hikon C, Bilaniuk L. Pneumatosis intestinalis in systemic lupus erythematosis. *Radiology.* 1975;116:563–564.

212. Braunstein EM, White SJ. Pneumatosis intestinalis in dermatomyositis. *Br J Radiol.* 1980;53:1011–1012.

213. Jaffe N, Carlson DH, Vawter GF. Pneumatosis cystoides intestinalis in acute leukemia. *Cancer.* 1972;30:239–243.

214. O'Connell DJ, Thompson AJ. Pneumatosis coli in non-Hodgkin's lymphoma. *Br J Radiol.* 1978;51:203–205.

215. Navari RM, Sharma P, Deeg HJ, et al. Pneumatosis cystoides intestinalis following allogenic marrow transplantation. *Transplant Proc.* 1983;15:1720–1724.

216. Maile CW, Frick MP, Crass JR, et al. The plain abdominal radiograph in acute gastrointestinal graft vs. host disease. *Am J Roentgenol.* 1985;145:289–292.

217. Day DL, Ramsay NKC, Letourneau JG. Pneumatosis intestinalis after bone marrow transplantation. *Am J Roentgenol.* 1988;151:85–87.

218. Borns PF, Johnston TA. Indolent pneumatosis of the bowel wall associated with immune suppressive therapy. *Ann Radiol.* 1973;16:163–166.

219. Yale CE, Balish E, Wu JP. The bacterial etiology of pneumatosis cystoides intestinalis. *Arch Surg.* 1974;109-89–94.

220. Olmsted WW, Madewell JE. Pneumatosis cystoides intestinalis: A pathophysiologic explanation of the roentgenographic signs. *Gastrointest Radiol.* 1976;1:177–181.

221. Kressler HY, Koehler RE, Holcroft J. Loculated pneumoperitoneum simulating gas in the bowel wall. *Radiology.* 1977;123:30.

222. Boijsen E, Kaude J, Tylen U. Radiologic diagnosis of ileal carcinoid tumor. *Acta Radiol (Diag).* 1974;15:65–83.

223. Case records of the Massachusetts General Hospital. Case 34-1973. *N Engl J Med.* 1973;289:419–424.

224. Kaude JV. Calcification in carcinoid tumors. *N Engl J Med.* 1973;289:921.

225. Noonan CD. Calcified carcinoid of the small bowel: A case report. *Radiol Clin Biol.* 1972;41:115–120.

226. Marine R, Lattomus WW. Cavernous hemangioma of the gastrointestinal tract: Report of case and review. *Radiology.* 1958;70:860–863.

227. Rosenfield AJ. Widespread calcified metastases, from adenocarcinoma of the jejunum. *Am J Dig Dis.* 1975;20:990–993.

228. Gemmell NI: Calcification within a gastric carcinoma. *Am J Roentgenol.* 1964;91:779–783.

229. Staple TW, McAlister WH. Roentgenographic visualization of iron preparations in the gastrointestinal tract. *Radiology.* 1964;83:1051–1056.

230. Hinkel CL. The significance of opaque medications in the gastro-intestinal tract with special reference to enteric coated pills. *Am J Roentgenol.* 1951;65:575–581.

231. Nathan MH, Newman A. Conjugated iopanoic acid (Telepaque) in the small bowel. An aid in the diagnosis of gallbladder disease. *Radiology.* 1973;109:545–548.

232. Shapiro JH, Rubinstein B, Jacobson HG, et al. Enteroliths in the small intestine. *Am J Roentgenol.* 1956; 75:343–348.

233. Grettve S. A contribution to the knowledge of primary true concrements in the small bowel. *Acta Chir Scand.* 1947;95:387–410.

234. Blix G. Contribution to chemistry of primary calculi of the small intestine. *Acta Chir Scand.* 1935;76:24–34.

235. Crummy AB Jr, Juhl JH. Calcified gastric leiomyoma. *Am J Roentgenol.* 1962;87:727–728.

236. Katz I, Fischer RM. Enteroliths complicating regional enteritis. A report of two cases. *Am J Roentgenol.* 1957; 78:653–660.

237. Brettner A, Euphrat E. Radiological significance of primary enterolithiasis. *Radiology.* 1970;94:283–288.

238. Bery K, Virmani P, Chawla S. Enterolithiasis with tubercular intestinal strictures. *Br J Radiol.* 1964; 37:73–75.

239. Gundersen AL, Kreiter RL. Cecal lithiasis. Secondary to cecal stenosis. *JAMA.* 1968;205:462–463.

240. Enge I, Frimann-Dahl J. Radiology in acute abdominal disorder due to Meckel's diverticulum. *Br J Radiol.* 1964;37:775–780.

241. Dovey P. Calculus in a Meckel's diverticulum—A preoperative radiological diagnosis. *Br J Radiol.* 1971; 44:888–890.

242. Feldman MI. Calculi in Meckel's diverticulum. *Radiology.* 1966;86:541–54.

243. Bischoff ME, Stampfli WP. Meckel's diverticulum with emphasis on the roentgen diagnosis. *Radiology.* 1955;65:572–577.

244. Altaras J. Calculi of the small intestine. *Br J Radiol.* 1956;29:684–686.

245. Maglinte DDT, Taylor SD, Ng AC. Gastrointestinal perforation by chicken bones. *Radiology.* 1979; 130:597–599.

246. Bunker PG. The role of dentistry in problems of foreign bodies in the air and food passages. *J Am Dent Assoc.* 1962;64:782–787.

247. Katz I, Arcomano J. Roentgen findings in a case of perforation of the cecum by a bone. *Radiology.* 1954; 63:411–414.

248. Berk RN, Reit RJ. Intra-abdominal chicken bone abscess. *Radiology.* 1971;101:311–313.

249. Zbornik RC. Large fecal stones—The sigmoid. *Am J Roentgenol.* 1971;113:355–359.

250. Harland D. A case of multiple calculi in the large intestine with a review of the subject of intestinal calculi. *Br J Surg.* 1965;41:209–211.

251. Thompson R, Barry WF Jr. Rectal calculus. *Radiology.* 1970;96:411–412.

252. Spitzer A, Caruthers SB, Stables DP. Radiopaque suppositories. *Radiology.* 1976;121:71–73.

253. Fletcher BD, Morreels CL, Christian WH III, et al. Calcified adenocarcinoma of the colon. *Am J Roentgenol.* 1967;101:310–305.

254. Van Patten HT, Whittirk JW. Heterotopic ossification in intestinal neoplasia. *Am J Pathol.* 1955;31:73–91.

255. Hall CW. Calcification and osseous metaplasia in carcinoma of the colon. *J Can Assoc Radiol.* 1962;13:135–139.

256. Engel S, Dockerty MD. Calcification and ossification in rectal malignant processes. *JAMA.* 1962;179:345–350.

257. Shockman AT. Calcified carcinoma of the colon superimposed on chronic ulcerative colitis. *Am J Dig Dis.* 1969;14:683–687.

258. Bell GA, McKenzie AD, Emmons H. Diffuse cavernous hemangioma of the rectum. Report of a case and review of the literature. *Dis Colon Rectum.* 1972; 15:377–382.

259. Bailey JJ, Barrick CW, Jenkinson EL. Hemangioma of the colon. *JAMA.* 1956;160:658–659.

260. Hollingsworth G. Haemangiomatous lesions of the colon. *Br J Radiol.* 1951;24:220–222.

261. Lehmann JS Jr, Farid Z, Bassily S, et al. Colonic calcifications and polyposis in schistosomiasis. *Radiology.* 1971;98:379–380.

262. Fataar S, Bassiony H, Hamed MS, et al. Radiographic spectrum of rectocolonic calcification from schistosomiasis. *Am J Roentgenol.* 1984;142:933–936.

263. Berg RM, Berg HM. Coproliths. *Radiology.* 1957; 68:839–844.

264. Carey LS. Lead shot appendicitis in northern native people. *J Can Assoc Radiol.* 1977;28:171–174.

265. Maglintie DDT, Bush ML, Aruta EV, et al. Retained barium in the appendix: Diagnostic and clinical significance. *Am J Roentgenol.* 1981;137:529–533.

266. Felson B, Bernhard CM, The roentgenolic diagnosis appendiceal calculi. *Radiology.* 1947;49:178–179.

267. Weisflog. X-ray diagnosis of enteroliths in the appendix. *Fortschr Geb Roentgenstr.* 1906;10:217–219.

268. Faegenburg D. Fecaliths of the appendix: Incidence and significance. *Am J Roentgenol.* 1963;89:752–759.

269. Thomas SF. Appendiceal coproliths: Their surgical importance. *Radiology.* 1947;49:39–49.

270. Brady BM, Carroll DS. The significance of the calcified appendiceal enterolith. *Radiology.* 1957;68:648–653.

271. Bunch GH, Adcock DF. Giant faceted calculus. *Ann Surg.* 1939;109:143–146.

272. Bogren HG, Billing L. Multiple calculi in a Meckel's

diverticulum. Report of a case. *Acta Radiol (Diagn)*. 1977;18:669–671.

273. Athey GN. Unusual demonstration of a Meckel's diverticulum containing enteroliths. *Br J Radiol*. 1980; 53:365–368.

274. Bigongiari LR, Wicks JD. Gas-filled appendix with meniscus: Outline of the appendicolith. *Gastrointest Radiol*. 1978;3:229–231.

275. May LM, O'Neill FE, Allen SW. Cecal ileus—An undescribed and helpful sign in acute appendicitis. *Tex Med*. 1958;54:92–95.

276. Soteropoluos C, Gilmore JH. Roentgen diagnosis of acute appendicitis. *Radiology*. 1958;71:246–256.

277. Killen DA, Brooks DW Jr. Gas-filled appendix: A roentgen sign of acute appendicitis. *Ann Surg*. 1965; 161:474–478.

278. Fisher MS. A roentgen sign of acute appendicitis. *Am J Roentgenol*. 1959;61:637–639.

279. Samuel E. Gas-filled appendix. *Br J Radiol*. 1957; 30:27–30.

280. Lim MS. Gas-filled appendix: Lack of diagnostic specificity. *Am J Roentgenol*. 1977;128:209–210.

281. Soter CS. The contribution of the radiologist to the diagnosis of acute appendicitis. *Semin Roentgenol*. 1973;8:375–388.

282. Casper RB. Fluid in the right flank as a roentgenographic sign of acute appendicitis. *Am J Roentgenol*. 1970;110:352–354.

283. Meyers MA, Oliphant M. Ascending retrocecal appendicitis. *Radiology*. 1974;110:295–299.

284. Harris S, Rudolph LE. Mechanical small bowel obstruction due to acute appendicitis: Review of ten cases. *Ann Surg*. 1966;164:157–161.

285. Melamed M, Melamed JL, Rahishka SF. Appendicitis: "Functional" bowel obstruction associated with perforation of the appendix. *Am J Roentgenol*. 1967; 99:112–117.

286. Chavez MC, Morgan BD. Acute appendicitis with pneumoperitoneum. Radiographic diagnosis and report of five cases. *Amer Surg*. 1968;32:604–608.

287. Rucker CR, Midler RE, Nay HR. Pneumoperitoneum secondary to perforated appendicitis. *Am Surg*. 1967; 33:188–190.

288. Farman J, Kassner EG, Dallemand S, et al. Pneumoperitoneum and appendicitis. *Gastrointest Radiol*. 1976;1:277–279.

289. McCort JJ. Extra-alimentary gas in perforated appendicitis. Report of six cases. *Am J Roentgenol*. 1960; 84:1087–1092.

290. Norman A, Leider LS, del Carman J. Mucocele of the appendix. *Am J Roentgenol*. 1957;77:647–651.

291. Euphrat EJ. Roentgen features of mucocele of the appendix. *Radiology*. 1947;48:113–117.

292. Peyton Barnes J. Calcified mucocele of the appendix. *Am J Surg*. 1948;76:323–327.

293. Bonann LJ, Davis JG. Retroperitoneal mucocele of the appendix. A case report with characteristic roentgen features. *Radiology*. 1948;51:375–382.

294. Douglas MJ, Cameron DC, Niyon SF, et al. Intussusception of a mucocele of the appendix. *Gastrointest Radiol*. 1978;3:97–100.

295. Ferris EJ, Shauffer IA. Hydrocele of the spermatic cord: With roentgenographic findings simulating a mucocele of the appendix. *Am J Roentgenol*. 1965; 94:395–398.

296. Milliken G, Poindexter CA. Mucocele of appendix with globoid body formation. *Am J Pathol*. 1925; 1:397–402.

297. Probstein JG, Lassar GM. Mucocele of the appendix with myxoglobulosis. *Ann Surg*. 1948;127:171–176.

298. Miller D. Mucocele and myxoglobulosis of the appendix. *Surg Clin N Am*. 1947;27:337–343.

299. Felson B, Wiot JF. Some interesting right lower quadrant entities. *Radiol Clin N Am*. 1969;7:83–95.

300. Dachman AH, Lichtenstein JE, Friedman AC. Review. Mucocele of the appendix and pseudomyxoma peritonei. *Am J Roentgenol*. 1985;144:923–930.

301. Mayer GB, Chuang VP, Fisher RG. CT of pseudomyxoma peritonei. *Am J Roentgenol*. 1981;136:807–808.

The Plain Film of the Liver, Bile Ducts, and Spleen

LIVER

The liver shadow occupies a broad area of the upper abdomen. Its homogeneous density and fixed position below the diaphragm provide a reliable background for the detection of subtle lucencies and opacities in the biliary tract, the gastrointestinal tract, the peritoneal cavity, and the retroperitoneal spaces. Yet, despite being the largest solid organ in the abdomen, most liver abnormalities cannot be seen on plain films. It does not alter its size or shape rapidly and its vast volume can accommodate growing masses without significant modification of contour. Moreover, many pathological processes in the liver result from cellular or subcellular derangements that produce profound metabolic effects but little spatial change. Nonetheless, some hepatic diseases are associated with distinctive signs on abdominal radiographs that are often readily recognizable and occasionally even pathognomonic.

Contour of the Liver

No plain film projection of the abdomen allows for a complete depiction of the entire margin of the liver. Much of its border abuts on structures of similar density, thus preventing a clear outline of the liver edge. The delineation of the hepatic contour must be assessed by an evaluation of its relationship with the diaphragm, and adjacent fat interfaces and by the location of nearby gas-filled structures.

The diaphragm tightly caps the liver, and its interface with air in the lung provides a good marker of the upper extent of the right hepatic lobe. Nevertheless a subphrenic abscess that separates liver from diaphragm and a subpulmonic pleural effusion that insinuates itself between diaphragm and lung can each give a false impression of the position of the superior hepatic margin. The close apposition of the heart with the medial aspect of both diaphragmatic leaves restricts a precise demarcation of all but

the most lateral extent of the superior surface of the left lobe.[1]

The relatively lucent properitoneal fat often provides adequate contrast for direct visualization of the lateral liver edge (Fig 2–58). Controversy exists about the exact location of the border-forming fat along the inferior hepatic margin. Whalen et al assert that the posterolateral margin of the liver is seen in juxtaposition with the properitoneal fat stripe at the hepatic angle.[2] Gelfand maintains that divergence of the radiological beam requires that the most lateralward edge of the liver be relatively ventral, in the plane of the anterior axillary line.[3] Hence, a more posterior fat–liver interface must be too medial to form the outer hepatic margin on supine films.

The location of adipose tissue delimiting the medial aspect of the hepatic angle is also a matter of dispute between these two investigators. Whalen et al have shown on autopsy studies that the perivisceral extraperitoneal fat is a bed upon which rests both sides of the inferior margin of the liver.[2] The frequent loss of the hepatic angle on prone films is caused by the falling away of the liver from this retroperitoneal cushion. Gelfand believes that intraperitoneal fat situated in the omentum and around the colon is abundant enough beside the liver to bring the hepatic edge into relief (Fig 3–33).[3] Both claims probably have validity. In some patients, a medial extension of properitoneal fat lies against the inferior hepatic margin whereas in others intraperitoneal adipose deposits afford sufficient contrast.

The anterior–inferior hepatic margin is not usually in contact with fat as it courses toward the midline, but its position can be estimated by the location of the gas-filled hepatic flexure. The undersurface of the liver has a variable contour. In mesomorphic individuals it often presents a horizontally directed face whereas in more asthenic patients it assumes a more oblique orientation. Occasionally, the undersurface of the liver can describe a complex undulation that may reveal a double liver edge as it abuts on adipose tissue in two planes (Fig 6–1). Near the midline, the inferior margin of the caudate lobe is in direct contact with the duodenal bulb and the stomach lies just beneath the left lobe.

Enlargements of the liver can be focal or generalized. The most readily discernible focal variation is Reidel's lobe, a downward overgrowth of the inferolateral right lobe. Reidel's lobe may reach far inferiorly as a tonguelike extension superimposed over the iliac crest (Fig 6–2). Almost always, the hepatic angle that defines its inferolateral border is maintained. Herniation of the liver upward through a diaphragmatic rent appears as a sharply defined rounded density projecting into the lung. The most common contour anomalies of the left and caudate lobe impinge upon the stomach and duodenal bulb, respectively.[4]

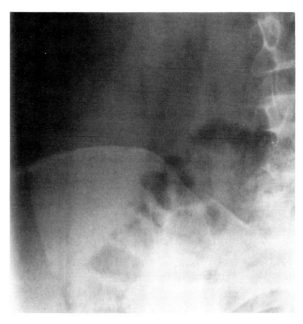

Figure 6–2. Reidel's lobe. A thin inferior extension of the right lobe abuts on the hepatic flexure.

Generalized enlargement of the liver is easy to diagnose if there is massive hepatomegaly. In such cases the liver shadow appears as a homogeneous opacity occupying the right upper and mid abdomen, with its lower margin superimposed upon the iliac fossa (Fig 6–3). The inferior liver edge crosses

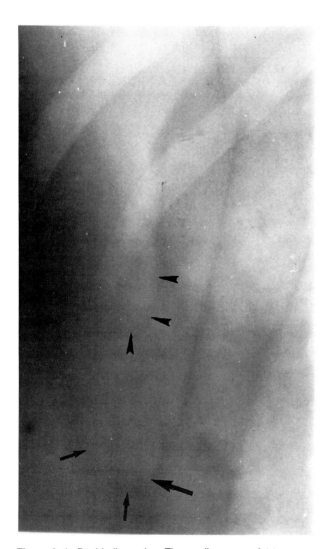

Figure 6–1. Double liver edge. The small arrows point to a posterior interface with retroperitoneal fat. The large arrows outline a more anterior liver–fat border. An undulating inferior hepatic surface enabled fat to cradle the liver in two planes.

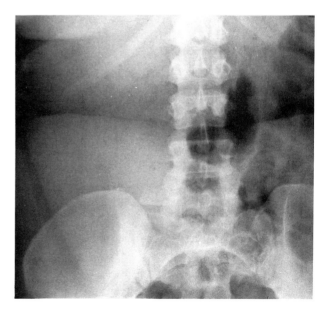

Figure 6–3. Hepatomegaly. The liver extends deep into the iliac fossa. No colon or small-bowel gas occupies the right abdomen. The horizontal liver lucency crossing the mid-abdomen is air trapped between skin folds in the back of this obese patient.

the right psoas muscle and deviates the stomach laterally as it pushes the duodenum inferiorly.[5] Often, a prompt and accurate assessment of marked hepatic enlargement can be accomplished by a rapid scan of the plain film (Fig 6–4). Lesser increases in volume demand more careful and deliberate assessment of specific radiological signs, however. Gelfand uses the relative position of the gas filled hepatic flexure and the right kidney as a measure of the orientation of the inferior liver edge.[3] He maintains that a vertical separation indicates an oblique hepatic undersurface. We have found that displacement of the hepatic flexure below the right kidney is not only evidence of a variation in the shape of the liver but also a good sign of hepatic enlargement. This finding is especially sensitive if previous films indicate a change in the relative positioning of the inferior pole of the right kidney and the gas-filled hepatic flexure (Fig 2–79).

Rounding of the hepatic angle suggests increasing size of the inferior liver (Fig 6–5). This sign has limited usefulness in the recognition of moderate hepatomegaly because of the wide range of appearances of the angle in normal patients. Upward displacement of the diaphragm is uncommon except in massive livers. Lateral deviation of the stomach is helpful in assessing growth of the left lobe, but gas-

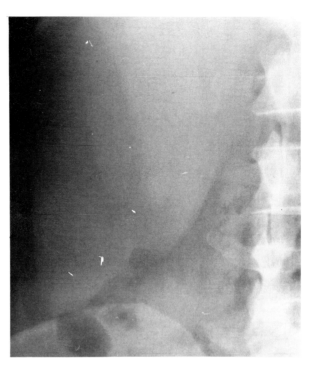

Figure 6–5. Rounding of the hepatic angle in a patient with an enlarged liver. The inferomedial edge of the liver overlies the right psoas muscle.

tric displacement usually implies marked general hepatic expansion (Fig 6–6). Downward relocation of the fundus of the stomach is another sign of left lobe enlargement (Fig 2–80). It is often difficult, to discern, however, especially if a dilated heart obscures clear definition of much of the left hemidiaphragm. In some cases displacement of the duodenal bulb to the left of the midline or below the L2 vertebral body accompanies hepatomegaly.[6,7] Movement of the bulb is too insensitive to reveal subtle increase in liver mass. Downward migration of the right kidney can be caused by a big liver but is seldom seen in the absence of the other plain film evidence of hepatic enlargement.

Assessment of reduced liver size by survey films is generally unreliable. Plain radiograph correlates of a small liver include deviation of the stomach towards the midline,[8] elevation of the duodenal bulb above the 12th rib, and upward migration of the right kidney. Considerable variability in the normal location of these structures, however, limits the ability of the plain film to denote a shrunken liver.

Any evaluation of the liver size presupposes a normal abdominal configuration. The depression of the diaphragm by inelastic lungs in chronic obstructive pulmonary disease can push an unenlarged liver inferiorly. Less commonly, chronic elevation of the diaphragm may accommodate superior migra-

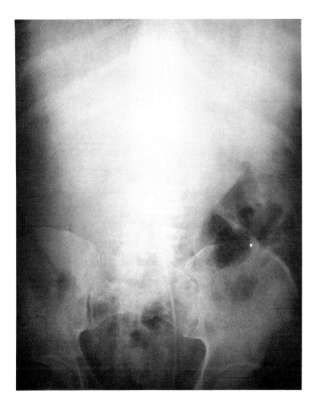

Figure 6–4. Massive hepatomegaly. A huge liver fills most of the abdomen above the pelvis.

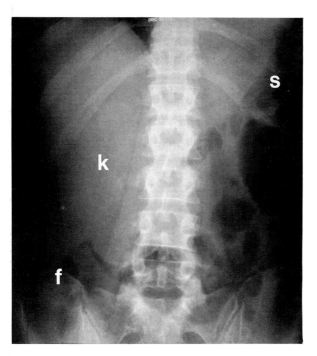

Figure 6–6. Hepatomegaly. The hepatic flexure (f) is displaced well below the right kidney (k). The stomach filled with air (s) has been pushed laterally.

single case of a diffuse increase in hepatic density simulating iron overload has been seen after the ingestion of an excessive amount of thallium sulfate.[12]

Thorotrast is a colloidal suspension of thorium dioxide that has been used as a contrast agent. It was first available for diagnostic radiology in 1928[13] but was banned in the early 1950s except for experimental studies, which continued until 1964.[14] Its predominant roentgenographic application was in cerebral angiography.[15] Almost from the outset thorium-232 was a controversial agent because it is radioactive, with a physical half-life of 1.4×10^{10} years, a biologic half-life of 200 years, and 90% of its emitted radiation is alpha particles.[15] Moreover, several of the daughter products of thorium are also radioactive. Between 50,000 and 100,000 individuals have received Thorotrast and many are still alive today.[16]

The untoward effects of thorium-232 have been well documented. After an intra-arterial injection, thorium accumulates in the liver, spleen, and nearby lymph nodes. In the liver, Thorotrast causes hepatic fibrosis and cirrhosis and predisposes to hepatic malignancies. Half the tumors resulting from Thoro-

tion of the liver. Foreshortening of the abdomen by multiple vertebral body fractures, severe angulation of the upper abdomen consequent to a thoracolumbar gibbus, and marked displacement of normal landmarks by a severe lumbar scoliosis all can cause a rearrangement of abdominal viscera, invalidating the plain film signs of hepatomegaly.

Diffuse Opacification of the Liver

There are several conditions that may give an opaque cast to the liver. The brightness of the liver shadow is dependent upon both the inherent density of the hepatic substance and the relative lucency of surrounding structures. Consequently, a normal liver may appear conspicuously and homogeneously radiodense if it is in close apposition with abundant retroperitoneal adipose tissue. In such instances, the lateral margin of the liver is displaced away from the right lateral ribs by a broad band of properitoneal fat (Fig 6–7).

Iron overload results in the diffuse accumulation of hemosiderin in the liver and spleen. In primary hemochromotosis, faint opacification of retroperitoneal nodes may also be seen, as these, too, are sites for iron deposition (Fig 3–60).[9,10] Any disease that requires treatment by frequent blood transfusions can result in excessive deposition of iron within the liver parenchyma (Fig 6–8).[11] Finally, a

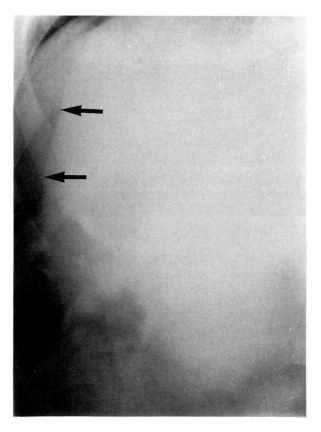

Figure 6–7. Abundant retroperitoneal fat makes this normal liver appear dense. Its lateral edge (*arrow*) is displaced toward the midline.

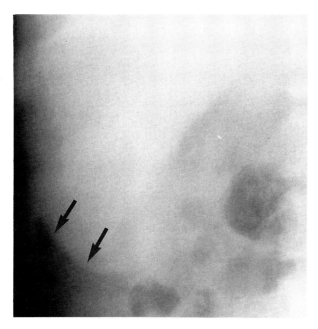

Figure 6–8. A patient with hemoglobin S-C disease who has received repeated transfusions for many years to treat his anemia. Excess iron has accumulated in the liver, rendering it radiodense. The lower hepatic margin is outlined by arrows.

trast injection are cholangiocarcinomas and hepatic cell carcinomas.[17] The other half are the otherwise rare hepatic angiosarcomas.[18] Soon after administration thorium concentrates in the liver and spleen, rendering both organs diffusely dense (Fig 6–9). Over the course of several years, there is a gradual transport of thorium from the liver to draining lymph nodes. The liver decreases in opacity, and a feathery or lacy pattern is seen along with dense, well-defined peripancreatic lymph nodes and a very dense small mottled spleen (Fig 6–10).[19] The association of densities in the liver, spleen, and peripancreatic lymph nodes is pathognomonic for Thorotrast retention (Fig 6–11).

Calcifications in the Liver

Compared with adjacent organs, calcification in the liver is unusual. In fact, unless a right upper quadrant opacity has an appearance highly specific for an intrahepatic entity, it should be presumed to be outside the liver. Single stones in this area are more likely to be in the gallbladder or kidney. Multiple concretions that cross the midline are almost always pancreatic in origin. Cystic lesions, with the exception of the cysts of *Echinococcus granulosis*, are very rare, as are calcifications in intrahepatic vessels. The vast majority of poorly defined opacities superimposed upon the hepatic shadow are calcifications in costal cartilage. Solid calcifications overlying the

liver may also be in the skin, abdominal wall, lower lung fields, peritoneal cavity, spleen, stomach, or adrenal glands. Intrahepatic solid calcification is quite uncommon and often very faint, and therefore may be missed if not searched for carefully.

There is, however, a wide spectrum of hepatic disorders that can present with radiodense lesions on plain films. Often their appearance is sufficiently characteristic to suggest a histologic diagnosis before additional imaging studies are done. The calcifications are mostly a manifestation of a quiescent condition of long standing, but, on occasion, plain film recognition is of diagnostic and prognostic importance because it can reveal a rapidly progressive disease.

Multiple Solid Calcifications in the Liver

Infectious Disease. Several conditions produce multiple calcifications in the liver, but tuberculosis and histoplasmosis are by far the most common

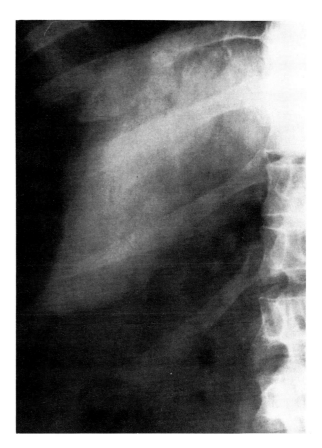

Figure 6–9. Early appearance of Thorotrast in the liver. Soon after intra-arterial administration, colloidal thorium is deposited diffusely in the liver. The liver appears homogeneously dense. This appearance is of historical interest only because the use of thorium has been discontinued.

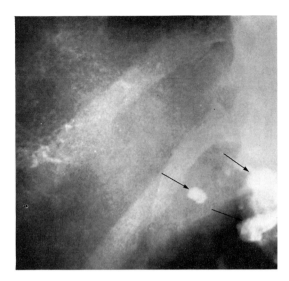

Figure 6–10. The appearance of thorium in the liver long after the administration of Thorotrast. This 45-year-old man had received Thorotrast 29 years previously. The findings of a fine linear pattern of radiodensity in the liver and dense opacification of peripancreatic lymph nodes (*arrows*) are characteristic.

worldwide. In endemic regions, a collection of well-defined matchhead-sized densities in the liver, seen with similar calcifications in the lungs and the spleen, suggest histoplasmosis (Fig 6–12). In most other locales, small, rounded opacities in the liver, even in the absence of radiographic changes in the lung or spleen, point to tuberculosis. These calcifications are often uniformly dense but may have a laminated or even a mottled appearance. Typically, hepatic tuberculomas are associated with radiodense granulomas in the spleen.

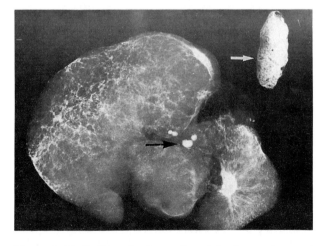

Figure 6–11. Radiograph of a section of the liver, spleen and peripancreatic nodes removed at autopsy from a patient who received Thorotrast. Observe the feathery linearity of densities in the liver, the dense nodes (*black arrow*), and the mottled opacity of the spleen (*white arrow*).

Although there be may only a few tubercular opacities in the spleen, in the liver they are often too numerous to count (Fig 6–13). Nevertheless, not all tuberculous granulomas are very small and some may be greater than 1 cm in diameter, with shaggy borders and dense granular interiors. Tuberculous nodes in the porta hepatis calcify occasionally and can be seen in the absence of other intrahepatic densities (Fig 6–14).[20,21]

Brucellosis is another chronic inflammatory disease that may calcify in the liver. All three species of brucellosis—*Br abortus, Br melitensis,* and *Br suis* can cause infection, but only with *Br suis* are there also radiodense lesions. Characteristically, the intrahepatic abscesses in brucellosis infection are multiple rounded densities, 1 to 2 cm in diameter, that are almost always associated with calcifications of similar size and configuration in the spleen.[22]

Armillifer armillatus is a parasite found in the rain forests of West Africa and the Philippines. The adult parasite lives in the respiratory tract of pythons and other snakes. Eggs are released in snake saliva and may be inadvertently ingested by humans. The larvae migrate to the peritoneal cavity and liver, where they become encysted and calcified. This infestation causes no symptoms, and its only interest is its pathognomonic appearance on plain films of the abdomen. The parasites appear as C-shaped or incomplete ring shadows, 4 by 6 mm in length by 1.5 mm in width. Seen on end, the calcified worms look like dash marks, but almost always, enough C-shaped forms are observed to permit a diagnosis (Fig 6–15).[23,24]

Metastatic Tumor Calcification. An ever-lengthening list of metastatic tumors have been reported with multiple calcifications in the liver. The radiographic appearance ranges from dense, well-defined masses to faint multifocal calcific agglomerations that may be missed on cursory examination. Calcification in metastatic disease usually occurs in large livers and in patients in whom the presence of a primary tumor is already known, but, on occasion, the recognition of hepatic calcifications may be the first sign of malignancy. Although an abdominal radiograph can reveal distinctive and even dramatic manifestations of liver metastases, its lack of sensitivity in most cases must be acknowledged. For example, plain films are only one third as effective as computed tomography in demonstrating calcified liver masses.[25]

Colonic Carcinoma Metastases. The most common primary tumors with multiple calcified metastatic deposits in the liver are adenocarcinoma of the

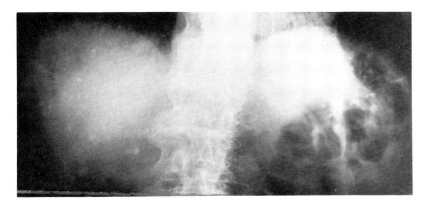

Figure 6–12. Histoplasmosis. Multiple punctate calcifications in the liver and spleen.

colon and papillary serous cystadenocarcinoma of the ovary. Metastatic colonic tumors appear as faint amorphous masses of closely arrayed punctate or stippled calcifications. Sometimes the calcifications are so close together that they impart a granular appearance to areas of the liver. Calcium deposition may be a consequence of tissue necrosis, but histological specimens have shown calcification in colonic metastases in the absence of cell death. Another explanation for calcification in colonic tumors is that mucin-producing masses have an avidity for calcium. This proposed mechanism does not account for all cases of radiopaque colonic metastases, however. In a series of 21 patients reported by Green, the presence of calcium in hepatic metastases from colon malignancy was found to be unrelated to the duration of the tumor or the maturity of the malig-

nant cells.[26] Calcified metastasis may appear along with calcification in the primary mass, but in many cases, only the hepatic metastases are radiodense. The finding of finely speckled or punctate calcifications in the liver and the absence of calcifications elsewhere should suggest colonic malignancy more than any other condition.[27-29] Care must be taken in

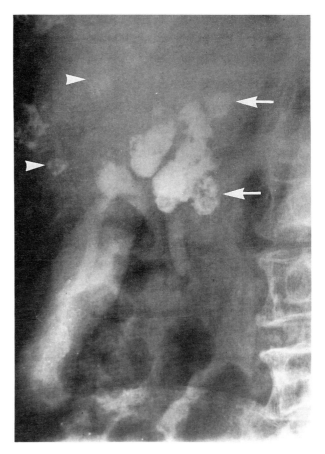

Figure 6–14. Large calcified porta hepatic nodes (*arrows*) in a patient with a history of tuberculosis. The arrowheads point to costal cartilage calcification. The gallbladder is opacified by contrast material.

Figure 6–13. Tuberculous granulomas in the liver. A film from an oral cholecystography shows a contrast-filled gallbladder and multiple calcified granulomas in the liver.

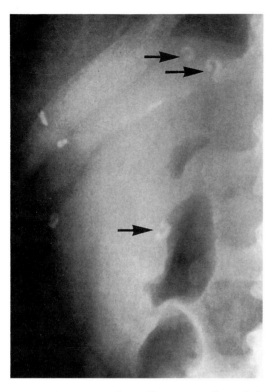

Figure 6–15. Armillifer armillatus. The arrows point to C-shaped encysted larvae within the liver—a pathognomonic finding. (*Courtesy of Dr. Esmond Mapp.*)

the observation of faint calcifications, for they can be simulated by feces coated with opaque material in the adjacent hepatic flexure or transverse colon. Sequential films taken 1 day apart may show a change in the pattern of intraluminal densities in the large intestine, but calcific metastases in the liver should be unchanged on multiple films taken within an interval of a few days.

Metastatic Ovarian Carcinoma. Metastatic serous cystadenocarcinoma calcifies in 20% to 30% of cases, and, infrequently, calcification is seen overlying the liver on plain films.[30] Metastatic deposits can be found in the substance of the liver, on the liver capsule, or in the peritoneal cavity adjacent to the liver. Ovarian carcinoma calcification occurs in intracellular psammoma bodies and is not related to tissue necrosis. The radiographic appearance of individual metastasis is similar, however, or even identical to that of colon carcinoma. Calcific densities in the tumor may be speckled, smudgy, and are sometimes barely perceptible (Fig 6–16). Calcification of the liver from serous cystadenocarcinoma of the ovary almost never occurs without coincident calcification elsewhere, usually in the peritoneal cavity or in the primary tumor (Fig 6–17). This is an important di-

agnostic consideration because few other conditions produce simultaneous calcified peritoneal and liver metastases. Occasionally, ovarian metastases in the liver become more opaque after radiotherapy.

Other Metastatic Tumors to the Liver. Calcification in metastatic tumors to the liver is usually an insidious process, with gradual intensification of radiopacity and visualization of an increasing number of foci on sequential films. Calcium deposition may occur rapidly, however, with the liver becoming diffusely dense within a few weeks (Fig 6–18). There are a number of tumors that, although rarely associated with calcific hepatic densities, can produce a characteristic picture of nodules scattered throughout the hepatic mass. Some of the nodules may be well-defined and markedly opaque, but often they have indistinct margins and may have central lucencies. Generally both lobes of the liver are involved. Included in this group of neoplasms are metastatic islet cell tumors of the pancreas,[31,32] carcinoma of

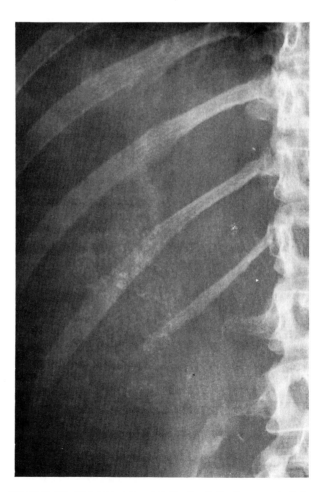

Figure 6–16. Psammomatous calcification in the liver—metastatic ovarian cystadenocarcinoma. Multiple faint, speckled opacities occupy the right lobe of an enlarged liver. The primary tumor in the pelvis was also calcified.

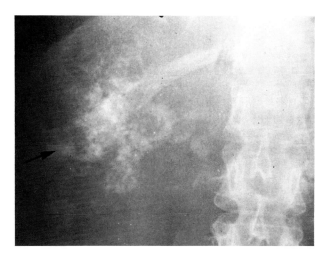

Figure 6–17. Dense psammomatous calcification in the peritoneal cavity (*small arrow*) and the liver (*large arrow*) from an ovarian cystadenocarcinoma. Calcified peritoneal deposits, in addition to liver densities, are characteristic of this tumor.

the breast,[33,34] malignant melanoma,[35,36] and mesothelioma.[31,37]

Calcification in Primary Tumors. There is no reliable criteria that helps to distinguish between primary and metastatic disease on the basis of the pattern of intrahepatic calcification. Neither the extent

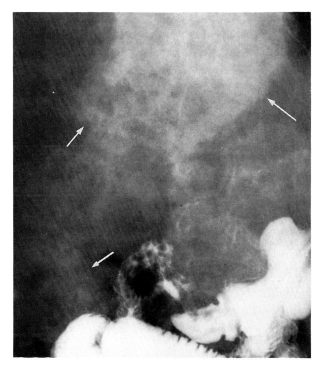

Figure 6–18. Multifocal, cloudlike calcified metastases in the liver (*arrows*) from a retroperitoneal mesenchymoma. One month before, there were no opacities in the liver.

nor the multiplicity of opacities can differentiate an indigenous tumor from a secondary deposit. In Northern America and Europe, primary tumors are much less common than colonic or even ovarian metastases. Hepatocellular carcinoma and cholangiocarcinoma may be unifocal or can appear as several separate masses in the hepatic parenchyma. A rare tumor with a propensity to calcification is mixed malignant tumor of the liver. This neoplasm, which contains both hepatocellular and mesenchymal elements, often presents with pulmonary osteoarthropathy.[38] Mixed malignant tumors are slow-growing masses, seen on plain films as calcified globular densities up to 2 cm in diameter scattered throughout the liver.[39] If a calcified primary hepatic cancer is identified, there should be a strong suspicion of this histological type. For example, in a series of 23 cases of calcified primary carcinomas, 13 were mixed malignant tumors.[40] Occasionally, fibrolamellar hepatoma, a tumor with a relatively favorable prognosis affecting young patients with no history of liver disease may have faint calcification detectable on plain films.[41]

Solitary Solid Calcification in the Liver

Inflammatory Lesions. Several inflammatory processes can calcify in the liver as a single solid mass. Although many of these entities are encountered often in clinical practice, roentgenographically visible calcification in the liver is very infrequent. An intrahepatic tuberculous granuloma can accumulate calcium salts, with the focus of opacity usually situated in an area of caseation.[42] A single granuloma may be found in the porta hepatis, deep within the liver parenchyma, and even in the peripheral, subcapsular location (Fig 6–19). There have been only a few reports of calcified hepatic gummas, each of which appeared as a well-defined mottled density several centimeters in diameter.[43,44] The liver is the organ that most often harbors luetic masses, but calcification within them is exceedingly rare. Even less common are calcified healed pyogenic and amebic abscesses.[45,58] A parasitic disease that may cause a single focus of hepatic calcification is fascioliasis, caused by *Fasciola gigantica,* a liver fluke found in equatorial Africa and Southeast Asia. Calcification in the liver may be the result of a tissue response to migrating larvae passing into the parenchyma of the liver. Usually a single lobulated mass with irregular lucencies is seen on plain films.[47]

Metastatic Disease. Most single solid hepatic calcifications are calcified metastases. Again, the most common primary sites are the colon and the ovary (Fig 6–20). A solitary focus of calcification, in fact,

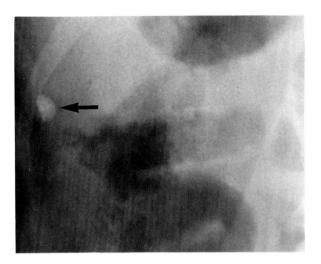

Figure 6–19. The arrow points to a discrete solid density in a subcapsular location in the periphery of the liver. Histological examination revealed a tuberculous granuloma.

may be more common than multiple calcifications in the liver from these tumors. A primary hepatic tumor can also be seen as a single radiodense lesion. Included in this group are bile duct and hepatocellular carcinomas,[48] but, once more, the rare mixed malignant tumor of the liver is the most common primary liver carcinoma presenting as a single focus of calcification.[40]

Benign Tumors. The cavernous hemangionia has the highest incidence of all benign hepatic tumors.

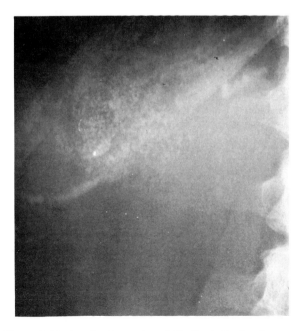

Figure 6–20. Localized granular calcification in the liver from carcinoma of the colon. The primary tumor was not calcified. (*Courtesy of Dr. Larry Oliver.*)

For the most part, hemangiomas are clinically silent and radiographically inconspicuous. Infrequently, however, they do calcify. First reported by Aspray in 1945,[49] only a few additional cases have been recorded. Most calcified hemangiomas are dense masses with irregular projections extending from the main radiopaque agglomeration.[50,51] Several cases have shown more than one focus of calcification. Usually, the radiographic features are not sufficiently characteristic of hemangioma to differentiate it from other solid lesions. Although hemangioma calcification in other organs such as the spleen, stomach, and colon is manifested by discrete opacification in the form of phleboliths, this pattern has not yet been observed in the liver.

Cystic Calcification

Echinococcus granulosis. Hydatid disease should be the first consideration for any calcified cystic lesion within the liver. The more common type of hydatid disease is caused by the larva of *Echinococcus granulosus*, a parasite with a global distribution but found most often in the Mediterranean basin in the Middle East. Humans are accidental and intermediate hosts and acquire the infestation by ingestion of the echinococcal ova. The parasites penetrate the small intestinal wall and enter the portal circulation. They may remain in the liver parenchyma or migrate to the hepatic veins and from there pass into the heart and other organs. In the liver they form a cyst composed of two walls: the endocyst or inner wall, containing the germinal layers, scoleces, and daughter cysts; and the encircling pericyst, composed of compressed hepatic tissue. The rimlike calcifications, seen on plain films in approximately 15% of patients, are due to calcium deposition in the pericyst.[52]

Echinococcus granulosis can infest any solid abdominal organ but by far the liver is the most common site. Calcification usually appears 5 to 10 years after initial exposure and is often associated with liver enlargement. The presence of calcium strongly suggests an inactive cyst,[53] and the heavier the calcific rim, the more likely the parasites have died. Multiple calcified cysts may be observed, but solitary calcification is more common. Nevertheless, the recognition of one calcified cyst by no means suggests the absence of one or several noncalcified cysts in other sections of the liver.

Radiographic Appearance. Like cystic calcification elsewhere, the marginal opacities are arclike but need not be continuous (Fig 2–111). Usually, the outer wall of a cyst of *E granulosis* is smooth but, at times, a portion of the wall may be irregularly calcified. Most often, one wall of the cyst appears slightly flattened, and a perfectly circular contour of rimlike calcification is unusual (Fig 2–110). Even densely calcified lesions can be deformed by adjacent structures. On occasion, focal intracystic densities are seen within the cyst and the presence of pericystic and smaller daughter cyst calcifications gives the density a complex inner architecture (Fig 6–21).[54]

Calcified hydatid cysts may collapse, with infolding of their arcuate walls (Fig 6–22). Surgical evacuation of cyst contents is a potentially hazardous procedure because spill of hydatid fluid into the peritoneal cavity can incite an anaphylactoid reaction. In such cases, the tip of a large tube is retained within the cyst for several days, allowing air to fill the cavity (Fig 6–23). In view of the high likelihood of parasite death in calcified cysts, they are best left alone unless they impinge on adjacent organs or on a major bile duct.

The radiographic configuration of *E granulosis* must be distinguished from a rarer but more aggressive form of hydatid disease due to *E multilocularis*. This parasitic infestation is found in Canada, Alaska, and Central Europe, and the definitive host is the fox or the wolf. *Echinococcus multilocularis* does not present as a cystic lesion. Rather, the pattern of calcium deposition resembles that seen in metastatic disease, with multiple solid densities throughout the liver. Individual opacities are usually dense and amorphous but in severe cases, calcium deposits with arcuate and solid components can be observed. Calcification occurs in two thirds of cases, most often confined to either the right or left lobe. Multiple poorly defined solid densities scattered throughout the liver in an ill patient from an endemic region with known exposure should strongly suggest the diagnosis.[55,56]

Other Cysts. Benign noninflammatory cysts occur in the liver frequently but hardly ever calcify.[57] Metastases from ovarian mucinous cystadenocarcinoma may have both cystic and solid components. Usually, calcification is also present in the peritoneal cavity (Fig 9–33). There have been a few reports of arcuate calcification in polycystic disease[58] and in amebic abscess.[46] Rimlike calcification in a biliary cystadenoma was noted in one patient, where it closely resembled a calcified echinococcal cyst.[59]

Conduit Calcification

Calcification of the vascular conduits supplying and draining the liver are very uncommon. The liver is unique among intra-abdominal organs in that venous opacities exceed arterial calcification in frequency and extent.

Calcification in the Portal Vein and Its Branches. Portal vein calcification detectable on plain films is a rare finding, with only 19 cases reported.[60] All have appeared in patients with portal hypertension and most of them have had histological confirmation of cirrhosis. Portal vein calcification is more frequent in men, corresponding to the higher incidence of cirrhosis in adult males.[61]

The main portal vein arises at the junction of the splenic and superior mesenteric veins and describes a superolateral course before it splits into right and left branches, which enter the liver. Usually, the vein has a straight or slightly curved path as it courses diagonally in the right upper quadrant (Fig 6–24). The vein is much wider than an undilated hepatic artery and its origin is located more inferiorly. Calcification in the portal vein may be localized in the wall or within an intraluminal thrombus.[62–66] If the calcification is limited to a small segment of the vein wall it may be overlooked or considered as an artifact or as an ingested foreign substance (Fig 6–25). More extensive intramural calcification appears as discontinuous lines of radiodensity, reflecting the nonuniform deposition of calcium. Sometimes, the venous walls are not parallel but appear to converge slightly as they near the point of bifurcation in the porta hepatis (Fig 6–26). Intraluminal thrombus calcification lacks the marginal accentuation of mural opacities as calcium is laid down diffusely in the clot.

The degree of vascular dilatation is remarkable in severe, long-standing portal hypertension, with some veins attaining a diameter of several centimeters. Dilatation may extend into the splenic and superior mesenteric veins and in some patients, cavernous transformation of collateral vessels also calcify. These dilated vessels can have a bizarre configuration both in the right upper quadrant and across the midline in the upper abdomen (Fig 6–27).[67–70]

Hepatic Vein. Hepatic vein calcification is exceedingly unusual. We have observed one case in which the calcified clot filled the lumen of the vein (Fig 6–28).

Hepatic Artery. Calcification in a nondilated hepatic artery detectable on plain films has not yet been reported. Hepatic artery aneurysm, a very rare abnormality, can result from trauma, mycotic infection of the vascular walls or arteriosclerosis. In 5% to 10% of cases the aneurysm can rupture either into the peritoneal cavity or into the biliary tract. Plain film evidence of a calcified hepatic artery aneurysm has been reported on only a few occasions and in all instances, the extrahepatic segment of the artery

254

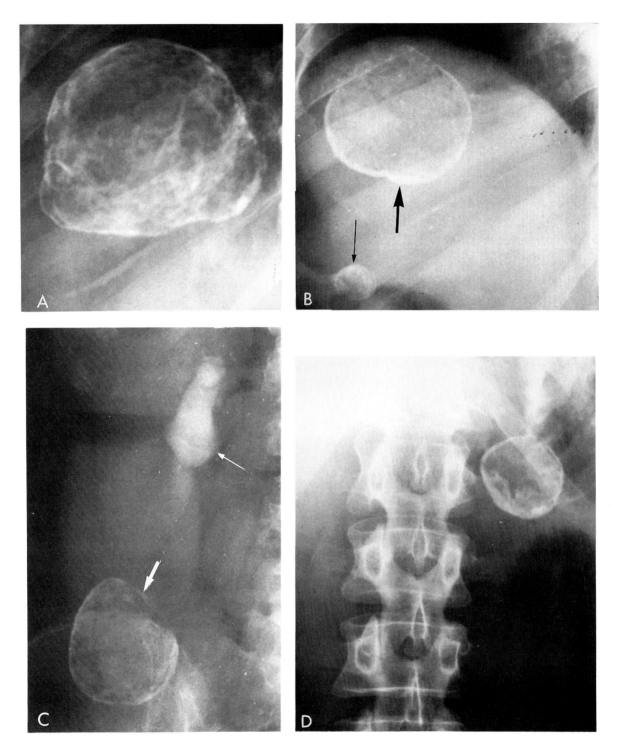

Figure 6–21. A spectrum of *Echinococcus granulosis* calcification. **A.** Dense calcification of a cyst in the liver, with slight irregularity of its inferior border. **B.** Two hepatic echinococcal cysts. The larger one (*upper arrow*) is not calcified circumferentially. **C.** A single echinococcal cyst attached to the capsule of the liver (*lower arrow*). The gallbladder is filled with contrast material (*upper arrow*). Sometimes an echinococcal cyst resembles a calcified gallbladder. **D.** A cyst in the left lobe of the liver. There is dense calcification throughout the wall of the cyst.

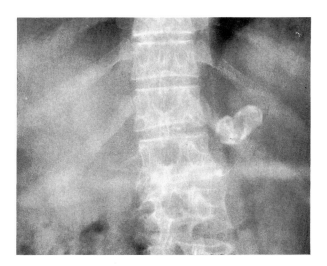

Figure 6–22. A collapsed *Echinococcus* cyst of the left lobe of the liver.

was dilated. The location and configuration of these aneurysms resemble small calcified hydatid cysts.[71–73]

Lucencies in the Liver

The hepatic shadow provides a featureless background upon which lucencies in other abdominal structures can be seen with special clarity. As discussed in Chapter 3 the right outer quadrant is the place to look for subtle signs of pneumoperitoneum and pneumoretroperitoneum. Air or gas in the duodenum, colon, gallbladder, and right kidney also stand out in relation to the homogeneous liver density. Although much less common, intrahepatic lucencies encompass a broad range of abnormalities, each with distinctive plain film findings (Table 6–1).

Fatty Liver. Diffuse fatty infiltration of the liver is a frequent pathological finding in alcoholic patients. The plain film demonstration of a fatty liver has been described only once in adults, however. In that case, the hepatic shadow of a middle-aged woman appeared more lucent than the lateral abdominal muscles, and the left kidney and the greater curvature of

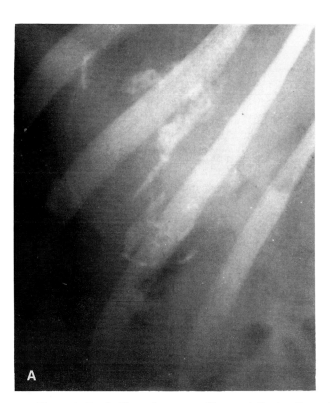

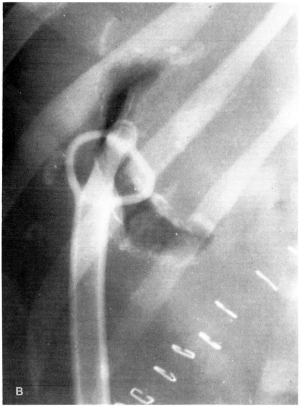

Figure 6–23. A. Discontinuous curvilinear calcific densities outline an echinococcal cyst. Calcified costal cartilage is superimposed upon it. **B.** After drainage, air occupies the collapsed cyst, which now has a crescentic configuration.

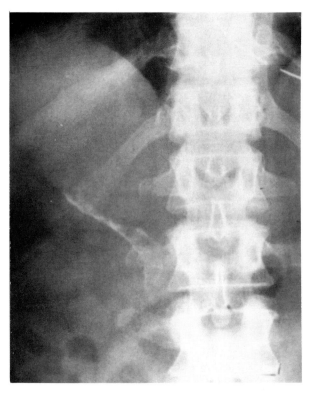

Figure 6–24. Extensive calcification of a portal vein of normal width.

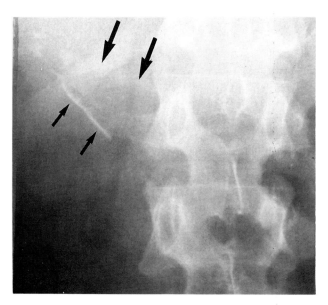

Figure 6–26. Mural calcification in a dilated portal vein. The sharp inferior calcification (*small arrows*) and the faint superior calcification (*large arrows*) converge as the vein courses laterally.

the stomach stood out in contrast to the density of the left lobe.[74] Plain film evidence of fatty liver in children has been observed more often, having been reported in many conditions, including various malabsorption syndromes, glycogen storage disease,

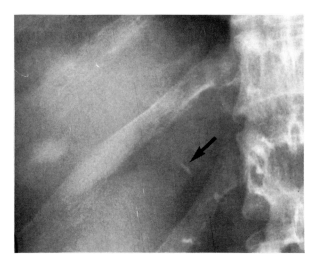

Figure 6–25. Portal vein calcification limited to one wall of the vein (*arrow*). The short line of radiodensity is oriented along the expected direction of the vein.

Reye's syndrome, and cystic fibrosis. Additional radiographic evidence of a diffusely lucent liver in children are obscuration of the medial edge of the properitoneal fat stripe and the presence of a fat–fluid interface, with ascitic fluid having a greater density than the adjacent hepatic shadow.[75]

Hepatic Gas

Liver Abscesses. Pyogenic liver abscesses are uncommon lesions observed in approximately 1% of autopsies. The most frequent causes are ascending cholangitis, often induced by ductal obstruction, seeding from another abdominal site either by direct extension or through the portal venous system, and septicemia from a distant or obscure focus. Inadvertent ligation of an hepatic artery at surgery can be an unfortunate predisposing factor. Gas-containing abscesses also are complications of such hepatic artery catheter procedures as infusion therapy and gelatin sponge embolization.

The most common organisms associated with hepatic suppuration are *Klebsiella aerogenes*, *Escherichia coli*, *Clostridium perfringens*, and *Staphylococcus aureus*, all of which can produce gas within the abscess cavity.[79] Worldwide, amebic abscesses have a much higher incidence than pyogenic abscesses, but they are rarely demonstrated on plain films because they seldom produce gas. On the other hand, gas in hydatid infestations is not rare.[80] In a series of 105 patients with hepatic *Echinococcus*, Gonzales et al ob-

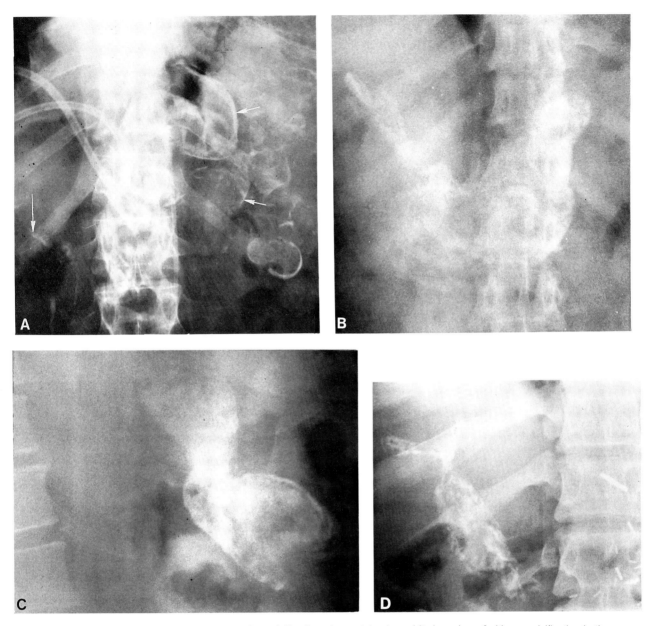

Figure 6–27. Three cases, each with extensive calcification of a portal vein and its branches. **A.** Linear calcification in the portal vein (*vertical arrow*). The horizontal arrows point to two segments of a markedly tortuous calcified splenic vein that wandered through the left upper quadrant. (*Courtesy of Dr. Jon Adler*) **B, C.** The frontal and lateral films of a patient with calcified and dilated portal and splenic vein walls which extend across the midline. **D.** A calcified clot occupies the portal vein and its right and left intrahepatic branches. (*Courtesy of Dr. Gregg Gaylord.*)

served ten cases with intraparenchymal air, six with a single large collection and four with a localized area of small bubbles.[52] They surmised that bacterial superinfection of the cyst or communication with the biliary tree was the source of the lucencies.

Prompt diagnosis of a pyogenic hepatic abscess is essential because affected individuals, usually very ill with high fever and debilitation, will succumb unless appropriate treatment is instituted without delay. Mild hepatomegaly is a frequent but not a definitive finding on plain films, but gas within the abscess is a highly specific sign, although it is present in only one sixth of cases.[1] The patterns of gas accumulation vary widely on supine views, ranging from numerous closely bunched bubbles (Fig 6–29) to an irregularly configured single lucency (Fig 6–30) to a large round unilocular collection (Fig 6–31) that sometimes has an air–fluid level on upright or decubitus views. Gangrene of the liver can involve the entire hepatic substance, appearing as a

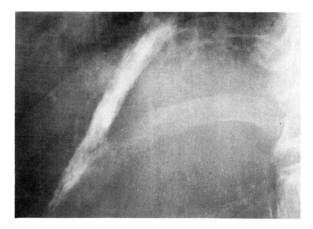

Figure 6–28. Dense calcification in a thrombosed hepatic vein.

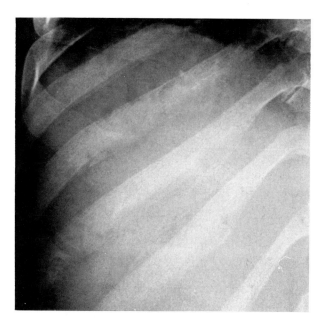

Figure 6–29. Hepatic abscess. Numerous small lucencies of varying diameter in the periphery of the right lobe of the liver.

diffusely mottled pattern of lucency throughout the liver.[81]

Pyogenic abscess can be mimicked by other gas-containing processes both within and near the liver. Diffuse aggregations of small air bubbles have been noted after both penetrating and blunt trauma. They tend to collect in the hepatic periphery,[82] close to other plain film signs of trauma, including loss of the hepatic angle due to hemoperitoneum and localized obliteration of the properitoneal fat pad caused by infiltration of blood into the adjacent retroperitoneal space.[83] The mechanism of formation of posttraumatic intraparenchymal bubbles is obscure. One theory maintains that upon impact gas is forced into the biliary tract from the duodenum through an open sphincter of Oddi and comes to lie in the hepatic periphery.[82] Such a notion does not account, however, for the absence of gas in the larger bile ducts, which is a hallmark of pneumobilia.

TABLE 6–1. LUCENCIES IN THE LIVER

I. Hepatic Gas
    A. Parenchymal lucencies
        1. Pyogenic abscess
        2. Hydatid infestation gas
        3. Gangrene of the liver
        4. Tumor necrosis
        5. Nonsuppurative gas formation
        6. Blunt trauma
        7. Penetrating trauma
    B. Conduit lucencies
        1. Portal vein gas
        2. Pneumobilia
        3. Hepatic artery gas
II. Hepatic fat
    A. Fatty liver
    B. Peribiliary fat (pseudopneumobilia)
    C. Fat in the intrahepatic fissure (ligamentum teres hepatis)

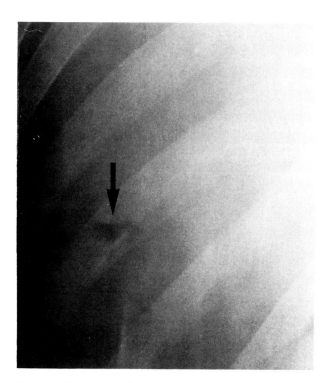

Figure 6–30. Hepatic abscess. An irregular lucency (*arrow*) in a patient with a single abscess. (*Courtesy of Dr. Chusilp Charnsangavej.*)

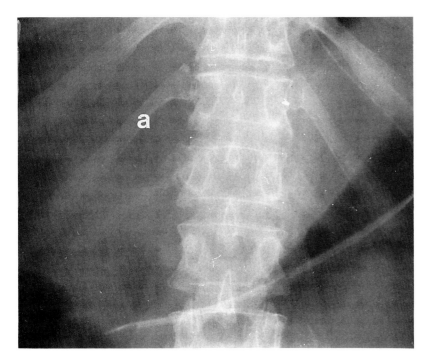

Figure 6–31. Hepatic abscess. A large, round gas collection (a) with well-defined margins inferiorly. (*Courtesy of Dr. Jutta Greweldinger.*)

Another cause of multiple lucencies within the liver is nonsuppurative tumor necrosis after hepatic artery embolization. It may not be a rare phenomenon, as Hennessey and Allison found intrahepatic gas in 44% of patients undergoing this catheter procedure.[84] Appearing as a patchy area of decreased density, the gas forms quickly after embolization and persists for up to 4 to 8 weeks.[85] It is apparently a benign phenomenon unrelated to signs or symptoms of infection. Similar findings have been seen after therapeutic infarction of renal tumors[86] and enlarged spleens.[87]

Gas within necrotic tumors consists primarily of carbon dioxide and oxygen. Carbon dioxide is derived from bicarbonate produced by the anaerobic metabolism of reticulocytes and oxygen is liberated from trapped oxyhemoglobin.[88] The extent of gas reflects the volume of infarcted tumor. With occlusion of a vessel feeding a large malignant deposit, the zone of necrosis may occupy much of the liver shadow. The plain film findings can be spectacular, resembling gangrene of the liver despite the fact that patients usually remain free of fever and pain during and after the procedure (Fig 6–32).

Hepatic abscesses can be mimicked by a diverse group of abdominal conditions. They can resemble subphrenic abscesses both clinically and radiographically, but subphrenic collections are more common and also more likely to contain gas. They almost always induce a pleural effusion whereas hepatic abscesses, even when situated just below the dia-

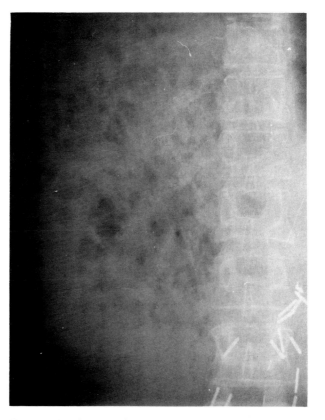

Figure 6–32. Innumerable foci of gas scattered throughout the right upper quadrant. The gas is not in the liver parenchyma but in metastatic hepatic deposits from an intestinal leiomyosarcoma. The huge tumor was treated by catheter embolization. (*Courtesy of Dr. Chusilp Charnsangavej.*)

phragm, often have little effect on the nearby pleura (Fig 6–33). A single featureless lucency in the right upper quadrant is a good sign of a pneumoperitoneum, with a pocket of free air situated in the subphrenic space (Fig 3–13) or in Morison's pouch (Fig 3–15). Almost always, the signs and symptoms of spontaneous pneumoperitoneum are distinctly different from hepatic abscess. Gas accumulates in the gallbladder lumen in emphysematous cholecystitis but is often associated with a curvilinear streak representing gas in the gallbladder wall. Chailaditi's syndrome (Fig 3–22) and duodenal diverticulum (Fig 4–45) both may appear as a single gas collection superimposed on the liver. Generally, neither of these two abnormalities of the gastrointestinal tract cause discomfort, and their recognition on supine films is most often an incidental finding.

Gas in Hepatic Conduits

Biliary Tract Gas. Gas in the biliary ducts is associated with a heterogenous list of abnormalities (Table 6–2). In most cases, the gas is not native to the biliary tract but enters through a communication either with the gastrointestinal tract or the skin. Pneumobilia is increasing in frequency because of the widespread adoption of surgical and endoscopic procedures that disrupt the anatomy of the biliary tree. Choledochoenterostomy eventuates in a permanent communication between the common bile duct and the small intestine. Because the sphincter of Oddi is bypassed there is no barrier to the entry

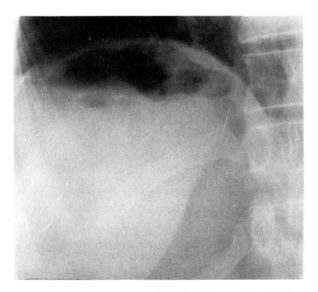

Figure 6–33. Hepatic abscess. An upright film reveals a fluid level within the liver just below the right hemidiaphragm. There is no pleural effusion.

TABLE 6–2. CAUSES OF PNEUMOBILIA

I. Surgery
   A. Choledochoduodenostomy
   B. Choledochojejunostomy
   C. Cholecystoenterostomy
   D. Percutaneous cholecystotomy
II. Endoscopic sphincterotomy
III. Trauma
   A. Communication with the skin
   B. Communication with the bowel
IV. Biliary–enteric fistulae
   A. Cholecystoduodenal
   B. Choledochoduodenal
   C. Cholecystojejunal
   D. Cholecystocolic
V. Infestation—*Ascaris lumbricoides*
VI. Infections
   A. Oriental cholangitis
   B. Emphysematous cholecystitis
VII. Atrophic pancreatitis
VIII. Choledochal abnormalities
   A. Anomalous insertion of the common bile duct
   B. Patulous sphincter of Oddi
   C. Recent passage of a stone

of intestinal gas into the biliary tract. Similarly, after endoscopic sphincterotomy, duodenal air has unrestricted access to the common bile duct, so that pneumobilia is an expected finding. Percutaneous cholecystotomy promises to become an important means of treatment of gallstones. If the cystic duct is patent, air in the biliary tree should be a frequent occurrence with this procedure.

A fistula between the biliary and gastrointestinal tracts is the most common nonsurgical cause of pneumobilia.[89] Most cholecystoenteric fistulas are due to the erosion of a gallstone into the intestines. If the stone is larger than 2.5 cm in diameter it is likely to lodge in the distal small bowel, obstructing the flow of gas and succus entericus. The classic radiographic triad of gallstone ileus seen in a small minority of patients includes air in the biliary tree, small bowel obstruction, and an ectopic calcified gallstone. Trauma, peptic ulcer penetration into the common bile duct, and direct extension of a malignancy of the pancreas, duodenum, stomach, or colon can also produce a biliary intestinal fistula. Emphysematous cholecystitis, unlike other forms of acute gallbladder inflammation, sometimes results from an ischemic event. As the cystic duct remains patent, gas in the gallbladder lumen is free to enter the common bile duct and intrahepatic biliary radicles.[90]

Infrequent causes of pneumobilia include anomalous insertion of the common bile duct, a patulous sphincter of Oddi, recent passage of a stone, and atrophic pancreatitis.[1] *Ascaris lumbricoides* can migrate through the ampulla of Vater, accompanied by a transient entry of gas into the biliary tree.[91] Infection of the bile ducts without fistulae are rarely associated with pneumobilia. Wastie and Cunningham reported a patient from Malaysia with recurrent Oriental cholangitis who had gas in the bile ducts.[92] In North America and Europe, however, there have been no well-documented cases of intrinsic ductal inflammation with plain film evidence of pneumobilia.

Small amounts of gas in the bile ducts are not often detected on survey abdominal films. Grant et al, using computed tomography as a standard, found plain radiographic signs in only 40% of patients with a biliary enteric fistula.[93] Nevertheless, the plain film findings of pneumobilia are so specific that no other pattern of lucency in the liver or in adjacent organs should be mistaken for it.

Pneumobilia collects centrally, never extending close to the liver margin. The branching pattern reflects the anatomy of the biliary tree, with the common bile duct as the trunk. Oriented obliquely inferiorly, with its distal end near the midline, the common bile duct appears as a smooth lucent channel varying from a few millimeters to 2 cm in width (Figs 2–46, 6–34). Usually both the right and left hepatic ducts are seen. In the supine position, however, gas tends to fill the less dependent left ducts first. Therefore, a truncated lucent biliary tree with absence of visualization of the right ducts should

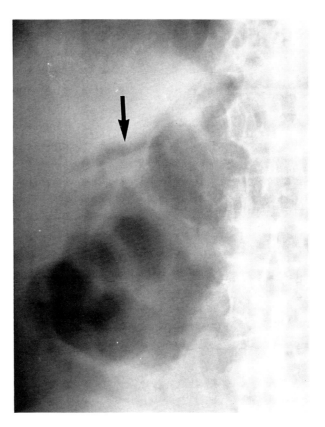

Figure 6–35. The arrow points to a slit of gas overlying the liver above the colon. This was the only plain film finding of pneumoperitoneum in a patient with a perforated duodenal ulcer.

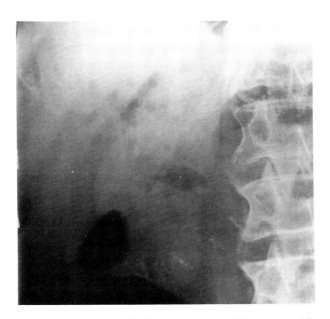

Figure 6–34. Pneumobilia. Gas in the lumen of the common bile duct and its intrahepatic branches. The patient had a cholecystojejunostomy to redirect bile flow because the distal common bile duct was occluded by a carcinoma of the pancreas.

not necessarily suggest a plain film diagnosis of focal occlusion or stenosis. In these patients, a remarkable redistribution of pneumobilia into the right lobe can be observed if a repeat film is done in the prone position.

Occasionally, gas in a superiorly positioned retrocecal appendix can extend above the hepatic flexure (Fig 2–140).[94] Also, a lucent slit in the right upper quadrant may be the only supine film evidence of pneumoperitoneum (Fig 6–35). Both of these tubular gas collections can be distinguished from biliary air because they lack branches and do not have the oblique orientation of the common bile duct.

Fat often envelops the ducts in the porta hepatis, with the amount of surrounding adipose tissue generally related to total body fat. On plain films, peribiliary fat can be visualized as a poorly defined, slightly lucent stripe oriented along the course of the common bile duct (Fig 6–36). Its roentgenographic appearance has been termed pseudopneumobilia because of its similarity in direction and density to biliary tract air. In most cases, it is clearly distinguishable from the sharp lucency of air in the biliary tree.[95,96] Another right upper quadrant linear

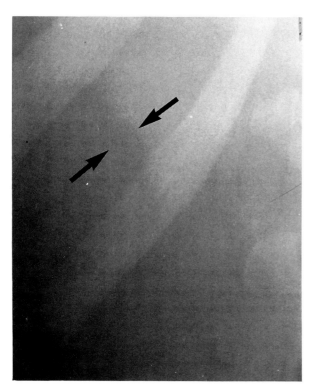

Figure 6–36. Pseudopneumobilia due to peribiliary fat. A faint oblique lucency (*arrows*) is fat, which accompanies the common bile duct in the porta hepatis.

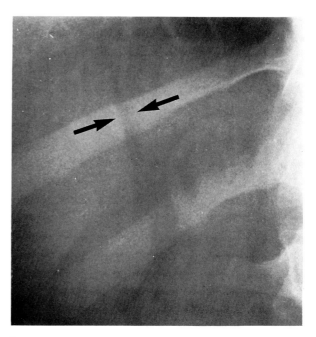

Figure 6–37. Fat in the falciform ligament (*arrows*). The lucency is more vertically directed than the common bile duct.

fat deposit accompanies the ligamentum teres hepatis as it enters the intrahepatic fissure that separates the left lobe from the quadrate lobe. Visible in up to 30% of patients, this faint sliver of decreased density is oriented vertically and lacks branches. Its superior margin is well above the usual position of the common bile duct (Fig 6–37).[97,98]

Portal Venous Gas

Gas in the portal vein was first described in children in 1955,[99] and the initial adult cases were reported 5 years later.[100] Since then numerous additional reports have appeared, and the list of causes of this distinctive radiographic finding continues to grow (Table 6–3).

Early on, the radiographic features of hepatic portal venous gas were accurately described and little has been added since then to augment plain film recognition. The arborizing pattern of portal venous gas extends almost to the capsule of the liver (Fig 6–38).[101] If there is doubt about the presence of these lucent channels on supine films a left lateral decubitus projection allows them to stand out more sharply.[102] In contrast, biliary tree gas is restricted to the central hepatic zones at or near the porta hepatis. The main portal vein and the dilated common

TABLE 6–3. CAUSES OF HEPATIC PORTAL VENOUS GAS IN ADULTS

I. Mesenteric ischemia
  A. Arterial insufficiency
  B. Venous thrombosis
II. Inflammation of the intestinal tract
  A. Gastroenteritis
  B. Diverticulitis
  C. Inflammatory bowel disease
  D. Abdominal abscess with pylephlebitis
III. Colonic tumors
  A. Obstructive
  B. Nonobstructive
IV. Bowel distension
  A. Gastric
  B. Intestinal
V. Pneumatosis
  A. Gastric emphysema
  B. Pneumatosis cystoides intestinalis
VI. Ingestion of corrosives
  A. Hydrochloric acid
  B. Antifreeze
VII. Peroxide enema—through intact mucosa
VIII. Diagnostic procedure in patients with inflammatory bowel disease
  A. Single-contrast barium enema
  B. Double-contrast barium enema
  C. Colonoscopy
IX. Miscellaneous—Bronchopneumonia

bile duct may have a similar diameter and orientation, but the peripheral portal venules are much narrower and more numerous than the smallest of gas-filled biliary ducts. A plausible explanation for the differentiation of gaseous distribution of these two conduit systems was offered by Susman and Senturia.[100] They pointed out that the centrifugal flow of blood in the portal venous system carries embolized gas peripherally into the fine venous radicles of the liver, but the centripetal flow of bile away from the liver retards the diffusion of biliary gas beyond the major lobar ductal branches.

There are two mechanisms for the production and propagation of hepatic portal venous gas. In children, especially, infection of the bowel by either C perfringens or E coli produces intramural gas, which then enters draining mesenteric veins and is carried to the liver.[103] In the absence of infection, when there is no intrinsic source of intramural lucency portal venous gas can only be derived from intestinal intraluminal air, which is able to traverse a damaged bowel wall.[104] Mesenteric ischemia, either from arterial insufficiency or venous thrombosis, results in a hypoxic or necrotic intestine that no longer restrains the transmural passage of bowel gas. On occasion, gas can be seen on plain films in the mural margin alone or in conjunction with gas in draining intestinal veins (Fig 1–5). Rarely, a lucent superior or inferior mesenteric vein is identified.[105] In most patients, however, only hepatic portal venous gas is observed, and intramural penetration from a luminal source can be surmised but not recognized on plain films.

Gas in the portal vein and its intrahepatic branches consists primarily of carbon dioxide and oxygen and is absorbed rapidly. Therefore, visualization of these vessels reflects a dynamic balance between formation in the intestine and resorption in the liver. McClandless noted the gradual disappearance of portal venous gas shortly before death in a young woman, suggesting that bowel gas production was decreasing as the patient became increasingly moribund.[106] Other possibilities for the absence of hepatic portal venous gas with persistence of mesenteric venous gas is obstruction to flow due to thrombosis of the portal vein[107] or blockage of venous return to the liver at the site of a small-bowel volvulus.[108]

Until the late 1960s all cases of hepatic portal venous gas in adults eventuated in rapid death, as nearly every patient had acute mesenteric vascular insufficiency or necrotizing intestinal infection. Even today, an ischemic etiology for hepatic venous gas portends an almost certain and imminent demise despite the heightened awareness of this condition by surgeons and radiologists. The overall mortality of hepatic portal venous gas is now only 75%, however, primarily because several benign conditions have been shown to be associated with it.[102] Portal venous gas, per se, is a transient and innocuous finding, the morbidity and mortality being related to the precipitating cause. Dilatation of the intestine may permit temporary egress of air from the lumen into the bowel wall. In these patients, hepatic portal venous gas resolves promptly with decompression of the lumen. Survival has been reported after gastric dilatation[109,110] and gastric emphysema.[111] Mucosal disruption in the absence of intestinal distention also affords an opportunity for gas to enter the portal circulation. Reversible hepatic portal venous gas has been noted in sigmoid diverticulosis,[105,112] nonobstructed splenic flexure carcinoma,[113] and ulcerative colitis.[114] Corrosive substances such as hydrochloric acid and antifreeze (ethylene glycol plus xylol) also produce hepatic portal venous gas by chemical digestion of the gastric mucosa.[115]

Recently, portal venous gas has been cited as an incidental finding after diagnostic procedures in patients with inflammatory bowel disease. Either single- or double-contrast barium enema can force gas through damaged intestinal mucosa in ulcerative colitis[116] or granulomatous colitis sufferers.[117] Haber reported linear lucencies in the liver after colonoscopy in an individual with ulcerative colitis.[118] In all of these cases, the gas resolves spontaneously. Also, benign portal venous gas has been noted soon after peroxide enema in a patient with intact colonic mucoa.[119] Finally, venous gas superimposed on the liver shadow has been observed as a complication of diseases seemingly unrelated to the bowel such as bronchopneumonia.[120] The reasons for intrahepatic lucencies in these cases is unclear.

Hepatic Artery Gas. Marks and Filly demonstrated hepatic artery gas on plain films and computed tomography in a patient with an unresectable hepatic adenoma who underwent operative ligature of the major vessel feeding the tumor.[21] The scout film after the procedure showed a collection of interconnected linear lucencies in the liver. The gas-filled hepatic arterial branches were less numerous than portal venous radicles and the shadow of the main hepatic artery was narrower than the lumen of either the portal vein or a dilated common bile duct. They concluded that gas was liberated in the artery from anaerobic metabolism of red cells.[121] More cases of hepatic artery gas will probably be reported in the future, as aggressive tumor vessel occlusive techniques gain popularity.

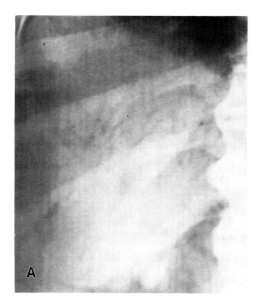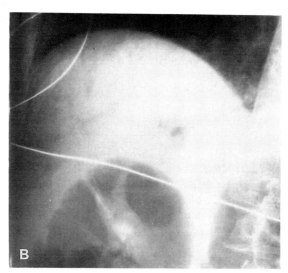

Figure 6–38. Two cases of hepatic portal venous gas. **A.** Many thin channels are seen within the liver shadow. **B.** The lucencies extend near the lateral hepatic margin. Both patients had suffered an acute mesenteric infarction.

GALLBLADDER

Gallbladder Enlargement
The gallbladder is a distensible viscus that can change its volume and configuration rapidly. Nevertheless, its location next to the liver, a large organ of similar roentgenographic density, and its lack of a border forming envelope of fat hides it from view on plain abdominal radiographs. In the absence of lucencies or densities within their walls or lumen, the location and dimensions of most gallbladders can be ascertained only by the addition of contrast material.

Only a markedly distended gallbladder can be seen on plain films as it impinges upon adjacent fat or gas-containing structures. Rarely, abundant fat in the gastrocolic ligament is displaced by the fundus of an enlarged gallbladder. More commonly, hydrops of the gallbladder affects the radiographic hepatic flexure and proximal transverse colon (Fig 2–81).[122] These intestinal segments can be compressed from above and even displaced inferiorly. Also, extension of inflammation beyond the walls of a distended and infected gallbladder may narrow and distort the lumen of the subadjacent colon (Fig 6–39).

Cholelithiasis
Most gallstones are caused by the precipitation of cholesterol salts, bilirubin pigments, or a combination of the two. Much less often, a patient may have numerous stones composed entirely of calcium carbonate. Roentgenographically visible calcification in gallstones almost always indicates the presence of bilirubin pigments within the calculi. Only 10% of gallstones are radiopaque. Considering the high incidence of cholelithiasis in the general population, however, it is not surprising that calcified stones are observed often on plain films.[123]

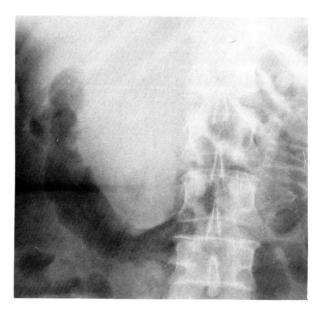

Figure 6–39. Acute cholecystitis with extension of inflammation to the colon. The large gallbladder has depressed the proximal transverse colon. The air-filled bowel lacks haustral outpouchings on its superior surface.

The radiographic appearance of calcified gallstones is variable, but in nearly every case it meets the criteria of concretion calcification. Multiple calculi may be small, sometimes almost punctate in size (Fig 2–90), whereas a single opaque stone can become very large. When many are present they are often faceted and tend to be similar in size. Occasionally, however, large and small concretions may be found together (Fig 6–40). Characteristically the margin of a gallstone is smooth, and, if only an opaque rim is seen, its width is constant throughout the entirety of its perimeter (Fig 2–95). Sometimes, in obese patients or in those with faintly calcified stones, a complete rim of calcification is not appreciated on plain films but tomographic cuts reveal a continuous opaque border. Gallbladder calculi are often laminated with alternating concentric bands (Fig 6–41). Less frequently, they have irregularly mixed dense and lucent centers (Fig 6–42). A rare stone, accumulating calcification on only one surface appears as an amorphous density with spicular contours. Irregularly calcified stones are most often situated in the cystic duct rather than free in the gallbladder lumen (Fig 2–96).

Calculi in Biliary Ducts

Stones in both the intrahepatic and extrahepatic portions of the biliary tree, exclusive of the gallbladder, are rarely seen on plain films of the abdomen. The incidence of calculi in the biliary ducts varies from less than 1% to 6% in patients with coincident cholelithiasis. Although most calculi in the biliary ducts are not radiopaque, on occasion a stone in the common hepatic or common bile duct can be seen on plain films. Generally, these concretions are similar in size and shape to the coexistent calculi in the gallbladder (Fig 6–43). At times, after cholecystectomy a calcified stone is retained in the common bile duct and can be observed on noncontrast films of the abdomen (Fig 6–44).

Very infrequently, there can be calcified stones in the intrahepatic radicles without cholelithiasis. In Caroli's disease, which is a congenital dilatation of the bile ducts, calculi may be seen within the dilated ductal system.[124] There have also been isolated reports of calcified stones in biliary conduits in the absence of structural abnormalities in the ducts.[125]

Gallstones should be readily distinguishable from other concretions of the right upper quadrant. Calculi in the renal pelvis and proximal ureter are usually more dense and seldom have both a thin margin of calcification and a central lucency. Except for very large stones in obstructed renal pelves, concretions in the genitourinary tract are not often laminated. Renal stones are more posterior and stay near the spine on a right posterior oblique film, whereas the gallbladder moves far anteriorly in this projection. An appendicolith in a high-riding retrocecal appendix can simulate a gallstone both radiographically and clinically. At times, costal cartilage calcifications can look exactly like gallbladder concretions on supine radiographs (Fig 6–45). They can be distinguished by oblique or inspiratory and expiratory films, which help to demonstrate the fixation of costal cartilage calcification to the expected contour of the anterior ribs.

The Movement of Gallstones

The movement of gallstones during one examination or on serial films may provide diagnostic clues. A wide excursion of gallstones on recumbent and upright films or on sequential supine films suggests a large gallbladder.[126] When a stone becomes fixed in the cystic duct it can precipitate an attack of acute cholecystitis. Occasionally the lodgment of a calculus in the cystic duct can be inferred on plain films from a lack of movement of previously mobile gallstones or from migration of a calculus superiorly and medially (Fig 6–46). Stones less than 5 mm in diameter can readily pass through the cystic duct into the common bile duct and then into the duodenum. Although this phenomenon is observed infrequently on plain radiographs, calculi up to 12 mm in diameter have been known to traverse the ductal

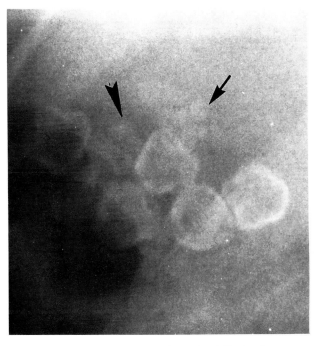

Figure 6–40. There are several faceted calcified gallstones as well as fainter, smaller calculi (*arrows*).

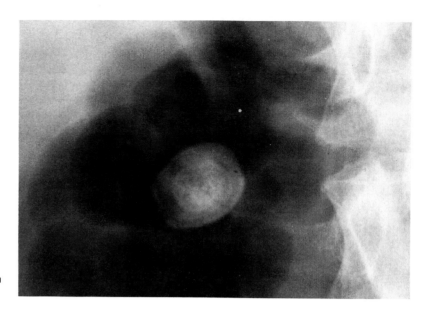

Figure 6–41. A single smooth gallstone with concentric laminations.

system without causing obstruction.[127,128] Rarely, stones perforate the gallbladder and can be found in a number of unusual locations, including the peritoneal cavity, anterior abdominal wall, and the pleura and pericardial spaces.[129] The most common location of an ectopic gallstone, however, is in the small or large intestine, where it can cause obstruction, the stone having passed into the bowel through a cholecystoenteric fistula.

Sometimes, a gallstone has an irregular lucent center. The interior of the stone is less dense than

the surrounding soft tissues because it contains gas. The appearance of gas in a gallstone is labeled the Mercedes-Benz sign, so-called because radiating lucencies from a central focus suggest the emblem of the motorcar. Many gallstones have a crystalline structure, which is subject to fissuring. As the stone ages, the crystalline lattice is broken and gas present in solution in the small amount of fluid within the stone may then be released by shearing forces to enter newly created internal crevices. The Mercedes-Benz sign is observed most often in noncalcific cholesterol stones (Fig 6–47), but occasionally a faint margin of calcification may accompany the linear lucencies in the interior of the calculus (Fig 6–48).[130–133]

Cholelithiasis occurs more frequently in elderly and obese patients and has a distinct female preponderance. Pregnant and multiparous women have a higher incidence of gallstones than women with no children. There are also a few conditions in which the incidence of calcific stones is increased relative to gallstones of all types. In chronic hemolytic anemias, red blood cell destruction leads to an elevated concentration of bilirubin in the bile and a greater risk for the development of bilirubin stones in the gallbladder. Phillips and Gerald found that 48% of patients with sickle cell anemia had cholelithiasis, and in 41% of this group the stones were opaque.[134] Thus, in their series, 20% of all patients with sickle cell disease had calcified gallstones visible on plain films.

Milk-of-Calcium in the Gallbladder. Milk-of-calcium or limy bile is an intraluminal opacity but its appearance is different from that of single or multiple calculi. It may occupy the whole of the lumen and on

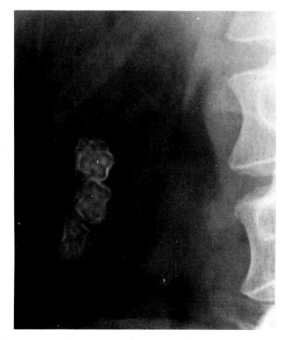

Figure 6–42. Three gallstones of irregular shape and mottled internal architecture. Note that in each stone the marginal calcification is uninterrupted.

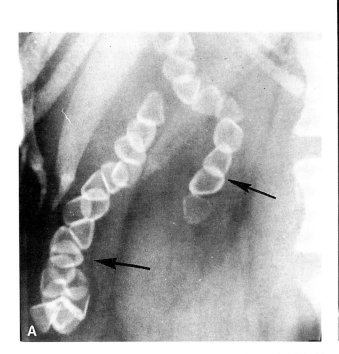

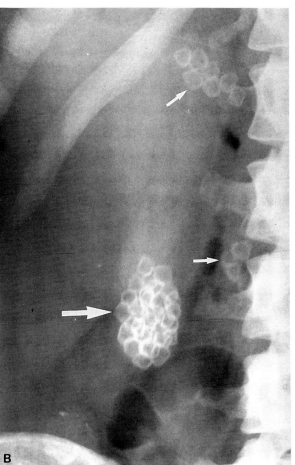

Figure 6–43. **A.** Stones in the common bile duct and gallbladder. The lateral arrow points to numerous gallbladder stones. The medial arrow points to multiple similar calculi in the common bile duct. **B.** Stones in the gallbladder fundus (*large arrow*), cystic duct (*upper small arrow*), and common bile duct (*lower small arrow*). The distance between fundal and cystic duct calculi suggests hydrops of the gallbladder.

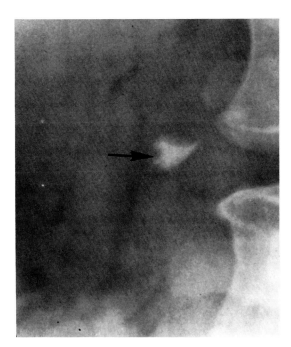

Figure 6–44. An irregularly shaped calcific stone in the common bile duct. This patient had his gallbladder removed 5 years previously. (*Courtesy of Dr. Murray Rosenberg.*)

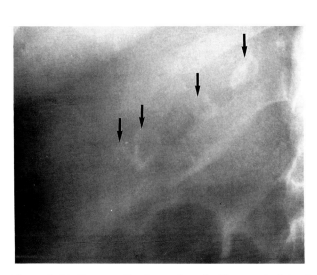

Figure 6–45. Four opacities (*arrows*), each with a marginal rim of density simulating cholelithiasis. All are focal calcifications of costal cartilage oriented along the course of an anterior rib.

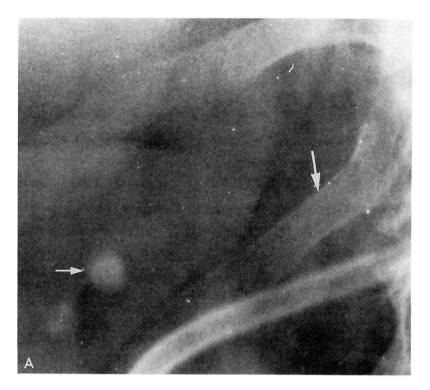

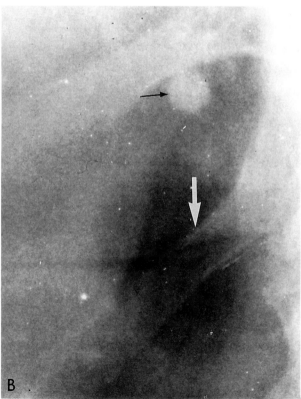

Figure 6–46. A. The horizontal arrow points to a gallbladder calculus and the vertical arrow indictes the 12th rib. **B.** One month later, the calculus has moved medially and superiorly and the patient has acute right upper quadrant pain. At operation an inflamed gallbladder and a single stone in the cystic duct were found. The impaction of the stone had precipitated an attack of acute cholecystitis.

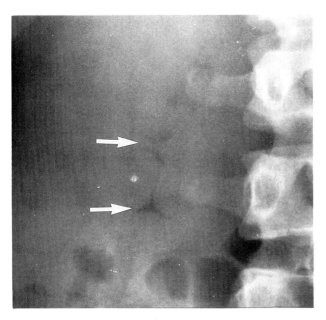

Figure 6–47. Two noncalcified stones with lucent clefts in their centers (*arrows*). Not all gas collections within stones have the pattern of the Mercedes-Benz emblem.

supine films can conform to the shape of the gallbladder (Fig 6–49). There are no laminations in milk-of-calcium bile, but rounded densities representing lucent cholesterol stones may be contained within it (Fig 6–50). The retention of milk of calcium stones within the gallbladder is usually accompanied by cystic duct blockage, but limy bile may persist even without ductal obstruction.[135,136]

The calcareous material in milk of calcium consists of myriad minute stones of calcium carbonate held in suspension in bile. Cross-table lateral and upright films frequently demonstrate a fluid level, as the heavier calcium carbonate calculi sink to a more dependent position in the gallbladder while clear bile layers superiorly (Fig 6–51). Not all cases of limy bile show free mobility with change in position. Sometimes the calcifications have a puttylike consistency and therefore no fluid level is observed in upright or decubitus positions.[137] Typically, milk-of-calcium has a distinctive appearance on plain films, seldom resembling other right upper quadrant opacities. If there is marked hepatomegaly and the gallbladder is therefore situated more inferiorly than normal, however, the opaque bile could simulate a solitary calcified mesenteric lymph node.

Milk-of-Calcium in the Bile Ducts. Milk-of-calcium of the common bile duct, much less common than limy bile confined to the gallbladder, occurs predominantly in women. Most patients are jaundiced and present with right upper quadrant pain.[138,139] The cystic duct can be patent and milk-of-calcium in the gallbladder may be seen along with the diffuse opacity in the common bile duct. The classic appearance is a homogeneous oblong density conforming to the expected location of the duct. It can be easily distinguished from the tracklike configuration of mural calcification of the portal vein or the irregular densities of a calcified venous thrombus. Occasionally, a point of narrowing at the distal duct is suggested by a tapering of the milk-of-calcium density (Fig 6–52).[140]

Limy bile need not be a permanent finding if there is no persistent obstruction to flow in the bil-

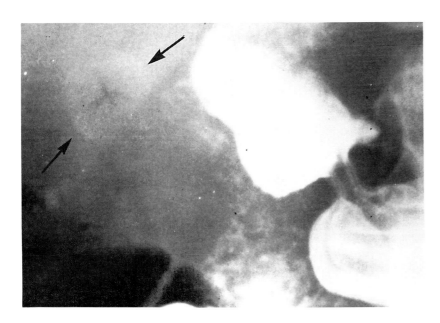

Figure 6–48. Mercedes-Benz sign. A faintly calcified gallstone (*arrows*) has central linear lucencies. The stone is lateral to the barium-filled duodenal bulb.

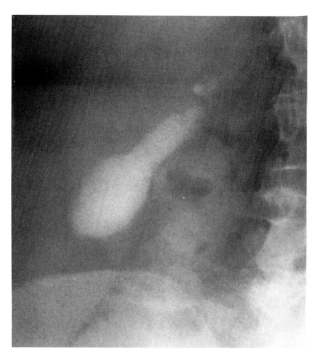

Figure 6–49. Milk-of-calcium. The entire lumen is filled with innumerable calcium carbonate stones. The appearance resembles a gallbladder filled with contrast material.

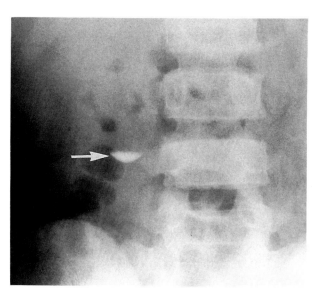

Figure 6–51. Upright view in a patient with limy bile demonstrates a clearly demarcated level caused by calcium carbonate calculi in the dependent position (*arrow*) and nonopaque bile above.

iary tract. Thus, milk-of-calcium can pass from the gallbladder and the common bile duct and be absent on successive plain films.[141–144]

Calcification in the Gallbladder Wall

Roentgenographically observable calcification in the gallbladder wall is not rare. We have collected 20

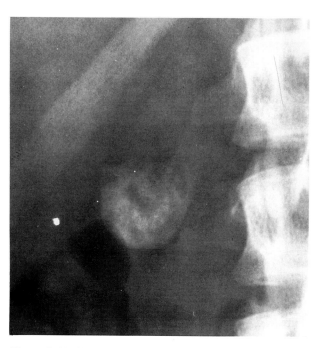

Figure 6–50. Limy bile with many filling defects caused by the coexistence of lucent cholesterol stones.

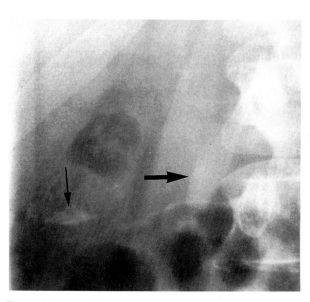

Figure 6–52. Milk-of-calcium in the common bile duct. Limy bile fills the common bile duct, which is narrowed inferiorly (*large arrow*). The small arrow points to a remnant of limy bile which has settled in the gallbladder fundus.

cases over a 10-year period at our institution. One retrospective review of cholecystectomy specimens revealed calcification in the gallbladder wall in 0.07% of patients.[145] Grossly, a calcified gallbladder is easily fractured and has a translucent bluish tint, hence the term "porcelain gallbladder." Other appellations for this condition are calcifying cholecystitis and cholecystopathia chronica calcarea. The precise mechanism for the deposition of calcium in the gallbladder wall is not known, but in all instances the gallbladder is chronically inflamed, the wall is thickened, the mucosa is irregularly denuded, and nearly always the cystic duct is obstructed.[146] Calcification occurs most often as strips or plaques in the muscular coat, but occasionally small concretions form in the Rokitansky–Aschoff sinuses.[147] Analysis of the dystrophic calcification in the porcelain gallbladder reveals calcium phosphate mixed with lesser amounts of calcium carbonate. Increased intraluminal pressure as a result of cystic duct obstruction and the local trauma of coexistent gallstones leads to focal tissue necrosis with the laying down of calcium salts. Chronic inflammation and hemorrhage may also play a part in the calcifying process. Histologically, calcium is deposited extracellularly in areas of hyaline degeneration.

In a large series of patients with porcelain gallbladders, the mean age of the first appearance of calcification was 54 years, with a range of 38 to 70 years.[148] In our cases, the average age of onset was 65 and one 94-year-old patient was known to have had a calcified gallbladder for 20 years. The youngest reported patient was a 24-year-old woman with no history of hematological or gallbladder disease.[149] Five times as many women as men are affected, a fact that may reflect the higher incidence of cholecystitis in females.

For the most part, despite pathological evidence of inflammation and obstruction, affected individuals are usually asymptomatic. In 1928, Robb stated, "The calcified gallbladder is so quiescent, so unproductive of symptoms that the existence of many must never be known or even suspected and they are cast upon the rubbish heap of treasures whose only signpost is senile decay."[150]

Another feature of this entity is its relationship to the later development of gallbladder carcinoma. Etala reviewed 1,786 consecutive operations upon the biliary tract during a 23-year period.[148] Seventy-eight patients had primary gallbladder carcinoma and 26 had calcified gallbladders. Sixteen of these, or 61% of patients with porcelain gallbladders, had concomitant gallbladder carcinoma. Thus, of the total of 78 malignancies of the gallbladder in this series, 16 (20%) were associated with a calcified gall-

bladder. All tumors were invasive, and only 2 of 78 patients survived 5 years.[148] In another study, Cornell and Clark evaluated the pathological reports of 4,271 cholecystectomies. There were 16 porcelain gallbladders, and 2 of these (12.5%) had primary carcinoma within them.[151]

In light of the putative association between cancer and calcification in the gallbladder wall, it has been suggested that a patient with a porcelain gallbladder should undergo prophylactic cholecystectomy. Although this appears to be good advice in general, two caveats must be heeded. First, there is little known about the temporal relationship of mural calcification to carcinoma. It is not clear how long after the gallbladder calcifies the cancer appears or if some calcified gallbladders are destined never to harbor a malignant neoplasm. The fact that some individuals live with a calcified gallbladder for a long time suggests that there may be a differential susceptibility to carcinoma. Second, many patients with a calcified gallbladder are elderly and may not be candidates for an elective operation whose value has not been proved conclusively.

The plain film appearance of a calcified gallbladder is usually distinctive, consisting of an ovoid or pear-shaped conglomeration of flakes or plaques of calcium in the right upper quadrant or right mid abdomen (Fig 6–53). The cystic duct may sometimes be seen also as a rounded or tubular opacity, medial and superior to the gallbladder. Unlike the appearance of cysts, both the inner and outer borders of the flakes of mural calcification in a porcelain gallbladder can be irregular. A well-defined double track of calcium may be noted, representing opacification in both the mucosa and in the muscle layer. Some calcified gallbladders appear rounded, whereas others have a more complex shape, especially if the gallbladder contains a Phrygian cap or is otherwise folded upon itself.

Sometimes the differentiation between a porcelain gallbladder and a cyst in other organs is difficult to make on a single supine film. The normally situated gallbladder moves far anteriorly on a right posterior oblique film. A calcified cyst in the liver may also be ventrally positioned. A cystic calcification is smooth at its outer border, however, whereas the margins of the gallbladder wall may be irregular. It is also important to distinguish a single large calculus in the gallbladder from a calcified gallbladder wall because of the link between a porcelain gallbladder and carcinoma. Almost always a gallstone is calcified continuously throughout the entirety of its circumference, whereas gallbladder wall calcification is discontinuous. If the gallbladder is densely calcified, however, the differentiation between these

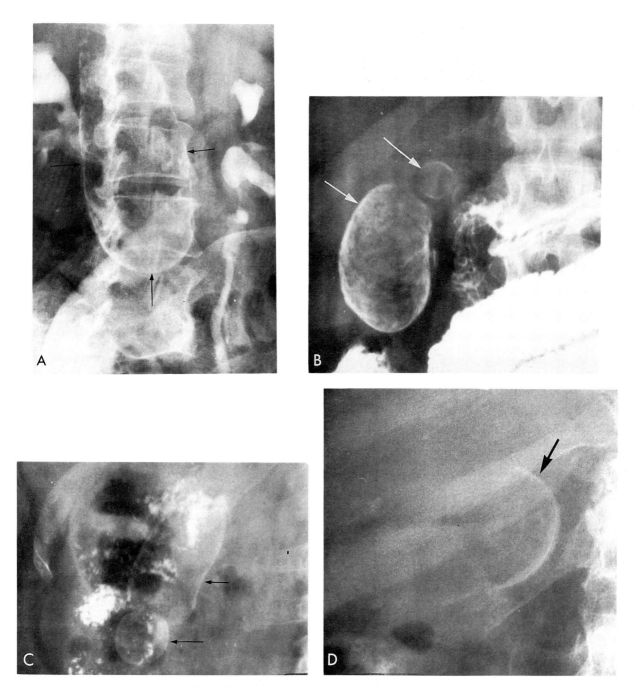

Figure 6–53. A spectrum of calcified gallbladders: **A.** An oblique film shows an enlarged porcelain gallbladder (*arrows*) projected over the lumbar vertebrae. **B.** Calcification in a gallbladder (*lower arrow*), and the cystic duct (*upper arrow*). **C.** Calcification in a gallbladder (*upper arrow*) with a Phrygian cap (*lower arrow*). Note the narrowing of the lumen near the fundus. The density overlying the gallbladder is unconjugated Telepaque in the large bowel. **D.** Curvilinear calcifications occupying only a part of the gallbladder wall (*arrow*).

two entities on plain films may be difficult or even impossible.

That is not to say that patients with calcified gallbladders do not have coincident cholelithiasis. In fact, almost all of them do have at least one stone.[152] Surprisingly, it is very uncommon to ob-serve a calculus in a calcified gallbladder. Usually, such gallbladder calculi are either radiolucent or, if calcified, much less dense than the radiodense gall-bladder wall and are therefore not seen on plain films. Occasionally, only a part of the gallbladder wall becomes radiopaque.[153,154] A carcinoma growing in a porcelain gallbladder may be recognized by the resorption of calcification at the site of the enlarging tumor (Fig 6–54).

Calcification in Gallbladder Carcinoma

Carcinoma of the gallbladder is not rare; several thousand cases are reported each year. In women it is the fifth most common malignancy of the gastrointestinal tract, following cancer of the colon, pancreas, stomach, and esophagus. The tumor is seldom resectable because it has almost always spread beyond the gallbladder before it is detected. Plain film studies hardly ever give an inkling of its presence because this neoplasm rarely calcifies. A few case reports have noted fine punctate calcification in the region of the gallbladder fossa.[155,156] Scattered calcification overlying a portion of the liver shadow is not, however, specific for a gallbladder carcinoma as it may also be found in primary hepatic tumors and in metastatic disease to the liver.

Lucencies in the Gallbladder and Bile Ducts

Biliary Enteric Fistula. A biliary enteric fistula is the abnormal opening of the gallbladder lumen or a bile duct into a segment of the tubular gastrointestinal tract. Most often a complication of cholelithiasis or cholecystitis, it is not a rare occurrence, developing eventually in 3% to 5% of patients with gallstones.[157] Perforation of the gallbladder wall occurs in 2% to 20% of patients with cholecystitis, and in one fifth of these a communication is formed with bowel.[39] Typically, fistulae are unassociated with pain or fever. Signs of infection are absent because there is no obstruction to bile flow. In fact, the majority of biliary enteric fistulae are transient and the abnormal aperture rapidly seal over. Some may remain patent for an extended period, however, especially if the rent in the gallbladder wall is large. If the cystic duct is not obstructed, gas from the bowel enters the biliary tree, enabling plain film recognition.

In 90% of patients, a biliary enteric fistula is the result of gallbladder inflammation.[158] Penetration of a duodenal ulcer through an adherent gallbladder accounts for only 5%.[159] Nearly all the remainder are due to extension of malignancies from the pancreas, stomach, duodenum, or colon. Rare causes include trauma, biliary and intestinal surgery, and inflammatory bowel disease.[160] One half[161] to three fourths[162] of biliary enteric fistulae involve the gallbladder and the duodenum. The next most frequent are cholecystocolic connections (10% to 20%),[163,164] followed by fistulae from the gallbladder to the stomach and jejunum. Choledochoduodenal fistulas are very uncommon, comprising no more than 1% of cases.[165,166]

Fistula formation is often accompanied by the extrusion and passage of a gallstone. Most calculi are too small to block the bowel lumen and harmlessly traverse the small bowel. Hence, biliary enteric communications are far more frequent, even if less symptomatic, than gallstone ileus. In fact, nonobstructive, uncomplicated fistulae[167,168] may outnumber gallstone intestinal obturation by as much as 18 to 1.

Gallstone Ileus. Obstruction of the intestine by ectopic gallstone was first noted by Bartholin in

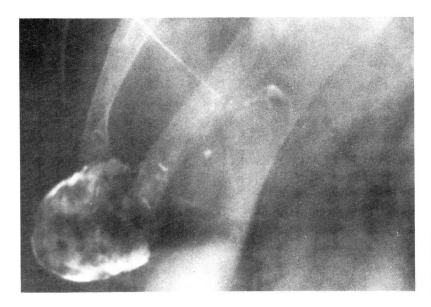

Figure 6–54. A porcelain gallbladder that at operation contained carcinoma in its proximal portion. The tumor was invasive, extending into the second portion of the duodenum. (*Courtesy of Dr. Harry Miller.*)

1654.[163] In the initial large series reported in 1890, gallstone ileus was found to be a disease of late middle age and the elderly.[163] Today, it accounts for 2% of bowel obstruction overall but up to 25% of small intestinal mechanical blockage in patients over age 70.[163] Women are affected 7 to 8 times more often than men.[166]

The typical patient is an obese elderly female, often diabetic, who complains of vague and poorly localized symptoms.[169] Palpation of the right upper quadrant frequently reveals no tenderness. Affected individuals experience vague discomfort, which is often intermittent and unassociated with abdominal distension. After a while, the variable and poorly defined constellation of clinical findings becomes confusing to the patient and may be dismissed by the examining physician. The changing nature of signs and symptoms betokens the migration of the ectopic calculus, at one time occluding the lumen entirely and then later passing more distally only to block the bowel once again (Fig 6–55). Such a slow progression of the gallstone may span several weeks. In many cases, the calculus freely negotiates the entire bowel, but if its diameter is greater than 3 cm the likelihood is remote for spontaneous passage through the ileocecal valve.[162]

In 70% of cases the obstruction is in the ileum. The small-bowel lumen is most narrowed there and peristalsis is often least active near the terminal ileum.[170] The jejunum is the next most common site of obstruction, and duodenal and pyloric gallstone blockage by gallstone is found in only 5%.[171,172] The

relatively wide diameter of the large bowel permits the passage of even very large calculi. Only 3% to 5%[164,170] of ectopic gallstones lodge in the large intestine, usually in the sigmoid colon in patients with extensive diverticulosis.[173,174]

The plain film triad of small-bowel obstruction biliary tract air and an opaque concretion was first described by Rigler et al in 1941 (Figs 1–7, 6–56).[175] Unfortunately, the classic appearance is found in less than 10% of cases.[165] Therefore, it is important to consider gallstone ileus even if only one sign is present (Fig 6–57). The absence of plain film findings by no means excludes gallstone ileus, however. In approximately one third of patients, the diagnosis is first made at laparotomy.

On plain films, small bowel obturation by an ectopic gallstone resembles mechanical obstruction by any other cause. The pattern of dilated ileal and jejunal loops out of proportion to distension of colonic segments is the hallmark of distal small bowel obstruction. The more proximal the luminal occlusion the more difficult the plain film diagnosis, as fewer loops become dilated. In the absence of an opaque calculus, gallstone obstruction of the duodenal bulb is especially difficult to recognize on plain films because only the stomach is blocked and frequent vomiting prevents its dilatation.[176]

Eisenmann noted that fluid-filled intestinal loops were more common in gallstone ileus than other types of mechanical small bowel obstruction.[177] Bryk et al confirmed this observation and offered an explanation for the frequency of a gasless

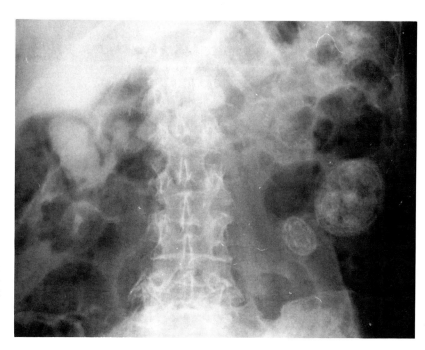

Figure 6–55. Gallstone ileus. Two calcified gallstones, one very large, in the jejunum. There is no evidence of bowel obstruction. The patient had intermittent symptoms over several weeks. At the time this film was taken, the abdomen was not distended.

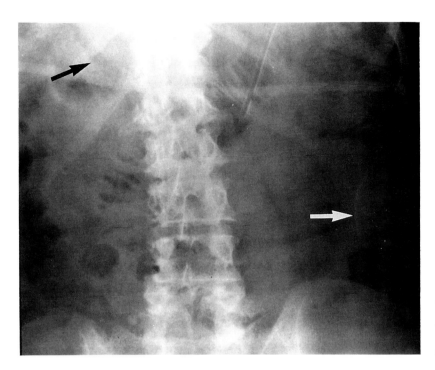

Figure 6–56. Gallstone ileus—Rigler's triad. A large calcified stone in the left mid-abdomen (*white arrow*) has obstructed the jejunum. Note the dilated air-filled small-intestinal loop crossing the midline. Gas is also in the common bile duct (*black arrow*).

abdomen in ectopic gallstone obturation.[178] In experimental studies with dogs, they showed that the biliary tree provides a venting mechanism for the swallowed gas that accumulates proximal to an intestinal obstruction. The communication of the bowel with the bile ducts makes available a large surface area for the resorption of ingested air, leaving only fluid behind in the intestinal lumen.[178]

The rapid absorption of gas across the ductal mucosa requires constant replenishment from the bowel. Therefore, in order to visualize biliary tract lucency there must be a continual diversion of gas or ingested air from the small intestine through the fistula. Consequently, pneumobilia is seen in only one half of patients with gallstone ileus. If the cystic duct is blocked, a common occurrence in patients with a history of cholecystitis, air has no other access to the biliary tree as long as the sphincter of Oddi is functioning normally. Air can be retained in the gallbladder lumen, however. In these patients, upright films can reveal adjacent fluid levels to the right of the midline—with air filling both the gallbladder and the duodenal bulb.[179]

A radiodense stone is found in one fourth[177] to one third[165] of supine abdominal films in patients with gallstone ileus. These large concretions are more likely to calcify than a smaller stone in an intact gallbladder. Typically, they have a thin margin of calcium that makes detection difficult if they overlie the spine or the bones of the pelvis. Occasionally, an ectopic calculus has an opaque central nidus in addition to a continuous rim of density. The diagnosis of gallstone ileus also can be suggested if a previous film demonstrated a stone in the expected position of the gallbladder and a present study reveals no calculus in the right upper quadrant.

Ectopic gallstones are apt to change their location and orientation on successive studies (Fig 6–58). When situated in small bowel loops, they tend to occupy a position in the periphery of the abdomen (Fig 6–59), outside the predictable location of most large calculi, which are confined to either the genitourinary tract or the gallbladder lumen.

Enteroliths, which are endogenous calculi of the small bowel, should not be confused with ectopic gallstones. Intestinal stone calcification must take place in an alkaline medium, and thus enteroliths are not seen in the acidic environment of the duodenum or proximal jejunum (Figs 5–102 and 5–103). Moreover, they are usually smaller than ectopic gallstones and are frequently multiple and faceted. Enteroliths form within diverticula or proximal to preexisting obstruction of the large bowel or distal ileum whereas in gallstone ileus the site of luminal occlusion is frequently more proximal. Coproliths, which are indigenous large bowel stones, are rare calculi and are almost always more irregularly marginated than ectopic gallstones that have passed into the colon.

Recurrent Gallstone Ileus. If gallstone ileus is treated by relief of obstruction alone there is a 5%

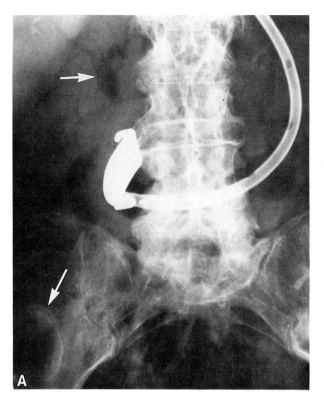

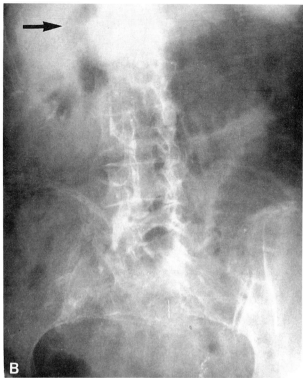

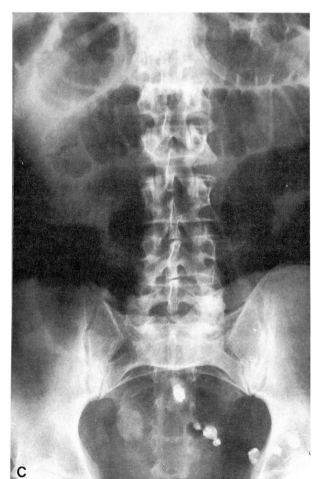

Figure 6–57. Combinations of two signs of gallstone ileus. **A.** Gas in the biliary tree (*upper arrow*) and a large calcified stone (*lower arrow*). The intestinal tube has decompressed the obstructed bowel. (*Courtesy of Dr. Jutta Greweldinger.*) **B.** Small-bowel obstruction and pneumobilia (*arrow*). Gas also occupies the gallbladder lumen. No opaque stone is seen. **C.** A calcified stone in the right pelvis and small bowel obstruction. There is no air in the biliary tract. (*Courtesy of Dr. Heribert Conradi.*)

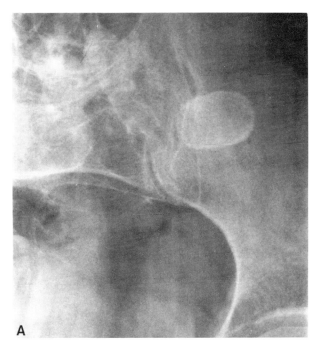
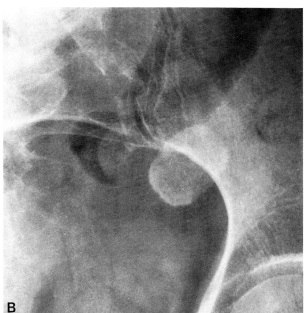

Figure 6–58. A, B. Changing location and orientation of a single large ectopic calculus is a feature of a stone in the intestinal lumen.

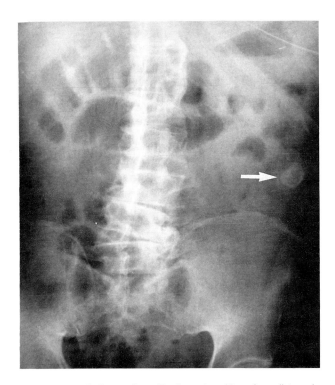

Figure 6–59. Gallstone ileus. Far lateral position of a gallstone in the jejunum (*arrow*), too peripheral to be in the urinary tract.

risk of a second obstruction by a retained stone. Recurrent gallstone ileus has been defined by Beutow et al as a "mechanical intestinal obstruction due to the intraluminal occlusion of the intestine by a second biliary calculus (calculi) which may have been present either in the gallbladder or intestines at the first surgical intervention; but is not the cause of the obstruction at that time."[180] The risk of a second obstructive episode is greater if the first stone was cylindrical or multifaceted, as both configurations imply the initial presence of a group of gallbladder calculi. The removal of the gallbladder at the initial operation decreases the risk of recurrent obstruction. The prolongation of operating time entailed by performing a cholecystectomy may not be a feasible option in elderly, ill patients, however. Therefore, a follow-up abdominal film should be carefully assessed for the presence of an opaque calculus even after apparent successful amelioration of symptoms by the initial surgery.[167,181,182] If clinical evidence of obstruction appears weeks or months later the diagnosis of recurrent gallstone ileus always should be entertained.

Emphysematous Cholecystitis

Emphysematous cholecystitis is an acute infection of the gallbladder caused by gas-forming bacteria. In 1908, in the first recorded case, Lobingier labeled it "gangrene of the gallbladder."[183] Because not all cases are caused by clostridial organisms, however, this term is a misnomer.[184] Moreover, some patients with emphysematous cholecystitis due to *E coli* infection have recovered without surgery despite gaseous penetration into pericholecystic tissues—a clinical outcome highly atypical for untreated gangrene.[185] Bacterial infection of bile is a necessary but not a sufficient condition for acute pneumocholecystitis. There must also be either obstruction to biliary flow by a blockage of the cystic duct or ischemia of the gallbladder wall before the clinical and radiological findings of the disease are manifested.

Emphysematous cholecystitis differs from the more common acute cholecystitis in several ways. The latter is found more often in women whereas emphysematous cholecystitis occurs in men in 70% to 80% of cases. The mortality rate from acute cholecystitis is 1.4% before age 60 and 8.4% in the elderly, compared to an age-independent fatality rate of 15% in emphysematous cholecystitis. Perforation is five times more common if the inflamed gallbladder contains gas.[186] Nearly all cases of acute cholecystitis have cholelithiasis whereas a stone-free gallbladder is found in 30% of patients with emphysematous cholecystitis.[187]

Usually, 1 to 2 days elapse between the onset of symptoms and radiographic evidence of gallbladder gas, but the minimal interval can be only 9 hours.[188] The pathogenetic role of ischemia was documented by Schoengerdt and Wiot in a patient who had a normal oral cholecystography just before undergoing aortography. Within 12 hours, he developed the stigmata of emphysematous cholecystitis, and at operation bile peritonitis and a gangrenous gallbladder was found.[189] Most probably small aortic plaques, dislodged during the angiographic procedure, had migrated to a cystic artery where they occluded the vessel lumen.

The progression of plain film abnormalities follows a well-defined sequence that can be observed in nearly all cases. At first gas fills the lumen alone, where it appears as a sausage- or pear-shaped lucency lacking internal markings (Fig 1–6). At this stage the gas-filled gallbladder can be mistaken for a distended duodenal bulb, a duodenal diverticulum, gas in a blind intestinal loop, an abscess in the liver, a focal collection of intraperitoneal air, or a gallbladder communication with the intestines through a fistula. Even a skin fold can simulate the ovoid shadow of gallbladder air (Fig 6–60).

Soon the gas infiltrates the gallbladder wall and becomes apparent as a single or double row of streaks encircling the lumen (Figs 2–43, 6–61).[190] If there is considerable fluid remaining in the gallbladder intraluminal gas may be less conspicuous than intramural gas on recumbent views (Fig 6–62). The

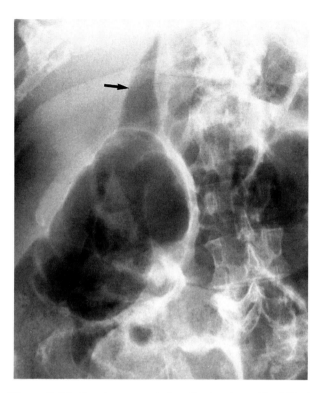

Figure 6–60. Pseudopneumocholecystis due to a skin fold. A pear-shaped lucency (*arrow*) above the hepatic flexure in an asymptomatic patient is air trapped between folds of skin. It was not present on a repeat film performed 1 hour later.

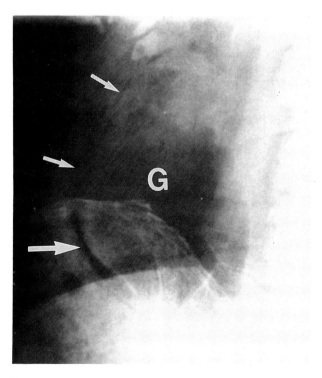

Figure 6–61. Emphysematous cholecystitis. Gas in the lumen (G) and in the gallbladder walls (*arrows*).

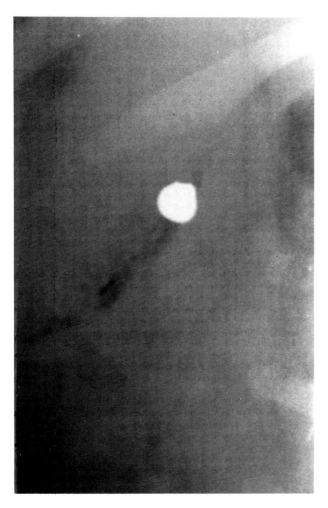

Figure 6–62. Emphysematous cholecystitis. Only mural streaks are seen, as fluid in the lumen obscures coexistent gas. The round density is barium in a colonic diverticulum.

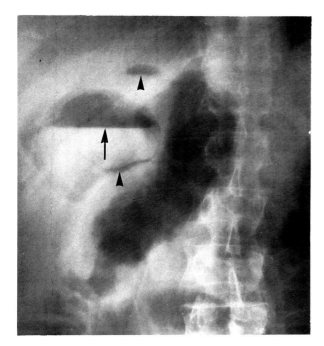

Figure 6–63. Upright film reveals a gas–fluid level in the gallbladder lumen (*large arrow*). Gas in the cystic duct (*small arrow*), gallbladder wall (*arrowhead*), and in the lateral pericholecystic tissues. The inflammation has caused an ileus of adjacent bowel.

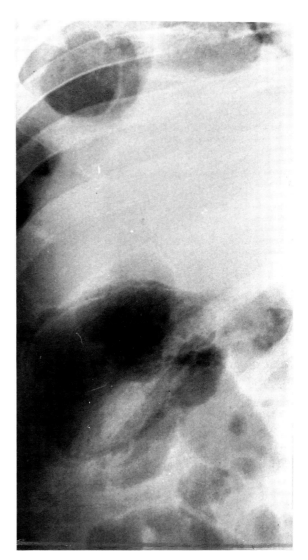

Figure 6–64. Emphysematous cholecystitis with right subphrenic abscess. The gallbladder lumen and wall contain gas. The multilocular gas collection superior to it is within a large abscess. (*Courtesy of Dr. Jon Adler.*)

interrupted circle of streaks quickly becomes an intact halo around the lumen. Gas then extends into the pericholecystic (Fig 2–47) tissues and is recognizable as bubbles or bands of lucency adjacent to the gallbladder wall.[191] If the advancing inflammation abuts on adjacent bowel it induces a localized ileus (Fig 6–63). Air in the biliary tree is surprisingly infrequent despite the relatively common finding of a patent cystic duct. If the perforated gallbladder is not treated promptly, a gas-containing abscess can develop in the right subphrenic space (Fig 6–64).[79]

SPLEEN

Normal Spleen

The normal-sized spleen varies greatly in configuration depending primarily on body habitus. The superior margin of the spleen usually lies just beneath the left hemidiaphragm, and its lateral edge is in contact with or close to the lateral abdominal wall. From these relatively constant landmarks, the non-enlarged spleen can extend medially to within 2 cm of the midline in hypersthenic individuals.[192] In asthenic persons the long axis of the spleen tends toward the vertical. Only when this solid organ reaches beyond the shadow of the stomach can it be seen as a separate soft tissue density.[193] Hence, only the lower pole of the normal sized spleen casts a distinct image on plain films. Brogdon and Cros observed the tip of the splenic shadow in only 44% of patients who had no evidence of splenomegaly.[194]

Splenic Enlargement

As the spleen grows, much of its accretion in volume takes place along its superior–inferior axis (Fig 6–65). Such a direction of expansion seems to be independent of body build. It is not an inevitable mode of enlargement, however, because, in a minority of patients, increases in size of the spleen are horizontally oriented. The slightly enlarged spleen is usually a posteriorly situated organ. As it extends inferiorly it tends to advance anteriorly as well because posterior enlargement is limited by the unyielding barrier of the left iliac bone. Thus, palpation of the splenic tip from an anterior approach is readily achieved with very big spleens but has lessened sensitivity in moderate and minimal splenomegaly.

Various numerical indeces of splenic volume by plain film assessment have been suggested, all of which depend upon the assumption of a vertically oriented spleen whose superior margin is closely related to the diaphragm.[194,195] These measurements are at best inexact. In fact, Reimenschneider and Whalen have shown that in most cases a subjective radiological interpretation is a good enough indicator of enlargement and is gauged best by noticing the location of the interface of fat with the splenic tip.[196] Inferior displacement of the radiographic splenic flexure can sometimes be misleading because this anterior structure may be situated far from the spleen. In patients with enlarging horizontal spleens unassociated with hepatomegaly or ascites, medial displacement of the stomach bubble and even lateral deviations of the descending duodenum are helpful plain film signs of splenomegaly (Fig 6–66).

Loss of Splenic Substance

A small or absent spleen is more difficult to appreciate on plain films. The high position of the splenic flexure just below the left hemidiaphragm is sometimes attributed to loss of splenic mass. There is a poor correlation, however, between the position of the colon and the presence of a spleen of normal or diminished size. A better sign is lateral deviation of the gastric air shadow, as the stomach is apt to migrate peripherally to occupy the space vacated by the spleen (Fig 6–67).

Wandering Spleen

The spleen develops in the left upper quadrant from mesenchymal cells in the dorsal mesogastrium. It is anchored primarily by the gastrolienal ligament and the lienorenal ligament, which contains the splenic vessels. A less important support inferiorly is the hammocklike phrenicocolic ligament. Incomplete fusion of the dorsal mesogastrium or lack of fixation of supporting ligaments can allow the spleen to wander within the peritoneal cavity.[197,198] This condition is seen most often in multiparous women, and it may be abetted by abdominal wall laxity and possibly by hormonal abnormalities secondary to pregnancy.[199,200]

The wandering spleen may remain asymptomatic throughout life. If it twists on its pedicle, however, it can become infarcted as its blood supply is cut off. Plain film findings include a mobile left abdominal mass, a medially and posteriorly displaced splenic flexure, an elevated left kidney that lacks a splenic hump, and a laterally deviated stomach.

Splenic Calcification

Radiodensities in the spleen occupy a narrower spectrum than those in the liver (Table 6–4). Although various entities may produce similar patterns of opacity in the hepatic parenchyma, the diagnostic choices are limited and usually clear-cut when one is confronted with a splenic density. Except for splenic cysts, where many different histological types can produce identical images, radiographic appearances are frequently characteristic or even pathognomonic. Thus, plain film recognition is usually informative and careful evaluation may obviate the necessity of further studies to reach a diagnosis.

Multiple Discrete Calcifications

Tuberculosis. Calcified tuberculous granulomas are the most common cause of splenic densities. In one series of patients with splenic calcifications, the underlying cause was tuberculosis in over 90%.[201] Sweany's observation in 1940 that "The spleen is affected more with tuberculosis calcification and perhaps less with nontubercular calcification than any other abdominal organ"[202] applies today in spite of the declining prevalence of this disease. Most often, calcified tubercles occur in a normal-sized spleen and in an asymptomatic patient. Infrequently, cal-

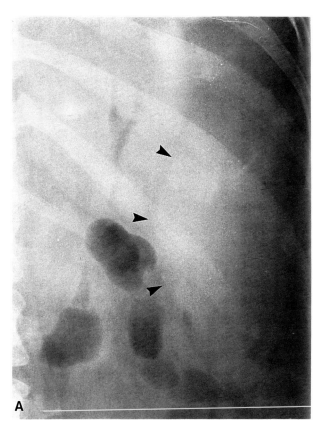

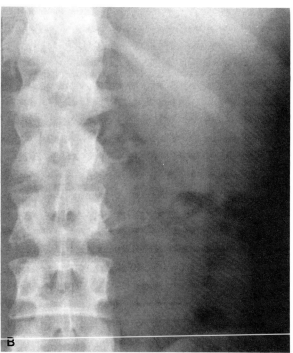

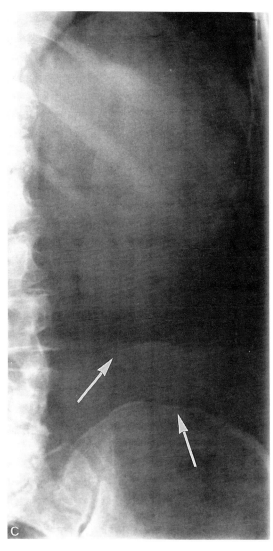

Figure 6–65. Splenomegaly extending inferiorly. **A.** Mild enlargement. The spleen extends below the left 11th rib. Its medial margin is delimited by the arrowheads. **B.** Moderate enlargement. The spleen depresses the distal transverse colon. **C.** Marked enlargement. The splenic tip extends to the iliac bone (*arrows*).

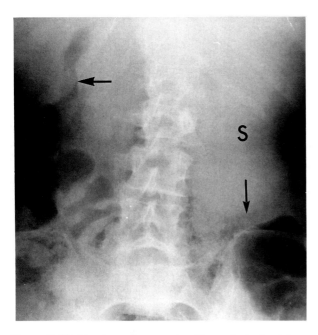

Figure 6–66. Massive splenomegaly with mostly horizontal enlargement. The spleen (S) does not reach the top of the iliac bone (*vertical arrow*), but its medial growth has displaced the air-filled duodenal sweep far from the midline (*horizontal arrow*).

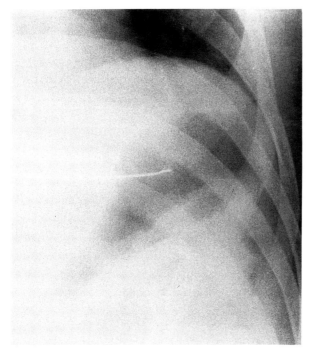

Figure 6–67. Postsplenectomy. The stomach, which contains the distal end of an opaque nasogastric tube, has moved laterally.

TABLE 6–4. RADIODENSITIES IN THE SPLEEN

I. Multiple Discrete Densities
  A. Common
      Tuberculosis
      Histoplasmosis
  B. Rare
      Brucella suis
      Hemangioma
      Hamartoma
II. Cystic calcification
  A. True cyst
      Epidermoid cyst
      Cystic hemangioma
  B. False cyst
      Hemorrhagic cyst
      Serous cyst
  C. Infestation—*Echinococcus granulosis*
  D. Splenic artery aneurysm
  E. Metastatic mucinous adenocarcinoma of the ovary
  F. Calcification of the splenic capsule
      Sickle cell disease
      Trauma
III. Solid calcification or opacification
      Sickle cell disease
      Hemosiderosis
      Thorotrast

cified granulomas may also be present in the liver. It takes several years for the calcification of splenic granulomas to be detected radiographically. Calcium is first laid down in the caseous center of the granuloma and then in the surrounding capsule. Consequently, younger granulomas may have irregular contours, but the more mature foci of inflammation have smoother outlines. Most calcifications in tuberculous infections of the spleen are approximately 5 mm in diameter, but the size of multiple opacities is not uniform. Generally, only a few calcifications are found in the spleen, but this is not an inviolate rule; in some cases, granulomas may be numerous (Fig 6–68).[203]

Histoplasmosis. In endemic areas, such as the Ohio Valley, the predominant cause of multiple discrete opacities in the spleen is histoplasmosis. Calcified granulomas were present in 44% of spleens observed at postmortem examinations in Cincinnati, Ohio, compared with 30% in splenic specimens removed at autopsy in New York City and 2% in specimens obtained in Rotterdam, The Netherlands.[204] Microscopic examination revealed evidence of histoplasmosis in most of the Cincinnati cases. The occurrence of well-defined multiple calcifications in the spleen correlates well with positive skin tests for histoplasmosis in regions where the disease is common.[205]

As in tuberculosis, the granulomas in the spleen

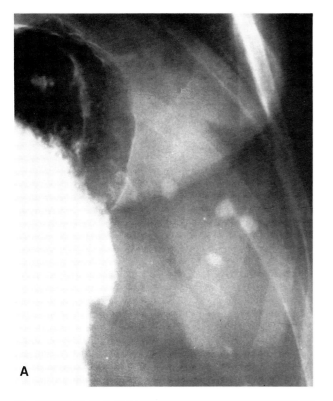

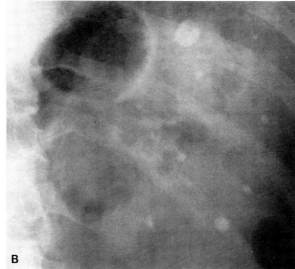

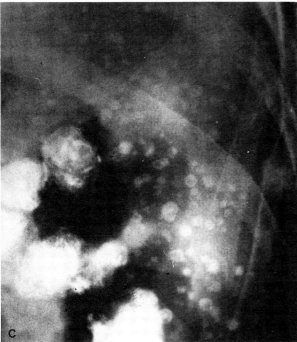

Figure 6–68. A spectrum of calcified tuberculous granulomata in the spleen. **A.** A few granuloma calcified foci of similar size. **B.** Scattered granulomas of varying diameters. **C.** Numerous granulomas. Many have central lucencies and resemble phleboliths.

caseate at their centers, and calcium is laid down within the central mass of necrotic and infected tissue. Calcium salts also may be deposited at the fibrous margins of the granuloma with a noncalcified band separating these two foci of calcification. Occasionally, the granuloma appears as a laminated concretion, which is a distinctive feature of histoplasmosis. In contrast to tuberculosis, there are almost always many calcifications in the spleen (Fig 6–69). Typically, they are round, smooth, less than 5 mm in diameter, and often associated with similar calcifications in the liver and chest.[206]

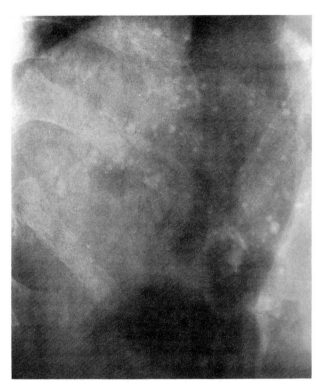

Figure 6–69. Histoplasmosis. Many calcified granulomas are scattered throughout the spleen.

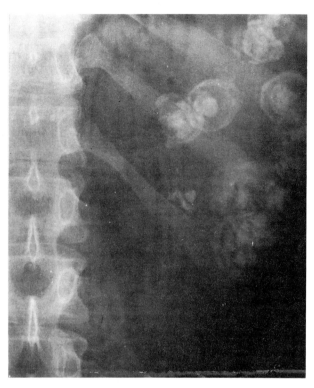

Figure 6–70. Calcified *Brucella suis* abscesses in the spleen. There are multiple "target" lesions with marginal calcifications and dense centers. (*Courtesy of K.C. Demetropoulos.*[82])

Brucellosis. Brucellosis is a third infectious disease with a predilection for splenic calcifications. Untreated patients have repeated episodes of fever and malaise, alternating with asymptomatic intervals. The disease is caused by one of three species of *Brucella*, but, as in the liver, only *B suis* engenders calcification. Interestingly, the calcifications are often so characteristic in brucellosis that a plain film diagnosis can be made with assurance. Granulomas contain a flocculent central nidus averaging 5 to 10 mm in diameter. Emanating from the central focus are irregular linear densities, and a separate encircling margin of calcification can be seen. In some cases the calcification represents a snowflake or a target (Fig 6–70). Calcified granulomas are multiple, never confluent, and usually associated with splenomegaly.[207–210]

Tumors of the Spleen. In the older literature, frequent mention was made of the presence of phleboliths in the spleen. Both tuberculosis and histoplasmosis can closely simulate the appearance of phleboliths. Histological examination almost always reveals that what mimic phleboliths roentgenographically are really granulomas. Thus, the presence of phleboliths in the spleen in the absence of a mass lesion should be considered very rare. Even in

hemangioma, which is the most common benign tumor of the spleen, the observation of radiographically visible phleboliths is uncommon (Fig 2–98). Most hemangiomas of the spleen are small and undetectable on plain films.[211] When phlebolithic calcification does occur, the multiple densities usually have central lucencies and are often greater than 5 mm in diameter. In these patients, the tumors are large and there is splenomegaly.

Hamartomas are very rare tumors of the spleen that are occasionally included with hemangiomas in a classification of splenic neoplasms, but they should really be considered as a separate entity. Because the reported cases of hamartomas are so few it is not clear if they have a characteristic pattern of calcification.[212]

Conduit Calcifications

Calcification of the Splenic Artery. The splenic artery ranks behind the aortic and the iliac arteries as a site for abdominal vascular calcification. Arising from the celiac axis and passing horizontally behind and adjacent to the pancreas, the splenic artery runs toward the hilus of the spleen, where it divides into several intrasplenic branches. The artery passes behind the stomach and may indent the posterior gastric wall below the cardia (Fig 6–71).[213] Calcification in the splenic artery can be seen as disconnected parallel arcuate lines of radiodensity. The pattern of calcification of the artery on plain films depends upon the extent of radiopacity, the degree of tortuosity, and the orientation of the vessel with respect to the X-ray beam. When the artery is both very convoluted and calcified, it appears as a disordered assemblage of irregular streaks. Sometimes, a markedly tortuous artery has a regular pattern of twists and turns, giving it an appearance akin to a folded hose (Figs 2–102,6–72). On the other hand, the finding of straight line calcification is rare because the splenic artery usually elongates before it calcifies.

Splenic Artery Aneurysms. Splenic artery aneurysms are not uncommon.[214–216] In one series, they were noted in 0.8% of all autopsies.[217] They are found most often in the elderly, where their incidence in men and women is equal.[217] Under age 50, they are two to three times more frequent in women.

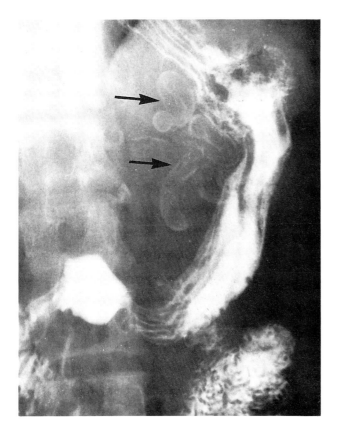

Figure 6–71. Calcified splenic artery (*arrows*) with impression upon the posterior wall of the stomach. Note the marked tortuosity of the splenic artery.

Usually, splenic artery aneurysms are asymptomatic, but occasionally, patients complain of left upper quadrant fullness or pain, and in approximately 50% of cases there may also be a significant splenomegaly. These aneurysms are susceptible to rupture; pregnant women are at greatest risk from this complication.[218]

Aneurysms appear anywhere along the course of the artery and can result from atherosclerosis, trauma, or infection.[219,220] In the aged, atherosclerosis is the leading cause and aneurysmal calcification is usually noted, along with intimal calcification in other parts of the artery (Figs 2–113,6–73). A congenital defect in the vascular wall appears to account for a significant minority of cases in younger females. Occasionally, aneurysms occur in patients with portal hypertension and splenomegaly.

At any place in the splenic artery, aneurysmal dilatation may be mistaken for a markedly tortuous artery of normal caliber. Annular calcification is a constant finding in calcified lesions. In most cases, the circle of calcification will be open at the junction of the normal artery and the aneurysm.

Many other calcified cystic structures resemble splenic artery aneurysms.[221] The differential diagnosis can be narrowed by dividing the artery into three segments. Near the origin of the splenic artery, a calcified cystic lesion of the superior or medial aspect of the left kidney, an aneurysm in the main left renal artery, a cystic retroperitoneal tumor, a left adrenal cyst, a calcified echinococcal cyst in the lateral segment of the left lobe of the liver, and a rare calcified pancreatic pseudocyst should be ruled out. Overlying the middle third of the artery can be a renal cyst, a renal artery aneurysm, and a mesenteric or an omental cyst. In the peripheral third, a splenic cyst should be considered, along with a cystic lesion in the lateral margin of the left kidney. A splenic artery aneurysm often has a complex configuration and consists of more than one annular rim of calcification (Fig 6–74). This is an important point because intrasplenic cysts are usually unilocular. With the help of lateral and oblique films (Fig 6–75), most aneurysms arising from any portion of the splenic artery can be differentiated from cystic lesions in adjacent structures. At times, however, the distinction between these aneurysms and other lesions cannot be made on plain radiographs alone, and contrast studies, including computed tomography and angiography, may be necessary to secure a diagnosis.

Cystic Lesions in the Spleen

There are many kinds of splenic cysts. A few, such as epidermoid cysts and cystic hemangiomas, are

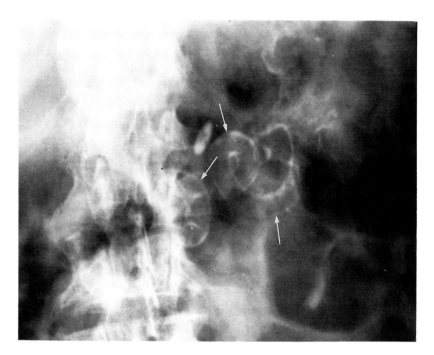

Figure 6–72. Tortuous and calcified splenic artery (*arrows*) with multiple twists and turns, an appearance suggesting a folded hose.

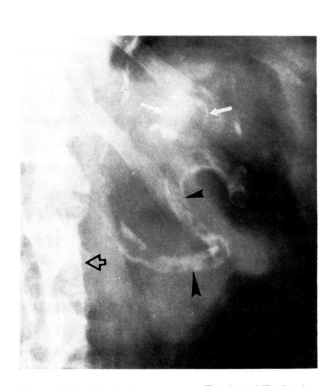

Figure 6–73. Splenic artery aneurysm. The rim calcification (*arrows*) represents an intrasplenic aneurysm. The main splenic artery is markedly calcified (*arrowheads*), as is the abdominal aorta (*open arrow*).

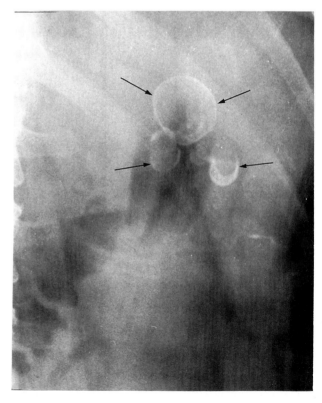

Figure 6–74. Multiple saccular aneurysms of the splenic artery. Note the several circular calcifications (*arrows*) in the splenic hilus. Multiple annular calcifications are more suggestive of an aneurysm than of a nonvascular cyst.

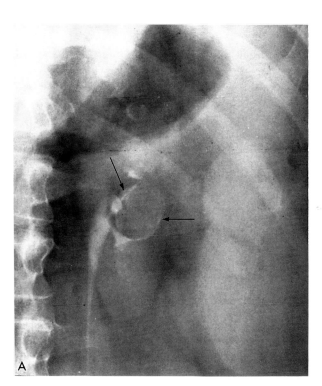

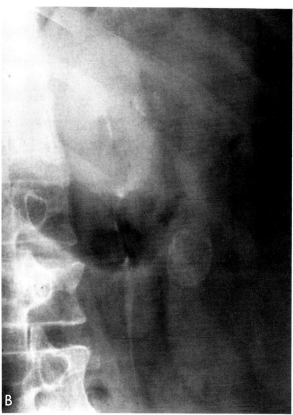

Figure 6–75. Splenic artery aneurysm. **A.** Anterior–posterior projection. Circular calcification (*arrows*) superimposed on the renal hilus. This can be mistaken for a calcified renal mass or renal artery aneurysm. **B.** Left posterior oblique projection. The calcification is clearly anterior to the kidney. There is also splenomegaly.

congenital.[222,223] Many are acquired either as a result of parasitic infestation or as a consequence of trauma. Several categorizations have been proposed, based on such factors as cytology, histology, or etiology. The classification offered in Table 6–4 considers only those entities that have been reported with calcification observable on plain films.

Two thirds of all reported splenic cysts are caused by *Echinococcus granulosus* (Fig 6–76).[224] They may occur in the spleen in the absence of cysts elsewhere, but most often the liver is also involved. The spleen is the second most common site of *E granulosus*. Usually, multiple cysts occupy an enlarged spleen, but, almost always, only one cyst calcifies.[225]

The remainder of calcified acquired cysts are the so called false cysts, all of which are believed related to trauma.[226] Eighty percent of these are hemorrhagic cysts whose formation is probably a result of the liquefaction of hematomas.[227] It is not known why some traumatized spleens rupture and others form cysts. Surprisingly, cystic degeneration is a rare event, considering the large number of cases of splenic trauma.[228] Serous cysts, which make up approximately 20% of all non-echinococcal-acquired

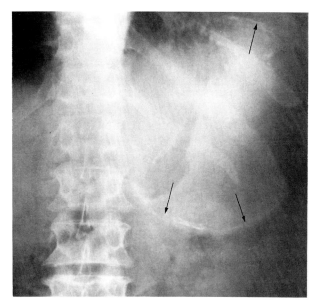

Figure 6–76. Large *Echinococcus granulosus* cyst (*arrows*) in the spleen. The etiology of a calcified splenic cyst usually cannot be determined by plain films alone in the absence of other lesions.

cysts of the spleen, also have a traumatic etiology (Fig 1–18). Like hemorrhagic cysts they have a fibrous lining.[229] Most probably, serous cysts are hemorrhagic cysts from which the blood had been totally resorbed leaving only a fibrous wall and clear fluid. Hemorrhagic and serous cysts are found most often in women of childbearing age for reasons which remain obscure.

A small percentage of cystic lesions are true cysts with epithelial or endothelial linings. Calcified epidermoid cysts and cystic hemangiomas have been observed on occasion but are much less common than radiodense, acquired cysts. Splenic cysts either are asymptomatic or cause vague sensations of discomfort or fullness in the left upper quadrant. Thus, they can grow to a large size before detection. Sometimes plain films of the abdomen, obtained for other reasons, demonstrate calcified cysts that were completely unexpected clinically.

A recent review of nonparasitic splenic cysts revealed that true cysts are usually first noted in adolescence whereas false cysts come to attention somewhat later. Both enlarge the spleen, and sometimes they produce a localized bulge in the splenic contour. Less than 5% of true cysts have radiodense walls on plain films but almost 30% of false cysts calcify.[230] In an area not endemic for *E granulosis* the finding of a single large annular calcification within the spleen is most likely a "false" cyst related to previous trauma.

The patterns of calcification in all the various types of splenic cysts are similar. Hydatid cysts look remarkably like hemorrhagic or epidermoid cysts. When small, splenic cysts tend to calcify circumferentially, with a continuous smooth outer wall and a less distinct and more irregular inner wall. Large cysts may appear only with interrupted arcs of opacity (Fig 2–108), but heavily calcified margins can also be seen in cysts of massive dimensions (Fig 6–77).[231]

The differential diagnosis of calcified splenic cysts is extensive. Understanding the principle of displacement by enlarging organs can help determine if a calcified mass in the left upper quadrant is indeed in the spleen. An echinococcal cyst of the left lobe of the liver may simulate a splenic mass. Enlargement of the liver can displace the stomach laterally, but a tumor of the spleen tends to deviate the stomach toward the midline. Calcified renal tumors are usually smaller than splenic cysts. Mesenteric and more posterior cysts elevate the transverse colon and splenic flexure whereas large splenic cysts depress the colon. Calcified pancreatic cysts are extremely rare but may not be differentiable from splenic cysts. On plain film examination, calcified aneurysms of the distal splenic artery can be misinterpreted as splenic cysts. Although splenic cysts are rarely multiple,[232] splenic artery aneurysms commonly have several contiguous annular calcifications.[233] The absence of splenomegaly and

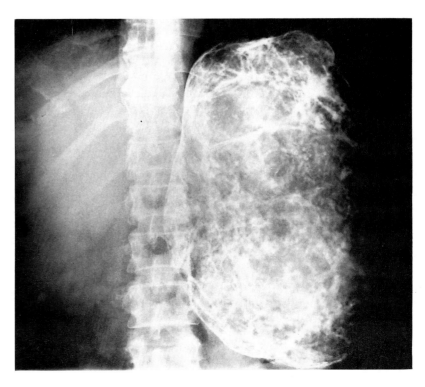

Figure 6–77. Enormous, heavily calcified splenic cyst of unknown etiology.

parts of the artery also suggest splenic artery aneurysms.

Metastatic mucinous adenocarcinoma of the ovary is one other type of arcuate calcification that is alway multiple in the spleen. This tumor may involve the spleen, with cystic deposits either on the surface or within the organ. Usually calcification is also present in metastases in the peritoneal cavity and in the liver.[234]

Calcification in the margin of the spleen can occur as a result of subcapsular hematoma formation, but it is sometimes seen in patients homozygous for sickle cell disease.[235] The radiographic appearance can simulate that of a calcified cyst if only a small portion of the capsule is radiopaque (Fig 6–78). If most of the splenic border is involved, however, smooth rimlike calcification will assume the configuration of the spleen itself (Fig 6–79).

Diffuse Opacification of the Spleen

Diffuse opacification of the spleen is seen in only a few conditions. In each of these, the appearance of the spleen is characteristic, and ancillary radiological findings in other organs usually permit a definitive diagnosis on plain films.

Sickle Cell Disease. Opacification of the spleen has been observed in 2% to 10% of adolescent and

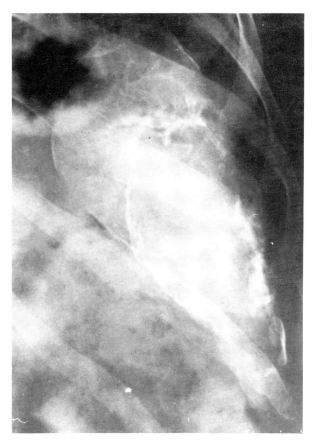

Figure 6–79. Extensive calcification involving the splenic capsule.

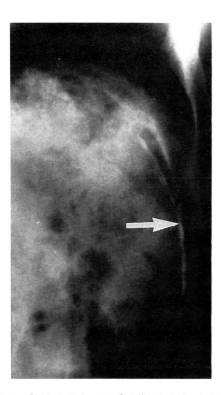

Figure 6–78. Sickle cell disease. Calcification of only a part of the lateral margin of the capsule of the spleen (*arrow*).

young adult patients, with homozygous sickle cell anemia.[236,237] Increased radiodensity in the spleen is probably due to a combination of hemosiderin deposition, which gives a generalized increased density to the spleen, and focal deposition of calcium in areas of hemorrhage, infarct, and fibrosis.

The precise relationship between the laying down of calcium salts and the presence of hemorrhage and scarring is unclear. The spleen may appear diffusely opaque, but most often multiple 1 to 2 mm punctate densities give it a coarsely granular appearance (Fig 6–80).[238–240] Opacification can occur initially in both large and small organs (Fig 6–81), but as the spleen decreases in size, it usually becomes more dense.[241] Rarely, in adults with mixed hemoglobinopathies such as thalassemia-S and S-C disease, the spleen becomes opaque but remains enlarged (Fig 6–82).[242] Almost always these splenic densities are associated with other changes characteristic of sickle cell anemia, including aseptic necrosis of the humeral heads, a generalized increase in bone density, central depression of the end plates of vertebral bodies, fibrotic streaks in the lungs, cardiomegaly, and calcified gallstones.

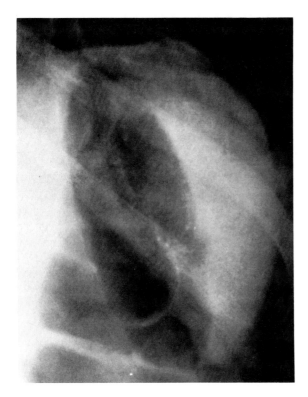

Figure 6–80. Dense, mottled calcification of the spleen in a patient with sickle cell anemia. Subsequent films revealed that the spleen had decreased in size and became denser.

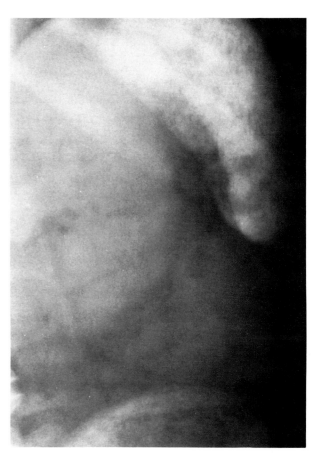

Figure 6–82. A 52-year-old patient with hemoglobin S-C disease. At this age, a patient homozygous for hemoglobin S should have autosplenectomized. The dense spleen is not reduced in size. Observe also the dense left iliac crest.

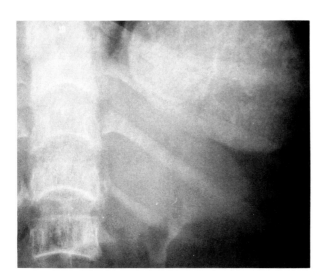

Figure 6–81. A young adult with SS disease. Severe osseous changes in the vertebra are seen, along with a horizontal, calcified spleen of normal dimensions.

Increased Density Due to Iron. In patients overloaded with iron because of idiopathic hemochromatosis, immoderate ingestion, or repeated transfusions, excess hemosiderin can be laid down throughout the spleen. The roentgenographic appearance is a diffuse and homogeneous density without the punctate granularity seen in sickle cell disease. Usually the spleen is enlarged at initial presentation and remains big. There is often a similar increase in density in the liver and retroperitoneal lymph nodes.

Thorotrast. After intravascular administration, Thorotrast, a colloidal substance, is retained by the spleen (Fig 6–83). The roentgenographic appearance is pathognomonic. Initially the spleen is homogeneously dense. After several years, the density becomes mottled and there are associated opacifications of peripancreatic lymph nodes as well as a very fine feathery density throughout the liver (Fig 6–84).[243]

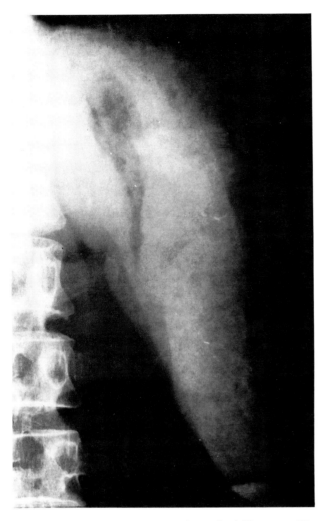

Figure 6–83. A patient who recently received Thorotrast. The spleen is enlarged and diffusely radiopaque.

Lucencies in the Spleen

Splenic Abscess. Splenic abscess is a serious and often fatal infection almost always associated with a hectic clinical course. In Africa, an idiopathic form also known as tropical splenic abscess, is most common. It is usually seen in patients with the gene for hemoglobin S and occurs more often in males.[244] In the United States, splenic abscess may be a complication of an abdominal operation, the result of a contiguous extension of a pus collection in adjacent organs, or an untoward outcome of a therapeutic infarction of the spleen by catheter occlusion of the splenic artery. By far the most common etiology, however, is blood-borne infection. The typical patient is an intravenous drug abuser with bacterial endocarditis.

Splenic abscess enlarges the spleen, displacing the stomach medially and deviating the colon infe-

riorly. Large collections can even depress the left kidney. Often the left hemidiaphragm is elevated and there is usually an effusion in the left pleural space. Gas formation is relatively common, appearing either as a collection of small bubbles or a single, large lucency (Fig 6–85).[245]

A gas-containing splenic abscess can be mimicked by a diverse group of lucencies in adjacent structures. Pus collections in the pancreas, left kidney, and left subphrenic space can overlie the spleen. Food in the stomach and feces in the splenic flexure may simulate intrasplenic bubbles. Even a left lower lobe pneumonia or abscess can resemble a splenic lucency, especially if it obscures the left hemidiaphragm and induces a pleural effusion (Fig 6–86).

Just as in the liver or kidney, nonsuppurative intrasplenic gas can be found after transcatheter splenic infarction. A benign condition, unassociated with clinical symptoms, it first appears 3 to 4 days after the procedure and persists for several weeks. The gas is seen as small bubbles scattered throughout the area of infarction.[87]

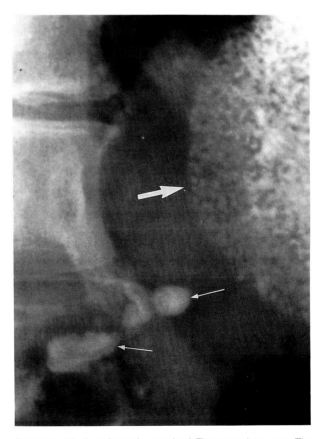

Figure 6–84. A patient who received Thorotrast long ago. The spleen is very dense and mottled (*large arrow*) and there is opacification of peripancreatic lymph nodes (*small arrows*).

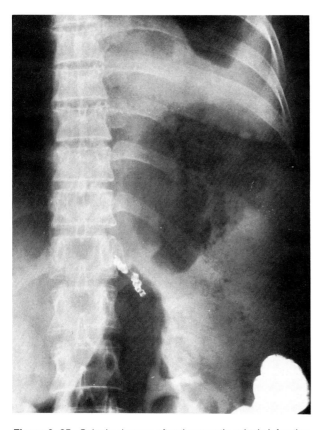

Figure 6–85. Splenic abscess after therapeutic splenic infarction. Radiodense coils were introduced into the splenic artery. One week later there is a large lucency overlying the stomach and numerous small bubbles extending more inferiorly. Both are in a huge splenic abscess. There is also a left pleural effusion.

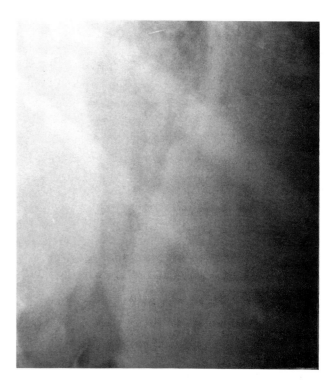

Figure 6–86. Scattered small bubbles superimposed over the gastric fundus and superior margin of the spleen simulate a splenic pus collection. In fact all were outside the abdomen in a left lower lobe lung abscess.

REFERENCES

1. Mindelzun R, McCort JJ. Hepatic and perihepatic radiolucencies. *Radiol Clin N Am*. 1980; 18:221–238.
2. Whalen JP, Berne AS, Riemenschneider PA. The extraperitoneal perivisceral fat pad. I. Its role in the roentgenologic visualization of abdominal organs. *Radiology*. 1969; 92:466–472.
3. Gelfand DW. The liver. Plain film diagnosis. *Semin Roentgenol*. 1975; 10:177–185.
4. Meyers HI, Jacobson G. Displacements of stomach and duodenum by anomalous lobes of the liver. *Am J Roentgenol*. 1958; 79:789–792.
5. Gore RM, Goldberg HI. Plain film and cholangiographic findings in liver tumors. *Semin Roentgenol*. 1983; 18:87–93.
6. Kattan KR, Moskowitz M. Position of the duodenal bulb and liver size. *Am J Roentgenol*. 1973; 119:78–84.
7. Chon H, Arger PH, Miller WT. Displacement of duodenum by an enlarged liver. *Am J Roentgenol*. 1987; 119:85–88.
8. Friedman E, Lewi Z. Gastric displacement in atrophic liver cirrhosis. A report of three cases. *Radiology*. 1967; 79:644–647.

9. Joffe N. Siderosis in the South African Bantu. *Br J Radiol*. 1964; 37:200–209.
10. Shambron E., Zheutlin M. Radiologic signs in hemosiderosis. *JAMA*. 1958; 168:33–35.
11. Smith WL, Quattromani F. Radiodense liver in transfusion hemochromatosis. *Am J Roentgenol*. 1977; 128:316–317.
12. Grunfeld O, Aldana L, Himostroza G. Radiologic aspects of thallium poisoning. *Radiology*. 1963; 80:847–849.
13. Mackenzie KGF, Preston CD, Stewart W, et al. Thorotrast retention following angiography. A case report with postmortem studies. *Clin Radiol*. 1962; 13:157–162.
14. Talley RW, Poznanski AK, Heslin JH, et al. Laminagrams of Thorotrast–opacified liver in evaluation of chemotherapy for metastatic cancer. *Cancer*. 1964; 17:1214–1219.
15. Janower ML, Sidel VW, Flynn MJ. A follow–up study of a large group of patients who received thorium dioxide for cerebral arteriography. *Radiology*. 1967; 88:1004–1006.

16. Levy DW, Rindsberg S, Friedman AC, et al. Thorotrast–induced hepatosplenic neoplasia: CT identification. *Am J Roentgenol.* 1986; 146:997–1004.

17. Lambrianides AL, Askew AR, Lefevre I. Thorotrast–associated mucoepidermoid carcinoma of the liver. *Br J Radiol.* 1986; 59:791–792.

18. Curry JL, Johnson WG, Feinberg DH, et al. Thorium induced hepatic hemangioendothelioma. *Am J Roentgenol.* 1975; 125:671–677.

19. Kuisk H, Sanchez JS, Mizuno N. Colloidal thorium dioxide (Thorotrast) in radiology with emphasis on hepatic cancerogenesis. *Am J Roentgenol.* 1967; 99:463–475.

20. Astley R, Harrison N. Miliary calcification of the liver. Report of a case. *Br J Radiol.* 1949; 22:723–724.

21. McCullough JAL, Sutherland CG. Intra–abdominal calcification: Interpretation of its roentgenologic manifestations. *Radiology.* 1941; 36:450–451.

22. Spink WW. Suppuration and calcification of the liver and spleen due to long–standing infection with *Brucella suis. N Engl J Med.* 1957; 257:209–210.

23. Bretland PM. *Armillifer armilatus* infestation— Radiologic diagnosis in two Ghanaian soldiers. *Br J Radiol.* 1962; 35:603–608.

24. Steinbach HL, Johnstone HG. The roentgen diagnosis of armillifer infection (porocephalus) in main. *Radiology.* 1957; 68:234–237.

25. Scatarige JC, Fishman EK, Saksouk FA, et al. Computed tomography of calcified liver masses. *J Comput Assist Tomogr* 1983; 7:83–89.

26. Green PA. Hepatic calcification in cancer of the large bowel. *Am J Gastroenterol.* 1971; 55:466–470.

27. Miele AJ, Edmonds HW. Calcified liver mestastases: A specific roentgen diagnostic sign. *Radiology.* 1963; 80:779–785.

28. Appleby A, Hackins DM. Calcification in hepatic metastases. *Br J Radiol.* 1958; 31:449–450.

29. Wells J. Calcified liver metastases. *N Engl J Med.* 1956; 253:639–640.

30. Fred AL, Eiband JM, Collins LC. Calcifications in intraabdominal and retroperitoneal metastases. *Am J Roentgenol.* 1964; 91:138–148.

31. Darlak JT, Moskowitz M, Kattan KE. Calcifications in the liver. *Radiol Clin N Am.* 1981; 18:209–219.

32. Zimmer FF. Islet-cell carcinoma treated with alloxan: Associated with calcified hepatic metastases and thyrotoxic myopathy. *Ann Intern Med.* 1964; 61:543–549.

33. Shonfeld ED, Guarino AV, Bessolo RJ. Calcified hepatic metastases from carcinoma of the breast. Case report and review of the literature. *Radiology.* 1973; 106:303–304.

34. Saghatoeslami M, Khodarghmi K, Epstein BS. Calcified intra-hepatic metastases from carcinoma of the breast. *JAMA.* 1962; 181:1139–1140.

35. Maddock WG, Lien RM. Calcified liver nodules from metastatic melanoma: Ocular primary 15 years previously. *Q Bull Northwester Univ Med School* 1955; 29:374–378.

36. Karras BG, Cannon AA, Zanon B Jr. Hepatic calcification. *Acta Radiol.* 1962; 57:458–468.

37. Persaud V, Bateson EM, Bankay CD. Pleural mesothelioma associated with massive hepatic calcification and unusual metastases. *Cancer.* 1970; 26:920–928.

38. Ludwig J, Grier MW, Hoffman HM, et al. Calcified mixed malignant tumors of the liver. *Arch Pathol.* 1975; 99:162–166.

39. Morgan AG, Walker WC, Mason MK, et al. A new syndrome associated with hepato-cellular carcinoma. *Gastroenterology.* 1972; 63:340–354.

40. Hall PM, Winkelman EI, Hauk WA, et al. Calcification in the liver, an unusual feature of ductal cell hepatic carcinoma. *Cleve Clin Q.* 1970; 37:93–105.

41. Adam A, Gibson RN, Soreide V, et al. The radiology of fibrolamellar hepatoma. *Clin Radiol.* 1986; 37:355–358.

42. Zipser RD, Rau JE, Ricketts RR, et al. Tuberculous pseudotumor of the liver. *Am J Med.* 1976; 61:946–951.

43. Alergant CD. Gumma of the liver with calcification. *AMA Arch Intern Med.* 1956; 98:340–343.

44. Haddow RA, Kemp-Harper RA. Calcification in the liver and portal system. *Clin Radiol.* 1967; 18:225–236.

45. D'Alessandro A, Leja J, Vera MA. Cystic calcifications of the liver in Colombia; echinococcus or calcified abscesses. *Am J Trop Med.* 1966; 15:908–913.

46. Rogers WF, Ralls PW, Boswell WD, et al. Amebiasis: Unusual Radiographic Manifestations. *Am J Roentgenol.* 1980; 135:1253–1257.

47. Grange D, Dhumeaux D, Couzineau P, et al. Hepatic calcification due to *Fasciola gigantica. Arch Surg.* 1974; 108:113–115.

48. Meyers MA. Calcifications in cholangio-carcinoma. *Br J Radiol.* 1968; 41:65–66.

49. Aspray M. Calcified hemangioma of the liver. *Am J Roentgenol.* 1945; 653:446–463.

50. Meuhlbauer MA, Farber MG. Hemangioma of the liver: Some interesting clinical and radiological observations. *Am J Gastroenterol.* 1966; 45:355–365.

51. Plachta A. Calcified cavernous hemangioma of the liver: Review of the literature and report of 13 cases. *Radiology.* 1962; 79:783–788.

52. Gonzalez LR, Marcos J, Illanos M, et al. Radiologic aspects of hepatic echinococcosis. *Radiology.* 1979; 130:21–27.

53. Bret PM, Fond A, Bretagnolle P, et al. Percutaneous aspiration and drainage of hydatid cysts in the liver. *Radiology.* 1988; 168:617–620.

54. Bonakdarpour A. Echinococcus disease: Report of 112 cases from Iran and a review of 611 cases from the United States. *Am J Roentgenol.* 1967; 99:660–667.

55. Thompson WM, Chisholm OP, Tank R. Plain film roentgenographic findings in alveolar hydatid disease—*Echinococcus multilocularis. Am J Roentgenol.* 1972; 116:345–358.

56. Heilbrun M, Klein AJ. Massive calcification of the liver: Case report with a discussion of its etiology on the basis of alveolar hydatid disease. *Am J Roentgenol.* 1946; 55:189–192.

57. Caplan LN, Simon M. Non-parasitic cysts of the liver. *Am J Roentgenol.* 1966; 96:421–428.

58. Kutcher R, Schneider M, Gordon DH. Calcification in polycystic disease. *Radiology.* 1977; 122:77–80.

59. Rutledge NJ, Pratt MC, Taupmann RE. Biliary cystadenoma mistaken for an echinococcal cyst. *South Med J.* 1983; 76:1575–1577.

60. Broker MH, Baker SR. Calcification in the portal vein wall demonstrated by computed tomography. *J Comput Assist Tomogr.* 1985; 9:444–446.

61. Baker SR, Broker MH, Charnsangavej C. Calcification in the portal vein wall. *Radiology.* 1984; 152:18.

62. Moberg G. Calcified thrombosis in portal system diagnosed by roentgen examination. *Acta Radiol.* 1943; 24:374–383.

63. Smallwood RA, Davidson JS. Calcification in the portal system. *Gastroenterology* 1968; 54:265–269.

64. Sherrick DW, Kincaid OW, Gambill EE. Calcification in the portal venous system. Unusual radiologic sign of portal venous thrombosis. *JAMA.* 1964; 187:861–862.

65. Haddow RA, Kemp-Harper RA. Calcification in the liver and portal system. *Clin Radiol.* 1967; 18:225–236.

66. MacKenzie RL, Tubbs HR, Laws JW, et al. Obstructive jaundice and portal vein calcification. *Br J Radiol.* 1978; 51:953–955.

67. Adler J. Venous calcifications associated with cavernous transformation of the portal vein: Computed tomographic and angiographic correlations. *Radiology.* 1979; 132:27–28.

68. Blendis LM, Laws JW, Williams R, et al. Calcified collateral veins and gross dilatation of the azygous vein in cirrhosis. *Br J Radiol.* 1968; 41:909–912.

69. Magovern GJ, Meuhsam GE. Calcification of the portal and splenic veins. *Am J Roentgenol.* 1954; 71:84–88.

70. Bleich AR, Kipen CS. Venous calcification in Banti's syndrome. *Radiology.* 1948; 50:657–660.

71. Jarvis L, Hodes PJ. Aneurysm of hepatic artery demonstrated roentgenographically. Case report. *Am J Roentgenol.* 1954; 72:1037–1040.

72. Quinn JL III, Martin JF. Hepatic artery aneurysm. A case report. *Am J Roentgenol.* 1962; 87:284–286.

73. Balthazar EJ. Hemobilia. Calcified hepatic artery aneurysm presenting with massive gastrointestinal bleeding. *Gastrointest Radiol.* 1977; 2:71–74.

74. Zammit AA, Wild SR. The radiographically visible fatty liver in an adult patient. *Br J Radiol.* 1980; 53:1018–1019.

75. Yousefzadeh DK, Lupetin AR, Jackson JH, Jr. The radiologic signs of fatty liver. *Radiology.* 1979; 131:351–355.

76. Thorley LL, Figiel LS, Figiel SJ, et al. Roentgenographic findings in accidental ligation of the hepatic artery. Case report. *Radiology.* 1965; 85:56–58.

77. D'Orsi CJ, Ensminger W, Smith EH, et al. Gas-forming intrahepatic abscess. A possible complication of arterial infusion chemotherapy. *Gastrointest Radiol.* 1979; 4:157–161.

78. Pueyo I, Guzman A, Fernandez F, et al. Liver abscess complicating embolization of focal nodular hyperplasia. *Am J Roentgenol.* 1979; 133:740–742.

79. Foster SC, Schneider B, Seaman WB. Gas-containing

80. Catto JVF. Multiple liver abscesses in hydatid disease. *Br J Radiol.* 1964; 37:859–860.

81. Elson MW. Antemortem radiographic demonstration of gas gangrene of the liver. *Radiology.* 1960; 74:57–60.

82. Wolfel DA, Brogdon BG. Intrahepatic air—A sign of trauma. *Radiology.* 1968; 91:952–953.

83. McCort JJ. Rupture or laceration of the liver by non-penetrating trauma. *Radiology.* 1962; 78:49–57.

84. Hennessey OF, Allison DJ. Intra-hepatic gas following embolisation. *Br J Radiol.* 1983; 56:348.

85. Siim E, Fleckenstein P. Gas formation following hepatic embolisation. *Br J Radiol.* 1982; 55:926–928.

86. Rankin RN. Gas formation after renal tumor embolization without abscess: A benign occurrence. *Radiology.* 1979; 130:317–320.

87. Levy JM, Wasserman PI, Weiland DE. Non-suppurative gas formation in the spleen after transcatheter splenic infarctions. *Radiology.* 1981; 139:375–376.

88. Stewart AM. The study of free gas in the foetus as a sign of intrauterine death. *Br J Radiol.* 1961; 34:187–193.

89. Balthazar EJ, Gurkin S. Cholecystoenteric fistulas: Significance and radiographic diagnosis. *Am J Gastroenterol.* 1976; 65:168–173.

90. Harley WD, Kirkpatrick RH, Ferrucci JT, Jr. Gas in the bile ducts (pneumobilia) in emphysematous cholecystitis. *Am J Roentgenol.* 1978; 131:661–663.

91. Cremin BJ. Biliary parasites. *Br J Radiol.* 1969; 42:506–508.

92. Wastie ML, Cunningham IGE. Roentgenologic findings in recurrent pyogenic cholangitis. *Am J Roentgenol.* 1973; 119:71–77.

93. Grant EG, Borts, F, Schellinger D, et al. Pneumobilia: A comparison of four imaging modalities. *J Comput Assist Tomogr.* 1980; 4:630–663.

94. Reilly HF Jr. Mosenthal W, Dyke Jr. Normal gas-filled appendix simulating biliary tree air in a case of acute cholecystitus. *Radiology.* 1967; 89:931–932.

95. Shaub MS, Birnbaum WN, Meyers HI. Peribiliary fat: A new roentgenographic finding. *Am J Roentgenol.* 1975; 123:330–337.

96. Govoni AF, Meyers MD. Pseudopneumobilia. *Radiology.* 1976; 118:526.

97. Halber MD, Daffner RH. Fat in the intrahepatic fissure. *Am J Roentgenol.* 1979; 132:842–843.

98. Haswell DM, Berne AS, Schneider B. Plain film recognition of the ligamentum teres hepatis. *Radiology.* 1975; 114:263–267.

99. Wolfe JN, Evans WA. Gas in the portal veins of the liver in infants: A roentgenographic demonstration with post mortem anatomic correlation. *Am J Roentgenol.* 1955; 74:486–489.

100. Susman N, Senturia HR. Gas embolization of the portal venous system. *Am J Roentgenol.* 1960; 83:847–850.

101. Sisk PB. Gas in the portal venous system. *Radiology.* 1981; 77:103–107.

pyogenic intrahepatic abscesses. *Radiology.* 1970; 94:613–618.

102. Liebman PR, Patten MJ, Manny J, et al. Hepatic-portal venous gas in adults: etiology, pathophysiology and clinical significance. *Ann Surg.* 1978; 107:281–287.

103. Wiot JF, Felson B. Gas in the portal venous systems. *Am J Roentgenol.* 1961; 86:920–929.

104. Barrett AR. Gas in the portal veins: Diagnostic value in intestinal gangrene. *Clin Radiol.* 1962; 13:92–95.

105. Graham GA, Bernstein RB, Gronner AT. Gas in the portal and inferior mesenteric veins caused by diverticulitis of the sigmoid colon. Report of a case with survival. *Radiology.* 1975; 114:601–602.

106. McClandless RL. Portal vein gas: A grave prognostic sign. *Am J Roentgenol.* 1964; 92:1162–1165.

107. Lefleur RS, Ambos MA, Rothberg M, et al. Angiographic demonstration of gas and thrombus in the portal vein. *Am J Roentgenol.* 1978; 130:1171–1173.

108. Cynn, WS, Hodes PJ. A new sign of small bowel volvulus. Gas in mesenteric vein without gas in portal vein. *Radiology.* 1973; 108:289–290.

109. Dell DM Jr. Gas in the portal vein. *Am J Roentgenol.* 1967; 100:424–425.

110. Benson MD. Case report. Adult survival with intrahepatic portal venous gas secondary to acute gastric dilatation with a review of portal venous gas. *Clin Radiol.* 1985; 36:441–443.

111. Haswell DM, Carsky EW. Hepatic portal venous gas and gastric emphysema with survival. *Am J Roentgenol.* 1979; 133:1183–1185.

112. Stein MG, Cruez JV, III, Hamlin JA. Portal venous air associated with barium enema. *Am J Roentgenol.* 1983; 140:1171–1172.

113. Gold RP, Seaman WB. Splenic flexure carcinoma as a source of hepatic portal venous gas. *Radiology.* 1977; 122:329–330.

114. Birnberg FA, Gore RM, Shragg B, et al. Hepatic portal venous gas. A benign finding in a patient with ulcerative colitis. *J Clin Gastroenterol.* 1983; 5:89–91.

115. Fink DW, Boyden FM. Gas in the portal vein. A report of two cases due to ingestion of corrosive substances. *Radiology.* 1966; 87:741–743.

116. Bull MJ, Kaye B. Portal vein gas following double-contrast barium enema. *Br J Radiol.* 1985; 58:1129–1130.

117. Sadler VK, Brennan RE, Madan V. Portal vein gas following air-contrast barium enema in granulomatous colitis: Report of a case. *Gastrointest Radiol.* 1979; 4:163–164.

118. Haber I. Hepatic portal vein gas following colonoscopy in ulcerative colitis—Report of a case. *Acta Gastroenterol. Belg.* 1983; 46:14–17.

119. Weinstein GE, Weiner M, Schwartz M. Portal vein gas. *Am J Gastroenterol.* 1968; 49:425–429.

120. Rovito V. Hepatic portal vein gas associated with bronchopneumonia. *Am J Gastroenterol.* 1982; 77:243–244.

121. Marks WM, Filly RA. Computed tomographic demonstration of intraarterial air following hepatic artery ligation. *Radiology.* 1979; 132:665–666.

122. McCort JJ. Acute hepatobiliary disease. *Semin Roentgenol.* 1973; 8:389–403.

123. McNulty JG. *Radiology of the Liver.* Philadelphia: WB Saunders Co; 1977.

124. Mathias K, Waldman D, Daikler G. Intrahepatic cystic bile duct dilatation and stone formation. A new case of Caroli's disease. *Acta Hepatotol Gastroenterol.* 1978; 25:30.

125. Bassler A, Peters AG. Hepatic calculi. *Am J Med Sci.* 1947; 214:427–430.

126. Young BR. Roentgen examination of the acute abdomen—The Carmen Lecture. *Radiology.* 1955; 64:481–497.

127. Richards P. Spontaneous migration of gallstones. *N Engl J Med.* 1962; 266:299–300.

128. Hansson K, Lundh G, Ranberg L. Spontaneous and total disappearance of stones from the gallbladder. *Acta Chir Scand.* 1964; 127:176–180.

129. Scanlan RL, Young BR. The roentgen diagnosis of gallbladder and biliary tract disease without cholecystography. *Am J Roentgenol.* 1954; 72:639–643.

130. Cancelmo JJ. Stellate fissuring in gallstones. *Radiology.* 1955; 64:420–423.

131. Hinkel CL. Fissures in biliary calculi further observations. *Am J Roentgenol.* 1954; 71:979–987.

132. Meyers MA, O'Donohue N. The Mercedes-Benz sign insight into the dynamics of formation and disappearance of gallstones. *Am J Roentgenol.* 1973; 119:63–70.

133. Wright FW. The "Jack Stone" or "Mercedes-Benz" sign—A new theory to explain the presence of gas within fissures in gallstones. *Clin Radiol.* 1977; 28:469–473.

134. Phillips JC, Gerald BE. The incidence of cholelithiasis in sickle cell disease. *Am J Roentgenol.* 1971; 113:27–28.

135. Phemister DB, Rewbridge AG, Rudisill H Jr. Calcium carbonate gallstones and calcification of the gallbladder following cystic duct obstruction. *Ann Surg.* 1931; 94:493–516.

136. Knutsson F. On limy bile. *Acta Radiol.* 1933; 14:453–462.

137. Ochsner SF, Orgeron EA. Opaque gallstones showing pliability during cholecystographic visualization. *Am J Roentgenol.* 1959; 82:1024–1026.

138. Simmonds HT. Milk-of-calcium in the common bile duct. *Am J Roentgenol.* 1957; 78:1020–1023.

139. Nolan B, Ross JA, Samuel E. Lime–water bile. *Br J Surg.* 1960; 40:201–204.

140. Morehouse HT, Roush G, Deshmukh S, et al. Milk-of-calcium in the common bile duct. *J Comput Assist Tomogr.* 1984; 8:177–179.

141. Marquis JR, Densler J. The disappearing limy bile syndrome. *Radiology.* 1970; 94:311–312.

142. Schwartz A, Feuchtwanger M. Radiographic demonstration of spontaneous disappearance of limy bile. *Gastroenterology.* 1961; 40:809–812.

143. Holden WS, Turner MJ. Disappearing limy bile. *Clin Radiol.* 1972; 23:507–509.

144. Gardner AMN, Holden WS, Monks PJW. Disappearing gallstones. *Br J Surg.* 1966; 53:114–120.

145. Ochsner SF, Carrera GM. Calcification of the gall-

bladder ("Porcelain Gallbladder"). *Am J Roentgenol.* 1963; 89:847–853.

146. Ochsner SF. Intramural lesions of the gallbladder. *Am J Roentgenol.* 1971; 113:1–10.

147. Berk RM, Armbruster TG, Saltzstein S. Carcinoma in the porcelain gallbladder. *Radiology.* 1973; 106:29–31.

148. Etala E. Cancer de la vesicula biliar. *Prensa Med Argent.* 1962; 49:2283–2299.

149. Baker SR, Buchbinder S. Porcelain gallbladder in a 24-year-old woman. *NY State J Med.* 1985; 85;609.

150. Robb JJ. Observations on calcification of the gallbladder-with the presentation of a case. *Br J Surg.* 1928; 16:114–119.

151. Cornell CM, Clarke R. Vicarious calcification involving the gallbladder. *Ann Surg.* 1959; 149:267–272.

152. Polk HC Jr. Carcinoma of the calcified gallbladder. *Gastroenterology.* 1966; 50:582–585.

153. Gunn A. Calcified cyst attached to the gallbladder. *Br J Radiol.* 1966; 39:68–69.

154. Lambert-Leder G, Lombard R. Diverticule calcie du bas fond vesiculaire. *Acta Gasterol Belg.* 1968; 31:175–181.

155. Rogers LF, Lastra MP, Lin KJ, et al. Calcifying mucinous adenocarcinoma of the gallbladder. *Am J Gastroenterol.* 1973; 59:441–445.

156. Parker GW, Joffe M. Calcifying primary mucus-producing adenocarcinoma of the gallbladder. *Br J Radiol.* 1972; 45:468–469.

157. Hricak H, Vander Molen RL. Duodenocolic fistula with gallstone ileus. *Am J Gastroenterol.* 1978; 69:711–715.

158. Calonge MA. Izenstark JL, Nice CM, Jr. Internal biliary fistula. *JAMA.* 1962; 179:198–200.

159. Rominger CJ, Canino CW. Internal biliary tract fistulae. *Am J Roentgenol.* 1965; 90:835–843.

160. Craig O. Hepato-colic fistula. *Br J Radiol.* 1965; 38:801–803.

161. Hoskins EOL. Gall-stone in the pyloric antrum. *Br J Radiol.* 1962; 35:355–357.

162. English RE, MacGuire MN, Guyen PB. Small bowel masses due to gallstones: Report of two cases. *Clin Radiol.* 1986; 37:153–154.

163. Day EA, Marks C. Gallstone ileus: Review of the literature and presentations of thirty-four new cases. *Am J Surg.* 1975; 129:552–558.

164. Griffths GC. Gall-stone obstruction of the descending duodenum. *Br J Radiol.* 1962; 38:869–870.

165. Balthazar EJ, Schecter LS. Gallstone ileus. The importance of contrast examinations in the roentgenographic diagnosis. *Am J Roentgenol.* 1975; 125:374–379.

166. Kirkland KC, Croce EJ. Gallstone intestinal obstruction: A review of literature and presentation of 12 cases, including 3 recurrences. *JAMA.* 1961; 176:494–497.

167. Levin B, Shapiro RA. Recurrent enteric gallstone obstruction. *Gastrointest Radiol.* 1980; 5:151–153.

168. Wolloch Y, Glanz I, Dinstman M. Spontaneous biliary enteric fistula. *Am J Surg.* 1976; 131:680–687.

169. Brockis JG, Gilbert MC. Intestinal obstruction by gall-

170. Fjermeros H. Gall-stone ileus. Case reports and review of 178 cases from Scandinavia and Finland. *Acta Chir Scand.* 1964; 128:188–192.

171. Lloyd TT, Jaques PF, Weaver PC. Gallstone obstruction and perforation of the duodenal bulb. *Br J Surg.* 1976; 63:131–132.

172. Argyropoulos GD, Velmachos R, Ayenidis B. Gallstone perforation and obstruction of the duodenal bulb. *Arch Surg.* 1979; 114:333–335.

173. Young WVB. Gallstone ileus of the colon. Report of an unusual type of colon obstruction. *Arch Surg.* 1961; 82:333–336.

174. Miller JDR, Costopoulos LB, Holmes CE, et al. Gallstone ileus of the colon. *Br J Radiol.* 1965; 38:960–961.

175. Rigler LG, Borman CN, Noble JF. Gallstone obstruction: Pathogenesis and roentgen manifestations. *JAMA.* 1941; 117:1753–1759.

176. Figiel LS, Figiel SJ, Wietersen FK, et al. Gallstone obstruction: Clinical and roentgenographic considerations. *Am J Roentgenol.* 1955; 74:22–38.

177. Eisenman JI, Finck EJ, O'Laughlin BJ. Gallstone ileus. A review of the roentgenographic findings and report of a new sign. *Am J Roentgenol.* 1967; 101:361–366.

178. Bryk D, Silverman MJ, Venugopal MK, et al. Fluid filled small bowel loops in gallstone ileus: clinical and experimental observations. *Invest Radiol.* 1977; 12:357–363.

179. Balthazar EJ, Schecter LS. Air in gallbladder: A frequent finding in gallstone ileus. *Am J Roentgenol.* 1978; 131:219–222.

180. Beutow GW, Glaubitz JP, Crampton RS. Recurrent gallstone ileus. *Surgery.* 1963; 54:716–724.

181. Ulreich S, Massi J. Recurrent gallstone ileus. *Am J Roentgenol.* 1979; 133:921–923.

182. Haq AU, Morris AH, Daintith H. Recurrent gallstone ileus. *Br J Radiol.* 1981; 54:1000–1001.

183. Lobingier AS. Gangrene of the gallbladder. *Ann Surg.* 1908; 48:72–73.

184. Friedman J, Aurelius JR, Rigler LG. Emphysematous cholecystitis. *Am J Roentgenol.* 1949; 62:814–821.

185. Blum L, Stagg A. Emphysematous cholecystitis. *Am J Roentgenol.* 1983; 89:840–846.

186. Hunter, ND, Macintosh PK. Acute emphysematous cholecystitis. An ultrasonic diagnosis. *Am J Roentgenol.* 1980; 134:592–593.

187. Mentzer RM, Golden GT, Chandler JG, et al. A comparative appraisal of emphysematous cholecystitis. *Am J Surg.* 1973; 129:10–15.

188. Ellis F. Acute pneumocholecystitis. *Br J Radiol.* 1961; 34:462,464.

189. Schoengerdt CG, Wiot JF. Emphysemtous cholecystitis following aortography. *Am Surg.* 1972; 38:274–277.

190. Heifitz CJ, Wyloge EK. Effect of distension of gallbladder with air and its relationship to acute pneumocholecystitis. *Ann Surg.* 1955; 142:283–288.

191. Esguerra-Gomez G, Arango O. Emphysematous

cholecystitis. Report of seven cases. *Radiology*. 1963; 80:369–373.

192. Rosch J. Roentgenologic possibilities in spleen diagnosis. *Am J Roentgenol*. 1965; 94:453–461.

193. Krell L, Mindell S. The radiographic positions of the spleen. *Br J Radiol*. 1969; 42:830–834.

194. Brogdon BG, Cros NE. Observations on the "normal" spleen. *Radiology*. 1959; 72:412–414.

195. Whitley JE, Maynard CD, Rhyne AL. A computer approach to the prediction of spleen weight from routine films. *Radiology*. 1966; 86:73–76.

196. Riemenschneider PA, Whalen JP. The relative accuracy of estimation of the liver and spleen by radiologic and clinical methods. *Am J Roentgenol*. 1965; 94:462–468.

197. Gordon DH, Burrell MI, Levin DC, et al. Wandering spleen. The radiological and clinical spectrum. *Radiology*. 1977; 125:39–46.

198. Isikoff MB, White DW, Diaconis JN. Torsion of the wandering spleen seen as a migratory abdominal mass. *Radiology*. 1977; 123:36.

199. Bosniak MA, Byck W. Wandering spleen diagnosed preoperatively by intravenous aortography. *Am J Roentgenol*. 1960; 84:898–901.

200. Salmonowitz E, Frick MP, Lund G. Radiologic diagnosis of wandering spleen complicated by splenic volvulus and infarction. *Gastrointest Radiol*. 1984; 9:57–50.

201. Gray EF. Calcifications of the spleen. *Am J Roentgenol*. 1944; 61:336–351.

202. Sweany HC. On the nature of calcified lesions with special reference to those in the spleen. *Am J Roentgenol*. 1940; 44:209–229.

203. Massoud MG, Shafei AXZ. Calcified miliary tuberculosis of the spleen. *Br J Radiol*. 1957; 30:101–102.

204. Schwarz J, Silverman FM, Adriano SM, et al. The relationship of splenic calcifications to histoplasmosis. *N Engl J Med*. 1955; 252:887–889.

205. Okudaira M, Straub M, Schwarz J. The etiology of discrete splenic and hepatic calcification in an endemic area of histoplasmosis. *Am J Pathol*. 1961; 39:599–611.

206. Serviansky B, Schwarz J. The incidence of splenic calcification in positive reactors to histoplasmosis and tuberculin. *Am J Roentgenol*. 1956; 76:53–59.

207. Yow EM, Brennan J, Nathan MH, et al. Calcified granulomata of the spleen in longstanding brucellar infection. *Ann Intern Med* 1961; 55:307–313.

208. Arcomano JP, Pizzolato MF, Singer R, et al. A unique type of calcification in chronic brucellosis. *Am J Roentgenol*. 1977; 128:135–137.

209. Demetropoulos KC, Lindenauer SM, Rapp R, et al. Target calcification of the spleen in chronic brucellosis (*Brucella suis*). *J Can Assoc Radiol*. 1974; 25:161–163.

210. Case Records of the Massachusetts General Hospital. Case (42461). *N Engl J Med*. 1956; 255:950–962.

211. Benjamin BI, Mohler DH, Sandusky WR. Hemangioma of the spleen. *Arch Intern Med*. 1965; 115:380–384.

212. Komaki S, Gombas OF. Angiographic demonstration of a calcified splenic hamartoma. *Radiology*. 1976; 121:77–78.

213. Rosenberg MA, Elkin M. Gastric deformity from extrinsic pressure by calcified splenic artery. *Radiology*. 1957; 69:735–738.

214. Owens JC, Coffey R. Aneurysm of the splenic artery, including a report of 6 additional cases. *Int Abstr Surg*. 1953; 97:313–335.

215. Spittel JA Jr, Fairbairn JF, Kincaid OW, et al. Aneurysm of the splenic artery. *JAMA*. 1961; 175:452–456.

216. Berger JS, Forsee JH, Furst JN. Splenic artery aneurysm. *Ann Surg*. 1953; 137:108–110.

217. Feldman M. Aneurysm of the splenic artery: An autopsy study. *Am J Dig Dis*. 1955; 22:48–50.

218. Lennie RA, Sheehan HL. Splenic and renal aneurysm complicating pregnancy. *J Obstet Gynecol*. 1942; 49:426–430.

219. Culver GJ, Pirson HS. Splenic artery aneurysm. *Radiology*. 1957; 68:217–223.

220. Yang J, Spinuzza SJ, Gilchrist RK. Aneurysm of splenic artery with calcification. *Arch Surg*. 1963; 87:676–681.

221. von Ronnen JR. The roentgen diagnosis of calcified aneurysms of the splenic and renal arteries. *Acta Radiol*. 1953; 39:385–400.

222. Greene WW, Goroughi E. Calcified epidermoid cyst of the spleen. *Am Surg*. 1963; 29:613–616.

223. Coleman WO. Epidermoid cyst of the spleen: Report of two cases. *Am J Surg*. 1960; 100:475–479.

224. Witter JA, Brekke VG. Solitary calcified cyst of the spleen. *Am J Surg*. 1948; 76:315–318.

225. Soler-Bechara J, Soscia JL. Calcified echinococcus (hydatid) cyst of the spleen. *JAMA*. 1964; 187:62–63.

226. Forde WJ, Finby N. Splenic cysts. *Clin Radiol*. 1961; 12:49–54.

227. Fowler RH. Collective review. Non-parasitic benign cystic tumors of the spleen. *Surg Gynecol Obstet*. 1953; 96:209–215.

228. Asbury GF. Calcified pseudocyst of the spleen. *AMA Arch Surg*. 1958; 76:148–150.

229. McClure RD, Altemeier WA. Cysts of the spleen. *Ann Surg*. 1942; 116:98–102.

230. Dachman, AH, Ros PR, Muran PJ, et al. Nonparasitic splenic cysts. A report of 52 cases with radiologic–pathologic correlation. *Am J Roentgenol*. 1986; 147:537–542.

231. Culver G, Becker C, Koenig ED. Calcified cystic tumor of the spleen. *Radiology*. 1942; 39:62–68.

232. Kierulf E. A calcified cyst of the spleen, demonstrated roentgenographically. *Acta Radiol*. 1946; 27:43–46.

233. Riemenschneider PA. Multiple large aneurysms of the splenic artery. *Am J Roentgenol*. 1955; 74:872–873.

234. Papavasiliou CG. Calcification in secondary tumors of the spleen. *Acta Radiol*. 1959; 51:278–281.

235. McCall IW, Vaidya S, Serjeant GR. Splenic opacification in homozygous sickle cell disease. *Clin Radiol*. 1981; 32:611–615.

236. Macht SH, Roman PW. Radiologic changes in sickle cell anemia. *Radiology*. 1948; 51:697–707.

237. Ehrenpreis B, Schwinger HH. Sickle cell anemia. *Am J Roentgenol.* 1952; 68:28–36.

238. Jacobson G, Zucherman SD. Roentgenographically demonstrable splenic deposits in sickle cell anemia. *Am J Roentgenol.* 1956; 76:47–52.

239. Henley SD, Mellins HZ, Finby N. Punctate calcifications in the spleen in sickle cell anemia. *Am J Med.* 1963; 34:483–485.

240. Seligman BR, Rosner F, Smulewicz JJ. Splenic calcification in sickle cell anemia. *Am J Med Sci.* 1973; 265:495–499.

241. Smith EH, Balthazar E, Moskowitz H. Roentgenographic signs of splenic atrophy in sickle cell disease. *J Can Assoc Radiol.* 1972; 23:133–135.

242. Whitley JE, Cooper HW, Hayes DM, et al. Radiodensities of the spleen associated with thalassemia-S disease. *Am J Roentgenol.* 1964; 91:900–902.

243. Samuel E. Thorotrast spleen. *Br J Radiol.* 1955; 28:204–205.

244. Kolawole TM, Bohrer SP. Splenic abscess and the gene for hemoglobin S. *Am J Roentgenol.* 1973; 119:175–189.

245. Zatzkin HR, Drazan AD, Irwin GA. Roentgenographic diagnosis of splenic abscess. *Am J Roentgenol.* 1964; 91:896–899.

CHAPTER SEVEN

Plain Film Radiology of the Pancreas and Adrenal Glands

PANCREAS

The pancreas is a small organ that is normally inconspicuous on supine films of the abdomen. Adjacent retroperitoneal fat does not help define its size or shape. Although it is situated just beneath and behind the stomach, contour changes in the gastric air bubble rarely reflect pancreatic expansion unless a pseudocyst, abscess, or neoplasm becomes very large. Furthermore, the intimate spatial relationship of the pancreas to the common bile duct and splenic vein permits even very small lesions to manifest clinical and laboratory findings well before roentgenographic detection.

Pancreatic abnormalities, however, especially acute and chronic inflammation, are associated with reliable plain film signs both within the gland itself and in nearby structures. Often, distinctive patterns of gas accumulation, organ displacement, and calcification are readily observable on abdominal roentgenographs. Careful attention to these plain film appearances may be very helpful in reaching a prompt diagnosis or in choosing the next best imaging examination.

Acute Pancreatitis

Usually, acute pancreatitis is diagnosed on the basis of history, physical examination and a serum amylase test. In a significant minority of patients, however, the typical clinical presentation is lacking; in others, the amylase determination may be misleading or unavailable. The plain film of the abdomen offers substantial assistance in these equivocal cases. Although roentgenographic evidence of acute pancreatitis is never definitive, a noncontrast abdominal roentgenogram can supply important diagnostic information. Also, it may reveal pathognomonic findings of other acute abdominal conditions, such as pneumoperitoneum, intestinal obstruction, and mesenteric ischemia, that can be confused with pancreatic inflammation.

Hollow Organ Signs. During the acute phase of pancreatitis, spread of the disease along tissue planes can affect the nearby tubular gastrointestinal tract. Most often involved are the colon, small intestine, duodenum, and stomach.

Colonic Signs. The pancreas and the large intestine, although not in contiguity, are connected by the transverse mesocolon—a peritoneal ligament attached dorsally to the anterior pancreatic surface and ventrally to the transverse colon. A frequent direction of dissemination of inflammation beyond the pancreas is along the course of this ligament. The predominant plain film manifestation of large intestinal involvement is gaseous dilatation. A long segment of the bowel may distend atonically, in a sense "paralyzed" by the extending inflammation, or a small segment may become severely narrowed either by spasm or stricture, with the proximal bowel dilating behind the point of obstruction.

The familiar term, the "colon cut-off" sign, is invoked when a distended, gas-filled colon is encountered on supine films in a patient with acute pancreatitis. Unfortunately, despite its popularity, this sign lacks precision, sensitivity, and specificity. The notion of an abrupt change in the caliber of the colon in response to inflammation was first reported by Baylin and Weeks, who observed increased width of the bowel proximal to an area of spasm in either the transverse colon or the splenic flexure in acute pancreatitis.[1] In 1956, Stuart noted dilatation of the hepatic and splenic flexures accompanied by a nondistended transverse colon in patients with acute inflammation.[2] In the same year, Price described another type of colon cut-off characterized by gaseous distension of the ascending colon and hepatic flexure with abrupt termination of the gas shadow in the proximal transverse colon.[3] The next year, Schwartz and Nadelhaft called attention to dilatation of the transverse colon as a feature of pancreatitis.[4] They cautioned that such a distribution of gas could closely simulate the roentgenographic appearance of a constricting carcinoma at the splenic flexure. The importance of this distal "colon cut-off sign" was emphasized in 1962 by Brascho et al, who found such a pattern in 28 of 54 patients with acute pancreatitis.[5]

Thus, the "colon cut-off" sign has been attributed to various configurations of large bowel dilatation. Today, it is applied most often to the settling of gas in the transverse colon alone or in both the ascending colon and transverse colon in the absence of distension beyond the splenic flexure. These two patterns of gas accumulation are also commonplace, however, in patients who are confined by their illness to bed rest, where they maintain a horizontal face-up or semierect position. Gas, normally present in the large intestine, preferentially seeks the transverse colon because it is the least dependent bowel segment when the patient is supine. In the immobile individual, gas may not progress beyond the distal transverse colon even as it accumulates proximally. Hence, in most cases, the most well-known of the "colon cut-off" signs is often just a consequence of prolonged recumbency rather than a unique reaction to pancreatic inflammation (Fig 7–1).

Several studies have shown that the colon cut-off configuration is infrequent. Cantwell and Pollock observed it in only 2 of 110 patients with acute pancreatitis.[6] Millward et al compared the bowel gas patterns in patients with pancreatitis to a control group who had either acute cholecystitis or a perforated duodenal ulcer.[7] The incidence of dilatation of the hepatic flexure, splenic flexure and transverse colon were nearly identical in the two populations. Davis et al assessed colonic signs in a cohort with pancreatitis against an equal number of nonacutely

ill individuals who were referred for intravenous urography.[8] No example of the "colon cut-off sign" was seen in either group, but a dilated transverse colon was present in 18% of acute pancreatitis sufferers and in only 2% of the controls. Most specific for pancreatitis, albeit very uncommon, is an abrupt termination of dilatation quite proximal to the splenic flexure (Fig 7–2).[9]

Splenic flexure narrowing induced by acute pancreatitis does have a pathophysiological explanation, however. The phrenicocolic ligament, the most lateralward extension of the transverse mesocolon, anchors the anatomic splenic flexure. Pancreatic inflammation can reach this fixed point, and consequent spasm of the colonic wall may create a functional obstruction with dilatation of the radiographic splenic flexure and transverse colon.[10]

Nearly all patients in whom the plain film reveals the "colon cut-off sign" initially have a transient deformity, with the bowel returning to normal as the inflammation subsides.[11] The development of a large-bowel constriction 1 week to 2 months after the onset of symptoms, however, often heralds a nonreversible and irregular stenosis that can be mistaken on barium enema for a colonic carcinoma. Most pancreatitis-induced large-intestinal strictures are due to the cicatrizing effect of postinflammatory necrosis encircling the bowel wall.[12,13] In a few patients, ischemic colitis, a direct result of pancreatitis on nearby splanchnic arteries, may be the cause of the focal narrowing.[14] Irregularities of the bowel wall after pancreatic inflammation occasionally resemble inflammatory bowel disease on plain films as they appear as fixed segments lacking haustra and septations.

Meyers and Evans have shown that colonic seg-

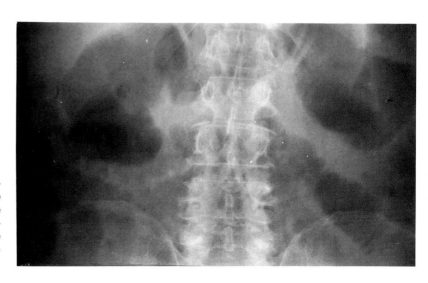

Figure 7–1. Severe pancreatitis. Gas has collected in many small bowel loops and in the transverse colon. There was no narrowing of the splenic flexure on barium enema. Prolonged recumbency allowed gas to accumulate in the transverse colon, the least dependent large intestinal segment.

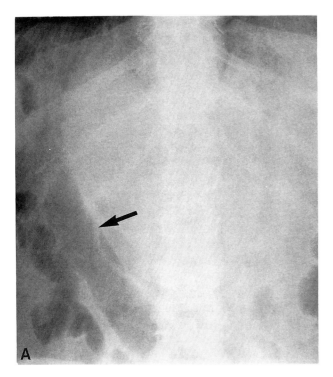
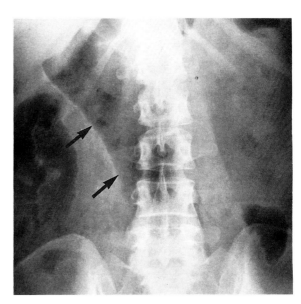

Figure 7–2. Two examples of the cutoff sign in the mid-transverse colon secondary to pancreatitis. **A.** The proximal U-shaped transverse colon is dilated but the distal end is nondistended (*arrow*). **B.** The two arrow points to a widened transverse colon. The air shadow ends abruptly at the midline.

ments remote from the pancreas may be disturbed by an advancing infection.[10] The small bowel mesentery is anchored posteriorly close to the pancreas and its interface with the transverse mesocolon. An additional route of intraperitoneal dissemination of inflammation is down this mesenteric pathway to the right lower quadrant where collections of pus can impinge upon the cecum and terminal ileum.

The widening of the distance between the transverse colon and the stomach has also been considered a plain film sign of pancreatic inflammation. Moreno and Rivera found a more than 3 cm separation of the gastric and colonic gas shadow in 49% of patients with pancreatitis.[15] Yet, in a controlled study, Seymour observed the distance from the stomach to large bowel to be greater than 3 cm in 36% of normal patients.[16] In some individuals the normal gastrocolic ligament may become lax and elongated, and consequently widening of the space between the stomach and large intestine has no pathological significance. What is more important is the contour of the greater curvature of the stomach and the superior margin of the transverse colon (Fig 7–3). Extrinsic impression and deformity should be regarded with suspicion whereas simple displacement without modification of stomach or bowel contour is an unremarkable finding.

Small Intestine (Sentinel Loop). Much of the jejunum is in close apposition to the body and tail of the pancreas, and the root of its mesentery originates from the peritoneal reflection adjacent to the ventral pancreatic surface. Thus, there is ample opportunity

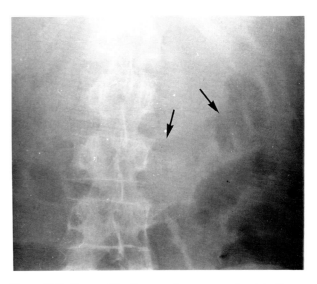

Figure 7–3. Pancreatitis. Pressure from a spreading infection on the superior haustral row of the transverse colon has narrowed the lumen from above (*arrows*).

for expanding inflammation to reach the proximal small bowel. The involved intestinal wall becomes atonic, and, as peristalsis decreases, swallowed air is not propelled distally. The bowel distends and is easily recognized on plain films. Since this finding may presage other roentgenographic evidence of abdominal inflammation it is known as the sentinel loop sign (Fig 7–4).

First reported in 1946 by Levitin, who noted the diagnostic value of dilated ileal segments on supine films of patients with appendicitis, the sentinel loop has now become closely identified with acute pancreatitis.[17] Grollman et al emphasized the importance of localized paralytic ileus in the early phases of pancreatic inflammation and demonstrated that the dilated intestinal loop could be in the mid abdomen as well in the left upper quadrant.[18] In a series of 73 consecutive patients with pancreatitis, Stein et al found a sentinel loop in 55%, by far the most frequent plain film sign of pancreatitis.[19] Benson[20] and Ranson et al[21] in separate later studies also found that a dilated segment of small bowel was the most common abnormality on a survey film of the abdomen.

The sentinel loop can be seen in other inflammatory diseases, including pyelonephritis of the left kidney and intrinsic infection of the small bowel. Moreover, a wide range of conditions can appear with air-filled proximal jejunal loops. It may be an incidental finding—a natural consequence of air swallowing. Normal air-filled jejunal loops rarely exceed 3 cm in diameter, but in many cases of pancreatitis, air fills the intestinal loops without marked distension occurring. Proximal small-bowel obstruction can present with only a few segments of dilated bowel, closely resembling a localized ileus. A helpful differentiating point is accentuation of the valvulae conniventes in mechanical obstruction due to hypertoxicity of their muscularis mucosa. In a localized paralytic ileus, the valvulae are often effaced because the muscle within them becomes flaccid in response to inflammation.

Duodenal Signs. The head of the pancreas sits snugly within the C-shaped duodenal loop. Therefore, the influence of pancreatitis on bowel configuration should be most evident in this intestinal section. Poppel evaluated duodenal changes in pancreatitis using barium as a contrast agent.[22] He found that the initial reaction to nearby inflammation is spasm and irritability, manifestations of disease that cannot be seen on plain films. As the infection proceeds, however, duodenal ileus ensues and the lumen becomes patulous. Soon after, the duodenum widens as it fills with intestinal juices and swallowed air. The duodenal bulb may also distend and the papilla of Vater can swell, indenting the medial margin of the descending duodenum. With enlargement of the pancreatic head, the C-loop describes a larger arc (Fig 7–5).

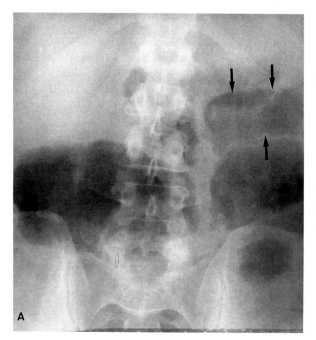 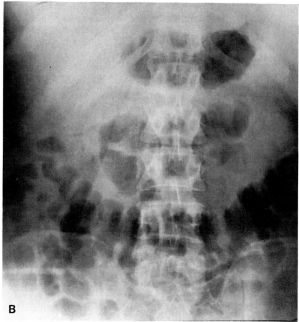

Figure 7–4. Sentinel loop sign. **A.** A single loop of jejunum (*arrows*) approaches the width of the transverse colon situated just below it. Note the absence of prominent valvulae conniventes. **B.** Several distended air-filled jejunal loops straddle the midline between the stomach and transverse colon.

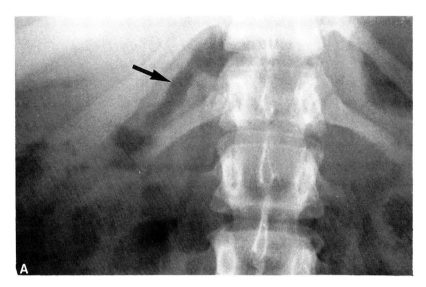

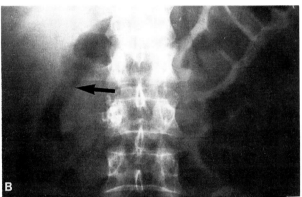

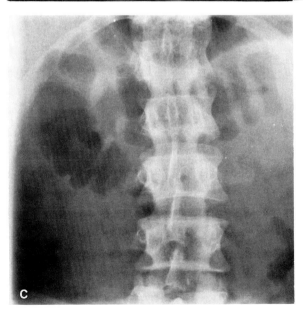

Figure 7–5. A spectrum of charges in duodenal ileus due to pancreatitis. **A.** The descending duodenum is not dilated but the lumen is filled with air (*arrow*). **B.** Ileus is revealed by a slightly distended lumen (*arrow*). Marked duodenal dilatation is seen in **C.** The duodenum is nearly as wide as the transverse colon.

Normally, the duodenum contains little air. The rate of inflow is precisely regulated by the pylorus, and transit of fluid within its lumen is rapid. In the supine position, overlying structures often prevent clear evaluation of duodenal gas. Frequently, the duodenum is projected over the bones of the spine, limiting appreciation of its luminal dimensions. A gas-filled transverse colon can obscure the contours of the distal descending duodenum. Also, a dilated stomach may be superimposed on the shadow of the duodenal bulb and the proximal descending portion of the duodenal sweep.

In pancreatitis, ileus leads to the accumulation of gas throughout the length of the C-loop. A left lateral decubitus projection is often the best view to demonstrate duodenal paralysis and gaseous distension (Figs 1–13, 7–6). With the right side elevated, intraluminal liquid contents drain distally, the transverse colon empties of gas and the duodenum is usually away from the spine as it projects within the homogeneously dense liver shadow. In the left lateral decubitus position the presence of gas within the duodenal lumen should be considered abnormal even if there is no dilatation.

At times, duodenal distension can be so marked on plain films that an impression of an enlarged pancreatic head can be noted as it indents the medial duodenal surface. Nonobstructive dilatation of the duodenum is not pathognomonic for acute pancreatitis, as it has been observed in acute cholecystitis and in pyeloanephritis of the right kidney.[23] Its frequency in pancreatic inflammation has been well established, however.[24] Millward et al found it to be the most reliable plain film sign of pancreatitis, observable in 42% of patients (Fig 7–7).[7] Barry noted duodenal changes in 19 patients with acute pancreatitis, but in 6 of these, the abnormalities could only be appreciated on the decubitus projection.[25]

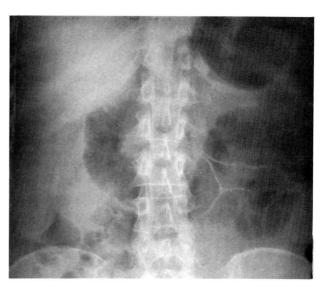

Figure 7–7. Duodenal ileus and sentinel loops. Pancreatitis has caused paralysis of the proximal small intestine, distending both duodenum and several jejunal segments.

Gastric Signs. In untreated patients gastric dilatation may be induced by acute pancreatic inflammation. Vomiting, however, which is a frequent and sometimes almost continuous problem in pancreatitis, prevents swallowed air from accumulating in the distended stomach. The treatment of moderately to severely ill patients includes the placement of a nasogastric tube to decompress the stomach and small bowel. Thus, an air-filled stomach is uncommon in pancreatitis. In fact, a totally gasless abdomen is a relatively frequent plain film finding in patients at bed rest receiving nasogastric suction.[26]

Extraintestinal Signs. Acute pancreatitis is associated with changes above the diaphragm in at least 20% of cases.[27] Pleural effusion, usually unilateral and more common on the left, is seen most often. Sometimes, basal atelectasis and small patches of pneumonitis in the lower lung fields accompanies the effusion and can be seen at the upper margins of a supine abdominal film.

Extension of inflammation to the retroperitoneal space has been well documented by computed tomography studies of acute pancreatitis. Approximately 50% of patients have fluid collections that reach beyond the pancreatic contours. The fluid may spread diffusely throughout the retroperitoneal compartments, displacing fat and connective tissue.[28] Despite the wide distribution of inflammatory effusions in the retroperitoneal spaces, plain films are not very good a defining their presence or dissemination.

Faint, patchy radiodensities scattered through-

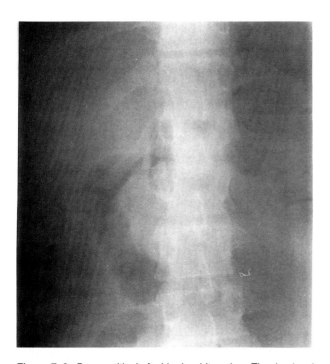

Figure 7–6. Pancreatitis. Left-side decubitus view. The duodenal sweep is clearly outlined by gas. The enlarged pancreas indents the medial wall. A mid-point indentation denotes the position of the ampulla of Vater. The medial duodenal contour resembles a reversed 3.

out the retroperitoneal spaces have been attributed to fat necrosis, with the lucency of adipose tissue replaced by the density of hemorrhagic infarction.[29] Nevertheless, fat necrosis need not be the only mechanism responsible for a mottled pattern of increased opacity. Infiltration of pus and/or blood through the tissue planes in the retroperitoneal space can also be seen as numerous relatively dense blotches of varying size. The "fat necrosis" sign is best seen on low-kilovoltage, coned-down oblique films.[30] It is rarely encountered on supine projections obtained with a standard radiographic technique and is especially hard to discern if there is gaseous distention in the small and large bowel. Retroperitoneal calcification can result from hemorrhage, abscess, or fat necrosis, but the demonstration of roentgenographically visible calcium salts in acute pancreatitis is exceedingly rare. In the only well-documented case, Baker and Glazer described faint bilateral calcification in both the anterior and posterior pararenal spaces in a patient with acute pancreatitis.[31]

Both kidneys are enveloped by perirenal fat, which, if abundant, can help outline the lateral, superior, and inferior renal margins on plain films. Normally, the perirenal fat blends imperceptibly with fat in the anterior and posterior pararenal spaces laterally. If an inflammatory effusion from pancreatitis occupies the anterior pararenal space without disturbing perirenal fat, the renal edge may stand out more clearly in contrast to the surrounding adipose tissue. Susman et al observed five patients with pancreatitis in whom fat sharply outlined the left kidney.[32] They labeled this phenomenon the "renal halo" sign. Although readily recognizable on computed tomography,[33,34] a renal halo is difficult to detect on plain films. In a retrospective review of 200 patients with pancreatitis, we have found no example of accentuation of the left kidney outline.

Demonstration of the psoas shadow depends upon the maintenance of an interface between the muscle and adjacent retroperitoneal fat. Infiltration and displacement of fat by spreading pancreatic inflammation can obscure the delineation of the psoas margin on supine roentgenograms. Furthermore, this sign is so undependable in otherwise normal individuals that loss of the psoas muscle should not be considered of diagnostic value in the plain film assessment of acute pancreatitis.

Pancreatic Abscess

Pancreatic abscess eventuates in 2% to 5% of patients with acute pancreatitis.[35,36] Typically, there is an interval of 1 to 2 weeks between seeming recovery from the initial attack and the recurrence of pain and fever.[37] Neither the etiology nor the severity of

pancreatitis is a good predictor of the likelihood of abscess formation. Necrotic pancreatic tissue appears to be an excellent substrate for suppurative bacteria originating from the blood, the transverse colon, or the bile or through lymphatics draining the gallbladder.[38] Prompt diagnosis is important because even today the mortality is very high, ranging from 30% to 67%.[35]

Pancreatic abscess can either remain confined to the pancreas or extend beyond its borders into the lesser sac anteriorly and the retroperitoneal spaces posteriorly.[39] Large lesions may displace the stomach, transverse colon, and small intestine.[40] The most characteristic roentgenographic abnormality is gas within the abscess, however. In the surgical literature, the finding of a gas-containing abscess on supine roentgenograms has been reported in 6% to 28% of cases of pancreatic abscess.[37,41,42] In a more recent report, however, Woodard et al noted plain film evidence of gas in 58% of affected patients.[43] Usually, the gas appears as an agglomeration of many closely packed small bubbles (Fig 7–8). On supine views, depending upon location it can resemble an abscess in the kidney, spleen, or liver. Careful attention to the position and distribution of lucency within the gastric and colonic borders can help distinguish pancreatic abscess from

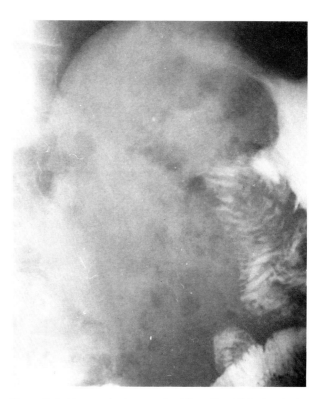

Figure 7–8. Pancreatic abscess. An oblique film with barium in the intestine. Numerous bubbles of varying diameters reside within a large pancreatic abscess that is displacing adjacent bowel loops.

food within the stomach or feces in the large intestine.

A single amorphous lucency, a much less common pattern of gas accumulation, can result from a large suppurative excavation within the pancreas itself but more often it indicates extension of infection to the lesser sac (Fig 7–9).[44,45] Rarely, gas may diffuse through the retroperitoneal space to enter the mediastinum or it may penetrate the greater peritoneal cavity, resulting in free air.[46]

Intrapancreatic gas is not necessarily diagnostic for abscess. Air can be introduced into the substance of the pancreas from fistulae with bowel or the skin. These abnormal communications can result from spontaneous decompression of a pancreatic abscess[38,47]) or pseudocyst[48] or may occur after operative drainage. Typically, patients with a pancreatic fistula are not hectically ill, as decompression through the bowel affords a respite from the symptoms of an enlarging infected mass (Fig 7–10). The most frequent termination of a pancreatic fistula is the transverse colon but communications with the duodenum, jejunum and skin also occur.

Pseudocyst

Pseudocyst formation is another serious complication of acute pancreatitis. Like pancreatic abscess, a pseudocyst takes several weeks to mature and usually becomes clinically apparent after the acute inflammation has abated. A pseudocyst may be situ-

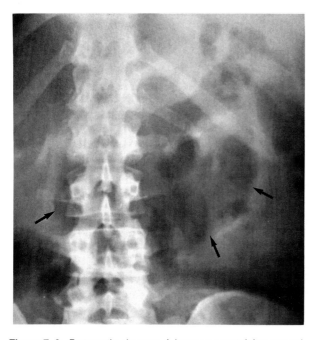

Figure 7–9. Pancreatic abscess. A large gas-containing pus collection appears as a giant lucency (*arrows*) and several smaller loculations. (*Courtesy of Dr. Jutta Greweldinger.*)

ated almost anywhere in the upper abdomen and can even be found as far inferiorly as the presacral space.[49] In review of 17 cases of pancreatic pseudocyst, 10 were clearly observable as a soft tissue mass on plain films. Often, the best roentgenographic clue is marked displacement of the stomach or transverse colon.[50]

Other plain film findings are much less common. Gas can enter a pseudocyst through a fistula from bowel or it may be produced endogenously by infection by a gas-forming organism. Lucencies within infected pseudocysts are larger and less numerous than the small bubbles in a typical pancreatic abscess (Fig 7–11). Occasionally, pseudocysts calcify with a rimlike opacity, characteristic of all cystic lesions. The calcification may be thin and incomplete or thick and circumferential (Fig 7–12). Calcified pseudocysts have a predilection for the tail of the pancreas, where they may be mistaken for a renal, adrenal, retroperitoneal, or mesenteric cyst, a renal or splenic artery aneurysm, or a tortuous splenic artery. The coexistence of pancreatic concretions raises the likelihood of pseudocyst calcification, but a definite diagnosis usually requires a computed tomography examination. Milk-of-calcium in a pancreatic pseudocyst has also been reported. Its radiographic appearance resembles milk-of-calcium in other cystic structures.[51]

Chronic Pancreatitis

By far the most frequently encountered plain film finding in pancreatic disease is multiple calcifications scattered throughout the substance of the gland. In nearly every case, this pattern is characteristic of chronic calcifying pancreatitis (Table 7–1). Long-standing ductal obstruction and inflammation promote the precipitation of protein and the denudation of mucosal cells, which serve as a nidus for the deposition of calcium. Small stones consist mainly of protein, but larger concretions contain increasing percentages of calcific compounds. Cut sections of pancreatic calculi usually demonstrate multiple, opaque laminae composed of calcium carbonate in the form of calcite.[52–55]

Common findings in pancreatitis are ductal narrowing and obstruction. Proximal to the point of stenosis, both the duct of Wirsung and tributary ducts may dilate and, after a period of time, more and more calculi can be accommodated within their larger lumens. On occasion, multiple calculi plug both large and small ducts, furthering the process of proximal dilatation. Atrophy of glandular tissue accompanies the increase in duct size. Frequently, calcifications progress to such an extent that the entire organ appears calcified. In the past, this was called

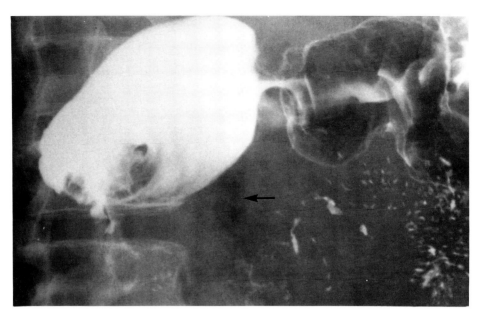

Figure 7–10. Pancreatic fistula. Bubbles of gas have entered the pancreatic bed (*arrow*) from a fistula with the large bowel resulting from perforation of the transverse colon by the spreading infection.

diffuse calcification of the pancreas and thought to represent opacification in acinar cells. Careful microscopic analysis has revealed that even in the most heavily calcified pancreases the small intralobular ducts contain stones, but parenchymal cells are free of calcium.[56–58] Fat necrosis, another feature of pancreatitis, has been considered a cause of calcification, but calcium deposition in this process is not

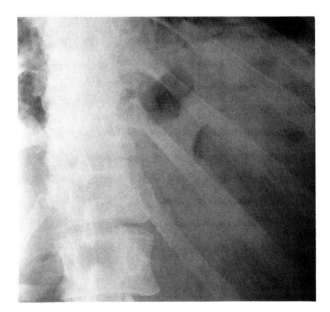

Figure 7–11. Several large gas pockets are confined within the margins of a pseudocyst that became infected by a gas-producing organism.

extensive enough to be seen on plain X-ray. Hence, the multiple pancreatic calcifications seen in chronic pancreatitis are exclusively concretions within ducts.

Radiographic Appearance. The typical appearance of chronic calcifying pancreatitis on abdominal films is numerous dense, discrete opacities that cross the midline at the level of L1–L2 and conform to the shape of the pancreas. On the right side, the densities are close to the midline, but on the left the limit of calcification may extend far peripherally, sometimes pointing upwards toward the left hemidiaphragm and in other instances traversing a horizontal course toward the lateral abdominal wall (Fig 7–13). Although the individual calcifications are distinct and separable, the chain of calcification is usually continuous. In approximately 25% of cases, opaque concretions are present in the head of the pancreas alone (Fig 7–14).[58] Calcification confined to the tail or body is much less common, appearing in no more than 5% of cases (Fig 7–15).[59] Occasionally, it may be difficult to discern concretions in the section of the pancreas that overlies the spine, but films taken in varying degrees of obliquity can move the vertebrae away from the pancreas and show the uninterrupted course of calcification. When only the pancreatic head contains calcification, the conglomeration of closely packed stones may simulate the configuration of a calcified mass. Here, again, oblique or lateral films can show that the pattern of calcification consists of multiple unconnected, sharply outlined densities.

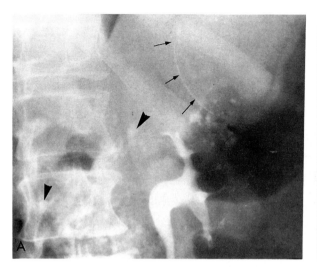 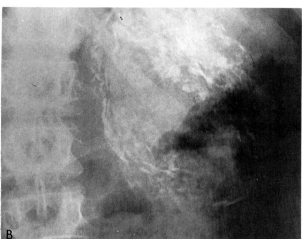

Figure 7–12. Two examples of calcified pancreatic pseudocyst. **A.** Thin-walled calcified pseudocyst of the pancreas (*arrows*). An oblique film from an intravenous urography also shows calculi in the pancreas (*arrowheads*). **B.** Thick-walled pancreatic pseudocyst. The margins are irregular because the cyst was partially drained.

Individual concretions often vary considerably in shape. In fact, it is unusual for pancreatic stones to have a monotonous appearance. Most often, they have rounded or irregularly angulated contours, but elongated and even branched stones may be seen. Almost without exception, stones are completely marginated and often they are very opaque. They may be laminated or contain small central or eccentric lucencies (Fig 7–16). Characteristically, multiple stones differ in size. It is common to see calculi of widely varying dimensions in the same gland, and, at times, individual stones may reach a diameter of

2 to 3 cm (Fig 7–17). Above 5 mm it must be presumed that the calculi are contained within an occluded main pancreatic duct.

The diagnosis of multiple pancreatic calculi is easy when stones extend from the head to the tail. There is no other entity consisting of numerous stones that cross the midline in the general location of the pancreas. Lymphangioma of the pancreas, a rare tumor, can have phlebolithic calcifications that are generally few and widely spread compared to the multiplicity of stones seen in chronic pancreatitis.[60] After a single intravascular injection of Thorotrast, colloidal thorium is gradually taken up in parapancreatic lymph nodes and remains there indefinitely. These nodes are observed on X-ray as multiple, large, very dense opacities arrayed along the course of the pancreas. Thorotrast deposition in parapancreatic nodes is almost always accompanied by Thorotrast in the liver and spleen, however, and should never cause confusion with the appearance of chronic calcifying pancreatitis (Fig 7–18).[61]

A less common pattern of chronic pancreatitis is the presence of only a few large stones. If the calculi are confined to a section of the pancreas and are of similar size and shape, they can be confused with gallbladder or urinary concretions (Fig 7–19).[62,63] The disappearance of stones has been noted in pancreatic carcinoma[64] and in chronic pancreatitis unaccompanied by a mass.[65–67] The mechanism for the dissolution of stones is unclear. A pseudocyst can also displace stones as it stretches and deforms the pancreas (Fig 7–20).

TABLE 7–1. PANCREATIC CALCIFICATION

Concretions
  Pancreatitis
    Chronic calcifying pancreatitis from alcohol abuse
    Nutritional pancreatitis
    Hyperparathyroidism
    Cystic fibrosis
    Hereditary pancreatitis
    Type 5 hyperlipoproteinemia
    Schistosoma haematobium
  Idiopathic pancreatic calculi
Solid calcification
  Microcystic adenoma
  Lymphangioma
  Islet cell tumor
  Adenocarcinoma
Cystic calcification
  Pseudocyst
  Macrocystic adenocarcinoma
  Zollinger–Ellison syndrome

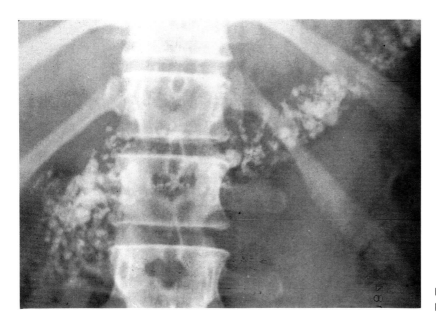

Figure 7–13. Innumerable dense calculi in the pancreas extending from head to tail.

Etiology. In North America, Europe, and the temperate regions of Latin America and South Africa, there is a close relationship between alcoholism and almost all cases of chronic calcifying pancreatitis. The other major cause of pancreatic inflammation, biliary tract disease, is rarely, if ever, a predisposing factor in the development of pancreatic lithiasis. At least 6 years of chronic alcohol abuse is necessary to develop calcifications in the pancreas, and calculi are usually first noted in the fourth decade.[54] It is not known why some alcoholics develop calcifica-

tions and others remain free of this complication. There appears to be no correlation between the development of stones and the type of alcohol consumed. Perhaps the propensity for both calculi formation and pancreatitis is related to the nutritional status of the alcoholic. At present, however, little has been established about the mechanism of chronic calcifying pancreatitis beyond the fact that there is a strong association with excessive ethanol intake.

In less developed regions of the world, pancre-

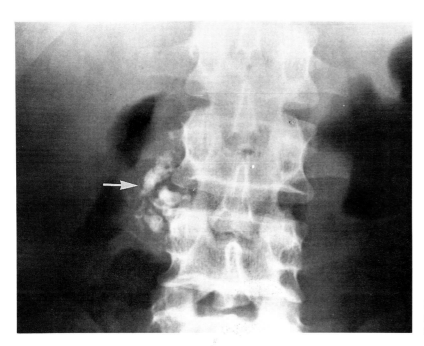

Figure 7–14. Calcification confined to the pancreatic head (*arrow*). Note that some of the concretions are elongated.

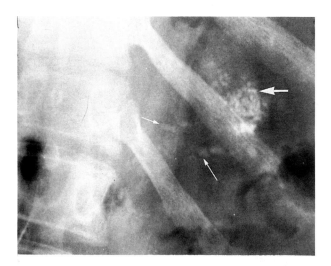

Figure 7–15. Most of the pancreatic calcifications in this 37-year-old alcoholic male are in the tail (*large arrow*). Scattered calculi are also present in the body (*small arrows*). The head is free of stones, however. This is an unusual pattern of pancreatic calcification.

atic calculi appear to be related to malnutrition. On a global scale, there may be more people with pancreatic stones as a result of protein deficiency than there are alcoholics with pancreatic stones. For example, pancreatic lithiasis is common in Marseilles, France, but its incidence is ten times higher in Kerala, India.[54] Calcification occurs at an earlier age in patients with nutritionally induced chronic pancreatitis. In a series of 45 patients from western Nigeria, the average age of onset of calculi was 20 years. Only two thirds of patients complained of abdominal pain but many had diabetes mellitus and their

presenting problem was often steatorrhea.[68,69] An investigation of 18 Indonesian adolescents and young adults with diffuse intraductal pancreatic calcification included none with a history of alcohol intake. Few complained of abdominal pain but 45% had diabetes and the majority presented with frequent, foul-smelling stools.[70] A recent report discussed a nonalcoholic patient in the United States who had celiac disease for several years and then developed pancreatic calculi.[71] The relationship between malnutrition and calcifying pancreatitis has not yet been given much attention in the Western medical literature, but the suggestively large group of patients with this disease in poorer regions of the world should provide the impetus for further research (Fig 7–21).

An association exists between hyperparathyroidism and chronic pancreatitis. In one investigation, 7 of 37 patients with primary hyperparathyroidism had pancreatic stones.[72] In a later study, only 9 of 155 patients had calcification in the pancreas.[73] The radiographic appearance of calcification induced by hyperparathyroidism is indistinguishable from that of the more common form of chronic calcifying pancreatitis.[74] Plain film recognition of pancreatic stones should raise the question of parathyroid disease (Fig 7–22). Nevertheless, these cases represent a very small percentage of all those with pancreatic concretions.

An uncommon cause of stones in the pancreas is cystic fibrosis. Here again, calcific densities are found only occasionally,[75,76] and almost always other clinical and radiographic features of the dis-

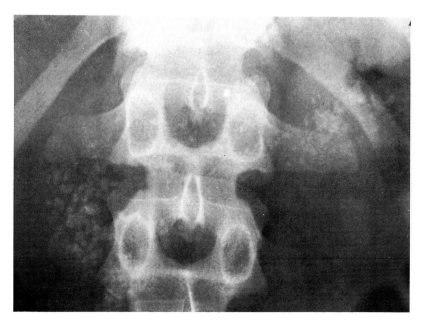

Figure 7–16. Multiple pancreatic stones of similar density and slightly varying size. Many have lucent centers.

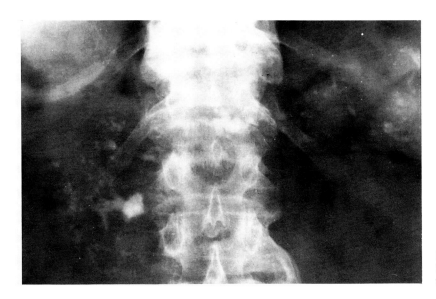

Figure 7–17. Pancreatic lithiasis of widely varying size. In the head, there is a very large stone with branching extensions.

ease are also present (Fig 7–23). Hereditary pancreatitis is a very rare but interesting entity that affects several Caucasian families in Appalachia. The disease, transmitted by an autosomal dominant gene, causes repeated episodes of abdominal pain. These patients may be at greater risk for the development of pancreatic carcinoma.[77] The calcifications are usually fewer but larger than those seen in other forms of pancreatitis. A recently recognized disease with pancreatic stones is type 5 hyperlipoprotenemia, a hereditary lipid abnormality characterized by frequent attacks of pancreatitis and elevated serum concentrations of circulating chylomicrons and triglycerides. Pancreatic lipase breaks down circulat-

ing triglycerides into fatty acids, which are directly damaging to the pancreatic ducts producing a toxic affect similar to that seen in alcohol-induced injury.[78] Calcifying pancreatitis has also been noted in one patient whose only pertinent history was trauma to the upper abdomen. Whether traumatic calcifying pancreatitis is a real entity remains an open question.[79] Moreover, pancreatic stones have been seen in infestation by *Schistosoma haematobium*.[68]

There remains a small group of patients who have calcifications without a history of pancreatitis and no apparent clinical predisposition for the de-

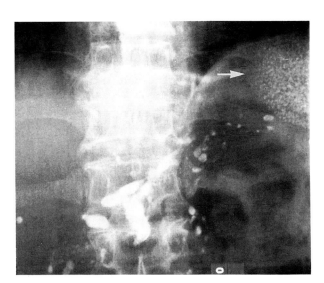

Figure 7–18. Thorotrast in peripancreatic lymph nodes. Very dense discrete opacities cross the midline in the upper abdomen. There is also Thorotrast in the spleen (*arrow*).

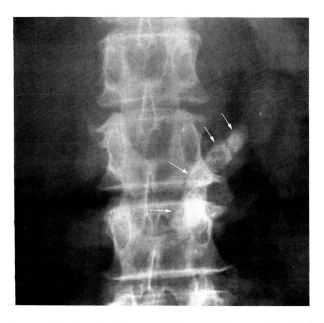

Figure 7–19. The arrows point to four faceted stones in the duct of Wirsung. The patient had a long history of alcoholic abuse.

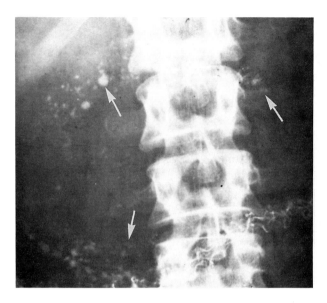

Figure 7–20. There is a pseudocyst of the pancreas which has displaced the head inferiorly and the body superiorly. The separation of calculi (*arrows*) suggests stretching of the pancreas.

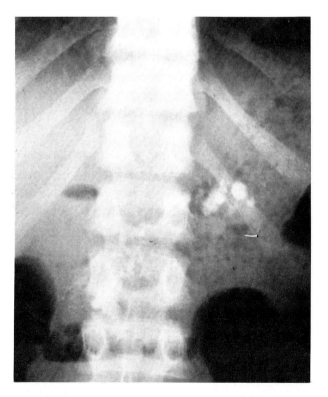

Figure 7–21. Multiple calcifications of varying sizes are noted throughout the pancreas in a 15-year-old Haitian female with a history of poor nutrition. (*Courtesy of Dr. William J McSweeny.*)

velopment of stones. Stobbe et al studied 130 patients with pancreatic lithiasis, of whom 22 had stones in localized sections of the pancreas.[80] Nineteen of these patients were over 70 years of age and none in the subgroup with focal stones ever had signs or symptoms of pancreatitis. Only one had a history of alcohol intake and none had evidence of hyperparathyroidism. At autopsy there are focal occlusions of distal pancreatic ducts with scarring and calculi.[80] The presence of asymptomatic pancreatic stones is still a poorly defined condition. Since only a few concretions are present it is easy to dismiss or misdiagnose them on plain films. When there are isolated stones in the pancreatic tail they may go unrecognized or be ascribed to the left adrenal gland, the left kidney, or even costal cartilage (Fig 7–24).

Tumors of the Pancreas

The most common neoplasm of the pancreas is adenocarcinoma. The incidence of this almost uniformly fatal tumor has been increasing gradually in the last 25 years and it now ranks fifth among all cancers as a cause of death in the United States.[81] In spite of its frequency, however, it is hardly ever diagnosed on plain films because, at the time of discovery, it is usually too small to displace adjacent solid organs or bowel segments. Moreover, calcification in the primary tumor is exceedingly rare (Fig 7–25).[82] The presumption should be that in an individual with suspected adenocarcinoma, a calcification is not within the tumor but is a manifestation of some other pancreatic process, most often chronic pancreatitis. Patients with chronic calcifying pancreatitis may be more likely to develop adenocarcinoma. In one series of 677 patients with pancreatitic calcification, 24 had coexistent pancreatic carcinoma.[83] In another report 417 patients with adenocarcinoma of the pancreas 1.4% had calcification consistent with chronic calcifying pancreatitis.[84,85] This is distinctly higher than the incidence of pancreatic calcifications in the general population.

Cystic Tumors. Cystadenoma and cystadenocarcinoma were the terms previously used to describe a group of slow-growing tumors predominantly affecting middle-aged and elderly women. They often attained a large size but individual lesions varied greatly in malignant potential. The accumulation of a large series of cases at the Armed Forces Institute of Pathology has led to a reclassification of these tumors into two well-defined groups on the basis of gross and microscopic appearance.[86]

Microcystic adenoma is an inevitably benign le-

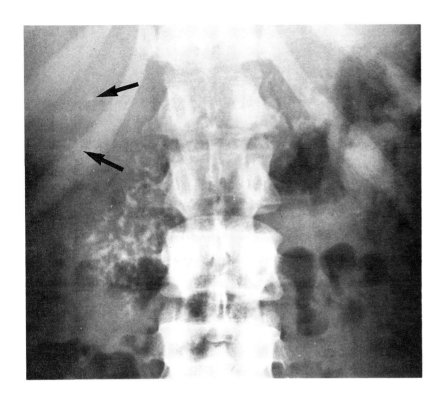

Figure 7–22. Calculi scattered throughout the pancreas in a patient with hyperparathyroidism. Renal calculi, another manifestation of the disease, are also present (*arrows*).

sion characterized by numerous tiny cysts within dense strands of connective tissue. The cysts are lined by flat or cuboidal cells that secrete a glycogen-rich substance. Microcystic tumors are more common in the body and tail of the pancreas and may grow silently, first coming to attention after physical examination or radiological study of the abdomen. Their mean diameter at the time of detection often

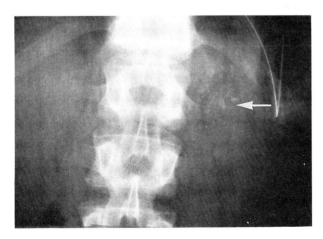

Figure 7–23. Finely granular flecks of calcification are present in the tail of the pancreas (*arrow*) in a patient with cystic fibrosis. (*Courtesy of Dr. William J. McSweeny.*)

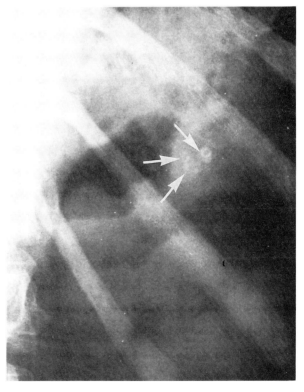

Figure 7–24. Several rounded calculi in the pancreatic tail (*arrows*). They look like phleboliths or isolated costal cartilage calcification. The patient had no history of pancreatic disease. Computed tomography confirmed their intrapancreatic location.

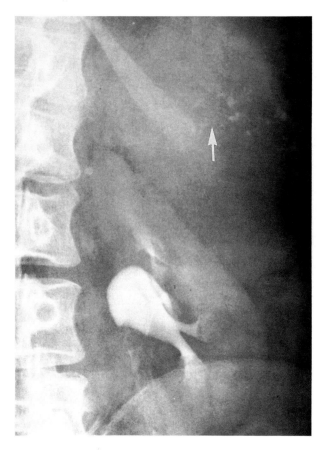

Figure 7–25. Calcifications within an adenocarcinoma of the tail of the pancreas. An oblique film obtained during an intravenous urography reveals scattered calculi in a large carcinoma of the pancreas (*arrow*). Histological examination demonstrated calcium within the tumor. (*Courtesy of Dr. Diane LoRusso.*)

exceeds 10 cm and they appear as a large, rounded density displacing nearby organs (Fig 7–26). In approximately two fifths of cases the glycogen-rich microcystic adenoma calcifies, with the opacity not at the margin of the cyst but deep within the stroma of the mass.[87] Patterns of calcific deposition vary, ranging from a large stellate density[88] to closely aggregated solid masses resembling radiodense lymph nodes[89] (Fig 7–27) to scattered clumps arrayed throughout the tumor (Fig 7–28).[90]

The other cystic tumor, the macrocystic adenoma, contains fewer but larger cysts, each lined by tall, columnar epithelia that produce mucin. This lesion has a definite malignant potential and should thus be called a cystadenocarcinoma. It, too, may attain a large size and be first detected on plain films as a soft tissue mass. Calcification occurs in less than 20% and is in a peripheral location, appearing as a plaquelike or arcuate density, which betokens its

cystic nature (Fig 7–29). Occasionally, flecks of increased density may be seen along with the more obvious curvilinear streaks of radiopacity.[86]

Calcification can also be found in endocrine tumors of the pancreas. In 23 malignant islet cell tumors reported by Imhof and Frank, 2 were calcified whereas none of 71 benign islet cell tumors contained opacities visible on plain films.[91] Another study revealed ten cases of calcification in endocrine tumors of the pancreas, seven of which occurred in malignant lesions.[92] Islet cell tumors of all types can calcify and in most cases the calcifications appear as irregular coarse, poorly defined densities. Occasionally, both the primary pancreatic lesion and hepatic metastases calcify in a similar way.[93,94] Jahnke et al noted cystic opacities in a patient with Zollinger–Ellison syndrome.[92] Calcifications in endocrine tumors of the pancreas are usually not as dense or as sharply marginated as other cystic neoplasms.

Arterial Calcification Near the Pancreas

Splenic Artery. The proximal splenic artery rests on the superior aspect of the pancreas. It frequently calcifies and its typical serpentine course in the left upper quadrant should cause no confusion with an intrapancreatic opacity. Splenic artery aneurysms

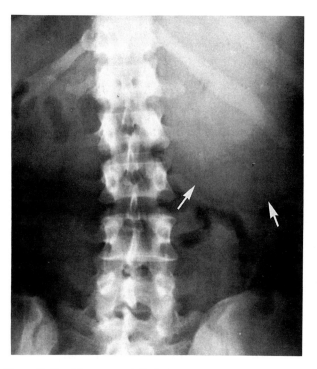

Figure 7–26. A large noncalcified microcystic adenoma. The lower margins of the mass are displacing bowel inferiorly (*arrow*).

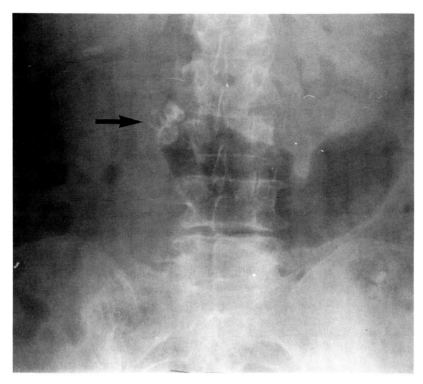

Figure 7–27. Calcifications in a microcystic adenoma (*arrow*) resemble lymph node opacification.

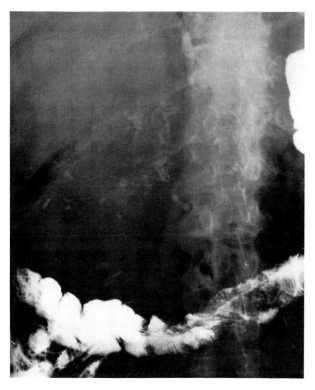

Figure 7–28. Scattered clumps of radiodensity scattered throughout a large microcystic adenoma. (*Courtesy of Dr. L. Berliner and Dr. P. Redmond.*)

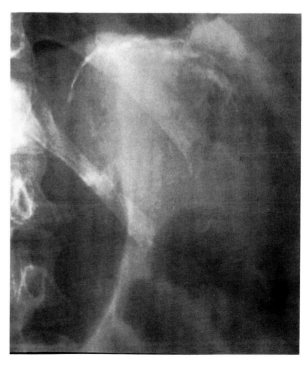

Figure 7–29. Curvilinear calcification in a macrocystic adenocarcinoma. The pattern of opacity closely resembles that seen in other cystic lesions.

316

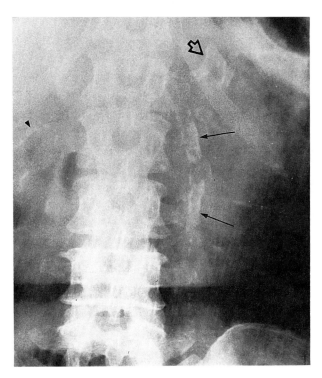

Figure 7–30. Superior mesenteric artery calcification. There is a tubular calcification to the left of the midline (*arrows*) running in a cephalocaudal direction. Also noted are calcifications in the right renal artery (*small arrowhead*) and splenic artery (*large arrowhead*).

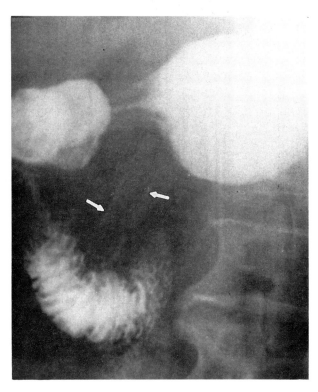

Figure 7–31. Superior mesenteric artery calcification. Note the relationship between the artery (*arrows*) and the third portion of the duodenum on this right posterior oblique projection.

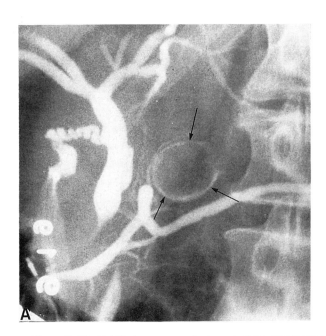

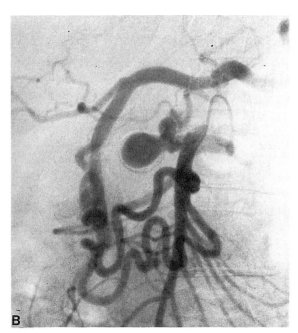

Figure 7–32. Calcified aneurysm of a branch of the dorsal pancreatic artery in a patient with stenosis of the celiac artery. **A.** An endoscopic retrograde cholangiopancreaticogram. The round calcification (*arrows*) was also noted on a plain film of the abdomen. The pancreatic duct and common bile duct are normal. **B.** A superior mesenteric arteriogram demonstrates the calcified aneurysm arising from the dorsal pancreatic artery (*Courtesy of Dr. Ronald Schliftman*).

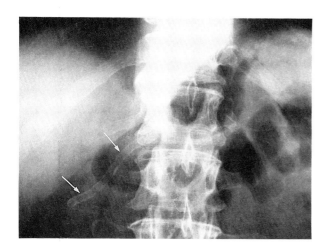

Figure 7–33. Gastroduodenal artery calcification (*arrows*).

are not rare but are usually much smaller than calcification in a pseudocyst or a cystic neoplasm of the pancreas. Moreover, they are almost always accompanied by calcification in nondilated portions of the artery (Fig 6–73).

Superior Mesenteric Artery. In patients with extensive atherosclerosis, the superior mesenteric arteries may calcify.[95] Appearing as a tubular opacity on either side of the spine, coursing vertically or obliquely from L1, it is almost always associated with marked aortic calcification and can be differentiated from that great vessel by its narrower caliber (Fig. 7–30). In diabetic patients, diffuse calcification of the tunica media may appear in the superior mesenteric artery.[96] On lateral or oblique films, the superior mesenteric artery runs slightly oblique to the course of the aorta anterior to the third portion of the duodenum (Fig 7–31).

Calcified aneurysms of the superior mesenteric artery are very rare.[97] As in other saccular aneurysms, circular rim calcification is a hallmark and, therefore, resembles the radiographic appearance of renal, pancreatic, or mesenteric cysts.

Gastroduodenal Artery. The gastroduodenal artery is a branch of the common hepatic artery, running caudally along the medial edge of the descending duodenum and then horizontally across the lumbar spine at the greater curvature of the stomach, where it becomes the gastroepiploic artery. Usually, calcification of this artery is associated with diabetes and presents as uniform tracks of calcification along the expected course of the artery (Fig 7–32). Calcification of aneurysms of the gastroduodenal artery and its branches (the pancreaticoduo-

denal arcades) have been reported in patients with stenosis or occlusion of either the celiac axis or the superior mesenteric artery (Fig 7–33).[98,99] With narrowing of one or both of these major vessels, the pancreaticoduodenal arcades and gastroduodenal artery can become the major collateral supply to the liver, spleen, and bowel. Increased flow through these arteries hastens the development of an aneurysm.

ADRENAL GLANDS

The adrenal glands, even more than the pancreas, are hidden from view on plain films of the abdomen. Although bordered by perirenal fat, much of their substance is superimposed on the renal shadow. The adrenal glands are rarely affected by acute or chronic inflammation and they do not contain gas. Their posterior position high up in the abdomen is far from the intestines and even when they are enlarged by an expanding tumor they tend not to deviate bowel loops. The stomach may be pushed forward by a left adrenal mass, but this direction of displacement is not readily seen on supine films.

It is only the varying patterns of calcification that allow inferences to be made about adrenal pathology on abdominal films. As in the pancreas, only a few diseases are associated with adrenal calcification. Yet, unlike the pancreas, where chronic calcifying pancreatitis is the leading cause of calcification and almost always presents with a characteristic roentgenographic appearance, clinically significant and innocuous adrenal entities can calcify similarly, resembling each other on plain roentgenographs. There are no lesions of this endocrine gland with a pathognomonic configuration of calcification. Almost all radiodensities are either of the cystic or solid morphological type, or occasionally a combination of the two. Hence, the finding of calcification on plain films often must be followed by other studies before a diagnosis can be established. Nonetheless, an abdominal roentgenogram can offer important clues which can narrow the range of diagnostic possibilities considerably.

Solid Calcification in a Normal-Sized Gland
The adrenal gland rests on the superior medial border of the adjacent kidney, with the right gland more caudally situated than the left. Normally, the adrenal glands are not longer than 3 cm or wider than 2.5 cm. If the extent of solid calcification describes an area and contour consistent with a normal-sized gland and there is no other evidence

of glandular enlargement, then it is unlikely that the calcification is caused by a malignant neoplasm.

In the adult, calcification in a normal-sized gland can be encountered in several conditions (Table 7–2). In many instances, adrenal calcification is observed as an incidental finding on abdominal plain films in individuals with no other evidence of adrenal disease. Many of these patients have had abnormal birth histories, with perinatal events that predispose to adrenal hemorrhage, eg, forceful delivery, prematurity, and newborn infection. Although a few infants succumb to adrenal hemorrhage, many others survive without symptoms of adrenal insufficiency. Either unilateral or bilateral calcifications have been shown to occur within 8 days of hemorrhage and may persist into adulthood.[100,101] Adrenal calcification by itself is asymptomatic and goes unnoticed until radiographs of the adrenal region are made at some later date (Fig 7–34). Mottled calcification ranging from faint to dense may occupy a portion of the adrenal gland or can extend throughout the entirety of the organ, and appear as a triangular clump of calcification (Fig 7–35).[102]

Adrenal calcification occurs in Addison's disease. In a study of 120 patients with adrenal insufficiency, Jarvis et al noted three forms of calcification: (1) gross mottled calcification of the gland, (2) multiple discrete deposits of calcium scattered throughout a normal-sized adrenal, and (3) a homogeneous increase in density of the gland.[102] However, only 23% of the patients in this group had adrenal calcification, and in no cases were the adrenal glands enlarged. The rarity of this disease and its association with radiodensities in just a minority of cases indicates that only a small percentage of patients with adrenal calcification suffer from adrenal insufficiency.[103]

In another study, 15 of 24 patients with adrenal calcification had evidence of tuberculosis and 7 had active disease.[104] Nine patients had both Addison's disease and active tuberculosis and seven of them had adrenal calcification[104] It appears that patients whose adrenal disease is caused by tuberculosis

TABLE 7–2. CALCIFICATION IN A NORMAL-SIZED GLAND

Neonatal hemorrhage
Tuberculosis, with or without Addison's disease
Histoplasmosis
Myelolipoma
Adrenal adenoma
Adrenal cortical carcinoma
Pheochromocytoma

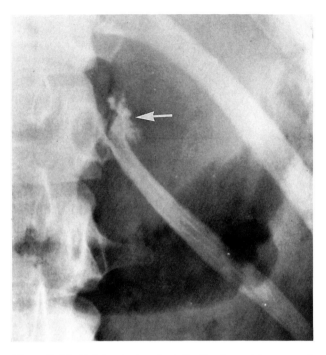

Figure 7–34. Unilateral adrenal calcification (*arrow*) in a normal-sized gland in a young adult with a history of difficult birth. There are no symptoms of adrenal disease or abdominal pain. The calcification is most likely a consequence of neonatal adrenal hemorrhage.

have a greater chance of developing calcification. The frequency with which tuberculosis alone produces calcification is not known, however. Less commonly, disseminated histoplasmosis involves the adrenal glands along with other solid organs, but, unlike its effect on the parenchyma of the liver and spleen, radiographically detectable granulomatous calcification is seldom noted.[105]

Small areas of punctate or mottled densities in the adrenal glands may be seen in patients over 50 and can be a source of puzzlement on plain flims. Usually they are either ignored or thought to represent a granuloma or old hemorrhage. On occasion, they are investigated further and may be surgically removed. In some patients, such calcifications are seen to lie within the substance of a myelolipoma, a benign tumefaction consisting of varying concentrations of fat and bone marrow elements. Myelolipoma, also known as choristoma, is a well-defined encapsulated mass, generally no more than a few millimeters in size, but some lesions may enlarge to 5 to 6 cm in diameter (Fig 7–36).[101] Not associated with endocrine dysfunction, it frequently goes unrecognized on most imaging modalities. Myelolipomas are identified on plain films by punctate calcification. Usually the tumor appears in the sixth

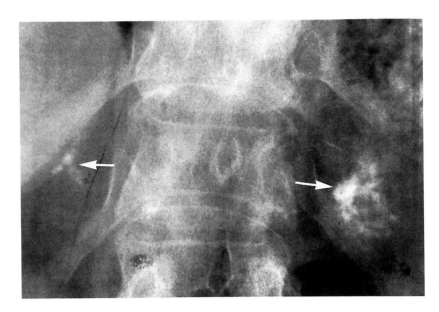

Figure 7–35. Bilateral adrenal calcification (*arrows*). There is no history of adrenal disease. Although calcifications are often bilateral, they need not be symmetrical.

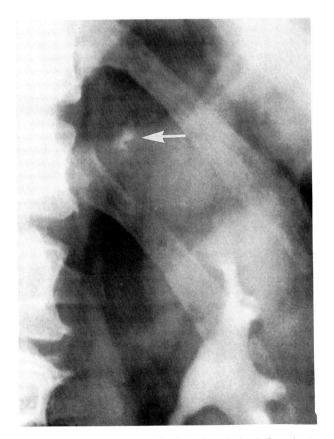

Figure 7–36. Myelolipoma of the left adrenal gland. Superior to the left kidney in a 62-year-old man are closely packed punctate calcifications (*arrow*). Because there was a coincident adrenal cyst, the left adrenal was removed and the calcification was shown to be within the myeloid stroma of the tumor.

and seventh decades, but the youngest reported example was in a 32 year old.[106] They are thought to arise from either embryonic rests in the adrenal gland or to represent metaplasia of glandular elements in fat and marrow tissue.[107] Calcification almost always occurs in areas of necrosis in the myeloid stroma.[108,109]

Less commonly, focal areas of calcification can be seen in both benign and malignant tumors of the adrenal gland. Often, the only clue to the presence of an enlarging mass on plain films is a nidus of mottled or speckled calcification, but the extent of calcification may not correspond to the actual size of the tumor.[110,111] Occasionally, adenocarcinoma of the adrenal cortex or pheochromocytoma appears only as a small area of radiopacity.[112] Although in most cases calcification in an apparently normal-sized gland indicates benign disease, in the appropriate clinical setting the possibility of a malignancy cannot be ruled out.

It is not always easy to sort out adrenal calcification from opacities in adjacent structures. Calcium deposition in costal cartilage may be mistaken for adrenal calcification, and an attempt should be made to see if the calcification lies along the course of a rib in more than one projection. Calcification of the aorta or splenic artery can look like the flecks of calcification in adrenal masses. The tail of the pancreas lies close to and in front of the left adrenal gland, but because isolated pancreatic calcifications are rare, they are not often a cause of confusion. Parenchymal calcification localized in the superior margin of the kidney or renal capsule may be indis-

TABLE 7–3. SOLID CALCIFICATION IN AN ENLARGED ADRENAL GLAND

Cortical carcinoma
Adenoma
Pheochromocytoma
Hibernoma
Hematoma
Myelolipoma
Intravascular papillary endothelial hyperplasia

tinguishable from adrenal calcification. Nevertheless, despite the fact that many nearby structures can contain foci of calcification, it is usually possible to recognize and localize small adrenal calcifications on plain films using frontal, oblique, and lateral projections.

Solid Calcification in Enlarged Adrenal Gland

When extensive suprarenal calcification is seen on plain films, an adrenal mass becomes a prime diag-

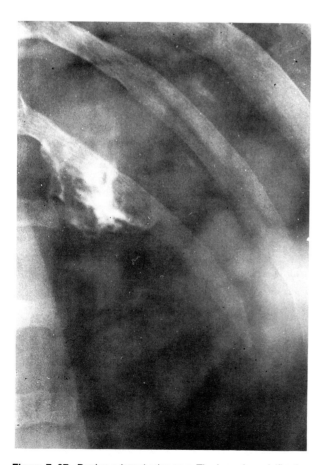

Figure 7–37. Benign adrenal adenoma. The irregular calcification is mostly in the inferior portion of the tumor. Carcinoma of the adrenal gland cannot be excluded on the basis of the radiographic appearance. (*Courtesy of Dr. Arthur Diamond.*)

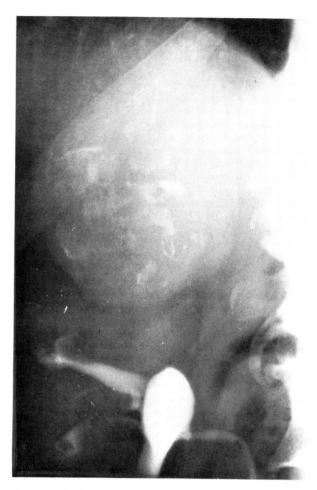

Figure 7–38. Calcification within an adrenal hematoma. There is curvilinear and amorphous calcification within a mass consisting mostly of old blood. A small adenoma was found at the periphery of the mass.

nostic consideration (Table 7–3). Many solid adrenal masses of large size are cortical carcinomas, with calcification deposited in areas of tumor degeneration and hemorrhage.[113–115] Calcification can be distributed throughout the tumor, but there is a

TABLE 7–4. ADRENAL CYSTS THAT CALCIFY ON PLAIN FILMS

Pseudocyst (cystic masses that result from hemorrhage or necrosis in a normal gland or adrenal neoplasm)
    Cystic adrenal hematoma
    Cystic benign tumor
    Cystic cortical carcinoma
    Metastases (melanoma)
True cysts with a calcified wall
    Epithelial-lined
    Endothelial-lined
Cystic pheochromocytoma
Parasitic cyst (*Echinococcus granulosis*)

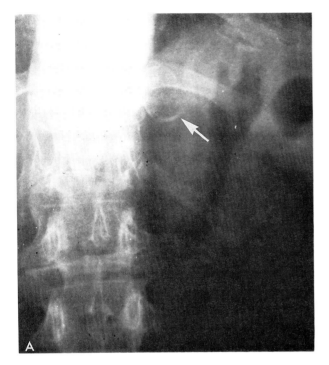

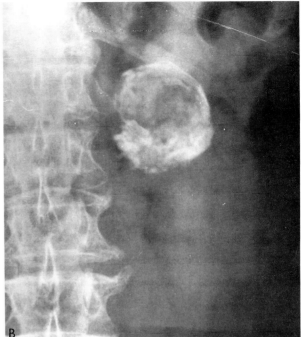

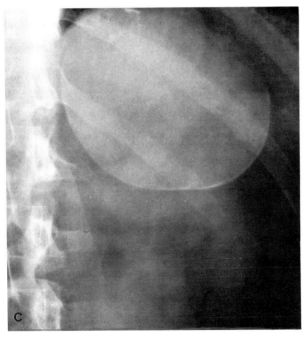

Figure 7–39. Three calcified cysts in the adrenal gland. **A.** Small cyst with smooth walls (*arrow*) simulating a calcified splenic artery aneurysm. **B.** Both cystic and solid calcifications are present in this calcified pseudocyst. **C.** A large smooth-walled pseudocyst of the left adrenal gland.

propensity for calcium to localize in its more necrotic portions. Up to 31% of all adrenal cortical malignancies contain radiologically visible calcification.[103,116]

On the other hand, adrenal adenomas rarely calcify. For the most part, benign cortical tumors have a pattern of calcification identical with that seen in adrenal malignancies, but only infrequently do they attain the dimensions of cortical carcinomas

(Fig 7–37).[116] A hibernoma, a rare benign tumor, which is akin to myelolipoma but lacks marrow elements, may become huge and calcify with multiple punctate radiodensities.[117] Hemangiomas of the adrenal can become very large and contain widely spaced calcified phleboliths with lucent centers[118] or more poorly defined discrete opacities.[119,120] Intravascular papillary endothelial hyperplasia of the adrenal gland, a benign simulator of angiosarcoma histologically, can contain calcification that resembles hemangioma roentgenographically. Solid calcification may also occur in an adrenal hematoma (Fig 7–38).[121]

Pheochromocytoma is a well-studied but uncommon tumor of the adrenal medulla. Calcification in pheochromocytoma is usually cystlike, but occasionally flecks or plaques of calcium are present within the substance of the tumor. Sometimes the opaque flecks are multiple and oriented at different angles, giving the calcification a stellate appearance.[122] Between 10% and 20% of pheochromocytomas involve both adrenal glands, but bilateral calcification is very rare.[123]

Cystic Lesions of the Adrenal Glands

Cystic lesions in the adrenal glands are infrequent (Table 7–4). Unless they become large or calcify, they may not be visible on plain films. Plain film visualization of radiodense margins in adrenal cysts varies widely, occurring in 15% to 50% of patients.[51,124] Cysts are found with equal frequency in either adrenal gland, and they are usually encountered in the fifth and sixth decades. The incidence of adrenal cysts of all types is 50% higher among women.[128]

Along with epithelial-lined single cysts, pseudocysts are probably the most common adrenal cyst that calcify.[125] Often part of the wall may be irregularly dense, suggesting coexistent calcium deposition in residual adrenal tissue or part of the solid tumor from which the cyst arises (Fig 7–39).[126] Cystic calcification can be the first manifestation of a benign tumor or a malignancy—either a primary cortical carcinoma or a metastatic deposit usually from melanoma.[127–129] Nonetheless, cystic lesions are nearly always benign. In a review of resected calcified adrenal masses, Kenney and Stanley encountered no calcified cystic lesions with malignant cells.[130] True cysts, which may have an endothelial or epithelial lining cannot be differentiated from pseudocysts on plain film appearance. Rarely, milk-of-calcium may occur in a benign adrenal cyst, appearing as a diffuse homogeneous opacity that layers out on upright or decubitis films.[131] Eggshell calcifications also can be a feature of pheochro-

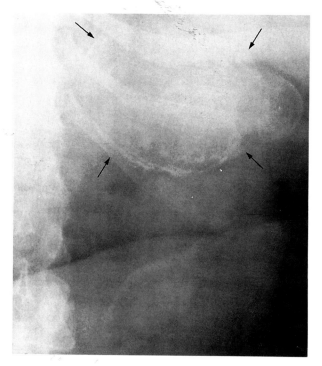

Figure 7–40. Calcified cyst (*arrows*) of *Echinococcus granulosus* in the left adrenal gland. (*Courtesy of Dr. Irwin Bluth.*)

mocytoma.[132–134] The arclike circumferential calcifications often have a relatively small diameter, sometimes no more than 3 to 4 cm. Most cystic pheochromocytomas are probably pseudocysts that have resulted from hemorrhage and necrosis in the tumor.[135,136] *Echinococcus granulosus* cysts in the adrenal are rare; the more common sites for hydatid cysts in the upper abdomen are the liver, spleen, and kidney (Fig 7–40).

Other abdominal cystic calcifications can simulate adrenal cysts. On the left, aneurysms of the splenic artery and the aorta, cysts of the spleen, pancreatic pseudocysts, and upper pole renal masses with rim calcification often look like adrenal cysts. On the right, calcification in hepatic artery aneurysms, gallbladder wall calcification, and cystic renal masses should be ruled out. Retroperitoneal and mesenteric cysts can be mistaken for adrenal cysts on either side.

REFERENCES

1. Baylin GJ, Weeks KD. Some roentgen aspects of pancreatic necrosis. *Radiology.* 1944;42:466–470.
2. Stuart C. Acute pancreatitis. Preliminary investigation of a new radiodiagnostic sign. *J Fac Radiol.* 1956;8:50–57.
3. Price CWR. The colon cut-off sign of acute pancreatitis. *Med J Aust.* 1956;1:313–314.
4. Schwartz S, Nadelhaft J. Simulation of colonic obstruction at the splenic flexure by pancreatitis: Roentgen feaures. *Am J Roentgenol.* 1956;78:607–616.

5. Brascho DJ, Reynolds TN, Zanca P. The radiographic "colon cut-off sign" in acute pancreatitis. *Radiology.* 1962;79:763–768.
6. Cantwell DF, Pollock AV. Radiology of acute pancreatitis. *J Fac Radiol.* 1959;10:95–99.
7. Millward SF, Breatnach E, Simpkins KC, et al. Do plain films of the chest and abdomen have a role in the diagnosis of acute pancreatitis. *Clin Radiol.* 1983; 34:132–137.
8. Davis S, Parbhoo SP, Gibson MJ. The plain abdominal radiograph in acute pancreatitis. *Clin Radiol.* 1980; 31:87–93.
9. Aronson AR, Davis DA. Obstruction near hepatic flexure in pancreatitis. A rarely reported sign. *JAMA.* 1961;176:451–452.
10. Meyers MA, Evans JA. Effects of pancreatitis on the small bowel and colon: Spread along mesenteric planes. *Am J Roentgenol.* 1973;119:151–165.
11. Thompson WM, Kelvin FM, Rice RP. Inflammation and necrosis of the colon secondary to pancreatitis. *Am. J Roentgenol.* 1977;128;943–948.
12. Katz P, Dorman MJ, Aufses AH. Colonic necrosis complicating post-operative pancreatitis. *Ann Surg.* 1974;179:403–405.
13. Mohiuddin S, Sakiyalak P, Gullick HD, et al. Stenosing lesions of the colon secondary to pancreatitis. *Arch Surg.* 1971;102:229–231.
14. Hunt DR, Mildenhall P. Etiology of strictures of the colon associated with pancreatitis. *Am J Dig Dis.* 1975; 20:941–946.
15. Moreno G, Rivera HH. Evaluation of the gastrocolic space in 100 cases of acute pancreatitis. *Radiology.* 1976;118:535–538.
16. Seymour EQ. Unreliability of an increased gastrocolic measurement in the diagnosis of acute pancreatitis. *Radiology.* 1977;123:527.
17. Levitin J. Scout film of the abdomen. *Radiology.* 1946; 47:10–29.
18. Grollman AI, Goodman S, Fine A. Localized paralytic ileus: Early roentgen sign in acute pancreatitis. *Surg Gynecol Obstet.* 1950;91:65–70.
19. Stein GN, Kalser MH, Sarian NM, et al. An evaluation of roentgen signs in acute pancreatitis, correlation with clinical findings. *Gastroenterology.* 1959;36:356–361.
20. Benson G. Plain film findings in acute pancreatitis. *J Natl Med Assoc.* 1974;66:148–159.
21. Ranson JH, Ritkind KA, Rose DF, et al. Objective early identification of severe acute pancreatitis. *Am J Gastroenterol.* 1974;61:443–451.
22. Poppel MH. Roentgen manifestations of pancreatitis. *Semin Roentgenol.* 1968;3:227–241.
23. Weens HS, Walker LA. The radiologic diagnosis of acute cholecystitis and pancreatitis. *Radiol Clin N Am.* 1964;2:89–106.
24. Balthazar EJ, Lutzker S. Radiological signs of acute pancreatitis. *CRC Crit Rev Radiol Nucl Med.* 1976;7:199–242.
25. Barry WF Jr. Roentgen examination of the abdomen in acute pancreatitis. *Am J Radiol.* 1955;74:220–225.
26. Felson B. Gasless abdomen. Letter from the editor. *Semin Roentgenol.* 1968;3:215–216.
27. Schultz EH Jr. Aids to diagnosis of acute pancreatitis by roentgenographic study. *Am J Roentgenol.* 1963; 89:825–836.
28. Siegelman SS, Copeland BE, Saba GP, et al. CT of fluid collections associated with pancreatitis. *Am J Roentgenol.* 1980;134:1121–1132.
29. Merner TB. Acute pancreatitis with peritoneal fat necrosis—Roentgen diagnosis. *Am J Roentgenol.* 1958; 80:67–72.
30. Berenson JE, Spitz HB, Felson B. The abdominal fat necrosis sign. *Radiology.* 1971;100:567–571.
31. Baker DE, Glazer GM. Bilateral pararenal calcifications resulting from pancreatitis. *Am J Roentgenol.* 1984; 143:51–52.
32. Susman N, Hammerman AM, Cohen E. The renal halo sign in pancreatitis. *Radiology.* 1982;142:323–327.
33. Fritzsche P, Toomey FB, Ta HN. Alteration of perirenal fat secondary to diffuse retroperitoneal infiltration. *Radiology.* 1979;131;27–29.
34. Dembner AG, Jaffe CC, Simeone J, et al. A new computed tomographic sign of pancreatitis. *Am J Roentgenol.* 1979;133:477–479.
35. Holden, JL, Berne TV, Rosoff SE. Pancreatic abscess following acute pancreatitis. *Arch Surg.* 1976;111:858–861.
36. Miller TA, Lindenauer SM, Frey LF, et al. Pancreatic abscess. *Arch Surg.* 1974;108;545–551.
37. Altemeier WA, Alexander JW. Pancreatic abscess. A study of 32 cases. *Arch Surg.* 1963;87:80–89.
38. Mendez G, Isikoff MB. Significance of intrapancreatic gas demonstrated by CT. A review of three cases. *Am J Roentgenol.* 1979;132:59–62.
39. Agnos JW, Holmes RB. Gas in pancreas as sign of abscess. *Am J Roentgenol.* 1958;80:60–66.
40. Bolooki H, Jaffe B, Gliedman ML. Pancreatic abscess and lesser omental sac collections. *Surg Gynecol Obstet.* 1968;126:1301–1308.
41. Evans FL. Pancreatic abscess. *Am J Surg* 1969;117:537–540.
42. Jones CE, Polk HC, Fulton RL. Pancreatic abscess. Am J Surg 1975; 129:44–47.
43. Woodard S, Kelvin FM, Rice RP, et al. Pancreatic abscess. Importance of conventional radiology. *Am J Roentgenol.* 1981;136:871–878.
44. Renert WA, Pitt MJ, Capp MP. Acute pancreatitis. *Semin Roentgenol.* 1973;8:405–414.
45. Felson B. Gas abscess of pancreas. *JAMA.* 1957; 163:637–641.
46. Fielding JA, Loughran LF. Sub-diaphragmatic gas in a case of acute pancreatitis. *Br J Radiol.* 1979;52:665–667.
47. Alexander ES, Clark RA, Federle WP. Pancreatic gas: indication of a pancreatic fistula. *Am J Roentgenol.* 1982;139:1089–1093.
48. Torres WE, Clements JL Jr, Sones PJ, et al. Gas in the pancreatic bed without abscess. Am J Roentgenol. 1981;137;1131–1133.
49. Rosenquist LJ. Pseudocyst of the pancreas. Unusual

radiographic presentations. *Clin Radiol.* 1973;24:192–194.

50. Komaki S, Clark JM. Pancreatic pseudocyst. A review of 17 cases with emphasis on radiologic findings. *Am J Roentgenol.* 1974;122:385–397.

51. Palubinskas AJ, Christensen WR, Harrison JH, et al. Calcified adrenal cysts. *Am J Roentgenol.* 1959;82:853–861.

52. Minagi H, Margolin FR. Pancreatic calcifications. *Am J Gastroenterol.* 1972;57:139–146.

53. Lagergren C. Calcium carbonate precipitation in the pancreas, gallstones, and urinary calculi. *Acta Chir Scand.* 1962;124;320–325.

54. Sarles H, Sahel J. Pathology of chronic calcifying pancreatitis. *Am J Gastroenterol.* 1976;66:117–139.

55. Snell AM, Comfort MW. Incidence and diagnosis of pancreatic lithiasis. *Am J Dig Dis.* 1941;8:237–243.

56. McGeorge CK, Widmann BP, Ostrum H, et al. Diffuse calcification of the pancreas. *Am J Roentgenol.* 1957; 78:599–606.

57. Peters BJ, Lubitz JM, Lindert MCF. Diffuse calcification of the pancreas. *AMA Arch Intern Med* 1951; 87:390–409.

58. Ring ER, Eaton SB Jr, Ferrucci JT Jr et al. Differential diagnosis of pancreatic calcification. *Am J Roentgenol.* 1973;117:446–452.

59. Galinsky MH, Leung JWC, Heron C, et al. Calcific pancreatitis. Calcification pattern and pancreatogram correlations. *Clin Radiol.* 1984;35:401–404.

60. Hanelin LG, Schimmel DH. Lymphangioma of the pancreas exhibiting an unusual pattern of calcification. *Radiology.* 1977;122:636.

61. Okuda K, Ichinohe A, Kono K, et al. Minimal Thorotrast deposition in parapancreatic lymph nodes. *Radiology.* 1976;119:25–26.

62. Gillies CL. Pancreatic lithiasis with report of a case. *Am J Roentgenol.* 1939;41:42–46.

63. Johnson RB, Baker HW. Solitary calculus of the duct of Wirsung. *Gastroenterology.* 1954;27:849–860.

64. Tucker DH, Moore IB. Vanishing pancreatic calcifications in chronic pancreatitis. A sign of pancreatic carcinoma. *N Engl J Med.* 1968;268:31–33.

65. Baltaxe HA, Leslie EV. Vanishing pancreatic calcifications. *Am J Roentgenol.* 1967;99:642–644.

66. Donowitz M, Stein SA, Keohane MF. Vanishing pancreatic calcifications. A non-specific finding in chronic pancreatitis. *JAMA.* 1974;228:1575–1576.

67. Andiole JG, Haaga JR, Bolwell BJ. Spontaneous pancreatic decalcification. *J Comput Assist Tomogr.* 1983; 7:534–535.

68. Olurin EO, Olurin O. Pancreatic calcification. A report of 45 cases. *Br Med J.* 1969;4:534–539.

69. Konstam P. Geographical pathology—West Africa. *Clin Radiol.* 1962;14:206–218.

70. Zuidema PO. Cirrhosis and disseminated calcification of the pancreas in patients with malnutrition. *Trop Geogr Med.* 1959;11:70–79.

71. Pitchumoni CS, Thomas E, Balthazar E, et al. Chronic calcific pancreatitis in association with celiac disease. *Am J Gastroenterol.* 1977;68:358–361.

72. Cope O, Culve PO, Mixter CG Jr. Pancreatitis. A diagnostic clue to hyperparathyroidism. *Ann Surg.* 1957; 145:847–852.

73. Mixter CG Jr, Keynes WM, Cope O. Further experience with pancreatitis as a diagnostic clue to hyperparathyroidism. *N Engl J Med.* 1962;266:265–272.

74. Schmidt A, Creutzfeldt W. Calciphylactic pancreatitis and pancreatitis in hyperparathyroidism. *Clin Orthop.* 1970;69:135–145.

75. Singleton EB, Gray PM Jr. Radiologic evaluation of pancreatic disease in children. *Semin Roentgenol.* 1968; 3:267–279.

76. Joffe N. Pancreatic calcification in childhood associated with protein malnutrition. *Br J Radiol.* 1963; 36:758–761.

77. Kattwinkel J. Lapey A, diSant'Agnese PA. Hereditary pancreatitis: Three new kindreds and a critical review of the literature. *Pediatrics.* 1973;51:55–69.

78. Hacken JB, Moccia RM. Calcific pancreatitis in a patient with Type S hyperlipoproteinemia. *Gastrointest Radiol.* 1979;4:143–146.

79. Batson JM, Law DH. Chronic calcific pancreatitis in a child. *Gastroenterology.* 1962;43:95–98.

80. Stobbe KC, ReMine WH, Baggenstoss AH. Pancreatic lithiasis. *Surg Gynecol Obstet.* 1970;131:1090–1099.

81. Beazley RM, Cohn I Jr. Pancreatic cancer. *Cancer.* 1981; 31:346–358.

82. Kendig TA, Johnson RM, Shackford BC. Calcification in pancreatic carcinoma. *Ann Intern Med.* 1966;65:122–124.

83. Johnson JR, Zintel HA. Pancreatic calcification and cancer of the pancreas. *Surg Gynecol Obstet.* 1963; 117:585–588.

84. Lundh G, Nordenstam H. Pancreas calcification and pancreas cancer. A discussion of two cases. *Acta Chir Scand.* 1970;136:493–496.

85. Paulino-Netto A, Dreiling PA, Baronofsky ID. The relationship between pancreatic calcification and cancer of the pancreas. *Ann Surg.* 1960;151:530–537.

86. Friedman AC, Lichtenstein JE, Dachman AH. Cystic neoplasms of the pancreas. *Radiology.* 1983;149:45–50.

87. Campagno J, Oertel JF. Microcystic adenomas of the pancreas (glycogen-rich cystadenomas). A clinico-pathologic study of 34 cases. *Am J Clin Pathol.* 1978; 69:289–298.

88. Freeny PC, Weinstein CJ, Taft DA, et al. Cystic neoplasms of the pancreas: New angiographic and ultrasonographic findings. *Am J Roentgenol.* 1978;131;795–802.

89. Swanson GE. A case of cystadenoma of the pancreas studied by selective angiography. *Radiology.* 1963; 81:592–595.

90. Parientes RA, Ducellier R, Lubrano JM, et al. Cystadenoma of the pancreas. Diagnosis by computed tomography. *J Comput Asst Tomogr.* 1980;4:364–367.

91. Imhof H, Frank P. Pancreatic calcifications in malignant islet cell tumors. *Radiology.* 1977;122:333–337.

92. Jahnke RW, Gnekow W, Harell S. Non-beta cell islet tumor calcification associated with Zollinger–Ellison

syndrome and multiple endocrine adenomatosis. *Gastrointest Radiol.* 1977;1:345–347.

93. Zimmer FE. Islet cell carcinoma treated with alloxan associated with calcified hepatic metastases and thyrotoxic myopathy. *Ann Intern Med.* 1964;61:543–549.

94. Bozymski EM, Woodruff K, Sessions JT Jr. Zollinger–Ellison syndrome with hypoglycemia associated calcifications of the tumor and its metastases. *Gastroenterology.* 1973;68:658–661.

95. Redman HC. Arterial calcification simulating aneurysm. *JAMA.* 1969;208:865–868.

96. Lackman AS, Spray TL, Kerwin DM, et al. Medial calcinosis of Monckeberg. A review of the problem and a description of a patient with involvement of peripheral visceral and coronary arteries. *Am J Med.* 1977;63:615–622.

97. Weidner W, Fox P. Brooks JW, et al. The roentgen diagnosis of aneurysms of the superior mesenteric artery. *Am J Roentgenol.* 1970;109:138–142.

98. Mora JD. Celiac axis artery stenosis with aneurysmal calcification of collateral supply. *Aus Radiol.* 1976;20:252–254.

99. West JE, Bernhardt H, Bowers RF. Aneurysm of pancreaticoduodenal artery. *Am J Surg.* 1968;115:835–839.

100. Gabrielle OF, Sheehan WF. Bilateral neonatal adrenal hemorrhage. *Am J Roentgenol.* 1964;91:656–658.

101. Martin JF. Suprarenal calcifications. *Radiol Clin N Am.* 1965;3:129–138.

102. Jarvis JL, Jenkins D, Sosman MC, et al. Roentgenologic observations in Addison's disease. A review of 120 cases. *Radiology.* 1954;62:16–29.

103. McAlister WH, Lester PD. Diseases of the adrenal. *Med Radiol Photogr* 1971;47:62–81.

104. Jarvis JL, Seaman WB. Idiopathic adrenal calcification in infants and children. *Am J Roentgenol.* 1959;82:510–520.

105. Schwarz E. Regional roentgen manifestations of histoplasmosis. *Am J Roentgenol.* 1962;87:865–874.

106. Giffen HK. Myelolipoma of the adrenals. Report of seven cases. *Am J Pathol.* 1947;23:613–619.

107. Tulcinsky DB, Deutsch V, Bubis JJ. Myelolipoma of the adrenal gland. *Br J Surg.* 1970;57:465–467.

108. McAlister WN, Koehler PR. Diseases of the adrenal. *Radiol Clin N Am.* 1967;5:205–220.

109. Costello P, Clouse ME, Kane RA, et al. Problems in the diagnosis of adrenal tumors. *Radiology.* 1977;125:335–341.

110. Verness M, Schour L, Jaffe ES. Calcification in benign, non-functioning adrenal adenoma: Report of a case with selective adrenal arteriogram. *Br J Radiol* 1972;45:621–623.

111. Drucker WD, Longo FW, Christy MP. Calcifications in a benign non-functioning tumor of the adrenal. *JAMA.* 1961;177:577–579.

112. Pendergrass HP, Tristan TA, Blakemore WS, et al. Roentgen technics in the diagnosis and localization of pheochromocytoma. *Radiology.* 1962;78:725–737.

113. Colapinto RF, Steed BL. Arteriography of adrenal tumors. *Radiology.* 1971;100:343–350.

114. Strittmatter WC, Brown CH, Tretbar HA. A large carcinoma of the adrenal. *Radiology.* 1957;68:23–232.

115. Boise CL, Sears WN. Calcification in adrenal neoplasms. *Radiology.* 1951;56:731–734.

116. McNulty JG, Lea Thomas M, Tighe Jr. Angiographic diagnosis of benign adrenal adenoma. *Am J Roentgenol* 1968;104:386–388.

117. Bosniak MA, Seigelman SS, Evans JA. *The Adrenal Retropritoneum and Lower Urinary Tract.* Chicago: Year Book Medical Publishers; 1976.

118. Rothberg M, Bastidas J, Mattey WE, et al. Adrenal hemangiomas. Angiographic appearances of a rare tumor. *Radiology.* 1978;126:341–344.

119. Nakagawa N, Takahashi M, Maeda K. Case report: Adrenal haemangioma coexisting with malignant haemangioendothelioma. *Clin Radiol.* 1986;37:97–99.

120. Lee WT, Weinreb T, Kumar S. Adrenal hemangioma. *J Comput Assist Tomogr.* 1982;6:392–394.

121. Kawashima A, Johnsen T, Murayama S. Intravascular papillary endothelial hyperolasia of the adrenal gland. *Br J. Radiol.* 1986;59:610–613.

122. Mori Y, Kiyohara H, Miki T, et al. Pheochromocytoma with prominent calcification and associated pancreatic islet cell tumor. *J Urol.* 1977;118:843–844.

123. Bosniak MA, Seigelman SS, Evans JA. *The Adrenal Retroperitoneum and Lower Urinary Tract.* Chicago: Year Book Medical Publishers. 1976:138.

124. Vezina CT, McLoughlin MJ, St. Louis EL, et al. Cystic lesions of the adrenal: Diagnosis and management. *J Can Assoc Radiol.* 1984;35:107–112.

125. Parker JM. Calcified cyst of the adrenal gland. *Milit Med.* 1970;138:791–792.

126. Anderson MY, Roberts HG, Smith ET. Calcified cyst of the adrenal cortex without endocrine symptoms. *Radiology.* 1950;54:236–241.

127. Wood JC. A calcified adrenal tumor. *Br J Radiol.* 1952;25:222–224.

128. Samuel E. Calcification in suprarenal neoplasms. *Br J Radiol.* 1948;21:139–142.

129. Twersky J, Levin DC. Metastatic melanoma of the adrenal. *Radiology* 1975;116:627–628.

130. Kenney PT, Stanley RT. Calcified adrenal cysts. *Urol Radiol.* 1987;9:9–15.

131. Moss AA. Milk of calcium of the adrenal gland. *Br J Radiol.* 1976;49:186–187.

132. Grainger RG, Lloyd GAS, Williams JL. Eggshell calcification. A sign of phaeochromocytoma. *Clin Radiol.* 1967;18:282–286.

133. Neilson J, Smith S McC. Eggshell calcification in phaeochromocytoma. *J R Coll Surg Edinb.* 1973;18:183–187.

134. Feist JE, Lasser EC. Pheochromocytoma with large cystic calcification and associated sphenoid ridge malformation. *Radiology.* 1961;76:21–26.

135. Meyers MA, King MC. Unusual features of pheochromocytoma. *Clin Radiol.* 1965;20:52–56.

136. Moser M, Sheehan G, Schwinger H. Pheochromocytoma with calcification simulating cholelithiasis. *Radiology.* 1950;55:855–858.

Plain Film Findings in the Urinary Tract

Stephen R. Baker and Milton Elkin

KIDNEYS

The kidneys, enveloped by perinephric fat and subject to calcification and even gas formation, are demonstrated often on survey radiographs of the abdomen. The renal contours can stand out because of the contrast afforded by adjacent adipose tissue in the retroperitoneal space. Distinctive patterns of lucency or opacity confined to either the renal collecting system or the kidney parenchyma frequently suggest specific diagnoses. For the most part, plain films help direct the choice of additional imaging examinations, but, in some cases, they provide definitive information. Hence, despite the wide availability of intravenous urography, computed tomography, and ultrasonography, the plain film still retains a rightful place in the repertoire of imaging studies for the evaluation of renal abnormalities.

The Renal Shadow

The size, configuration, and position of the kidneys can be ascertained on many plain films of the abdomen. Failure to observe the renal contours by no means indicates disease, however. A paucity of retroperitoneal fat—a normal finding in thin individuals—or overlying intestinal gas and feces can limit visualization of the renal perimeter. The right kidney, superimposed on the homogeneous density of the liver, is seen more often than the left kidney, which often lies posterior to the proximal small bowel and the transverse and descending colon. Since the medial border of the kidney abuts the edge of the soft tissue shadow of the psoas muscle, it is outlined less frequently than the lateral, superior, and inferior renal margins.

Generally, the two kidneys are situated at nearly the same level in the upper abdomen, with the upper pole of each rarely extending above the T11 vertebral body. A normally functioning kidney can, however, be found in the pelvis or even in the thorax, where it may migrate in fetal life through a congenital opening in the posterior diaphragm. The unilateral absence of one renal shadow on plain films should, of course, raise suspicion of agenesis, atrophy, or surgical removal but it may merely indicate an ectopic positioning of the kidney.

The long axis of the renal density has an oblique orientation, diverging from the midline inferiorly. A vertical or convergent direction of the axes of both kidneys in association with medial migration of at least part of the renal shadow over the psoas muscle is plain film evidence of a horseshoe kidney (Figs 2–8,8–1). Typically, the right and left "arms" of the conjoined organ are attached at the lower poles. The extension across the midline may consist of functioning renal tissue, a fibrous band, or a combination of parenchymal and supporting structures.

Renal masses are recognized by marginal distortions or enlargement of the kidney (Fig 8–2). Small cysts or tumors are best appreciated if they project beyond the lateral edge of the renal shadow. Sometimes an oblique projection can bring into relief a mass hidden on frontal views. Larger lesions not only widen and/or lengthen the homogeneous renal shadow, they also redirect the renal axis, displacing renal tissue as they grow. Occasionally, an expanding tumefaction with a primarily exophytic pattern of growth can be surrounded by fat to a greater extent than the kidney from which it arises. Consequently, a renal mass may be evident on plain films even if the parent kidney is not seen (Fig 8–3).

The presence of a soft tissue density in the expected location of the renal shadow need not be related to the urinary tract, however (Fig 8–4). Aneurysms of the abdominal aorta and its branches, pancreatic pseudocysts, intestinal tumors, mesenteric cysts, retroperitoneal sarcomas, and neoplasms of the muscles of the back can all resemble renal masses on plain films (Fig 8–5). Another confusing appearance is a very large, kidney-based tumor that

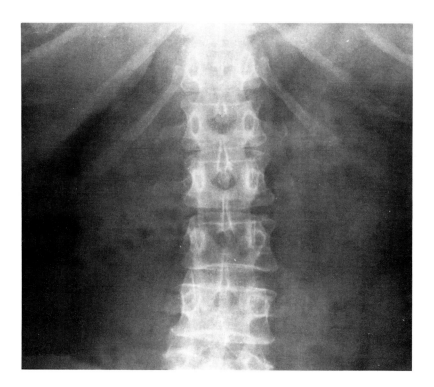

Figure 8–1. Horseshoe kidneys. The axis of each kidney is nearly vertical. Both renal shadows are medially positioned and their lower poles overlie the psoas muscles. They are joined at their lower poles.

occupies much of the upper or mid abdomen, compressing fat and displacing nearby organs. Such huge lesions can be mistaken for enlargements of other viscera or even fluid in bowel loops (Fig 8–6).

Renal and Perirenal Gas

Gas within or contiguous to the kidney is never normal; when first discovered a search should be undertaken promptly to determine its cause. In some cases, it is an innocuous finding that resolves quickly with appropriate treatment, whereas in others, it is a manifestation of a disease whose major consequences involve adjacent organs and, in a few patients, it is a crucial marker of a renal-based infection. Gas may accumulate in the pelvicalyceal system, the renal parenchyma, or surrounding retro-

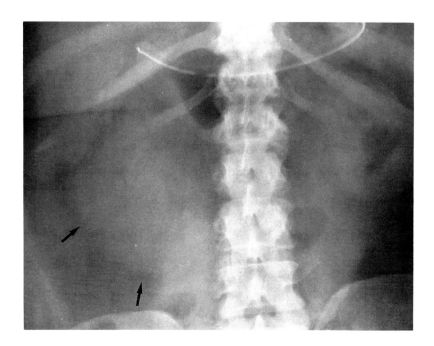

Figure 8–2. Renal mass. The right renal shadow has been lengthened by a hypernephroma arising from its inferior pole (*arrows*) Compare the size of the right kidney with the normal left kidney, which extends from T12 to L2.

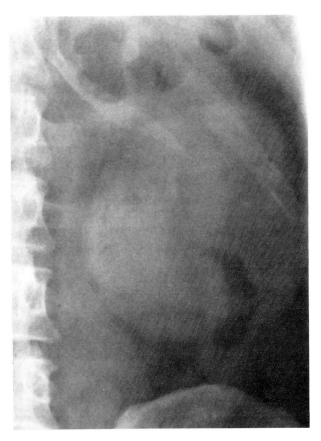

Figure 8–3. A larger anterior cyst of the lower pole of the left kidney. It is enveloped by retroperitoneal fat and is much more sharply demarcated than the remainder of the kidney above it.

peritoneal tissue. Each location has a range of distinctive appearances, easily recognizable on plain films of the abdomen. Moreover, intraluminal, intraparenchymal, and perirenal lucencies differ from one another in etiology, clinical presentation, treatment, and prognosis (Table 8–1).

Intraluminal Gas

Surgical Intervention. Entry of air into the pelvicalyceal system may be achieved through a percutaneous nephrostomy (Fig 8–7) or with retrograde instrumentation of the bladder and ureter. Today, with increasing reliance on interventional imaging procedures, iatrogenic investigation or treatment of the urinary tract is the most common cause of lucencies in the renal collecting system. Air may be confined to the pelvis and calyces or can extend distally if there is no blockage at the ureteropelvic junction. Usually, the air resolves gradually over several days. A surgical reimplantation of the ureters is apt to result in prolonged intrarenal lucencies. For example, ureteroileostomy permits access to the renal

pelvis by external air via the stomal opening on the skin, the interposed ileal segment, and the ureters.[1]

Fistula

Fistulas between the bladder or ureter and nearby hollow viscera can be associated with intrarenal lucencies, the air, or gas ascending from the vesical or ureteral lumen. The most frequent inciting lesions are carcinomas of the distal large intestine and rectum and diverticular abscesses of the sigmoid colon (Fig 8–8). Less common causes include bladder malignancy extending to adjacent bowel loops and cervical carcinoma, with the communication to the bladder resulting from the tumor itself or as a late complication of radiation therapy. Although patients with fistulae to the bladder often present with pneumaturia, the amount of intraluminal air is seldom more than a few milliliters, and thus extension of lucency to the ureter and renal collecting system is infrequently observed on plain films.

Renocolic fistulas are also very uncommon. They may eventuate from a pyonephrosis infiltrating in turn the kidney, the perirenal and pararenal spaces, and the bowel wall. Malignancies and pus collections originating from the colon can invade the kidney. The confluence of the perirenal fascia and the phrenicocolic ligament at the anatomic splenic

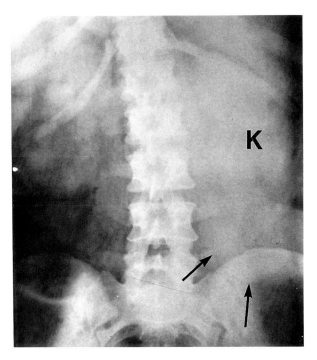

Figure 8–4. A retroperitoneal mass separate from the kidney. A nonenlarged left kidney (K) with normal axis lies behind a slow-growing paraganglioma in the anterior pararenal space (*arrows* on its inferior extent). It simulates a renal-based mass.

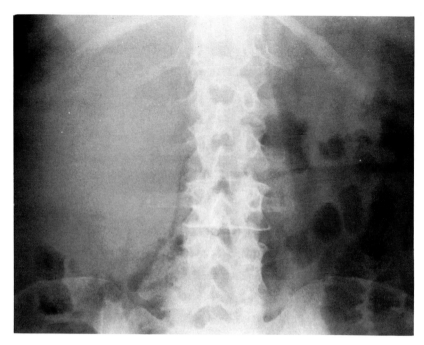

Figure 8–5. A mass in the right mid abdomen displaces bowel loops inferiorly. No separate renal shadow is seen. Operation revealed a paralumbar abscess involving the muscles of the back. The kidney was displaced medially and anteriorly.

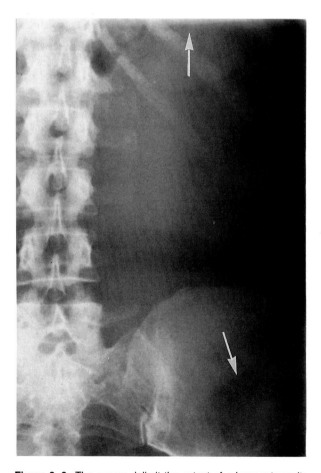

Figure 8–6. The arrows delimit the extent of a huge retroperitoneal mass that at operation was shown to be a sarcoma of the left renal capsule. Plain films could not localize the tumor to the kidney.

flexure makes it a favored site for the spread of colon carcinoma to the left kidney.[2]

Traumatic Connections. Air may reach the renal collecting system after an injury in which an object traverses the skin, intervening soft tissue, and the kidney. An indirect route from the skin to the kidney involves disruption of the bladder wall and retrograde passage of air through the ureter. A third traumatic pathway follows the formation of an abnormal communication between damaged kidney and bowel. In each instance, air in the collecting system may persist until the integrity of the urinary tract is restored.

Urinary Tract Infection. Most gas-forming infections of the renal collecting system occur in diabetic individuals. Usually, these patients have no obstruction and the gas reaches the renal pelvis by retrograde extension from the bladder lumen, where it is formed by bacterial digestion of glucose-rich urine. A spontaneous pneumopyelogram in a nondiabetic is rare, almost always occurring proximal to a ureteral or ureteropelvic obstruction.[3] A frequent concomitant in these patients is an opaque staghorn calculus that appears in marked contrast to the lucency that also occupies the pelvis and renal calyces. Even in the absence of opaque stones, hydronephrosis is commonplace and can be recognized by its

TABLE 8-1. RENAL AND PERIRENAL LUCENCIES

Intraluminal gas
  Surgical intervention
    Nephrostomy
    Retrograde instrumentation
  Fistula
    Intestine to bladder
    Intestine to ureter
    Intestine to kidney
  Trauma
    Direct renal trauma
    Bladder trauma
    Traumatic renocolic fistula
  Infection—gas-forming organism
Intraparenchymal
  Emphysematous pyelonephritis
  Intrarenal abscess
  Postembolization gas
Perirenal gas
  Renal origin
    Pyonephrosis
    Intrarenal abscess
    Emphysematous pyelonephritis
  Intestinal origin

specific pattern of gas accumulation. Occasionally, papillary necrosis ensues and gas may define the deformed calyces on plain films (Fig 8–9). Successful control of blood glucose in diabetics and relief of obstruction plus antibiotic therapy in nondiabetics are necessary to prevent dissemination of the infection into the renal parenchyma.

Intraparenchymal Gas

Emphysematous Pyelonephritis. Emphysematous pyelonephritis is a rare, fulminant, and often fatal infection of the kidney that can be diagnosed with assurance on plain films. A typical patient is a middle-aged diabetic woman with a history of urinary tract infections.[4] The disease is often heralded by the rapid onset of fever and flank pain. By the time air is recognized in the renal parenchyma, kidney function has been lost, and no consideration should be given to preserving the infected kidney. Emergency treatment, either incision and drainage or nephrectomy, must be directed towards preventing septicemia, a complication that is more likely if gas is observed beyond Gerota's fascia.[5]

Surprisingly, only about 50% of patients have urinary tract obstruction. The usual offending organisms are not rare pathogens but common intestinal microorganisms such as *Esherichia coli*, *Pseudomonas aerugenosa*, *Aerobacter aerogenes*, and *Klebsiella* species, all of which can metabolize carbo-

hydrates with the release of carbon dioxide and hydrogen peroxide.[6] Nearly all patients are diabetic but recent reports have documented emphysematous pyelonephritis in transplanted kidneys.[7,8]

It is not clear how gas enters the renal substance, but once the infection reaches the parenchyma, total kidney involvement is the rule. In almost every instance, the appearance of emphysematous pyelonephritis is striking and highly specific. Most often, the disease appears as myriad, tiny lucencies scattered throughout the kidney, giving it a lacelike pattern on plain films. Occasionally, one or two large confluent areas are seen along with the bubbles (Fig 8–10). The massive accumulation of gas enlarges the kidney, sometimes doubling or tripling its length.[9] When an arcuate gas shadow appears at the margin of the infected kidney it is highly suggestive of penetration into the perirenal space (Figs 8–11, 8–12).[6] More distant gas collections identify spread into the pararenal compartments.

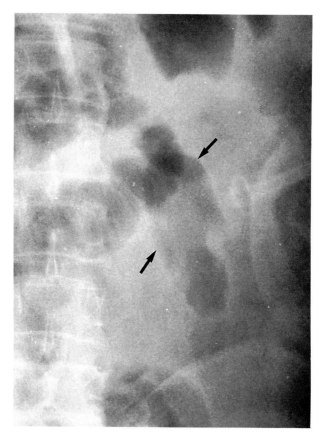

Figure 8–7. Air in the left renal pelvis (*arrows*), introduced during performance of a nephrostomy. A large-bore catheter is seen just lateral to the renal pelvis.

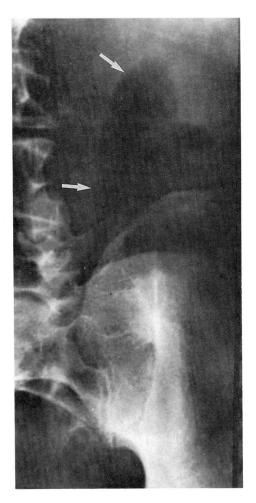

Figure 8–8. Gas in the ureter (*lower arrow*) and the left renal pelvis (*upper arrow*) secondary to fistula between the sigmoid colon and the bladder. The patient had an extensive sigmoid diverticular abscess.

Intrarenal Abscess. Most pus collections within the kidney are initially fairly discrete masses surrounded by normal renal tissue. These renal carbuncles may be multiple, and if left untreated, can enlarge within the kidney, invade adjacent tissues and spread through the bloodstream to distant sites. Although large lesions may distort the renal contour, most renal abscesses are undetected on plain films. Distinctly uncommon is focal accumulation of lucency within the abscess cavity as gas formation is infrequently encountered in this type of renal infection.

Postinfarction Gas. A benign, self-limited form of intraparenchymal gas accumulation occurs in some patients after renal tumor embolization.[10,11] This phenomenon is similar to that seen in embolization

of arteries supplying the liver,[12] spleen,[13] and adrenal gland.[14] At the same time gas is observed, the patient rarely complains of fever or discomfort. Typically, small bubbles appear approximately 1 week after the procedure and resolve in several days. The bubbles probably represent transient liberation of gas in infarcted tissues.

Perirenal Gas

Perirenal gas refers to a localized form of retroperitoneal emphysema confined to tissues adjacent to the kidney. It need not have a renal origin, with most cases occurring after colonic or small bowel perforations. An intestinal origin of perirenal gas usually engenders minimal discomfort and fever at first, the retroperitoneal space being notoriously quiet to the presence of bowel gas, feces, and succus entericus. A typical presentation is a feeling of fullness or crepitus in the back and side, often accompanied by mild tenderness.

Perirenal gas from a renal origin is seen almost always as a complication of a severe infection. Three causes are pyonephrosis extending beyond the collecting system into the perirenal space, intrarenal abscesses penetrating beyond the renal margins, and retroperitoneal contamination in the late stages of emphysematous pyelonephritis.[15] Perirenal gas

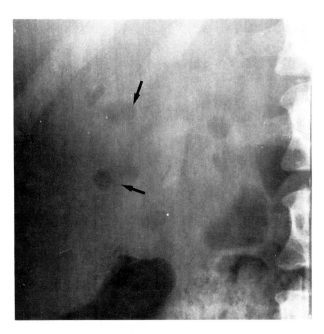

Figure 8–9. Renal papillary necrosis and pyonephrosis. A gas-forming microorganism is responsible for the infection in the renal collecting system. Gas bubbles (*arrows*) conform to the shape of the deformed calyces.

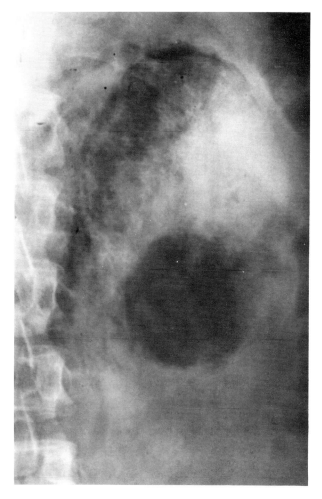

Figure 8–10. Emphysematous pyelonephritis of the left kidney. The enlarged renal shadow contains innumerable bubbles. A confluent lucency occupies part of the lower and middle zone of the kidney. Gas also extends into the left perinephric space.

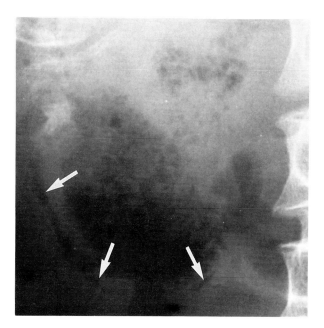

Figure 8–11. Emphysematous pyelonephritis of the right kidney. An arc of lucency (*arrows*) defines the lower margin of the kidney, suggesting perinephric space involvement.

essential components. Noted in only a few case reports,[18,19] it appears as a poorly marginated radiolucency confined within the borders of the renal shadow. Most angiomyolipomas, however, lack sufficient fat to be recognized on survey radiographs.

Concretions

Inasmuch as the urinary tract is a system of fluid-filled tubes subject to wide variations in pH and

bubbles can accumulate close to the kidney or collect far from the renal fossa (Fig 8–13).[16] They can be distributed as closely bunched lucencies or may be arrayed in a linear fashion resembling pneumatosis cystoides intestinalis. A potential mimic is an anomalous position of gas-filled colon that can simulate the lucent pattern of a perirenal infection.[17]

Intrarenal Fat

Fat is a normal constituent of the supporting tissues surrounding the pelvis of the kidney. Sometimes renal sinus fat is so abundant as to be visible on plain films as a faint area of decreased density occupying the medial aspect of the mid portion of the kidney (Fig 8–15). Fat within a renal mass has been observed on plain films in angiomyolipoma, a hamartoma with both muscle and adipose tissue as

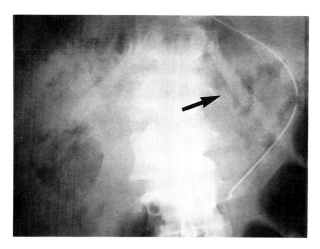

Figure 8–12. Bilateral emphysematous pyelonephritis. Extensive changes on the right, less advanced disease on the left (*arrow*). (*Courtesy of Dr. Murray Rosenberg*).

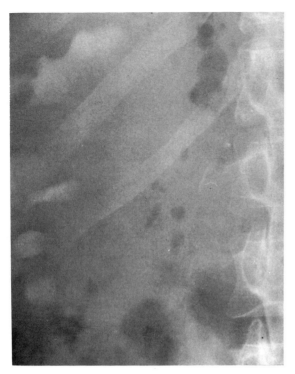

Figure 8–13. Right perinephric abscess. A film from an intravenous urography showing lateral displacement and stretching of the contrast-filled calyces. Medially positioned bubbles of gas are in a large perinephric pus collection.

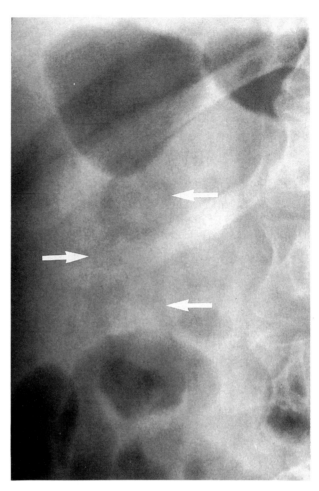

Figure 8–15. Fat in the right renal sinus. A poorly defined lucency (*arrows*) overlying the medial aspect of the kidney. It is less black than nearby gas-filled intestinal segments.

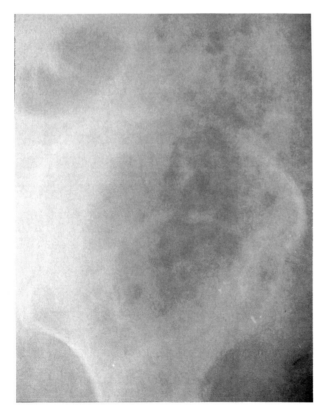

Figure 8–14. A mottled pattern of lucency suggests gas in the colonic wall. Actually, it is distant spread of a perinephric abscess originating from the left kidney.

chemical content, it is not surprising that urinary calculi are common. Concretions can form in tubules within the renal parenchyma or more often in the larger lumina of the collecting systems. They can be found within structures of normal configuration as well as in abnormal lumina.

Normal Lumina. Among the factors predisposing to the formation of calculi, most important are hypercalcemia and hypercalciuria, as may be present with hyperparathyroidism, renal tubular acidosis, bone dissolution secondary to immobilization or widespread metastases, excessive ingestion and absorption of calcium from the gastrointestinal tract, and idiopathic hypercalciuria. Increased urinary excretion of oxalic acid promotes the formation of calcium oxalate stones. Uric acid stones are associated with hyperuricosemia and hyperuricosuria. Cystine stones result from hypercystinuria.

The pH of the urine is also important, alkaline urine promoting the precipitation of triple phosphate stones, and acid urine, the formation of uric acid stones. Stasis of the urine in an obstructed lumen or puddling in an abnormal lumen promotes the formation of stones. Urinary infections also predispose to calculi, probably related to changes in pH.

In the United States, urinary calculi consist of calcium oxalate most commonly. These are usually homogeneously dense and sharply outlined. Next in frequency are the triple phosphate or struvite stones (ammonium–magnesium–phosphate hexahydrate), less dense than calcium oxalate and occurring often in infected urine of alkaline pH. Pure uric acid stones, having the same radiodensity as surrounding soft tissue, cannot be visualized on the abdominal radiograph. Cystine, containing two atoms of sulfur, with its relatively high atomic number, is more radiodense than soft tissues, and thus cystine stones are visualized on abdominal radiographs as faint opacities.

The growth and configuration of calculi accommodate to the dimensions of the lumen. Consequently, urinary concretions vary greatly in diameter and configuration. Concretions in the collecting

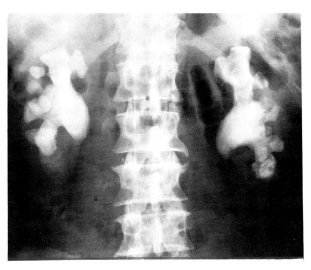

Figure 8–16. Bilateral staghorn calculi of distinctive shape.

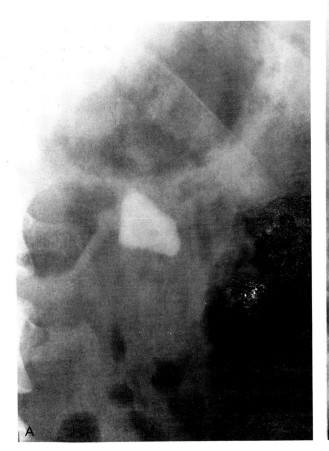
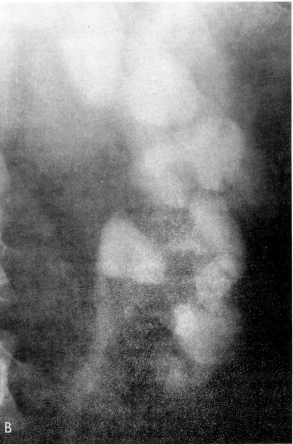

Figure 8–17. Triangular-shaped renal calculus, with a lucent center, the shape reflecting that of the renal pelvis in which the calculus formed.

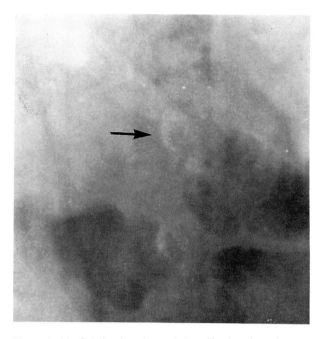

Figure 8–18. Calcification of extruded papillae in calyces in a patient with renal papillary necrosis. Scout radiograph shows faint rims of calcification. The arrow points to one such density, triangular in shape.

ducts are initially minute and rounded, and later, with growth, assume the linear shape of the duct and then increase in overall size, causing dilatation of the lumen and destruction of the enveloping tissues.

Sometimes, specific shapes betray the nature of a renal stone. The staghorn calculus, a triple phosphate stone, makes a cast of the pelvicalyceal system and is easily recognizable on an abdominal radiograph (Fig 8–16). On occasion, a urinary concretion has the configuration of a calyx of the renal pelvis in which it grew (Fig 8–17). The triangular-shaped extruded necrotic papilla of renal papillary necrosis, when calcified, appears on the abdominal radiograph as a rim of increased density, often with a shape distinctive enough to indicate the diagnosis (Fig 8–18).

Abnormal Lumina. A pyelogenic cyst (calyceal diverticulum), communicating with the pelvicalyceal system via a narrow isthmus, often contains concretions. There may be a single calculus occupying most of the lumen or an agglomeration of smaller calculi (Fig 8–19). Most distinctive is milk-of-calcium, consisting of a colloidal suspension of calcific granules so small that they appear as a finely

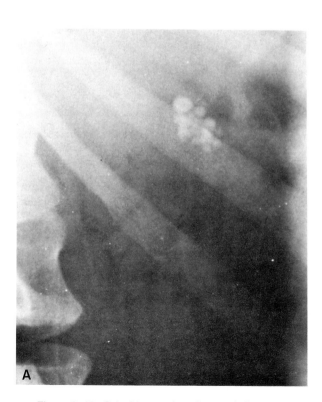
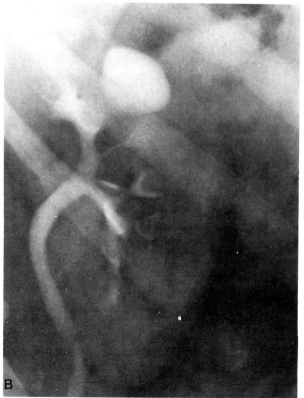

Figure 8–19. Calculi in a pyelogenic cyst. **A.** Scout radiograph shows a collection of concretions, in an oval configuration, at the upper pole of the left kidney. **B.** Urogram demonstrates that the calculi lie in a pyelogenic cyst.

opaque cloud on the abdominal radiograph.[20,21] The granules layer out dependently and are thus easily diagnosable by horizontal beam radiograph with proper positioning of the patient (Fig 8–20), the density maintaining a constant position within the kidney.[22] The chemical composition of the granules has been reported to include calcium carbonate, calcium hydroxyapatite, calcium oxalate, calcium phosphate, and ammonium phosphate with calcium phosphate.[23]

Concretions, including milk-of-calcium, occur less commonly in other types of renal cysts, either communicating or noncommunicating, such as simple cyst[24] or a cyst of adult-type polycystic kidney.[25]

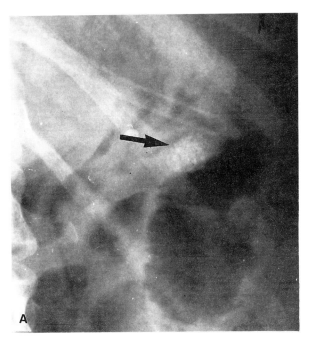

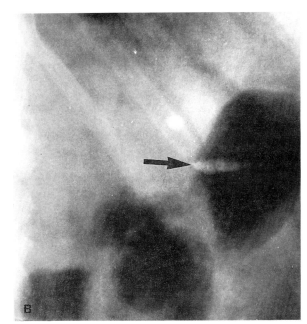

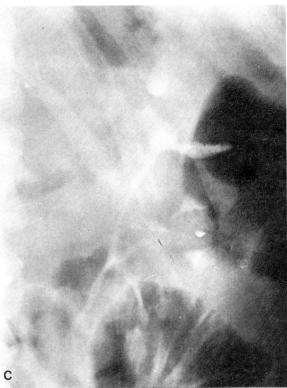

Figure 8–20. Milk-of-calcium in a pyelogenic cyst. **A.** Supine scout radiograph shows the oval granular opacity (*arrow*) in the left upper quadrant. **B.** Erect scout radiograph shows layering out of the calcific granules (*arrow*) in a pyelogenic cyst. **C.** Urogram, in erect position, demonstrates the relation of the pyelogenic cyst to an upper calyx.

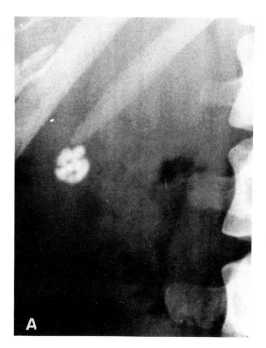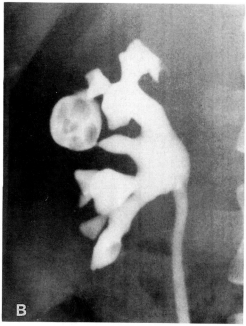

Figure 8–21. Multiple calculi in a hydrocalycosis. **A.** Scout radiograph shows multiple concretions in the right flank. **B.** Retrograde pyelogram demonstrates that the calculi are contained within a dilated calyx, secondary to stricture of the calyceal neck.

Similarly, the cystic spaces of a hydrocalycosis (Fig 8–21) or marked hydronephrosis can contain calculi of various sizes, as well as milk-of-calcium.[23,26] In a dilated pelvis and in a large cyst there can be innumerable small calculi, usually spherical and of uniform size, distinguishable on the abdominal radiograph as well-defined, separate concretions, referred to as seed calculi (Fig 8–22).

Medullary sponge kidney is characterized by ectatic collecting ducts and associated small cysts communicating with these ducts. Such abnormal lumina are common sites for stones. Initially the calculi are small, rounded, or sometimes linear in shape, and located in the region of the pyramids. The appearance is that of a nephrocalcinosis, the underlying anatomic abnormality becoming obvious on urography with demonstration of the dilated collecting ducts (Fig 8–23). Later the concretions can become larger and ulcerate into the pelvicalyceal system, obliterating the early distinctive plain film appearance.

Nephrocalcinosis. Nephrocalcinosis refers to roentgenographically demonstrable, diffuse, small concretions in the renal parenchyma, either cortical or medullary in location, occurring initially in the cells of the tubules as well as in tubular basement membrane and tubular lumina. Later, calcifications are also present in the interstitial tissues of the kidney, with focal scarring. Nephrolithiasis refers to calculi within the pelvicalyceal system. Patients with

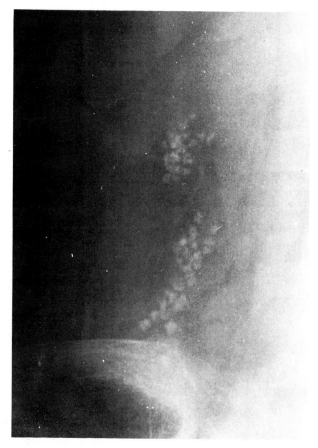

Figure 8–22. Seed calculi in a moderately dilated pelvicalyceal system of a 76-year-old woman with ureteropelvic junction obstruction.

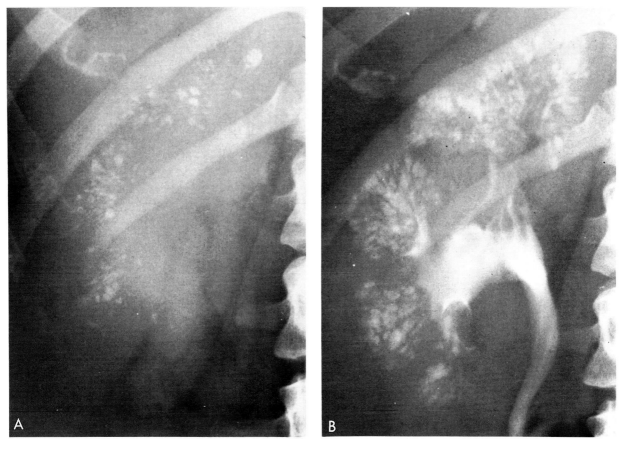

Figure 8–23. Medullary sponge kidney. **A.** Scout radiograph shows clusters of small calculi in the region of the renal pyramids. **B.** Urogram demonstrates that the calculi are in the pyramids, in association with streaks of contrast medium in dilated collecting ducts.

nephrocalcinosis frequently have coexistent nephrolithiasis, the underlying metabolic abnormalities favoring the formation of concretions in both the collecting system and in the parenchyma. Moreover, parenchymal calcifications can gain access to the pelvis and the calyces. Since the concentration of calcium is greater in the pyramids than in the cortex, nephrocalcinosis is more pronounced in the renal medulla, with cellular damage and calcification occurring first in the collecting ducts and long loops of Henle.

The typical radiological appearance consists of clusters of stippled calcifications in both kidneys, most pronounced in the pyramids (Fig 8–24) but, in more severe cases, also found in the cortex. Initially, punctate and diffuse, the calcifications can later become conglomerate and dense. Among the causes of nephrocalcinosis are the following:

1. Hyperparathyroidism. This is most often the primary type.
2. Renal tubular acidosis. In this abnormality there

is an inability or diminished ability to excrete acid urine in response to systemic acidosis. A defect in the proximal tubule results in loss of bicarbonate due to impaired tubular reabsorption of bicarbonate ions. With a distal tubular defect, impairment of the secretion of hydrogen ions leads to cation wasting, including the loss in the urine of calcium ions. Thus, nephrocalcinosis almost always occurs with a distal tubular defect, being rare in proximal renal tubular acidosis.[27]

3. Sarcoidosis. In most of the reported cases with nephrocalcinosis, hypercalcemia was also present. The mechanism for the occurrence of elevated serum calcium in sarcoidosis has not been established; there may be an increased tissue sensitivity to normal vitamin D levels.

4. Bone dissolution, as with patient immobilization, bone metastases, and excess steroids (endogenous or exogenous).

5. Hypervitaminosis D.

6. Idiopathic hypercalciuria.

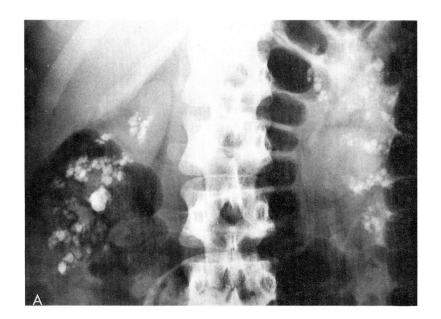

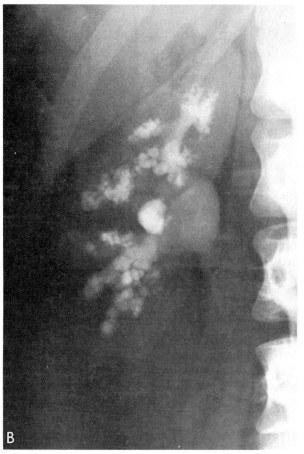

Figure 8–24. Nephrocalcinosis in a 55-year-old woman with renal tubular acidosis. **A.** Scout radiograph shows multiple concretions of varying sizes in both kidneys. **B.** Urogram (right kidney) demonstrates that the concretions occur in the pyramids.

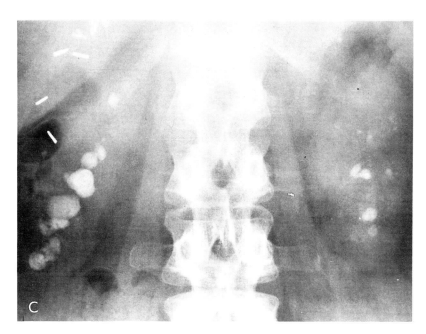

Figure 8–24. (cont.) C. Six years later, there are fewer calculi in each kidney, many having been passed. The remaining calculi are larger than in **A.**

7. Milk–alkali syndrome.
8. Hypothyroidism (Fig 8–25). In some of these patients there is apparently a hypersensitivity to vitamin D.[28]
9. Oxaluria. Increased amounts of oxalate in the urine can result from a primary metabolic defect. There is also an enteric hyperoxaluria, caused by excess ingestion of oxalic-containing substances secondary to derangements in the intestinal tract, such as regional enteritis, distal small bowel resection, and intestinal bypass operations for obesity, resulting in an increasing intestinal absorption of dietary oxalate.[29,30]
10. Wilson's disease (Fig 8–26). Some patients with Wilson's disease have subnormal urinary acidifying capacity.[31]
11. Idiopathic hypercalcemia.

Radiological Characterization of Urinary Tract Concretions. Opacities suspected of being concretions in the kidney can be assessed according to:

1. Location
2. Size
3. Shape
4. Density
5. Mobility

Location. A renal stone should overlie the expected site of the kidney. It must be remembered, however, that abnormalities of renal position can place a concretion in an unusual location, as may be seen with dilatation of the renal pelvis due to ureteropel-

vic junction obstruction or medial placement of inferior calyces in a horseshoe kidney (Fig 8–27).

Size. Concretions in the kidney vary greatly in size, from minute opacities to giant calculi. The largest intrarenal stones occur in proximal long-standing ureteropelvic junction obstruction (Fig 8–28).

Shape. With some renal stones, the shape is distinctive enough to be diagnostic. Examples are the staghorn calculus of the renal pelvis and the triangular calculus of renal papillary necrosis (Fig 8–18).

Density. In addition to its volume, the density of a calculus depends on its calcium content. For a given thickness, calcium oxatate stones are more radioopaque than triple phosphate calculi, and cystine stones are less opaque than calcium-containing concretions (Fig 8–29). A small percentage of uric acid calculi may be faintly opaque if they contain a significant amount of calcium urate.

Axis. If the calcification is linear or oval in shape, it is important to take account of its axis. The orientation of intrarenal stones can be another clue to malrotation of the kidney (Fig 8–27).

Mobility. A helpful plain film feature of some stones is their mobility with respect to the confines of the urinary tract as patient position changes. A calculus in an undilated renal calyx maintains a fixed position relative to the kidney, independent of gravity. On the other hand, a stone lying free in a hydro-

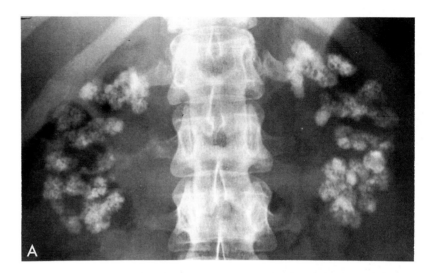

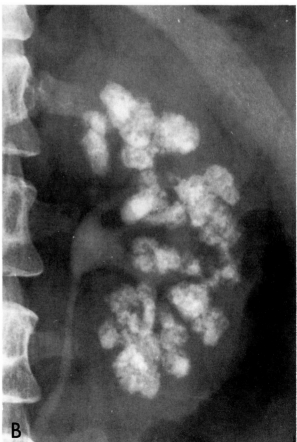

Figure 8–25. Nephrocalcinosis in 23-year-old woman with juvenile hypothyroidism. She has received thyroxine treatment for 14 years. **A.** Scout radiograph shows clusters of calculi in the renal parenchyma bilaterally. **B.** Urogram (left kidney) demonstrates that the calcifications are in the renal pyramids.

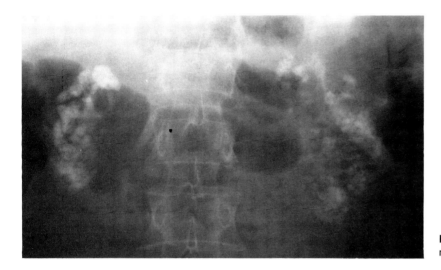

Figure 8–26. Nephrocalcinosis. A 23-year-old man with Wilson's disease.

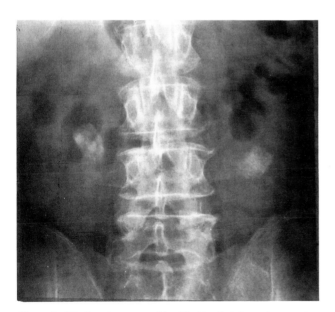

Figure 8–27. Struvite stones, identified by their irregular margins and incomplete calcification, are oriented inferiomedially and overlie the psoas shadow, indicating their location in a horseshoe kidney.

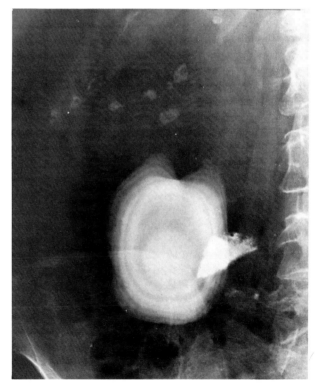

Figure 8–28. Giant, laminated calculus in a dilated renal pelvis secondary to ureteropelvic junction obstruction. There is a triangular collection of barium in the bowel overlying the calculus. The circular calcifications cephalad to the calculus represent calcifications of costal cartilages.

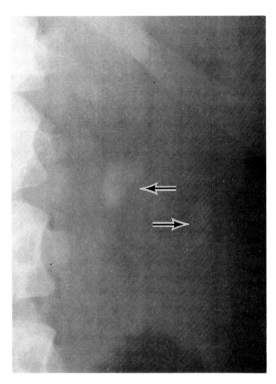

Figure 8–29. Faintly opacified cystine calculi (*arrows*) in the left kidney. A 22-year-old woman with cystinuria. Crystallographic analysis of the removed calculi showed 100% cystine.

nephrotic sac can move within the soft tissue density of the kidney.[32] Similarly, concretions enclosed in renal cysts usually move freely within the cyst, and multiple concretions (seed or milk-of-calcium) layer dependently when assessed by a horizontal beam radiograph (Fig 8–20).

Conduit Calcification

Renal Artery. The renal arteries arise from the abdominal aorta at or near L1 and run horizontally and posteriorly toward the hilum of the kidney, where they then divide into smaller segmental vessels that radiate through the renal parenchyma. Calcification can occur anywhere in the main artery and its branches. On supine films, opacities in the proximal right renal artery may be hidden by the vertebral structures. Placing the patient in the right posterior oblique position can reveal the calcification as the artery moves away from the spine.

Calcification in the walls of the renal arteries has the same radiographic characteristics as calcification in other major abdominal arteries. These linear opacifications are typically of tramline configuration, with the longitudinal plaques of radiodensity most often discontinuous due to separation by uncalcified segments. The calcifications often vary in width, some smooth and pencil thin (Fig 8–30), others appearing chunky and irregular (Fig 8–31).

The orientation of calcification in the renal arteries is a helpful distinguishing feature. Renal artery calcification is usually directed horizontally, unlike ureteral calculi, which follow the vertical course of the ureter. Often, several segmental renal arteries calcify and have a distinctive radiographic appearance as they cross the renal pelvis to enter the parenchyma (Fig 2–103). For the most part, calcification in the main renal arteries is a consequence of atherosclerosis and is accompanied by aortic calcification. If only segmental arteries are involved, it may be a result of either atherosclerosis or diabetes.[33,34]

Rarely, calcification occurs in the wall of a renal vein that has been "arterialized" as a result of a marked increase in its intraluminal pressure and blood flow, as with an ateriovenous fistula. Calcification in a renal vein segment can also accompany venous thrombosis (Fig 8–32).

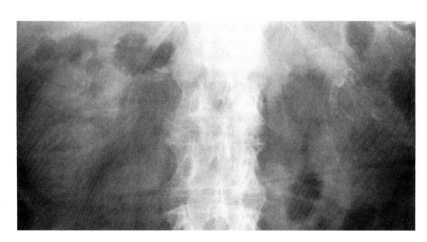

Figure 8–30. Both renal arteries and their branches are markedly calcified, showing the typical branching pattern of tramline calcification.

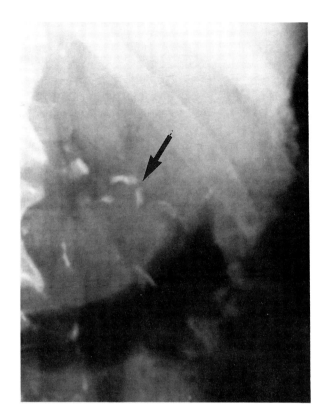

Figure 8–31. Scout radiograph shows discontinuous linear plaques of calcification, varying in width, in the aorta and left renal artery (*arrow*).

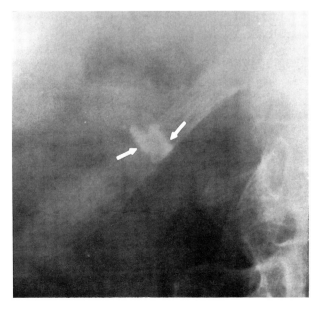

Figure 8–32. Localized calcification in a thrombosed segmental renal vein (*arrows*) draining the upper pole of the right kidney.

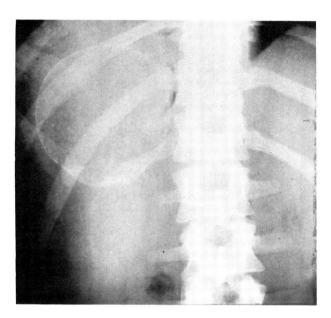

Figure 8–33. Renal cyst. Scout radiograph shows a large right upper quadrant mass with a continuous thin rim of calcification. At operation, this proved to be a renal cyst.

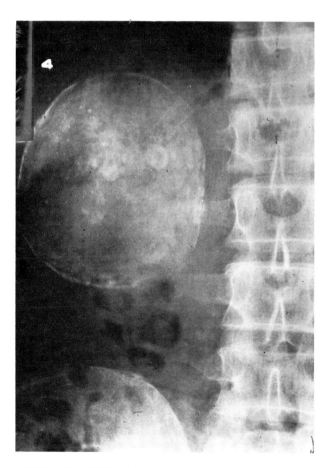

Figure 8–34. Renal adenocarcinoma with cyst wall type of calcification. Scout radiograph shows a large right upper quadrant mass with a thin, somewhat mottled rim of calcification. At operation, this proved to be a renal carcinoma.

Cystic Calcification

Neoplasms of the kidney, both benign and malignant, may show rimlike calcification. In simple cysts, calcium salts are deposited in the wall (Fig 8–33). If the calcification is extensive and of irregular thickness, the radiographic presentation can be deceptive, consisting of both a margin of increased opacity and mottled interior densities. In fact, the central mottling represents calcification of a part of the cyst surface that is not tangential to the X-ray beam but is sufficiently dense to be projected within its margins, thereby simulating the configuration of a solid mass. On the other hand, both carcinomas and adenomas of the kidney may have cystic components, sometimes so pronounced that they dominate the gross appearance of the tumor (Fig 8–34). Also, smooth, annular opacities can characterize primarily solid lesions with calcification in areas of fibrosis, necrosis, and hemorrhage (Table 8–2).

Phillips et al stated that any renal mass containing calcifications is probably a neoplasm rather than a cyst.[35] In their series of 225 cases of renal masses with pathologically proven diagnoses, 72 were cysts, of which 2 (3%) were calcified, and 66 were renal carcinomas, of which 9 (14%) were calcified. Kikkawa and Lasser found radiodensities in 1 of 51 renal cysts and in 11 of 60 hypernephromas, 9 of which had curvilinear calcification.[36] In cancer, the arcuate calcification is present most frequently within the soft tissue mass of the tumor whereas with simple cyst it is located at the very periphery (Figs 8–35, 8–36).[37,38] Daniel et al, reviewing a large series of renal masses, concluded that even though marginal eggshell calcification without interior densities was usually associated with benign simple cysts, the risk of malignancy was still about 20%.[39] Therefore, plain film interpretation cannot ascribe conclusively a cystic lucency to benign disease and corroborating imaging examinations must be done for a full evaluation.

Cystic calcification may be seen in various renal solid tumors. It has been described in oncocytoma,[40] benign papillary adenoma (Fig 8–37),[41] sclerosing lipogranuloma,[41] and even chondrosarcoma of the kidney.[42] There also are a diverse group of fluid-containing lesions with cystic calcification morphology. Rarely, one or more of the many cysts that occur in adult type polycystic kidney may calcify, mimicking the appearance of a radiodense simple cyst.[43] Rimlike opacities also occur infrequently in parapelvic cysts, pararenal pseudocysts, and multilocular cysts (Fig 8–38). Mural calcification and even ossification is sometimes seen in the walls of one or more of the cysts in the multicystic kidney in an adult patient. Calcification is frequent in the lining of a renal echinococcal cyst.[44] Occasionally, several of these calcific parasitic cysts can be confined within a single kidney (Fig 8–39).

Renal artery aneurysms are uncommon, occurring in only 0.01% of autopsies, and yet extensive calcification may be found in 25% of these lesions. Again, the leading cause is atherosclerosis but trauma and infection may also be responsible for aneurysmal dilatation of a renal artery. The aneurysms are almost always saccular and, when calcified, show an incomplete rim of density. Usually, they are between 1 and 3 cm in diameter[45] but may expand into a huge mass that even exceeds the kidney itself in length.[46] Both the main artery and its branches can be involved but most frequently the aneurysm is located near the renal hilus (Fig 8–40).[45]

A right renal artery aneurysm should be distinguished from a round gallstone or a urinary calculus. Stones have a complete margin of radiodensity and may be laminated. Aneurysms of the hepatic or gastroduodenal arteries should also be included in the differential diagnosis but they are both exceedingly rare lesions. On the left side, splenic and renal artery aneurysms are apt to look exactly alike on supine films. A left posterior oblique projection may be helpful because the splenic artery should move anteriorly while the renal artery stays close to the spine within the renal hilus.

Solid Mass Calcification

Hypernephromas comprise 90% of all solid mass type calcification in the kidney (Table 8–3). Streaky, mottled, speckled, or amorphous calcification without sharp margination characterizes the varied appearances of radiodensity in renal cell carcinoma. The opacities may be small and indistinct, easily missed on plain films, or can extend over a large area, occupying much of the kidney (Fig 8–41).

TABLE 8–2. CYSTIC LESIONS OF THE KIDNEY

Cysts
    Simple cysts
    Parapelvic cysts
    Pararenal cysts
    Multilocular cysts
    Adult multicystic kidney
    Polycystic kidney
    Echinoccus granulosis cysts
Tumors
    Hypernephroma
    Oncocytoma
    Papillary adenoma
    Sclerosing lipogranuloma
    Chondrosarcoma
Renal artery aneurysm

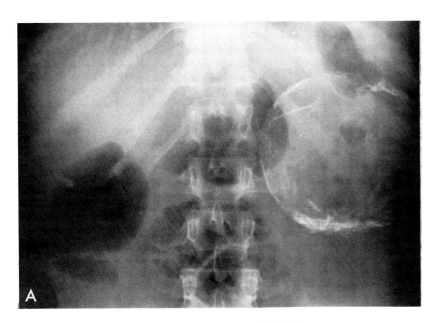

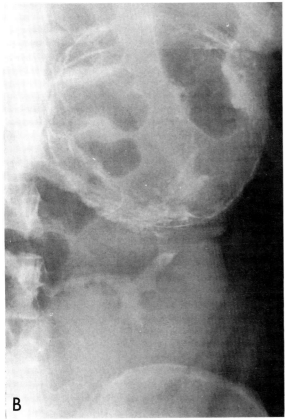

Figure 8–35. Renal cell carcinoma in a 47-year-old woman. **A.** Scout radiograph shows a large left upper quadrant mass with cyst type calcification. **B.** Urogram demonstrates the relationship of the mass to the left kidney. (*Courtesy of Dr. Noel Nathanson.*)

348

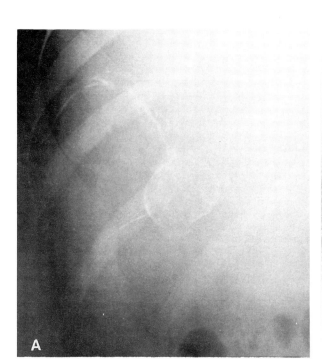
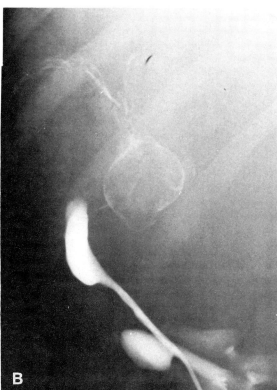

Figure 8–36. Renal cell carcinoma in a 32-year-old man. **A.** Scout radiograph shows linear and rimlike calcification in a right upper quadrant mass. **B.** Retrograde pyelogram demonstrates that the mass is in the right kidney and that the calcification is within the mass rather than at its periphery.

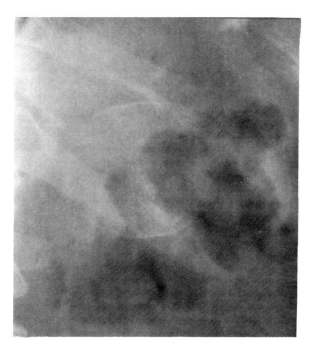

Figure 8–37. Papillary adenoma of the kidney in a 59-year-old man. Scout radiograph shows a thin rim of calcification in a mass in the left upper quadrant. Subsequent urography demonstrated the mass to be in the upper pole of the left kidney. Nephrectomy disclosed a cortical edenoma with cystic necrosis and hemorrhage.

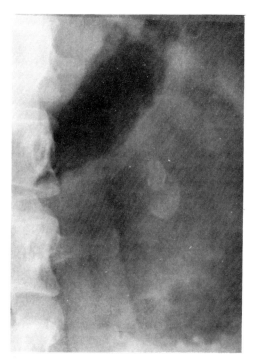

Figure 8–38. Multicystic kidney in a 39-year-old woman. Scout radiograph shows rims of calcification in two of the cysts.

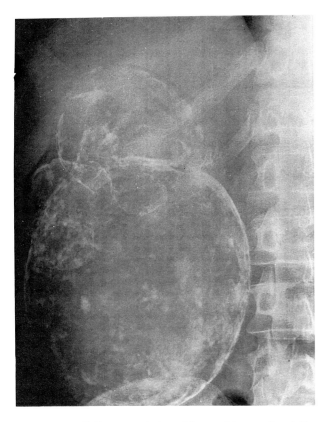

Figure 8–39. Echinococcosis in a 64-year-old man. Scout film shows rimlike calcifications in the walls of the large main cyst as well as of the daughter cysts, located in the right kidney.

Radiodensities discernible on plain films are very rare in transitional cell carcinoma of the kidney. Occasionally, solid type calcification is noted in adult Wilms tumor (Fig 8–42) and renal hamartoma (Fig 8–43). Osteogenic sarcoma, either arising de novo in the kidney (a disease of the middle-aged and elderly) or metastatic from a skeletal focus (a disease of adolescents and young adults), has a unique plain film appearance. The primary renal lesion may have a sunburst configuration (Fig 8–44) whereas renal metastases are more often smoothly rounded (Fig 8–45). In both tumors, the malignant deposits are very dense, much more opaque than nearby bone.[47,48]

The disordered new bone formation of renal osteosarcoma in no way resembles the clearly defined cortex and trabeculae of perirenal teratomas that grow between the adrenal gland and the adjacent kidney. These tumors are encountered at any age, most often in the middle years of life. They are often very large when discovered on physical or roentgenographic examination. Sixty percent of perirenal teratomas ossify and appear on plain films as bulky masses containing bone and even teeth (Figs 2–

120,8–46). The size of the lesion and the extent of calcification are not predictors of biologic activity. Both benign and malignant tumors have similar plain film appearances.[49,50] Metastases to the kidney from nonosseous primary sites are hardly ever radiodense. An exception is lymphoma of the kidney, especially Burkitt's tumor (Fig 8–47), which can calcify after treatment by radiation or chemotherapy.

Renal infarcts calcify infrequently. A characteristic configuration is a fine, mottled density in the infarcted zone.[51] Calcified posttraumatic renal pseudotumor has two patterns of density depending on location. Most often seen in hypertensive patients,[52] the more frequent perirenal hematoma is recognized by an arcuate rim reflecting increased density of the capsule (Fig 8–48) or the wall of a hematogenous cyst. Intrarenal pseudotumor calcification has a more complex roentgenographic appearance, with solid densities interspersed with curvilinear accentuations.[53] Solid mass type calcification has also been reported in a multilocular renal cyst that had been irradiated 3 months previously.[54]

Among inflammatory disease of the kidney, tuberculosis most frequently shows calcification. The radiodensities are first seen near collecting systems arising in necrotic, caseating granulomas. Discrete small calcifications resemble calyceal stones, but as the tuberculomas grow and adjacent lesions coalesce, the calcification assumes a solid mass configuration (Figs 8–49,8–50).[55] Most distinctive of tuberculosis are the amorphous opacities in lobar distribution, a reflection of the lobar type of parenchymal destruction around the calyces. In xanthogranulomatous pyelonephritis, opaque calculi usually predate and very likely produce the obstruction, which, when secondarily affected, leads to chronic infection and destruction of the renal parenchyma. In addition, dystrophic calcification of solid mass type can occur in the tissues damaged by xanthogranulomatous pyelonephritis (Fig 8–51). Calcification seldom occurs in a chronic abscess of the kidney and is very rare in chronic pyelonephritis.

Cortical Calcification. Diffuse cortical calcification is usually related to ischemia. Thrombosis and severe spasm of the intrarenal arteries both can cause much of the cortex to become necrotic except for a narrow zone at its periphery where perfusion is maintained by the capsular arteries and their perforating branches.[56] Central to the necrotic layer is the still viable medulla. Thus, calcium salts can be deposited at two interfaces of necrotic and viable tissue, one between the necrotic layer and the thin peripheral cortical rim and the other between the necrotic layer and the medulla.

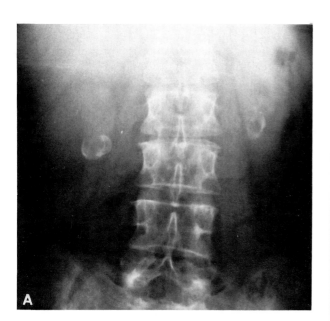

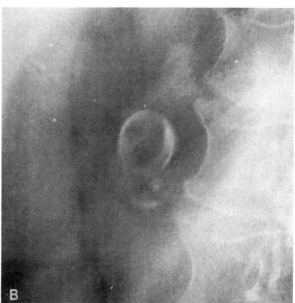

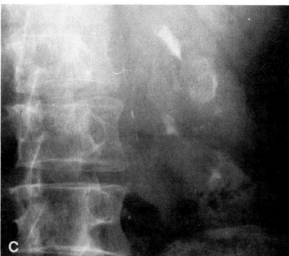

Figure 8–40. Calcified renal artery aneurysms are usually located in the distal main renal artery or in interlobar or segmental arteries. Thus, they remain close to the renal hilus. **A.** Anterior–posterior projection. Circular calcifications near the hila of both kidneys. **B.** Right posterior oblique projection. The calcification stays close to the hilus of the right kidney. **C.** Left posterior oblique projection. The calcification maintains its position within the left kidney.

The classic but rarely observed configuration of cortical calcification is a tramline of increased density encircling the kidney a few millimeters below its capsule.[57] After the acute ischemic episode the kidneys first enlarge, possibly owing to edema, and then gradually shrink.[58,59] It usually takes several weeks for calcium to be deposited in sufficient amounts to be detected on plain films. The calcifications may be either focal and scattered or diffuse (Fig 8–52) and extensive, sometimes extending into the septa of Bertin (renal columns). Ischemia-related cortical calcification has been reported in sickle cell disease,[60] rejected renal transplants (Fig 8–53),[61] and after ingestion of such renal toxins as ethylene glycol and methoxyflurane. It has also been observed in an Alport's syndrome[52] and primary hyperoxaluria,[62] both rare congenital diseases.

Widespread, mottled, or speckled calcification of the kidney located primarily in the cortex occurs rarely in chronic glomerulonephritis. Very few such instances have been described[63–65] since the first report in 1947 of a young man 28 years old at the time of death. Autopsy showed both kidneys to be small, with diffuse, finely nodular calcifications through-

TABLE 8–3. FOCAL SOLID RENAL CALCIFICATIONS

Tumor
  Hypernephroma
  Transitional cell carcinoma
  Adult Wilms' tumor
  Perirenal teratoma
  Osteogenic sarcoma
  Lymphoma (treated)
Infection
  Tuberculosis
  Xanthogranulomatous pyelonephritis
  Chronic renal abscess
Other
  Hamartoma
  Renal infarct
  Intrarenal posttraumatic pseudotumor
  Treated multiolocular cyst

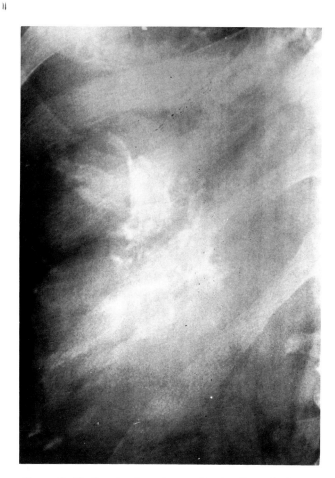

Figure 8–41. Renal cell carcinoma. Scout radiograph shows a large collection of streaky and amorphous calcification, without marginal calcification, in a large mass of the right kidney.

out the cortices. Calcified casts were widely present in the dilated convoluted and collecting tubules of the cortex.[66]

URETER

Ureteral Gas

Endogenous Production. The ureter can fill with gas originating from the renal pelvis or the bladder. Most cases of endogenous gas production result from bacterial metabolism of glucose-rich urine in the vesical lumen. Surprisingly, ureteritis emphysematosa is an unusual concomitant of cystitis emphysematosa. Constriction of the ureterovesical junction is a normal muscular response that prevents reflux and can occur even if gas occupies the bladder lumen. Also, intramural gas cysts in the trigone may narrow the ureterovesical junction, preventing passage of gas into the distal ureter. Moreover, cystitis emphysematosa is almost always a transient abnormality and coexistent intrauteral gas may be an even more evanescent finding.[67] Ureteritis emphysematosa is characterized by an irregular linear lucency, the slight widening and narrowing of the lumen caused by thickening of the ureteral wall (Fig 8–54). Isolated ureteritis emphysematosa is very rare. Its roentgenographic appearance of vertically arranged

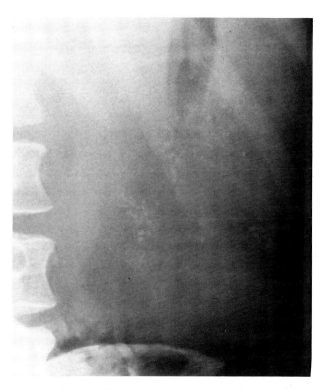

Figure 8–42. Adult Wilms' tumor in a 62-year-old man. Scout radiograph shows speckled calcification, without marginal calcifications, in a large mass of the left kidney.

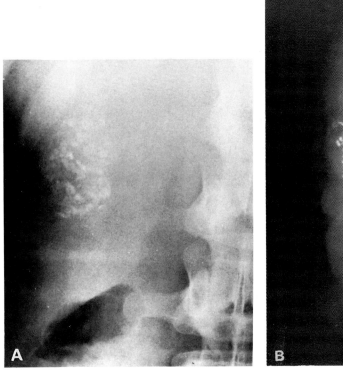
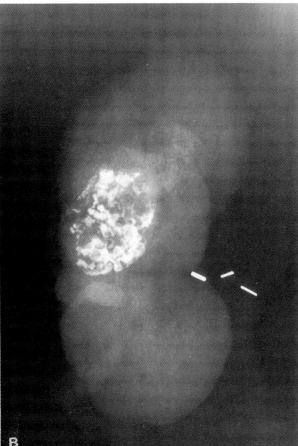

Figure 8–43. Renal hamartoma in a 27-year-old woman. **A.** Scout radiograph shows an oval collection of mottled calcification, without marginal calcification, in the right kidney. **B.** Nephrectomy was done because of the belief that the lesion was malignant. Radiograph of the specimen shows the nature of the calcification clearly. Pathological diagnosis was angiomyoma, a hamartoma containing vascular and muscular elements.

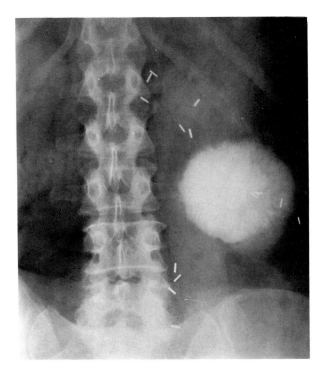

Figure 8–44. Recurrence of a primary osteogenic sarcoma of the left kidney after nephrectomy. The lesion is much denser than normal bone. (*Courtesy of Dr. Chusilp Charnsangavej.*)

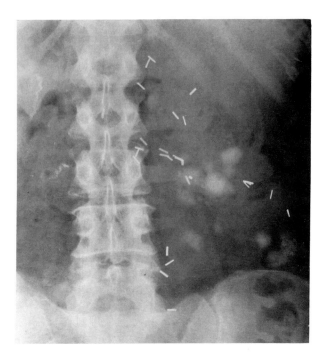

Figure 8–45. Metastases to the kidney from a distal osteogenic sarcoma that recurred after an initial operation. They simulate retained barium. (*Courtesy of Dr. Chusilp Charnsangavej.*)

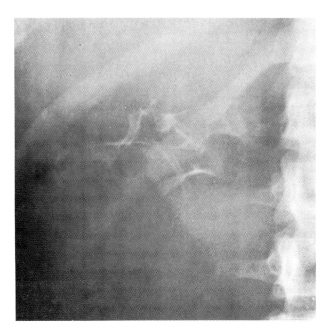

Figure 8–46. Benign teratoma growing between the right adrenal gland and the right kidney. Multiple foci of ossification occupy part of the mass.

intramural and intraluminal gas can simulate pneumatosis cystoides intestinalis.[68]

Fistula. The ureter as well as the bladder can be the terminus of a fistula resulting from communication with the sigmoid colon. Diverticulitis and carcinoma of the colon are the two principal causes of a ureterocolic fistula. Characteristically, the gas-filled lu-

men appears as a featureless, tubular lucency, with smooth margins often expanding superiorly as gas enters the renal pelvis (Fig 8–55). The classic configuration of pneumoureter can be mimicked by air in a rectal tube if it is directed vertically just lateral to the spine, a position sometimes seen after decompression of a sigmoid volvulus (Fig 8–56).

Ureteral Calcification

Nearly all opacities in the ureter are intraluminal calculi. Like stones elsewhere, they share the morphological characteristics of an intact perimeter of radiodensity and a homogeneous or geometric inner architecture (Fig 8–57). Most ureteral calculi have an angulated contour and are quite dense, casting a more opaque shadow than phleboliths or arterial wall calcification (Fig 8–58).

Stones can be seen anywhere along the course of the ureter. In most patients, the ureters run in a paramedian location as they cross the tips of the lumbar vertebral transverse processes and traverse the bony pelvis, overlying the sacroiliac joints and adjacent bones. Within the true pelvis, the ureters converge slightly as they enter the bladder wall at the lateral margins of the trigone (Fig 8–59). There are, however, numerous causes of ureteral deviation, including retroperitoneal fibrosis, retroperitoneal and pelvic masses (Fig 8–60), and longstanding lower urinary tract obstruction, which dilates and elongates the ureteral lumen. In each instance, ureteral stones can be seen some distance from their expected location.

Ureteral calculi can vary greatly in size, from

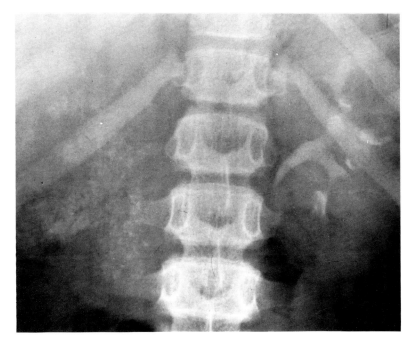

Figure 8–47. Burkitt's tumor of the kidney, treated. Urography shows mottled and speckled calcification in a mass of the right kidney, which is not excreting contrast medium. (*Courtesy of Professor L.R. Whittaker.*)

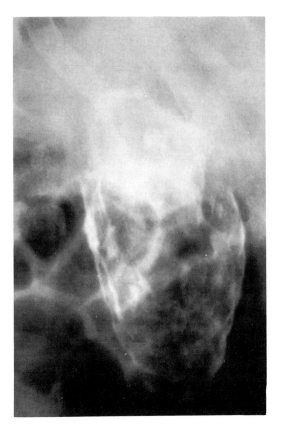

Figure 8–48. Calcification of renal capsule. Scout radiograph shows a peel of calcification surrounding the left kidney, probably the result of an old subcapsular hematoma.

tiny opacities to very large, concretions. Although most calculi lack protuberances, on occasion a stone may have a peculiar configuration, especially if it migrated from its origin in a renal calyx (Fig 8–61). If the calcification is linear or oval in shape it is instructive to take account of its axis. Giant ureteral calculi are often elongated, with the major axis conforming in orientation with the usual direction of the ureter (Fig 8–62). Exceptions can occur; a calculus in a dilated tortuous ureter may be seen with its axis quite askew from the expected vertical direction of the ureteral channel (Fig 8–63). Ureteroceles are mucosal outpouchings of the distal ureter contained within the bladder wall. Stasis of urine in these small sacs promotes the formation of stones that can be identified by their location near the midline and their oblique or horizontal orientation (Figs 2–93,8–64).

A comparison of present radiographs to previous abdominal plain films can be rewarding. If a concretion seen now has been observed, with little change in position or size, for weeks or months or years, it is not likely to be a urinary tract calculus. Conversely, an opacity currently appearing along

the course of the urinary tract but not observed on previous radiographs is apt to be an intraluminal calculus (Fig 8–65). Also, the demonstration of movement on a sequence of radiographs is a valuable sign. A stone overlying the lower segment of the ureter on a later study and shown to have been present earlier in the region of the kidney can be confidently diagnosed as a urinary tract concretion (Fig 8–66). In this regard, it is important to remember that a stone situated in the ureter anterior to the wing of the sacrum or a transverse vertebral process can be hidden by the denseness of bone (Fig 8–67). Hence, a calcification now located in the lower ureter or the ureter could have resided formerly in a proximal segment of a segment obscured by bone. A careful evaluation of the old films may disclose the previously overlooked concretion.

On a single abdominal radiograph it is often difficult to distinguish a calculus in the lower segment of the ureter from a pelvic phlebolith. Several considerations can help in this differentiation. A uri-

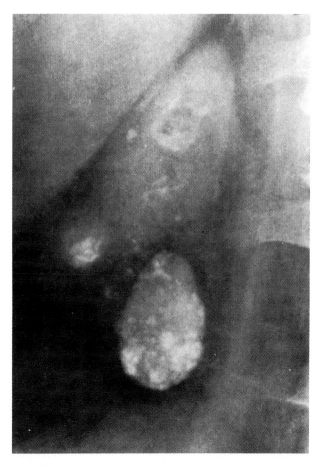

Figure 8–49. Renal tuberculosis. Scout radiograph shows a small right kidney with areas of amorphous and mottled calcification. Subsequent urography demonstrated no excretion of contrast medium by the right kidney.

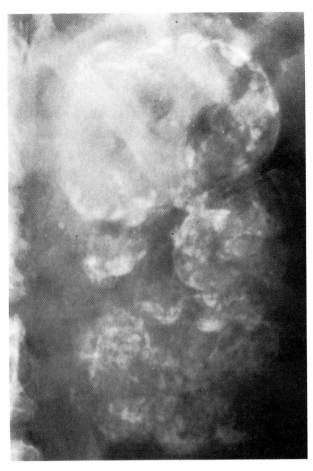

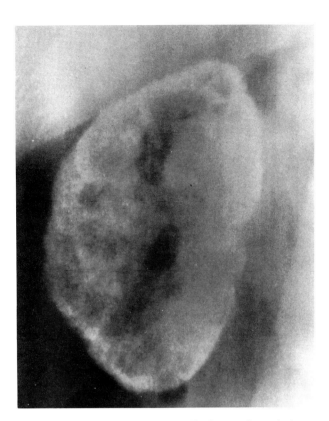

Figure 8–52. Chronic glomerulonephritis. Scout radiograph shows diffuse calcification in the cortex of the small right kidney. The left kidney had a similar appearance. The patient was a 46-year-old man with chronic renal failure.

Figure 8–50. Renal tuberculosis. A scout radiograph demonstrates a very large nonfunctioning left kidney with amorphous calcification in a lobar distribution.

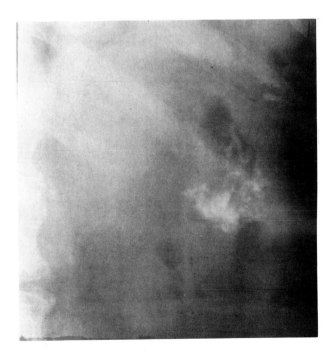

Figure 8–51. Xanthogranulomatous pyelonephritis. Scout radiograph shows a zone of amorphous and streaky calcification, without marginal calcification, in an enlarged left kidney. This kidney did not excrete contrast medium at urography. (*Courtesy of Dr. Robert Shapiro.*)

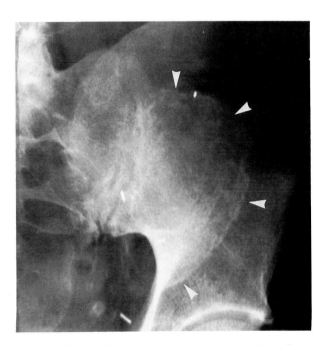

Figure 8–53. Calcification in a rejected renal transplant. Scout radiograph shows discontinuous linear calcifications of varying thickness in the cortex of the renal transplant (*arrowheads*). (*Courtesy of Dr. Arthur Graham.*)

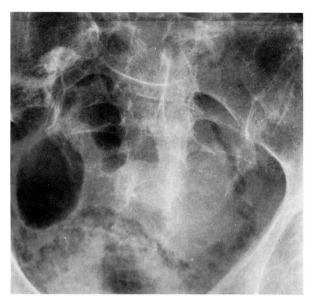

Figure 8–54. Cystitis and ureteritis emphysematosa. Gas is seen in the bladder wall as an irregular curvilinear lucency. The pelvic segment of the left ureter is similarly affected with mural gas.

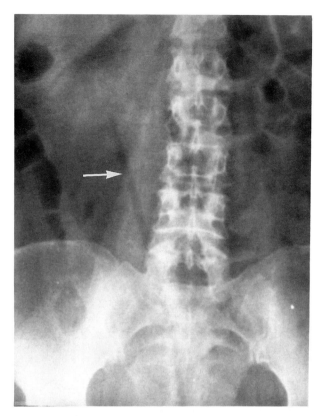

Figure 8–56. Gas in a rectal tube after decompression of a sigmoid volvulus. The gas-filled tube (*arrow*) is rigidly straight, unlike the gentle curves described by a ureter as it descends into the pelvis.

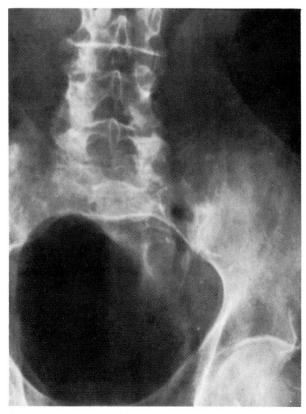

Figure 8–55. Fistula from the sigmoid colon fills the bladder lumen and the left ureter. The ureteral channel is nearly hidden by the lateral aspect of several lumbar vertebral bodies.

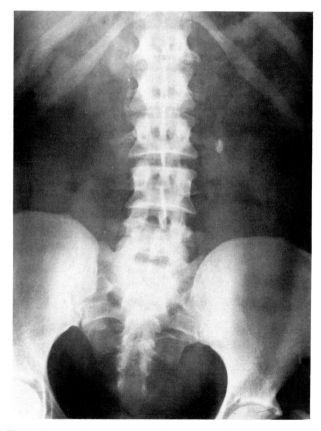

Figure 8–57. Ureteral stone just lateral to the L3 left transverse process. It has the morphological characteristics of a concretion and is oriented along the course of the ureter.

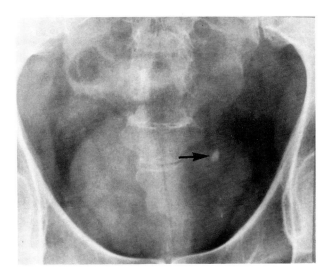

Figure 8–58. A single calcification (*arrow*), to the left of the sacrum is angular rather than round. Subsequent urography proved it to be a ureteral calculus.

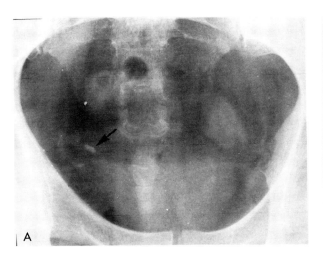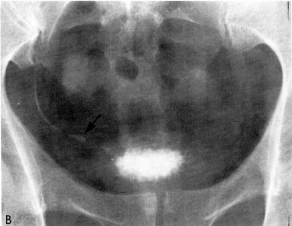

Figure 8–59. Ureteral calculus. **A.** Oval-shaped concretion (*arrow*) with its long axis approaching the horizontal, consistent with the course of the terminal segment of the pelvic ureter. **B.** Urography proves that the calculus is in the ureter (*arrow*).

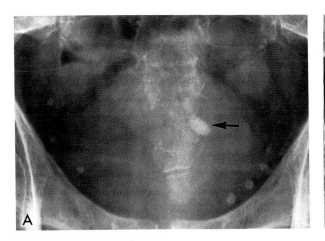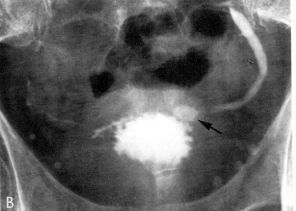

Figure 8–60. Ureteral calcification in unusual location and of unusual axis because of displacement of the ureter by prostatic enlargement. **A.** The ureteral calculus (*arrow*) is located much more medially and its axis is abnormal for the usual location of the ureter. The other rounded concretions are phleboliths. In addition, there are small linear flecks of calcification in pelvic arteries. **B.** Urogram demonstrates that the terminal segment of each ureter has been elevated by an enlarged prostate, the calculus (*arrow*) lying in the distal portion of the left ureter.

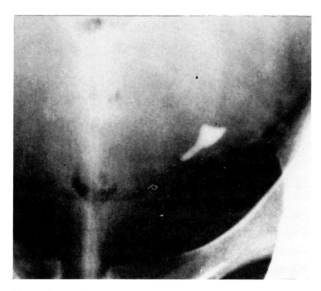

Figure 8–61. Calculus in the lower segment of the left ureter, with the configuration reproducing the shape of a calyx in which it had formed and the axis of the calculus conforming to that of the ureter.

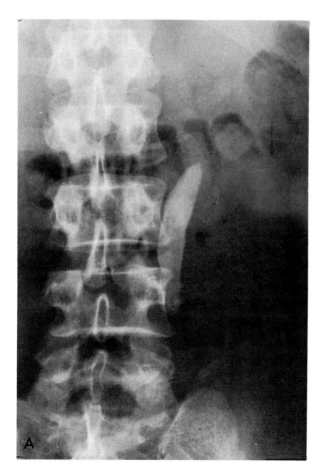

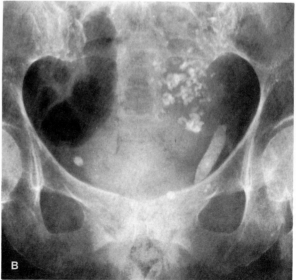

Figure 8–62. Two examples of giant ureteral calculi. **A.** An elongated stone in the proximal left ureter. **B.** A similar appearing concretion in the distal ureter in a woman who has uterine prolapse which is dragging the ureter inferiorly. Calcified phleboliths and a large calcified leiomyoma are also present.

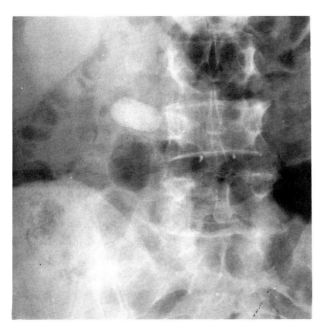

Figure 8–63. Horizontal orientation of a large right ureteral stone. The dilated ureter is elongated and deviated medially at the L4 level. The stone follows the course of the ureter.

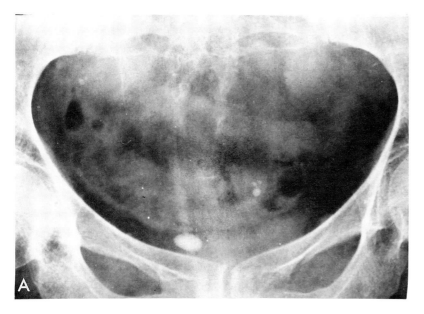

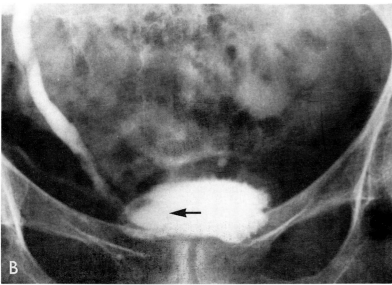

Figure 8–64. A 56-year-old woman with urinary infection. **A.** Scout radiograph shows an oval concretion just above the right pubic bone and at the right side of the soft tissue density of an emptied bladder. The smaller concretions are pelvic phleboliths. **B.** Urography shows the calculus to be in a simple ureterocele (*arrow*).

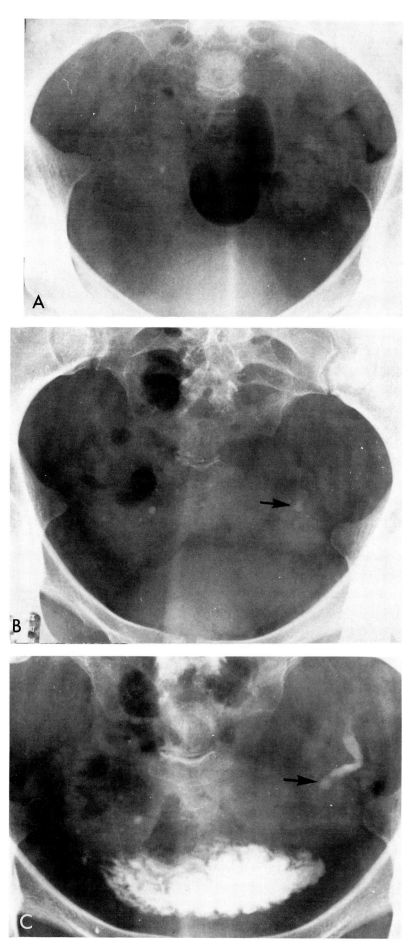

Figure 8–65. Ureteral calculus. **A.** Scout radiograph shows several small round concretions in the right side of the pelvis. These are phleboliths, most likely in a uterine vein. Note that there are no calcifications in the left side of the pelvis. **B.** Scout radiograph 9 days later shows a triangular calcification in the left side of the pelvis (*arrow*). **C.** Urography proves that this new calcification is a ureteral calculus (*arrow*).

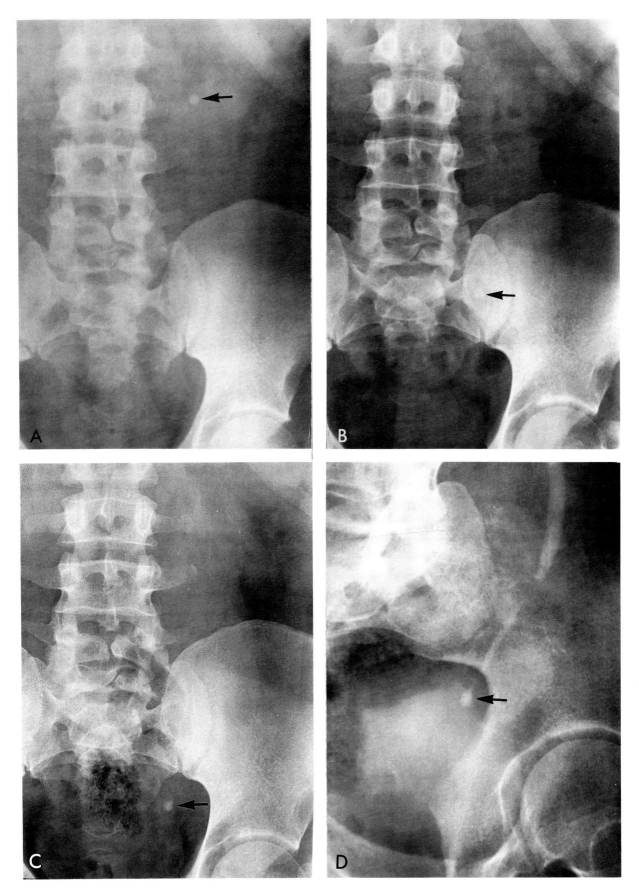

Figure 8–66. Ureteral calculus. **A.** Scout radiograph shows a round concretion (*arrow*) in the region of the left kidney. **B.** Scout radiograph 3 days later shows no calcification in relation to the left kidney. Note, however, that the calcification (*arrow*) overlies the sacrum and is hidden by the bone density. **C.** Scout radiograph, 7 days after **B,** demonstrates that the calcification (*arrow*) has moved caudally into the pelvis. **D.** Urography, in left posterior oblique position, proves the presence of a ureteral calculus (*arrow*).

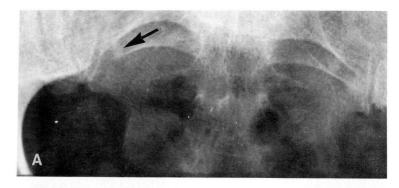

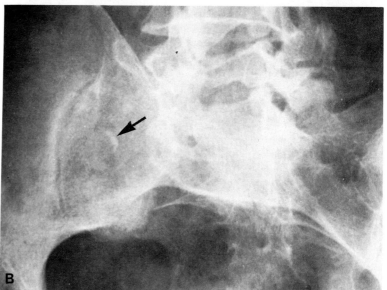

Figure 8–67. Ureteral calculus hidden by sacrum. **A.** There is a barely visible calcification (*arrow*) overlying the right wing of the sacrum, the long axis of the calcification conforming to the expected course of the ureter. **B.** With the patient in the right posterior oblique position, the calculus (*arrow*) is seen more clearly. Subsequent urography proved the calcification to represent a ureteral calculus.

nary tract calculus is almost always homogeneously dense; a venous stone is apt to have a lucent center or several interior lucencies. A phlebolith tends to be round while a ureteral calculus is typically angulated. Although calcified pelvic phleboliths are usually multiple, ureteral calculi are most often solitary (Fig 8–68).

Arising from the pelvis, each gonadal vein runs parallel and very close to its ipsilateral ureter. Phleboliths in the ovarian vein are not rare in middle-aged and elderly women.[69] Like those in the pelvis, they tend to be circular, with only a marginal rim of calcification, usually markedly different in appearance from the diffuse opacification of a ureteral stone (Fig 2–97). In some cases, however, an unequivocal identification of either a gonadal vein phlebolith or a urinary calculus cannot be made on plain films alone, and intravenous urography is required for a definitive determination.

The movement of ureteral stones is primarily

under the influence of hydrostatic pressure and peristalsis, which can be increased by diuretic medication and increased fluid consumption. Erect positioning may also hasten the passage of stones. Decubitus and upright views can demonstrate a layering of suspension of stones in a milk-of-calcium ureter, a rare finding seen much less often than milk-of-calcium in the collecting system or in a renal cyst.[70]

Almost all ureteral stones originate from the kidney. The successful passage of a calculus depends on its size. Concretions greater than 1 cm in diameter usually do not pass, becoming impacted in either the upper or middle third of the ureter. A stone must be at least 2 mm in its greatest diameter to be seen on plain film. Approximately 80% of calculi less than 4 mm in length negotiate the entire ureter and reach the bladder lumen. Ureteral concretions between 4 and 10 mm in diameter migrate with more difficulty. A serrated appearance to a dis-

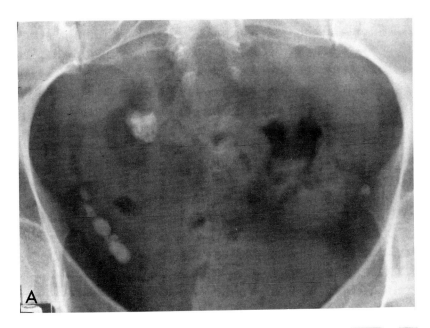

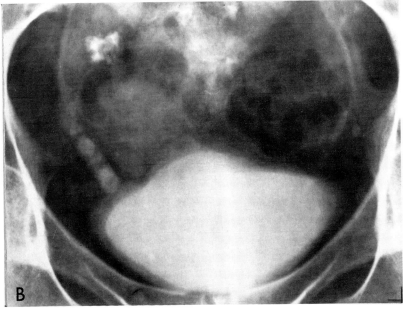

Figure 8–68. Ureteral calculi. **A.** Scout radiograph shows a line of homogeneously dense calculi, of different sizes and shapes, in the region and alignment of the lower segment of the right ureter. The triangular shape of some of the calculi would be most unusual for phlebolith. The concretion near the left ischial spine is round and has a central lucency, characteristic of a phlebolith. The irregular, somewhat mottled calcification overlying the right border of the sacrum is in a uterine fibroid. **B.** Intravenous urogram demonstrates the relationship of the ureters to the various calcifications.

tal stone is a sign of impaction. The obstruction is not usually complete, as some urine usually manages to bypass the calculus.[71]

Calcification in the Ureteral Wall. By far the most common cause of calcification of the ureteral wall is schistosomiasis (*Schistosoma haematobium*), usually seen as a continuous layer of wall calcification. The lower ureteral segments are involved most frequently, but the opacity can extend the entire length of the ureter to the renal pelvis. The calcification, stimulated by the deposit of dead ova, occurs primarily in the submucosa but may also involve the

muscle layers and the adventitia. It appears on the radiograph as parallel thin, smooth lines defining the normal ureteral lumen, or, if the ureters are dilated, as converging curvilinear calcification (Fig 8–69, 8–87) or, occasionally, as mottled collections of calcification. Nearly always there is also calcification of the bladder wall.

Tuberculosis of the ureter results usually in fibrotic narrowing of the lumen, with wall calcification appearing only infrequently and then usually in the lower ureteral segment. Focal mural calcification of a granular pattern can be seen in any ureteral segment in amyloidosis of the urinary tract.[72]

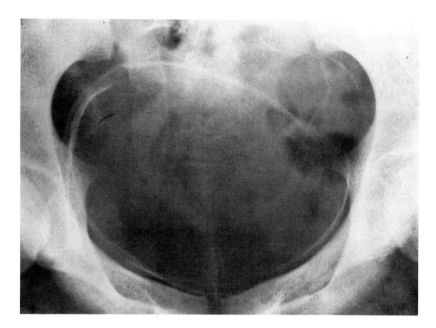

Figure 8–69. Schistosomiasis in a 16-year-old African female. Scout radiograph shows thin curvilinear calcification of the bladder wall. Thin lines of calcification define dilated and tortuous ureters. Because of fibrosis and distortion of the trigone, the ureteral orifices may be close to each other, as in this patient.

BLADDER

Vesical Enlargement

A dilated, urine-filled bladder is a common finding, mostly a consequence of lower urinary tract obstruction, neurological impairment, or an obtunded sensorium. If this distended, hollow viscus is surrounded by sufficient pelvic fat, it can be discerned easily on radiographs of the abdomen, with its rounded lateral and superior margin clearly demarcated (Fig 8–70). In many cases of vesical dilatation, however, plain film evidence is surprisingly meager even when the bladder contains more than 2 L of fluid. In patients lacking a prominent envelope of pelvic adipose tissue, the lateral borders of the bladder may not be discerned clearly (Fig 2–87). Similarly, the water density of the cystic wall and its luminal contents do not stand out in relation to the anterior abdominal wall or to fluid-containing bowel loops. Displacement of anteriorly situated air-filled intestinal segments is a helpful sign but one that is seen only occasionally. In order not to miss massive bladder enlargement on plain films there must be a consideration of its likelihood in a particular patient (Fig 8–71). A homogeneous grayness to the soft tissue of the pelvis should be regarded with suspicion. In women, pelvic masses can be mistaken for vesical enlargement. Recognition of the location of the thin fat plane often separating the bladder wall from the uterus can help identify a nondistended bladder. This bordering fat stripe need not be present, however, even in normal patients.

Bladder Gas

Gas in the Bladder Lumen. The most frequent cause of lucencies within the bladder lumen is the spontaneous generation of gas by microorganisms in infected urine. Once called primary pneumaturia, it should now be considered as a manifestation of

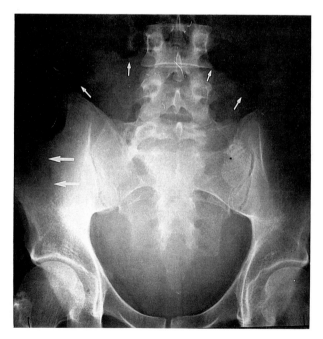

Figure 8–70. Distended bladder. The superior border abuts bowel loops (*small arrows*) and the right lateral border is seen next to fat (*large arrows*).

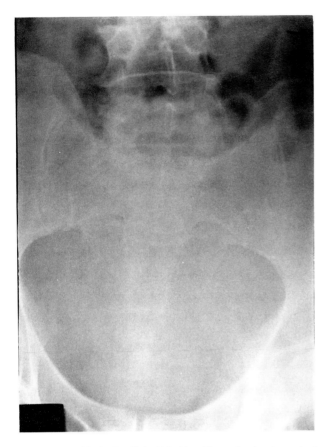

Figure 8–71. Markedly dilated bladder. The only clue to vesical enlargement is a homogeneous grayness to the pelvis.

cystitis emphysematosa—a response to infection in which gas may accumulate in either the vesical wall or lumen. The usual offending organisms are *Escherichia coli* and *Aerobacter aerogenes,* but *Staphylococcal aureus, Proteus mirabils,* and various *Streptococcus* species have also been implicated.[73] In most instances, the affected individuals are diabetics in poor control of blood sugar. Glycosuria is an excellent substrate for the proliferation of these bacteria, which are capable of splitting glucose into carbon dioxide and hydrogen. Absence of glycosuria can be expected in some cases, however, as all the sugar may be metabolized by the urinary pathogens.[74] *Candida albicans* also ferments sugar and the gas collects in the lumen, sometimes even within a growing intravesical fungus ball. *Candida* infection occurs in diabetics and in patients with immunodepression from debilitation, malignancy, or steroid therapy. Rarely, intraluminal gas can develop from the bacterial digestion of albumen.[75]

The risk of the spontaneous generation of intraluminal gas is increased with urinary retention. Hence, it is more common in individuals with neurogenic bladder, prostatic hypertrophy, cystocele,

and bladder diverticula. Women are affected about twice as often as men and the condition is usually found in the middle-aged and in the elderly. Typically, patients are unaware of pneumaturia, presenting instead with dysuria, fever, or, rarely, hematuria.[76] Therapy consists of relief of obstruction, treatment of infection, and control of blood glucose. In most cases, the intraluminal lucency resolves after a few days of medical management.

Air can be introduced into the bladder during instrumentation, but it is usually a temporary phenomenon, rarely persisting for more than a few hours. Gas can enter the vesical lumen from fistula with the intestines or the vagina, but only small amounts are present at any time, never enough to distend the bladder. Clostridial infection may fill the lumen and infiltrate the wall with gas, a rare and disastrous complication seen with long-term cyclophosphamide therapy.[77]

Gas within the bladder lumen appears as a featureless homogeneous lucency overlying the pelvis (Fig 8–72). It is easily distinguished from the rectal air shadow, which is delimited by the valves of Houston and further identified by the soft tissue density of retained fecal matter. Marked distension of the bladder by gas may extend the vesical lucency into the abdomen (Fig 8–73), where it can be mistaken for a cecal volvulus or a giant air-filled sigmoid diverticulum.[78]

Intramural Gas. Gas in the bladder wall, the other roentgenographic manifestation of cystitis emphysematosa, is about as common as intraluminal gas, and in many patients the two appear together (Fig 8–74). Interstitial and intraluminal gas have the same prognostic implications, and a combination of these two findings does not indicate a more complicated course or a more advanced infection. Intramural gas is nearly pathognomonic for urinary tract infection. It may, however, be seen infrequently and for several hours only as an innocuous finding immediately following transurethral resection of the prostate. Gas, either carbon dioxide, carbon monoxide, or sulfur dioxide, is probably induced by the high temperature at the cutting edge of the resectoscope and enters the bladder wall through destroyed mucosa in the prostatic urethra.[79]

Interstitial gas appears en face as a collection of small bubbles each no more than 1 cm in diameter. Such an agglomeration of rounded lucencies often has a cobblestone configuration. In profile, gas in the bladder wall is recognized by an arcuate or ring-like accumulation of bubbles or as a curvilinear streak confined to the edge of the bladder shadow (Fig 8–76).

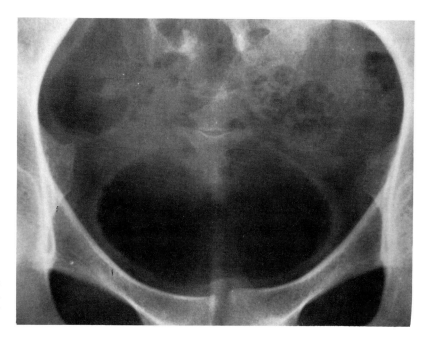

Figure 8–72. Air in the lumen of the bladder. The ovoid lucency is featureless with a smooth, nonindented border. It is bisected by the midline.

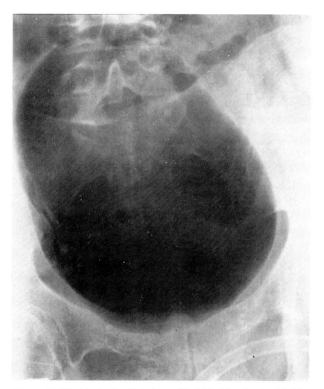

Figure 8–73. Markedly dilated gas-filled bladder. As the bladder ascends into the abdomen it often loses its oval or circular configuration, becoming more elongated like a distended colonic loop.

Cystitis emphysematosa should be distinguished from other lucencies in the pelvis. Gas-forming abscesses typically appear as contiguous, rounded lucencies. Vaginitis emphysematosa, a rare disease occurring most often in pregnancy and in the puerperium, can be recognized as a collar of bubbles in the mid pelvis situated well above the symphysis pubis (Fig 9–4). Emphysema of the uterine wall is characterized by large bubbles located in the upper pelvis conforming to the shape of a distended uterus (Fig 2–50). Gas in sigmoid diverticula and in pneumatosis cystoides intestinalis of the distal colon both follow the course of the large bowel and are not usually positioned astride the midline in the lower pelvis. Finally, a layer of adipose tissue abutting on the lateral or superior vesical wall may mimic the streaky lucency of mural gas (Fig 8–77). The fatty lucency does not change on sequential films whereas gas in the wall should disappear over a few days.

Calcifications in the Bladder

Bladder Calculi. Stones may enter the bladder lumen as migrants from the upper urinary tract. Such calculi are rarely seen on plain radiographs because of their small diameter, which enables them to pass through the ureterovesical junction, and promptly transit through the bladder into the urethra. Occasionally, they may remain in the vesical lumen for some time, where they can be distinguished from phleboliths or distal ureteral stones by their mobil-

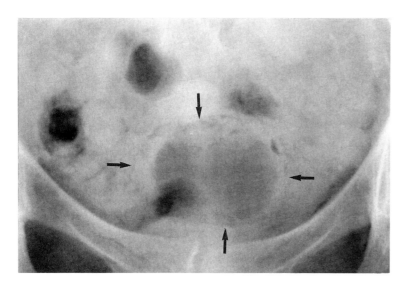

Figure 8–74. Gas in the vesical lumen and wall. The central round lucency represents luminal gas. A faint strip of decreased density, concentric with the lumen (*arrows*), is intramural gas.

ity, as demonstrated on supine, prone, and decubitus views.

In the Middle East and the Orient, primary bladder calculi are often seen in children, especially boys, who are free of obstruction, infection, or congenital abnormalities in the urinary tract. These concretions, when radiopaque, contain calcium oxalate or calcium phosphate. They come to attention with the presenting complaints of dysuria or interruption of the urinary stream. More common among the poor, primary bladder calculi may be related to a specific but as yet undetermined dietary deficiency.[80]

In the United States, almost all bladder concretions occur in the presence of stasis. Ninety-eight percent of affected patients are elderly men, but on occasion stones may be seen in women with large cystoceles.[75] Urinary retention, resulting from prostatic enlargement or neuropathic bladder dysfunction are the most usual predisposing factor in calculi formation.

Single bladder calculi vary in appearance from barely perceptible radiodensities to brightly opaque concretions. Usually, they are situated at or close to the midline near the center of the bladder shadow.

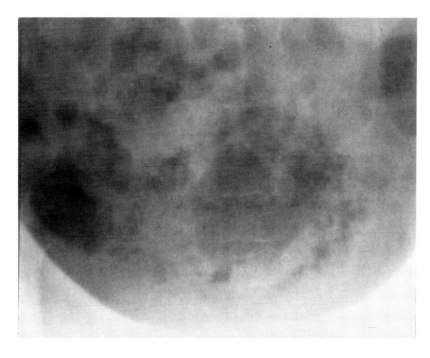

Figure 8–75. Intramural bladder gas. A ring of tiny bubbles outlines the wall of a nondistended bladder.

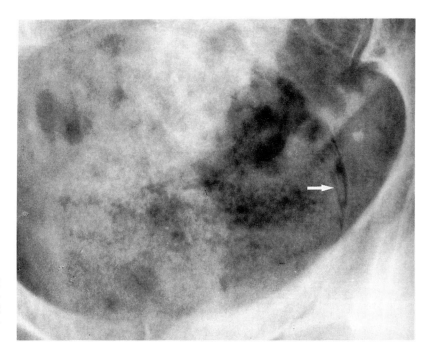

Figure 8–76. Focal accumulation of vesical wall gas. The patient also has a feces-filled distended rectum. The curvilinear streak at the left lateral bladder wall (*arrow*) identifies cystitis emphysematosa.

Most are smoothly rounded and diffusely calcific but sometimes a few laminations are seen near the stone periphery (Fig 8–78). Occasionally, a calculus may continue to grow in the bladder, eventually becoming huge, nearly filling the entire lumen.[81] Rarely, a solitary bladder concretion has a peculiarly distinctive shape. The stellate or jackstone stone, a large calcium oxalate density, is easily recognizable by its spiculations radiating in all directions from the center of the calculus (Figs 2–9,8–79). The dumbbell-shaped stone occurs in the urinary bladder, with the waist of the dumbbell at the bladder outlet, the

cephalad, expanded portion at the bladder base, and the caudal portion in the postprostatectomy urethral fossa (Fig 8–80).

Multiple vesical concretions are usually of similar shape and radiographic density. They can vary in size but generally the majority of stones have similar dimensions. As they fill the vesical space, they are apt to develop faceted edges. Bladder stones are usually arrayed throughout the lumen, but with intravesical growth of an enlarging prostate gland, the calculi are displaced toward the superior and lateral zones of the vesical shadow, the

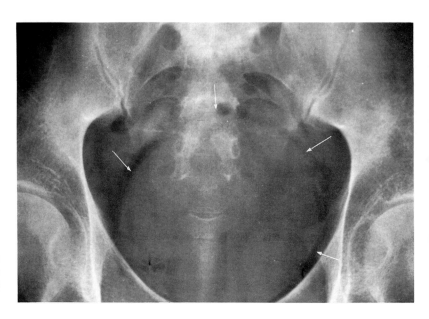

Figure 8–77. An encircling lucency (*arrows*) clearly outlines a distended bladder. Despite its narrow width, the lucency is not vesical wall gas but surrounding pelvic fat.

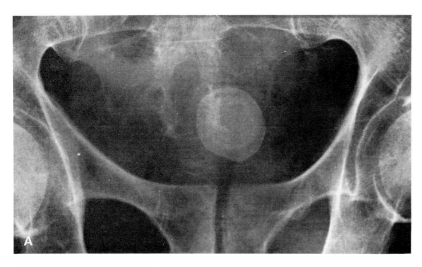

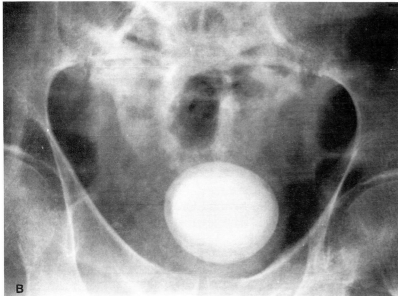

Figure 8–78. Two typical bladder stones. Both are round with a continuous rim of calcification and marginal laminations. The stone in **A** is faintly opaque while the stone in **B** is brightly radiodense.

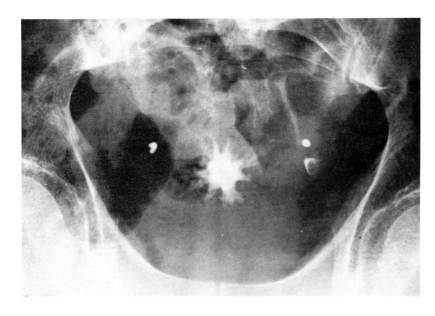

Figure 8–79. Stellate calculus in the urinary bladder. The three smaller opacities of metallic density represent barium in sigmoid diverticula.

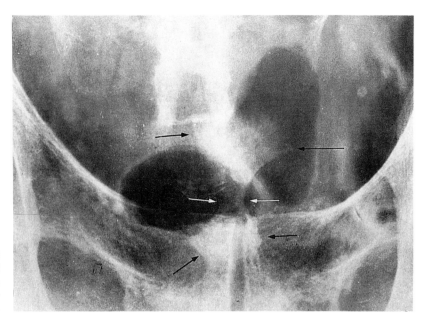

Figure 8–80. Dumbbell-shaped calculus at the bladder outlet. A 79-year-old man, who had had a prostatectomy in the past, now has hematuria. The white arrows point to the waist of the calculus and the black arrows to its expanded ends.

distribution resembling a corona beneath the bladder dome (Fig 8–81).

Vesical diverticula, subject to stasis and infection, are also likely sites for stone formation (Fig 8–82). Sometimes calculi are seen only in these outpouchings, with the bladder lumen free of concretions (Fig 8–83). A dumbbell-shaped stone may form here as well, with the diverticular neck confining its narrowest part.

A final type of endogenous bladder calculus has a foreign body core around which is deposited calcium phosphate. The nidus is most often a fragment of a ruptured Foley catheter balloon. Other sub-

stances implicated in stone formation include bone fragments from a pelvic fracture, metallic wires, indwelling nondilated catheters, nonabsorbable suture material,[80] and intact Foley balloons.[82] Even pubic hairs, introduced during intermittent catheterization in patients with neurogenic bladders, have been nidi, the stones having a serpentine configuration.[83]

Vesical Wall Calcification. In Europe and North America, bladder wall calcification is an unusual plain film finding occurring predominantly in malignant neoplasms (Table 8–4). Roentgenographi-

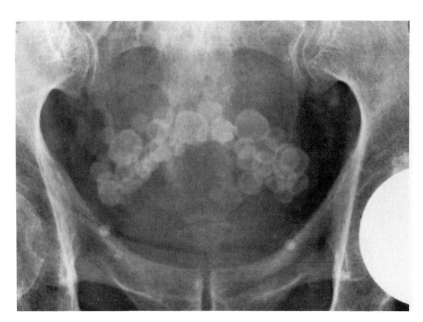

Figure 8–81. Multiple vesical calculi, the unusual configuration of the collection due to an enlarged prostate.

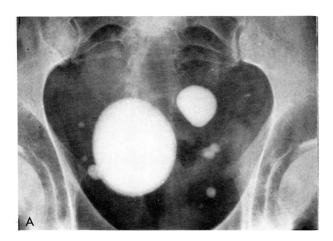

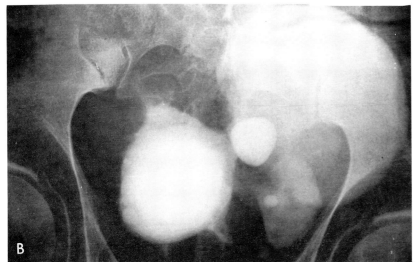

Figure 8–82. Calculus in the bladder and calculus in a vesical diverticulum. **A.** Scout radiograph shows two large dense concretions; both could be calculi in the bladder, but despite changes in the patient's position, such as decubitus projections, the calculi maintained a separation from each other. The other, smaller concretions are pelvic phleboliths. **B.** Cystogram demonstrates the larger dense calculus to be in the ladder and the other to be in a large vesical diverticulum, near the neck of the diverticulum. There is also a smaller diverticulum.

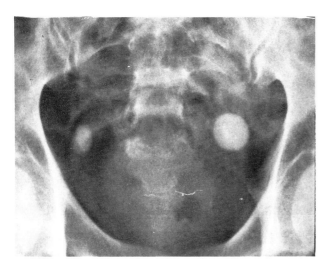

Figure 8–83. A single calcified stone in each of two superiolateral vesical diverticula. The bladder lumen contained no calculi.

TABLE 8–4. BLADDER CALCIFICATIONS

Calculi
  Migrant stones
  Primary bladder calculi
  Secondary calculi
  Foreign body nidus stones
Wall calcification
  Carcinoma
    Transitional cell
    Squamous cell
    Undifferentiated
  Other tumors
    Hemangioma
    Leiomyosarcoma
    Osteogenic sarcoma
    Pheochromocytoma
  Schistosoma haematobium infestation
  Tuberculosis
  Amyloidosis
  Bladder wall encrustation
    Infection (usually *Proteus*)
    Cyclophosphamide toxity
    Radiation cystitis

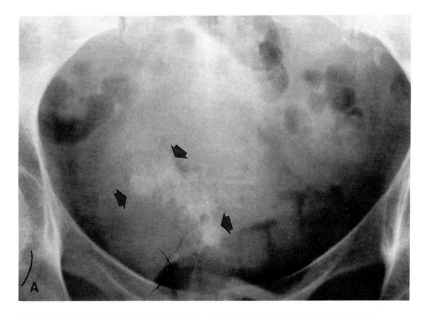

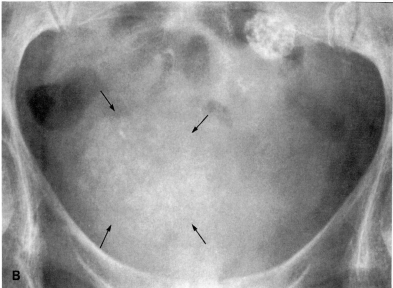

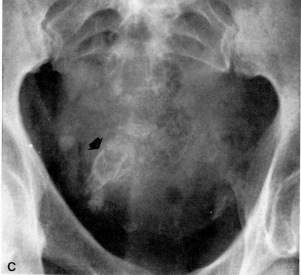

Figure 8–84. Three examples of calcifications in a bladder carcinoma. **A.** Squamous cell carcinoma of the bladder. Scout radiograph shows a poorly defined zone of hazy, amorphous calcification (*arrows*) in the region of the urinary bladder. (*Courtesy of Dr. Stanford Goldman.*) **B.** Undifferentiated carcinoma of the bladder. Scout radiograph shows a large collection of nodular, faint calcifications (*arrows*) in the region of the urinary bladder. The dense, mottled calcification at the brim of the pelvis is in a uterine fibroid. **C.** Keratinizing squamous cell carcinoma of the bladder. Scout radiograph shows several scattered zones of amorphous calcification, some with linear dense rims (*arrow*), in the region of the urinary bladder.

cally detectable calcification is seen in only 0.5% of bladder tumors,[84] although it is recognized with much greater frequency on specimen radiographs and histological sections.[85] Calcium salts can be deposited in both sessile and papillary sections of a tumor either as surface encrustations or as dystrophic agglomerations deeper in the lesion.[80] Calcification has been noted in transitional cell, squamous cell, and undifferentiated carcinoma;[86] in each type of tumor it has several roentgenographic patterns, including fine speckling, coarse nodular densities, and faint linear accumulations (Fig 8–84).[87] The opacities may be focal or extensive, appearing either de novo or after treatment by chemotherapy or radiation.

Bladder wall calcification has been noted in hemangioma,[88] leiomyosarcoma,[89] and even osteogenic sarcoma of the bladder.[89] A ringlike density can be a plain film manifestation of a bladder pheochromocytoma.[90] To be differentiated from tumor calcification in a bladder neoplasm is postoperative ossification occurring at the site of a scar in the soft tissues of the lower anterior abdominal wall. Heterotopic bone formation may occur following surgery on the urinary bladder via a suprapubic approach. On supine radiographs, it projects over the location of bladder, and thus can be confused with vesical calcification (Fig 8–85). The diagnosis can be made easily by physical examination, with the palpation of a stony hard mass or a plaque in the surgical scar. Radiographically, the opacity is much more dense and more sharply outlined than vesical neoplasm calcification. Also, a radiograph obtained in the oblique projection demonstrates that the calcification is not coterminous with the urinary bladder.

Worldwide, infestation by *Schistosoma haemato-*

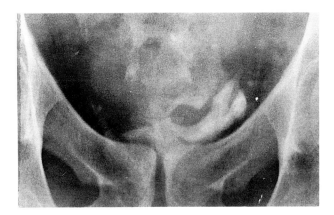

Figure 8–85. Ossification in abdominal surgical scars. Scout radiograph shows a zone of calcification (ossification), just above the symphysis and left pubic bone. The patient, a 58-year-old man, underwent cystostomy and two-stage urethroplasty for urethral stricture, about 6 months before.

bium is the most common cause of mural calcification of the bladder. The roentgenographic pattern is distinctive. Beginning at the base of the bladder, the calcification advances continuously, ultimately involving the entire vesical wall (Fig 8–86) and often extending into the ureters (Fig 8–69, 8–87).[91] It appears in the distended bladder as a thin, arcuate calcification, usually without focal interruptions, a configuration reminiscent of calcified cysts. Nevertheless, since the bladder wall retains pliability, the smooth cystic calcification of the full urinary bladder may appear irregular and corrugated once the bladder is evacuated (Fig 8–87). With the development of carcinoma, a well-recognized complication of vesical schistosomiasis, a plain radiograph may show a discontinuity of the rim of calcification, the break resulting from invasion of the bladder wall by the malignant neoplasm. Uncommonly, calcification in the trigone is of flocculent type. The intensity of bladder calcification in schistosomiasis is related directly to the number of dead ova in the venules of the submucosa, muscularis, and adventitia. Approximately 50% of patients with vesical bilharziasis have roentgenographically demonstrable bladder wall calcification.[92]

With urinary tract tuberculosis, renal calcification is relatively common, ureteral calcification is infrequent, and bladder calcification is rare. In the bladder, the calcification can appear as dense clumps scattered diffusely in the wall, possibly representing calcification in a zone of caseation in the mucosa (Fig 8–88). Tuberculosis can also produce a faint and irregular rim of mural calcification.[93]

Necrosis of the bladder mucosa from any cause in the presence of urine of high pH can result in calcium deposits on the mucosa of the bladder wall, a condition known as alkaline encrusting cystitis.[33,34] The cause of mucosal necrosis may be radiation therapy, cytoxan-induced cystitis, severe urinary infection, or chemical toxins instilled directly into the bladder. The opacity consists of calcium phosphate or struvite.[94,95] Urine of high pH can be due to infection by a urea-splitting organism, usually a species of *Proteus*, a high alkaline dietary load, an isolated renal acidification defect, or chronic pyelonephritis in association with nonrespiratory acidosis.[96] The patterns of calcification are protean, with flocculent, nodular, and curvilinear configurations having been noted.

A rare cause of bladder calcification is amyloidosis. The submucosal accumulation of amyloid in branches of the vesical arteries can promote ischemia and the dystrophic deposition of calcium salts in a nodular or coarsely granular pattern in the bladder wall.[72]

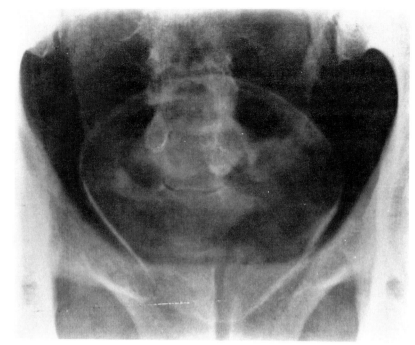

Figure 8–86. *Schistosoma haematobium* infestation. Continuous marginal calcification in a distended bladder.

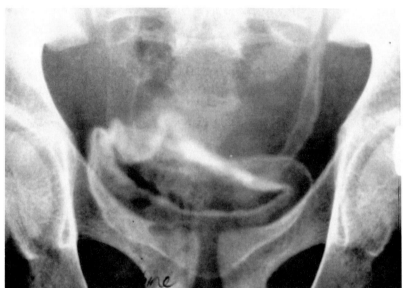

Figure 8–87. Schistosomiasis. Scout radiograph shows a continuous, partly wrinkled rim of calcification in the wall of the empty bladder of a 16-year-old male with schistosomiasis. Note the conduit type of calcification in the walls of the ureters.

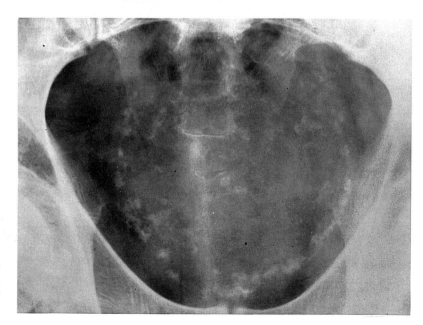

Figure 8–88. Tuberculosis of the urinary bladder. Scout radiograph shows scattered, poorly marginated calcific nodules of varying sizes in the wall of the bladder. (*Courtesy of Dr. Joseph Toth.*)

URETHRA

Except for their presence in diverticula, urethral calculi occur infrequently and then much more often in men than in women. The calculi, almost always calcium oxalate, have been classified as primary, originating in the urethra (Fig 8–89), and secondary, having migrated to the urethra from elsewhere in the urinary tract (Fig 8–90). The primary urethral calculus results from urinary stagnation and infection in a urethral recess, such as from a prostatic or a periurethral abscess or from mucosal ulceration. A foreign body in the urethra can act as a nidus for the formation of a calculus. More than 90% of urethral calculi are of the secondary type.[80]

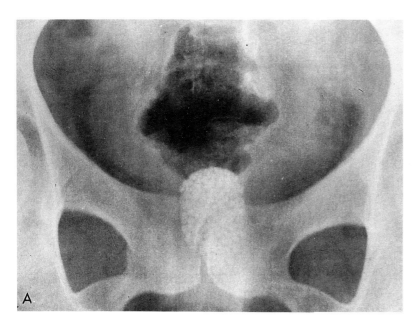

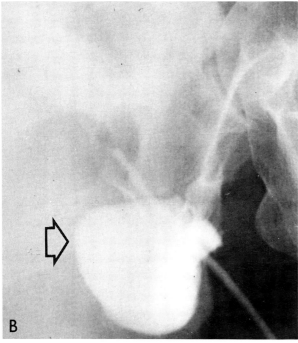

Figure 8–89. Seed calculi in a urethral diverticulum. This 58-year-old woman underwent transurethral resection of a ladder neoplasm 1 year ago, at which time the urethra was apparently injured. **A.** Scout radiograph shows many seed calculi overlying the symphysis pubis and collected in a smoothly oval configuration. **B.** Retrograde urethrogram shows the large urethral diverticulum (*arrows*).

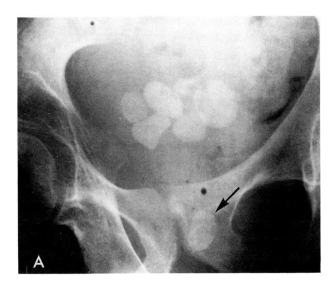 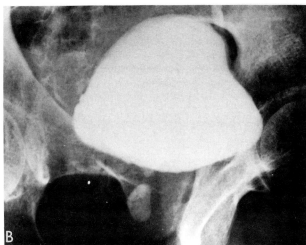

Figure 8–90. Urethral calculus and bladder calculi in a 27-year-old paraplegic man. **A.** Several round and faceted calculi in the urinary bladder, one of which (*arrow*), now in the region of the symphysis pubis, has passed into the urethra (a secondary urethral calculus). **B.** Urography shows the relationship of the urethral calculus to the bladder outlet.

REFERENCES

1. Rittenberg GM, Warren E. Air in the pelvicalyceal system: A normal finding in patients with ureteroileostomies. *Am J Roentgenol.* 1977;128:311–312.
2. Meyers MA, Whalen JP, Peelle K, et al. Radiologic features of extraperitoneal effusions: Anatomic approach. *Radiology.* 1972;104:249–257.
3. Sheshanarayana KN, Keats TE. Spontaneous pneumopyelogram in a non-diabetic patient. *Am J Roentgenol.* 1969;107:760–762.
4. Clifford NJ, Katz I. Subcutaneous emphysema complicating renal infection by gas-forming coliform bacteria: Report of two cases in diabetic patients. *N Engl J Med.* 1962;266:437–439.
5. Bliznak J, Ramsey J. Emphysematous pyelonephritis. *Clin Radiol.* 1972;23:61–64.
6. Langston CS, Pfister RC. Renal emphysema. A case report and review of the literature. *Am J Roentgenol.* 1970;110:778–786.
7. Norman A, Brenbridge AG, Buschni AJ, et al. Renal emphysema of the transplanted kidney. Sonographic appearance. *Am J Roentgenol.* 1979;132:656–658.
8. Parameswaran R. Gas nephrogram: An unusual complication of renal transplantation. *Br J Radiol.* 1977; 50:438–440.
9. Kim DS, Woesner ME, Howard TF, et al. Emphysematous pyelonephritis demonstrated by computed tomography. *Am J Roentgenol.* 1979;132:287–288.
10. Rankin RN. Gas formation after renal tumor embolization without abscess: A benign occurrence. *Radiology* 1979;130:317–320.
11. Wilms G, Baert AL, Marchal G, et al. Demonstration of gas formation after renal tumor embolization. *J Comput Assist Tomogr.* 1979;3:838–839.
12. Siim E, Fleckenstein P. Gas formation following hepatic embolisation. *Br J Radiol.* 1982;55:926–928.
13. Levy JM, Wasserman PI, Weiland DE. Nonsuppurative gas formation in the spleen after transcatheter splenic infarctions. *Radiology.* 1981;139:375–376.
14. Long JA, Jr., Dunnick NR, Doppman JL. Noninflammatory gas formation following embolization of adrenal carcinoma. *J Comput Assist Tomogr.* 1979;3:840–841.
15. Yu SF. Spontaneous renal and perirenal emphysema. *Br J Radiol.* 1966;39:466–467.
16. Levy AH, Schwinger HN. Gas-containing perinephric abscess. *Radiology.* 1953;60:720–723.
17. Fisher, MS. Pseudo-abscess: Anomalous colon simulating peri-renal infection. *Br J Radiol.* 1974;47:288–289.
18. Khilnani MT, Wolf BS. Hamartolipoma of the kidney: Clinical and roentgen features. *Am J Roentgenol.* 1961; 86:830–841.
19. Sheshanarayana KN, Keats TE. Angiomyolipoma of the kidney: Diagnostic roentgenographic findings. *Am J Roentgenol.* 1968;104:332–334.
20. Berg RA. Milk of calcium renal disease. Report of cases and review of the literature. *Am J Roentgenol.* 1967;101:714–718.
21. Rosenberg MA. Milk-of-calcium in a renal calyceal diverticulum. Case report and review of literature. *Am J Roentgenol.* 1967;101:714–718.
22. Healy T, Way BG, Grundy WR. Milk of calcium in calycine diverticula. *Br J Radiol.* 1980;53:845–852.
23. Herman RD, Leoni JV, Matthews GR. Renal milk-of-calcium associated with hydronephrosis. *Am J Roentgenol.* 1978;130:572–574.
24. Freed TA. Hemorrhagic cyst aspirate in milk of cal-

cium renal cyst. A diagnostic dilemma. *J Can Assoc Radiol.* 1971;22:83–85.

25. Benendo B, Litwak A. "Milk-of-calcium" in a renal cyst. *Br J Radiol* 1964;37:70–71.
26. Ziter FMH Jr., Wurster RE. Renal milk-of-calcium associated with hydronephrosis. *J Can Assoc Radiol.* 24:48–50, 1973.
27. Courey WR, Pfister RC. The radiographic findings in renal tubular acidosis: Analysis of 21 cases. *Radiology.* 1972;105:497–503.
28. Bateson EM, Chander S. Nephrocalcinosis in cretinism. *Br J Radiol.* 1965;38:581–584.
29. Chikos PM, McDonald GB. Regional enteritis complicated by nephrocalcinosis and nephrolithiasis: Case report. *Radiology.* 1976;121:75–76.
30. Dowling RH, Rose GA, Sutor DJ. Hyperoxaluria and renal calculi in ileal disease. *Lancet* 1971;1:1103–1106.
31. Fulop M, Sternlieb I, Scheinberg IH. Defective urinary acidification in Wilson's disease. *Ann Intern Med.* 1968; 68:770–777.
32. Pantoja E, Pagan Saez H, Gonzalez Flores B. The wandering staghorn calculus betraying the hydronephrotic nature of a renal mass. *Am J Roentgenol.* 1971; 113:732–734.
33. Azimi F, Cameron DD. Calcification of the intrarenal branches of the renal arteries. *Clin Radiol.* 1977;28:217–219.
34. Sheshanarayana KN, Keats TE. Intrarenal arterial calcification: Roentgen appearance and significance. *Radiology.* 1970;95:145–147.
35. Phillips TL, Chin FG, Palubinskas AJ. Calcification in renal masses: An eleven-year survey. *Radiology.* 1963; 80:786–794.
36. Kikkawa K, Lasser EC. "Ringlike" or "rimlike" calcification in renal cell carcinoma. *Am J Roentgenol.* 1969; 107:737–742.
37. Shockman AT. The significance of ring-shaped renal calcification. *J Urol.* 1969;101:438–442.
38. Cannon AH, Zanon B Jr, Karras BG. Cystic calcification in the kidney. Its occurrence in malignant renal tumors. *Am J Roentgenol.* 1960;84:837–848.
39. Daniel WW Jr, Hartman GW, Witten DM, et al. Calcified renal masses: A review of ten years experience at the Mayo Clinic. *Radiology.* 1972;103:503–508.
40. Wasserman NF, Ewing SL. Calcified renal oncocytoma. *Am J Roentgenol.* 1983;141:747–479.
41. Jonutis AJ, Davidson AJ, Redman HC. Curvilinear calcifications in four uncommon benign renal lesions. *Clin Radiol.* 1973;24:468–474.
42. Pitfield J, Preston BJ, Smith PG. A calcified renal mass: Chondrosarcoma of kidney. *Br J Radiol.* 1981;54:262.
43. Kutcher R, Schneider M, Gordon DH. Calcification in polycystic disease. *Radiology.* 1977;122:77–80.
44. McAfee JG, Donner ME. Differential diagnosis of calcification encountered in abdominal radiographs. *Am J Med Sci* 1962;243:609–650.
45. Salik, JO, Abeshouse BS. Calcification, ossification and cartilage formation in the kidney. *Am J Roentgenol.* 1962;88:125–143.
46. Charnsangavej C, Baker SR, Adler J, et al. Giant vas-

cular malformation of the kidney: Computed tomographic and angiographic appearances. *Urol Radiol.* 1985;7:8–11.
47. Chambers A, Carson R. Primary osteogenic sarcoma of the kidney. *Br J Radiol.* 1975;48:316–317.
48. Nelson JA, Clark RE, Palubinskas AJ. Osteogenic sarcoma with calcified renal metastases. *Br J Radiol.* 1971; 44:802–804.
49. Engel RM, Elkins RC, Fletcher BD. Retroperitoneal teratoma. Review of the literature and presentation of an unusual case. *Cancer* 1968;22:1068–1073.
50. Bruneton JN, Diard F, Drouillard JP, et al. Primary retroperitoneal teratomas in adults. Presentation of two cases and review of the literature. *Radiology.* 1980; 134:613–616.
51. Hicks CE, Evans C. Renal infarction as a cause of a calcified renal mass. *Br J Radiol.* 1984;57:840–842.
52. Lalli AF. Renal parenchymal calcifications. *Semin Roentgenol.* 1982;17:101–112.
53. Loughran CF, Ehmke FM. Calcified post-traumatic renal pseudotumor. *Br J Radiol.* 1986;59:515–518.
54. Brown RC, Cornell SN, Culp DA. Multilocular renal cyst with diffuse calcification simulating renal cell carcinoma. *Radiology.* 1970;95:411–412.
55. Tonkin AK, Witten DM. Genitourinary tuberculosis. *Semin Roentgenol.* 1979;14:305–310.
56. Hipona FA, Park WM. Calcific renal cortical necrosis. *J Urol.* 1967;97:961–964.
57. Lloyd-Thomas HG, Balme RH, Key JJ. Tram-line calcification in renal cortical necrosis. *Br Med J* 1962; 1:909–911.
58. McAlister WH, Nedelman SH. The roentgenographic manifestations of bilateral renal cortical necrosis. *Am J Roentgenol.* 1961;86:129–135.
59. Whalen JG Jr, Ling JT, Davis LA. Antemortem roentgen manifestations of bilateral renal cortical necrosis. *Radiology.* 1967;89:682–689.
60. Riesz PB, Wagner CW Jr. Unusual renal calcification following acute bilateral renal cortical necrosis: A case report. *Am J Roentgenol.* 1967;101:705–707.
61. Harrison RB, Vaughan ED Jr. Diffuse cortical calcifications in rejected renal transplants. *Radiology.* 1978; 126:635–636.
62. Wilson DA, Wenzl JE, Altschuler LP. Ultrasound determination of diffuse cortical nephrocalcinosis in a case of primary hyperoxaluria. *Am J Roentgenol.* 1979; 132:659–661.
63. Arons WL, Christensen WR, Sosman MC. Nephrocalcinosis visible by x-ray associated with chronic glomerulonephritis. *Ann Intern Med.* 1955;42:260–282.
64. Palmer FJ. Renal cortical calcification. *Clin Radiol.* 1970;21:175–177.
65. Esposito WJ. Specific nephrocalcinosis of chronic glomerulonephritis. *Am J Roentgenol.* 1967; 101:688–691.
66. Vaughan JH, Sosman MC, Kinney TD. Nephrocalcinosis. *Am J Roentgenol.* 1947;58:33–45.
67. Soteropoulos C, Kawashima E, Gilmore JH. Cystitis and ureteritis emphysematosa. *Radiology.* 1957; 68:866–868.
68. Imray TJ, Hubert LH. Isolated ureteritis emphysema-

tosa simulating pneumatosis intestinalis. *Am J Roentgenol.* 1980;135:1082–1083.

69. Berlow ME, Azimi, Carsky EW. Gonadal vein phlebolith simulating a midureteral stone. *Am J Roentgenol.* 1979;133:919–920.

70. MacMillan BG, Fritzhand MD, Spitz HB. Milk-of-calcium in the ureter. *Radiology.* 1978;127:376.

71. Thornbury JR, Parker TW. Ureteral calculi. *Semin Roentgenol.* 1982;17:133–139.

72. Thomas SD, Sanders PW III, Pollack HM. Primary amyloidosis of urinary bladder and ureter. *Urology.* 1977;9:586–589.

73. Holesh S. Gas in the bladder. Cystitis emphysematosa. *Clin Radiol.* 1969;20:234–236.

74. Bailey H. Cystic emphysematosa. 19 cases with intraluminal and interstitial collections of gas. *Am J Roentgenol.* 1961;86:850–862.

75. Imray TJ, Kaplan P. Lower urinary tract infections and calculi in the adult. *Semin Roentgenol.* 1983;18:276–287.

76. Wilson GF. Haemorrhagic cystitis emphysematosa. *Br J Radiol.* 1985;58:899–900.

77. Galloway NJM. Gas gangrene of the bladder complicating cyclophosphamide cystitis. *Br J Urol.* 1984;56:100–101.

78. Fetterman LF. An unusually large gas-containing bladder. *Br J Radiol.* 1972;45:67–69.

79. Sanders RC, Textor JH Jr, Bowerman JW. Bladder intramural gas following transurethral prostatectomy. *Br J Radiol.* 1972;45:902–904.

80. Banner MP, Pollack HM. Urolithiasis in the lower urinary tract. *Semin Roentgenol.* 1982;17:140–148.

81. Dahniya MH, Gordon-Harris L. Giant urinary bladder calculi. *Clin Radiol.* 1985:36:313–314.

82. Lome LG, Navani S. Foley calculus formation. *Br J Radiol.* 1970;43:487–488.

83. Amendola MA, Sanda LP, Diokno AC, et al. Bladder calculi complicating intermittent clean catheterization. *Am J Roentgenol.* 1983;141:171–173.

84. Miller SW, Pfister RC. Calcification in uroepithelial tumors of the bladder. Report of 5 cases and survey of the literature. *Am J Roentgenol.* 1974;121:827–831.

85. Lang EK. *Roentgenographic Diagnosis of Bladder Tumors.* Springfield, Ill: Charles C Thomas Publishers; 1968: 18–19.

86. Braband H. Incidence of urographic findings in tumours of urinary bladder. *Br J Radiol.* 1961;34:625–629.

87. Ferris EJ, O'Connor SJ. Calcification in urinary bladder tumors. *Am J Roentgenol.* 1965;95:447–449.

88. Gross BH. Bladder and ureteral calcifications. *Semin Roentgenol.* 1979;14:261–262.

89. Davidson HD, Witten DM, Culp OS. Roentgenographically demonstrable calcification in tumors of the bladder: Report of three cases. *Am J Roentgenol.* 1965; 95:45–454.

90. Kolawole TM, Nkposong EO, Abioye AA. Ring calcification in a bladder phaeochromocytoma. *Br J Radiol.* 1975;48:931–932.

91. Al-Ghorab MM. Radiological manifestations of genitourinary bilharziasis. *Clin Radiol.* 1968;19:100–111.

92. Umerah BC. The less familiar manifestations of schistosomiasis of the urinary tract. *Br J Radiol.* 1977; 50:105–109.

93. Holman CC. Urinary tuberculosis with extensive calcification of the bladder. *Br J Surg.* 1952;40:90.

94. Harrison RB, Stier FM, Cochrane JA. Alkaline encrusting cystitis. *Am J Roentgenol.* 1978;130:575–577.

95. Francis RS, Shackelford GD. Cyclophosphamide cystitis with bladder wall calcification. *J Can Assoc Radiol.* 1974;25:324–325.

96. Pulvertaft R, Hurst C. Bladder calcification related to end-stage renal failure. *Br J Radiol.* 1984;57:335–336.

CHAPTER NINE

Plain Film Radiology of the Female and Male Genital Tracts

FEMALE GENITAL TRACT

Vagina

Normally, the vagina cannot be visualized on plain films of the abdomen. Its radiographic density is similar to adjacent soft tissues and it lacks a bordering layer of fat to distinguish it from other pelvic organs. The vaginal vault is usually empty and its walls never calcify. Therefore, it is only when its lumen is filled with air or another relatively lucent substance that the location and contour of the vagina can be discerned by conventional radiography. Tampons contain sufficient air to be seen on X-ray. They appear as oblong shadows, more dense than gas, forming the configuration of the vagina (Fig 2–49). A sharply curving or apparently foreshortened vagina, as evidenced by the tampon shadow, is a clue to the orientation of the uterus (Fig 9–1).

Occasionally, a pelvic film is obtained when a vaginal speculum is in place. The distended, gas-filled lumen has a quadrilateral shape with an indistinct inferior margin and roughly parallel sidewalls markedly different from the rounded margin and indistinct superior border of a gas-filled rectum (Fig 9–2). After a pelvic examination, a small residual volume of air remains for a few minutes in the vaginal fornices around the cervix. If a roentgenogram is obtained at that time a transient crescentic lucency may be seen in the mid pelvis. It should not be confused with intrauterine air (Fig 9–3).

Vaginitis emphysematosa is a benign, self-limited condition characterized by numerous gas-filled cysts confined to the subepithelial layer of the ectocervix and the upper two thirds of the vagina.[1,2] The cysts, varying from a few millimeters to 3 cm in diameter, usually encircle the vaginal vault and extend laterally into the parametrium. Most cases occur during pregnancy or in the puerperal period but these cysts may form even if the uterus is in a nongravid state. Generally, vaginitis emphysematosa is accompanied by mild discomfort and almost always resolves without specific treatment. Gas-forming bacterial infection has been implicated but *Trichomonas vaginalis* infestation may also be an important predisposing factor, as it has been shown to liberate gas in experimental animals.[1]

The radiographic appearance is distinctive, with the cysts describing a corona of lucencies in the mid pelvis (Fig 9–4).[3,4] Their marginal location around the cervix sets them apart from abscesses, which usually appear as a rounded focus of contiguous bubbles. Mural emphysema of the uterus is characterized by larger lucent spaces in the pelvis and appears in acutely ill patients. Feces within the colon follow the course of the large intestine and lack the symmetrical arrangement of vaginitis emphysematosa.

Air can enter the vaginal cavity from a fistula with the rectum. There is almost always too little gas in the vagina to be discerned on plain films, however.

A colpolith or calcified concretion in the vagina is a stone whose formation requires either a vesicovaginal fistula or bladder incontinence which allows urine to enter the introitus. Vaginal stones are found exclusively in bedridden patients in whom stasis abetted by prolonged recumbency permits the precipitation of calcium salts if the urine pH is alkaline. Vaginal stones may form de novo or they can coat a retained foreign body.[5] The primary stones are often large, smooth, round, and laminated, exactly simulating a bladder calculus on frontal films.

Cervix

The margins of the cervix are not seen on plain films of the abdomen. On occasion, however, the consequences of cervical carcinoma and its treatment can be recognized. Infrequently, calcification takes place in iliac lymph nodes involved by metastases from cervical carcinoma (Fig 9–5).[6] Roentgenographically detectable nodal opacification usually follows radiotherapy but may occur in the absence of treatment.[7] Calcium deposition can be seen in the pelvis after injections of radioactive gold (^{198}Au) administered

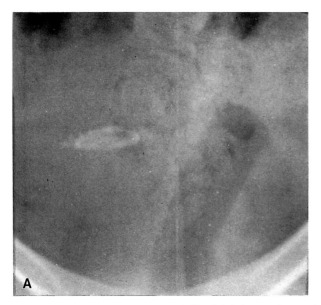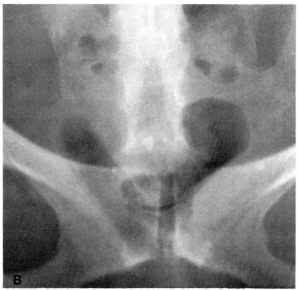

Figure 9–1. Vaginal tampons. **A.** The faintly lucent elongated rectangular shadow of the tampon bends gently to the left. An opaque intrauterine device demonstrates the position of the anteverted uterus, which projects slightly inferior to the junction of the cervix and vagina. **B.** In the prone position a wide divergence from the midline is a normal variant for vaginal position as illustrated by the location of a tampon.

as adjunctive therapy for cervical carcinoma. First observable between 5 and 10 years after treatment, the calcifications are limited to the region of the gold injections, which are typically close to the lateral walls of the bony pelvis along the course of the external iliac and hypogastric lymph nodes but usually not within the nodes themselves. The appearance varies from thin linear and laminated deposits to thick globular opacities that progress in density and extent. The calcifications are most likely due to tis-

sue necrosis secondary to the radiation from the isotope.[8]

Another complication of cervical carcinoma with radiation treatment is pelvic abscess consequent to parametrial tissue necrosis. Often, the abscess occurs in the context of radiation enteritis, which permits the transmural spread of gas-forming bacteria. The typical plain film appearance is a focus of bubbles often accompanied by dilatation and fixation of small bowel loops. A helpful sign, fre-

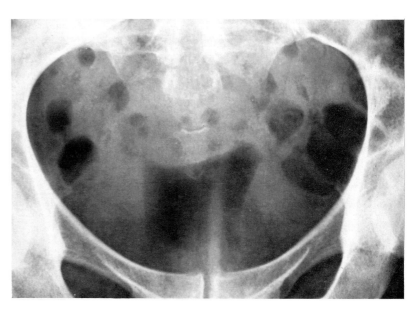

Figure 9–2. Air in the vaginal vault distended by a radiolucent speculum.

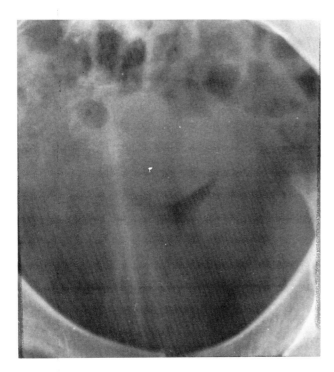

Figure 9–3. Air temporarily remaining in the vaginal fornices. This film, a scout roentgenograph taken as part of a hysterosalpingography, was obtained just after pelvic examination. The air left the vagina on subsequent films. Its position outside the uterine cavity was confirmed during fluoroscopic examination with the uterus filled with contrast material.

quently seen in these cases, is the presence of a single or several metallic clips in the pelvis that are affixed to the cervical lip before therapy commenced. The clip identifies the center of the treatment field for the radiation oncologist (Fig 9–6). For

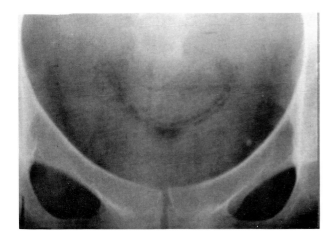

Figure 9–4. Vaginitis emphysematosa. Small bubbles arrayed as a double rim of lucencies surrounding the cervix. Bubbles also extend into the parametrium bilaterally.

the radiologist, its permanent retention is a handy marker of previous disease and its therapy.

Uterus

In addition to pregnancy, there are many causes of uterine enlargement. Expansion of the dimensions of the uterus may be due to distension of its cavity by blood or pus or by masses originating from its mucosa or muscular wall. The enlarged, nongravid uterus usually appears as a homogeneous soft tissue density indenting the superior wall of the bladder from above (Fig 9–7). Smaller uterine masses confined to the pelvis often have well-defined lateral and superior margins as they abut on extraperitoneal fat. As the uterus grows into the abdomen, however, its upper border is often indistinct as it comes to lie next to structures of similar soft tissue density (Fig 9–8). Noncalcified leiomyomata arising from the serosal surface tend to give the uterus an asymmetric configuration. Multiple tumors can impart a bumpy appearance superiorly and laterally.

Since all of these signs have limited specificity, the plain film designation of a uterine origin to a pelvic mass is unreliable. Superior indentation of the bladder can also be caused by an enlarged ovary or by other less common pelvic masses (Figs 2–88, 9–9). The confluent shadow of multiple ovarian tumors may simulate the eccentric location and lobular margin of uterine neoplasms (Fig 9–10). Moreover, the fat plane separating the bladder from the uterus may be absent or indistinct, and a diffuse pelvic density without a clearly defined inferior border may be a uterine or ovarian tumor as well as vesical distension (Fig 9–11).

Leiomyoma, the most common uterine neoplasm, can be identified with greater certainty if it calcifies. Myomatous calcification has a range of appearances the most typical being numerous, closely packed clumps of radiodensity distributed throughout the mass (Fig 2–115, 9–12). A calcified tumor may also have a mottled, speckled, or whorled configuration, sometimes admixed with plaques or streaks of increased density (Fig 2–116). In many cases, marginal accentuation predominates, often in association with less conspicuous central densities (Fig 2–117, 9–13). Occasionally, an arcuate rim is the only finding, and it may be so thin and smooth that it mimics cystic calcification (Fig 9–14).

A minimal focus of radiodensity in a uterine fibroid is sometimes poorly defined or punctate, occasionally closely resembling psammomatous calcification, which is found most often in ovarian papillary serous cystadenocarcinomas (Fig 9–15). Uterine leiomyosarcoma can also contain calcification, often indistinguishable from that of a benign

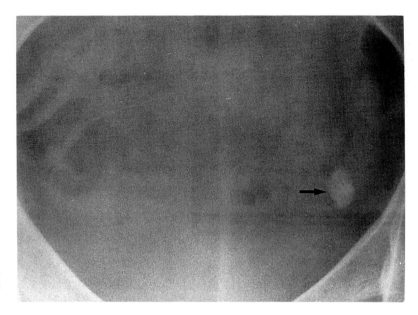

Figure 9–5. Unilateral iliac node calcification (*arrow*) in a patient with carcinoma of the cervix who received a full course of radiotherapy.

fibroid (Fig 9–16). A rapidly growing mass with flakes of radiodensity instead of cystic or solid opacities suggests malignant degeneration. Although leiomyomas are apt to be multiple in a given patient only a single tumor may be calcified. The soft tissue mass of an individual fibroid is frequently much larger than the volume of calcification, merely reflecting the fact that calcification may be limited to only a part of the tumor.

A mottled zone of calcification can sometimes resemble a radiodense lymph node (Fig 9–17). Lymph nodes in the pelvis are arranged along the course of the internal, external, and common iliac arteries. Hence, in general, nodal calcification occupies a more lateral site in the pelvis than does a calcified leiomyoma. A small focus of radiodensity can be mistaken for a confluent phlebolith. The perirectal and perivesical veins are also lateral structures situated outside the peritoneal cavity whereas the veins of the broad ligament, another site for phleb-

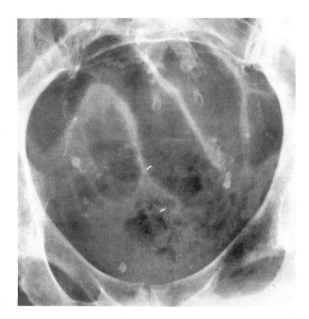

Figure 9–6. Pelvic abscess after radiation treatment for carcinoma of the cervix. Numerous bubbles in the left pelvis denote a large abscess cavity. The two metallic clips were inserted to localize the cervical lip to assist in radiotherapy portal positioning.

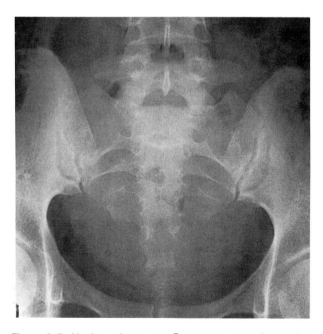

Figure 9–7. Uterine enlargement. Postpartum uterus impressing upon the roof of the bladder. A fat plane separates the two structures.

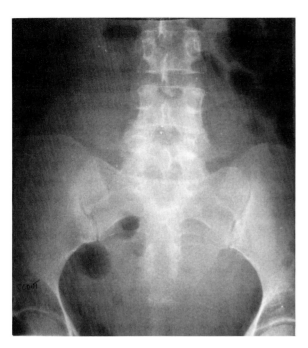

Figure 9–8. Large uterus containing a noncalcified leiomyoma. The uterus fills the pelvis but its upper extent into the lower abdomen is poorly defined.

oliths, are closer to the midline and may lie next to the uterine wall.

A large leiomyoma can extend from the pelvis into the abdominal cavity, sometimes to the level of kidneys or even higher. If such tumors calcify completely or diffusely, it is easy to determine that the calcified structure most likely originates in the pelvis and the type of calcification indicates the correct diagnosis. If only a portion of a huge fibroid calcifies, however, and that portion is in the abdomen, the nature of the abnormality may remain obscure unless note is made of the extent of the entire soft tissue component of the leiomyoma (Fig 2–118, 9–18). In addition, the position of the uterus varies with the degree of filling of the urinary bladder. Therefore, a uterine fibroid may appear in its expected location of the pelvis when the bladder is empty but can be displaced within the abdomen by a distended bladder (Fig 9–19).

Other Neoplasms

Among other types of uterine neoplasm, the most common is adenocarcinoma of the endometrium, which calcifies very rarely. Even after radiation therapy, deposition of calcium salts is seldom seen on plain films. It has the typical configuration of a solid mass, consisting of speckled or coarsely nodular densities occurring apparently in zones of necrosis, ischemia, and hemorrhage. Rarely, calcification may be observed in lymph nodes involved by metastases from uterine carcinoma following radiotherapy or even without prior treatment.[7] Calcification of a fine, punctate nature has been reported in malignant mixed uterine tumors.[9] These are neoplasms containing both sarcomatous and carcinomatous elements and account for about 6% of primary malignancies of the uterine corpus. The plain film findings of a localized zone of fine punctate calcification

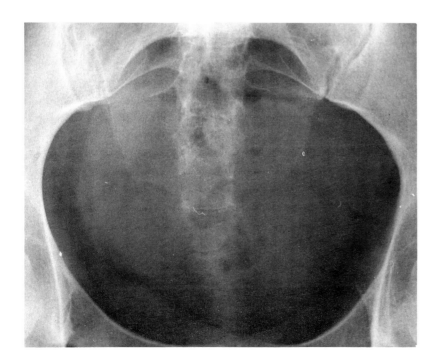

Figure 9–9. A granulosa cell tumor of the ovary confined to the pelvis. It displaces the bladder roof downward and is indistinguishable from a uterine mass.

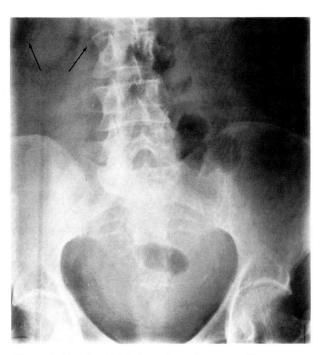

Figure 9–10. Mixed Müllerian cell ovarian tumor. The mass extends from the pubis to the right mid abdomen with a clearly outlined rounded upper border (*arrows*). Both uterine and ovarian masses can have this plain film appearance.

within an enlarging soft tissue mass located centrally in the pelvis of a postmenopausal woman should raise the suspicion of mixed malignant uterine tumor.

Pregnancy

Ossification in a normal third or late second trimester fetus is so distinctive as to require no further discussion. Faint calcification within the fetus in early pregnancy, however, can be confused with other types of pelvic calcification.

Lithopedion, the petrifaction or calcification of a retained dead fetus, is an end result of an extrauterine pregnancy. Three general patterns have been described[10]:

1. The membranes are calcified, forming a hard shell surrounding the fetus, which may be skeletonized but not involved in the process of calcification (lithokelyphos) (Fig 9–20).
2. The membranes and the fetus are both calcified (lithokelyphopedion) (Fig 9–21).
3. The fetus is infiltrated with calcium salts but calcification of the membranes is negligible (true lithopedion).

For a lithopedion to develop the patient must have had an extrauterine pregnancy that had not been diagnosed and thus not treated. The abdominal pregnancy must have survived for more than 3

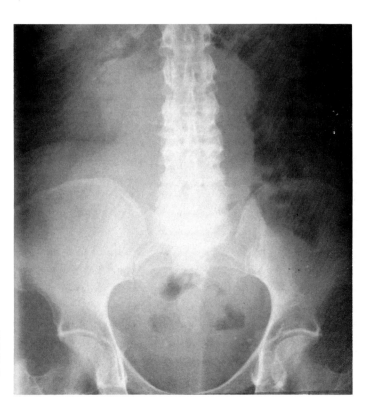

Figure 9–11. Large ovarian tumor extending from the pelvis to the level of L1. The fat plane between bladder and other pelvis organs is not seen. An enlarged bladder may also expand into the abdomen in a similar way.

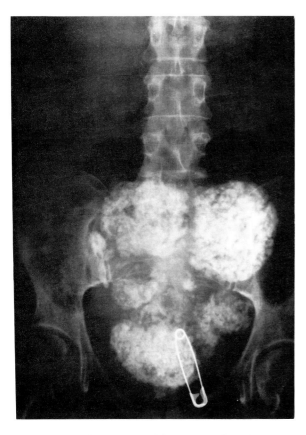

Figure 9–12. Multiple uterine leiomyomas. Densely packed opaque clumps are distributed throughout the tumor masses.

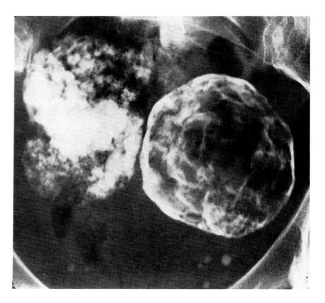

Figure 9–13. Uterine leiomyomas with different types of calcifications. The fibroid on the patient's right has coarsely mottled calcification with no rim. The fibroid on the patient's left has a well-defined dense rim with whorled internal calcification.

months; otherwise, it would have been absorbed.[11] Usually the configuration of a fetal part can be recognized on the abdominal radiograph along with the calcification, leading to the appropriate diagnosis. If the abdominal pregnancy had been implanted on the omentum, the lithopedion may show marked mobility with changes in patient position. The location of the lithopedion can be highly unusual. For example, an extrauterine pregnancy implanted on the liver can end up as a calcified mass in the right upper quadrant.

Uterine Artery

In elderly women, the uterine artery is often calcified. This vessel, a branch of the anterior division of the internal iliac artery initially follows the lateral

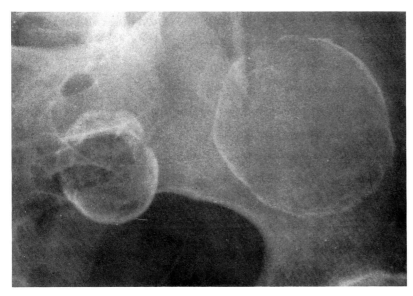

Figure 9–14. Two uterine leiomyomas with cystic morphology. Calcium has been deposited predominantly on the margin of the mass.

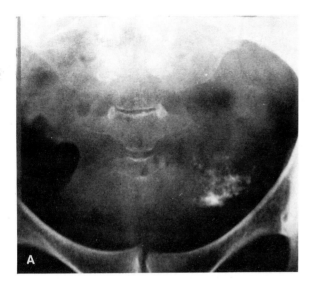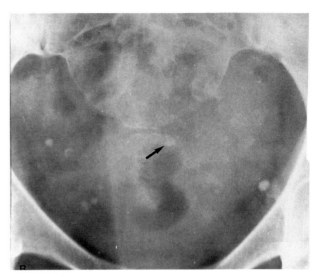

Figure 9–15. A. Punctate linear and globular calcifications occupy a portion of leiomyoma of the uterus. **B.** Faint calcifications scattered throughout a leiomyoma confined to the pelvis. Many of the calcifications are barely discernible. The overall picture is similar to psammomatous calcifications in ovarian malignancy. A larger density resembles a phlebolith but it, too, is within the tumor (*arrow*).

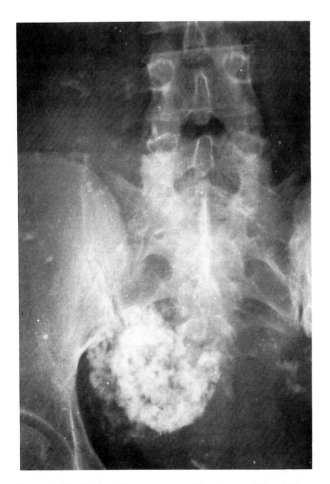

Figure 9–16. Uterine leiomyosarcoma. The large pelvic calcification resembles a fibroid. The diffusely scattered irregular calcifications in other parts of the tumor are atypical and should raise the suspicion of malignant change.

pelvic wall and then traverses medially and anteriorly along the broad ligament to the lateral margin of the uterus, where it may again turn in a longitudinal direction. Most often, calcification is recognized along the transverse portion of the artery. Linear, narrow tubular radiodensities extending horizontally for 3 to 4 cm from the lateral pelvic wall just above the ischial spines are characteristic of uterine artery calcification (Fig 2–104).[12,13] The artery may deviate from the horizontal plane if the uterus is situated away from the midline (Fig 9–22). The general direction of the uterine artery is straight, but slight undulations are to be expected. Less commonly, marked tortuosity of the intrauterine portion of a calcified artery can appear as an irregular, poorly defined structure simulating psammomatous calcification in ovarian neoplasms (Fig 9–23). Moreover, as is true of the uterus itself, the uterine artery can exhibit a wide excursion in position with varying extent of bladder dilatation (Fig 9–24).

Phleboliths in the veins or the broad ligament also attest to uterine position extending below the symphysis pubis with uterine prolapse (Fig 3–80), crossing the midline after hysterectomy (Fig 3–81), and most often occupying asymmetric positions in the pelvis as the uterus is displaced or tipped to one side (Fig 9–25).

Uterine Gas

Mural emphysema most often occurs in the puerperium, with dead fetal tissue being a good substrate for clostridial infection.[14,15] Fetal death is not essen-

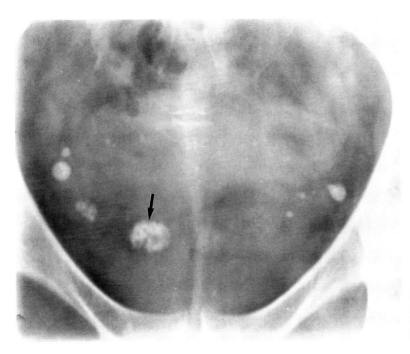

Figure 9–17. Dense mottled calcification in a uterine leiomyoma situated just to the right of the midline (*arrow*). It has the appearance of a lymph node but it is too medially situated.

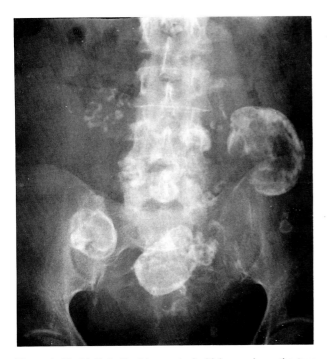

Figure 9–18. Multiple fibroids, most of which are above the true pelvis. The cystic lesions and the solid calcification to the right of the midline resemble lesions originating in other abdominal organs. Leiomyomas of the uterus should be considered in the differential diagnosis of upper and mid-abdominal calcifications in middle-aged and elderly women.

tial because gas in the uterus has been described even after delivery of a normal child.[16] If the gas-forming infection is limited to the fetus, the placenta, and the endometrium, it runs a benign course, especially if the uterine cavity is evacuated. The situation becomes more grave if the myometrium is involved, as the infection can spread rapidly to adjacent soft tissue structures, the peritoneal cavity, and the bloodstream.[2] Typically, uterine wall gas occupies an extensive area in the pelvis conforming to the enlarged uterus (Fig 2–50). It is usually configured as numerous, contiguous large bubbles, or bubbles and streaks confined within the uterine walls. There may also be gas in the uterine cavity and in retained fetal parts. The lower margin of the lucency is well above the symphysis pubis, which helps distinguish mural emphysema from gas in the bladder wall. The hectic course of the infection contrasts sharply with the benign nature of vaginitis emphysematosa. Also, vaginal wall gas is usually confined to a much smaller zone in the mid pelvis.

Leiomyomas that undergo cystic degeneration can then become infected by gas-forming bacteria.[2,17] In such cases *E coli, Staphylococcus,* and *Streptococcus,* as well as *Clostridium perfringens,* may be responsible. The gas collections can present as a large unilocular lucency that, depending on location, bears a resemblance to a distended air-filled bladder, a giant sigmoid diverticulum, a dilated cecum, or an extrauterine abscess.[18] Suppurating leiomyomas may also be seen on plain films as numer-

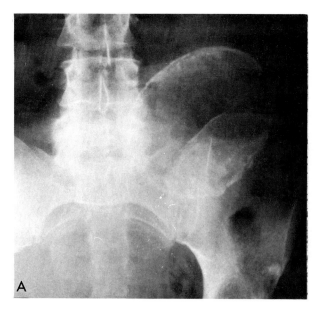

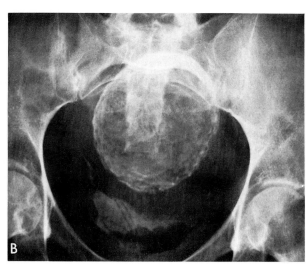

Figure 9–19. Change in position of uterine leiomyoma with extent of bladder distention. **A.** With a filled bladder, the calcified uterine leiomyoma is located in the lower abdomen. The patient is paraparetic, with bladder atony. **B.** With the bladder emptied, the leiomyoma is in the pelvis.

ous bubbles contained within the rounded mass of the degenerating leiomyoma.

Gross et al, in a computed tomography study, found intrauterine air more commonly in necrotic tumors than in abscesses.[19] The decline in the incidence of septic abortions and the frequency of uter-

ine tumors substantiates this observation. Plain film demonstration of a necrotic gas-containing intrauterine neoplasm has not yet been reported, however.

Uterine rupture can be a cause of a pelvic abscess. Such pus collections are recognizable on radiographs of the abdomen if they contain gas. Usually, they cannot be distinguished from other pelvic abscesses (Fig 9–26). Only the presence of intrauter-

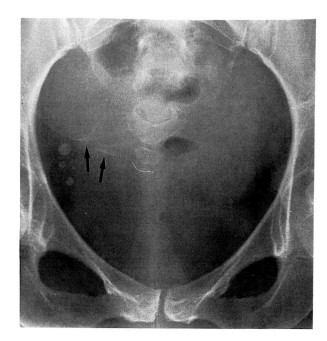

Figure 9–20. Lithopedion. Faint calcification of fetal membranes (*arrows*). This film was obtained 6 months after the birth of intrauterine twins. The extrauterine fetus was missed.

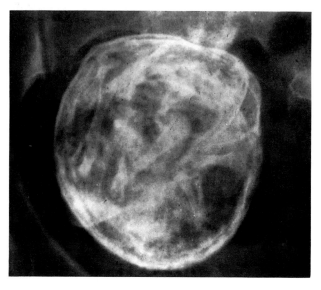

Figure 9–21. Lithopedion in the pelvis with major calcification of the membranes and well-formed fetal bones.

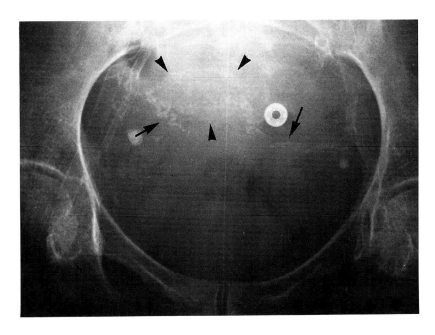

Figure 9–22. Marked vascular calcification in the pelvis. The markedly calcified uterine arteries (*arrows*) could be mistaken for fallopian tube calcification. The uterus is defined (*arrowheads*) by calcification of the intrauterine arteries.

ine air enables a definitive plain film identification of the origin.

Fallopian Tubes

The plain film rarely demonstrates masses or calcifications in the fallopian tubes. Neoplasms are infrequent and tubo-ovarian abscesses seldom produce a sufficient amount of gas to be discerned on survey radiographs. Calcified salpingolithiasis is distinctly unusual, as is opacification of the walls of the tubes. Uterine artery calcification is occasionally misinterpreted as a tubal opacity. The most common densities associated with the fallopian tubes

are the occlusion rings placed around the lumen during a ligation procedure (Fig 3–85).

Ovary

Tumors in the ovary may become very large before detection by either physical examination or plain roentgenographs, as the intraperitoneal location of the ovary favors silent extension via the flow of ascitic fluid in the peritoneal cavity. Noncalcified ovarian masses may cast a soft tissue shadow in the pelvis and lower abdomen, which often closely resembles uterine enlargement. The propensity for several types of ovarian tumors to calcify in a dis-

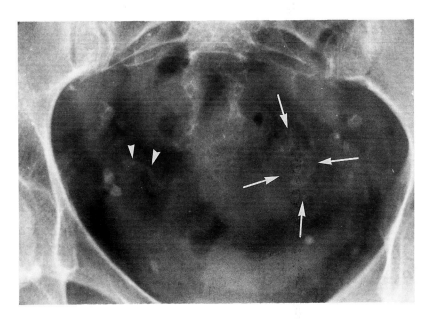

Figure 9–23. The right uterine artery has a typical configuration (*arrowheads*). The left artery is markedly tortuous (*arrow*), with the twists and turns of the calcified vessel, resembling the amorphous densities of a calcified serous cystadenocarcinoma of the ovary.

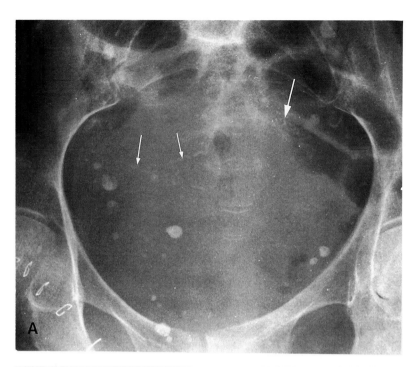

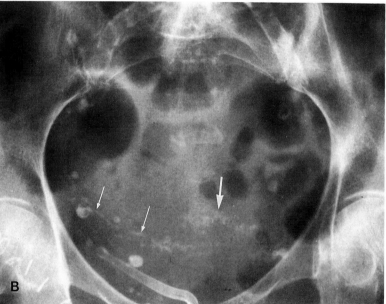

Figure 9–24. Movement of the uterine artery. **A.** With the bladder full the right artery (*small arrow*) and the tortuous left artery (*large arrows*) are high in the pelvis. **B.** After bladder evacuation, both vessels move inferiorly. Broad ligament phleboliths have migrated also.

tinctive way, however, allows for the presumption of a specific histological diagnosis in many cases on the basis of plain film appearance alone (Table 9–1).

Cystic Teratoma (Dermoid Cyst)

Not only do many cystic teratomas contain teeth and bone; they also often possess large quantities of fat. The presence of any of these distinguishing features is by itself sufficient to reach a diagnosis on a single film of the pelvis. Although the manifestations of cystic teratomas on plain X-ray are often obvious, in some cases the radiographic findings are more subtle and yet still pathognomonic. Therefore, it is important to scan the pelvis and lower abdomen carefully for roentgenographic evidence of these readily identifiable, and relatively common, benign ovarian lesions. Overall, in about 40% of patients, the findings on scout abdominal radiographs are characteristic enough to allow a specific diagnosis.

"Cystic teratoma" is preferable to "dermoid" because it indicates that the tumor contains derivatives of all three germ layers. Cystic teratomas ac-

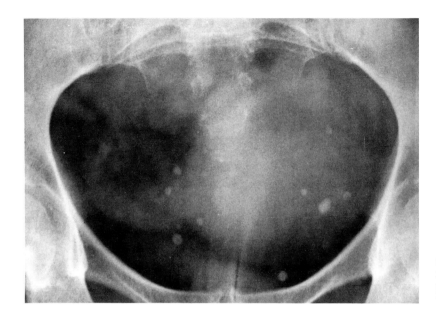

Figure 9–25. The uterus, well outlined by fat, is mostly to the left of the midline. Broad ligament phleboliths, located close to the uterine wall reflect uterine position.

count for 10% of all ovarian tumors and have a 10% to 20% bilateral incidence, occasionally being multiple in one or both ovaries.[20] Malignant transformation, usually a squamous cell carcinoma, is rare, occurring in less than 1% of the lesions. In a review of 1007 dermoid cysts, Peterson et al reported that 80% were between 5 and 15 cm in diameter, 13% were less than 5 cm, and 7% were larger than 15 cm.[21]

Cystic teratomas are the most common abdominal lesions with radiodensities appearing in the form of rudimentary teeth (Figs 1–11B, 2–21, 9–27). Sometimes there is a single tooth and in other instances several teeth are seen, almost all of them having a recognizable dentiform configuration. The

teeth are most frequently of the incisor and molar type and may be contained in a fragment of maxillary or mandibular bone (Fig 9–28). They can lie free within the cyst but more often are embedded in the cyst wall, usually in a raised nipple-like tissue protuberance, the dermal plug. A tooth may not be observed with initial recognition of the teratoma but, like the normal dentition, it can become radiodense at a prescribed time as the toothbud matures and calcifies within the cyst.[22,23] Teeth are seen in approximately 30% of dermoids.[24] A curvilinear cystic type calcification occurs in approximately 10% of cases (Fig 9–29). It may be confined to the entire wall or a segment of the border of the cyst. These arcuate densities occur in many other types of cysts

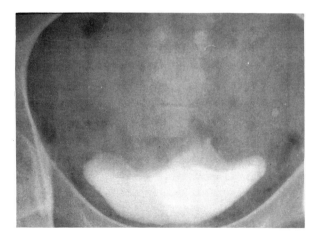

Figure 9–26. Pelvis abscess due to rupture of an infected uterus. The bladder has been filled with contrast material. Bubbles from the abscess are seen above the bladder extending to the right pelvic wall.

TABLE 9–1. CALCIFICATIONS IN THE OVARY

Cystic calcification
    Benign cystadenoma
    Cystic teratoma
    Mucinous cystadenocarcinoma (in peritoneal metastases)
Solid calcification
    Papillary serous cystadenocarcinoma
    Cystic teratoma
    Fibroma
    Thecoma
    Brenner tumor
    Virilizing lipid-laden tumor
    Gonadoblastoma
    Focal sclerosing stromal tumor
    Corpora albicantia
    Amputated ovary
    Tuberculosis of the ovary
Ossification and tooth formation
    Cystic teratoma

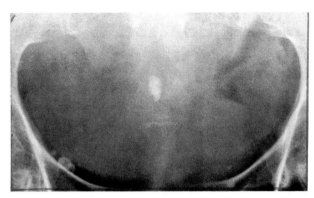

Figure 9–27. Dermoid cyst containing one tooth, having the appearance of an incisor. There is a poorly defined soft tissue mass without radiolucent contents.

and are not specific for a dermoid. In another 10%, the calcifications are structureless, not resembling teeth and thus not a differentiating plain film feature.[25] Rarely, they can mimic psammomatous calcifications.

The observation of a soft tissue mass, within which the presumed tooth or teeth is situated, is helpful in achieving a diagnosis. The mass appears smooth, round to oval in shape and is relatively radiolucent owing to its content of thick, lardaceous material formed by the sebaceous glands of the squamous epithelium lining the cyst wall. Fat within the lesion is present in 35% of cases, and in some patients it may be the only roentgenographic finding (Figs 2–72, 9–30).[26] If the cystic teratoma abuts pelvic fat, the similar lucencies both within and without the tumor can outline the thin soft tissue density of the cyst wall interposed between them. Fat in the

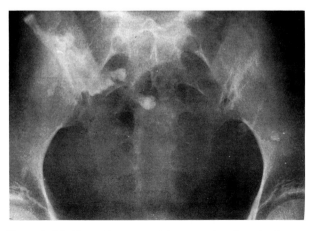

Figure 9–28. Dermoid cyst containing several teeth and rudimentary mandible. There is no radiolucent mass.

tumor is almost always distinguishable from bowel gas. Although the fat shadow is often wider than the bowel lumen, it appears less black than colonic gas or swallowed air in the small intestine (Fig 9–31). In almost every case, it is well confined in the tumor, not admixed with liquid material.[26] Hence, a fat–fluid level is a rare phenomenon and upright films obtained to look for this finding are almost always unrewarding.

Cystic teratomas are capable of extensive movement in the peritoneal cavity (Fig 9–32). In about 10% of cases, large tumors may twist upon themselves, producing an acute torsion characterized by severe unremitting abdominal pain.[21] Dermoids rarely obstruct or perforate bowel even if they attain large size.[27] Several examples of rupture into the urinary bladder have been reported, however.[28]

Papillary Serous Cystadenocarcinoma

Papillary serous cystadenocarcinomas constitute 15% to 35% of all cystic tumors of the ovary. They are, by far, the most common histological type of cancer, comprising two thirds of all ovarian malignancies. Occurring most often in women between 30 and 60 years of age they are frequently bilateral and often present with ascites.[29,30]

In approximately 10% of cases[29] the distinctive pattern of psammomatous calcification can be found in the papillary excrescences of the tumor, both in the primary site and in metastatic deposits in the peritoneal cavity, liver, and retroperitoneal nodes.[31–33] Psammoma bodies are small, discrete calcifications, fairly uniform in size and distribution. They have also been called corpora amylacea or calcospherites, and are composed of calcium carbonate arranged in a concentric organic framework. They are typically less dense than the calcification of lymph nodes or leiomyomas. Psammomatous calcification can vary from a flocculent, sharply demarcated focus to a less well-defined density consisting of punctate and squiggly opacities (Figs 2–119, 9–33). Their most characteristic form, a cloud of hazy density, is seen as a single large diffuse deposit or as multiple smudgy densities often scattered over a wide area.

Psammomatous calcification can be simulated by a diverse group of conditions (Table 9–2). Colon cancer presents, on occasion, with innumerable small densities representing calcification within the stroma of necrotic sections of the tumor (Fig 5–113).[34] Faint and diffuse opacification is sometimes seen in uterine leiomyomas and mixed malignant tumors (Fig 9–15B).[9] Chondrosarcoma of the ischial or pubic bone or chordoma of the sacrum may be revealed on plain films only as an irregular soft tissue calcifica-

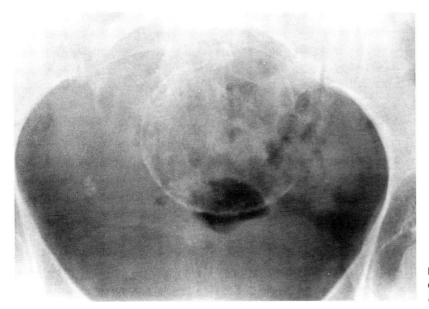

Figure 9–29. Dermoid cyst with curvilinear calcification in its wall. (*Courtesy of Dr. Erich Leichter.*)

tion superimposed on the pelvis, unaccompanied by demonstrable osseous destruction (Fig 9–34). Angiomatous lymphoid hamartoma (Castleman's disease) is a benign, self-limited condition that most often presents elsewhere in the body, especially in the mediastinum. If located in the pelvis, approximately half of the lesions calcify, sometimes as a diffuse density but, in other cases, with a highly specific arborizing pattern of increased opacity.[35]

Barium, conjugated oral cholecystography material, and bismuth compounds can each give a faint opaque cast to feces that, in some cases, is reminiscent of the amorphous densities of papillary serous

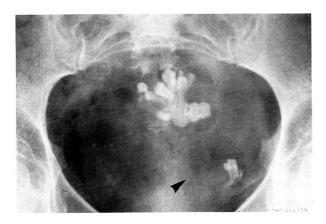

Figure 9–30. Two dermoid cysts with radiolucent (*sebaceous*) contents. The dermoid cyst on the patient's right contains multiple teeth and its border is not well defined. The dermoid cyst on the left contains a single tooth embedded in a small section of rudimentary jawbone; its border is well defined, with visualization of a thin wall (*arrowhead*).

cystadenocarcinoma (Fig 2–119). Ingested opacities may also cause confusion. There is a report of a young woman with punctate calcifications in the pelvis that were undigested fragments of bone meal residing in the colon.[36] A similar appearance can be seen with geophagy if the ingested soil is radiodense. Marked tortuosity of a calcified uterine artery wall can be mistaken for ovarian malignancy calcification (Fig 9–23). Occasionally, densities in the lower abdominal subcutaneous tissue simulate amorphous ovarian calcification. An example is a calcium deposition within the coiled section of a guinea worm (Fig 9–35).[37,38]

The ovary is notable for its long and diverse list of neoplasms. In recent years, there have been reports of calcification in several less common ovarian tumors, some of which closely mimic papillary serous cystadenocarcinoma on plain films. Fibromas represent approximately 5% of all ovarian tumors.[39] A neoplasm of older women, it may often become a large lesion accompanied by ascites. Ovarian fibromas are also a concomitant of the basal cell nevus syndrome.[40] Grossly detectable calcification, which occurs in 9% of tumors,[39] can occupy the entire lesion or be confined to a small peripheral focus. Diffuse opacification in fibromas resembles psammomatous calcification radiologically (Fig 9–36). More localized deposits are usually well-defined, often similar in configuration, size, and location to pelvic phleboliths (Fig 9–37).

A thecoma has a similar histological appearance to a fibroma, differing from it by the presence of intracellular and extracellular fat. Microscopic calcification in hyaline collagen is common, but exten-

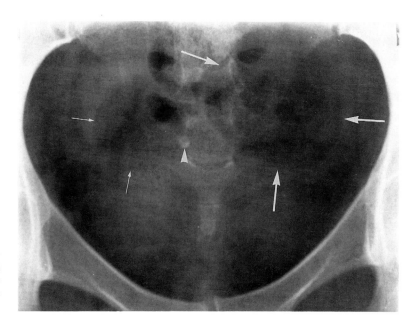

Figure 9–31. Bilateral fat-containing cystic teratomas (*arrows*). The arrowhead points to a small tooth. Despite their relatively large volume, they are only slightly more lucent than surrounding soft tissues.

sive calcification detectable on X-ray is rare. In one case, a fine granular opacity characterized the lesion on plain films.[41] A Brenner tumor is a benign ovarian lesion that may have diffuse dystrophic calcification, akin in configuration to a psammomatous pattern of radiopacity.[42] Sculley et al reported a calcified virilizing, lipid-laden tumor of the ovary that

also can be mistaken for serous cystadenocarcinoma on plain film.[43]

Two benign neoplasms affecting young women can calcify. Gonadoblastoma, formerly known as atypical dysgerminoma, contains cells from the three embryonal elements of the gonad—germ cells, cells of the sex chord, and cells of mesenchymal

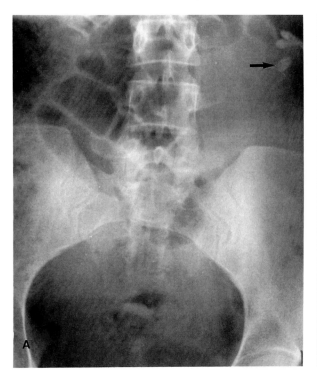

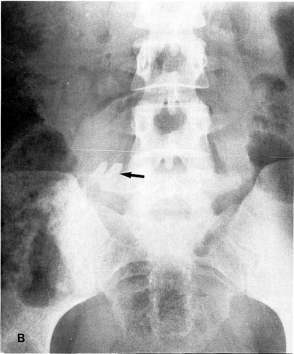

Figure 9–32. Wide excursions of an ovarian cystic teratoma. **A.** The tooth-containing mass (*arrow*) is in the lateral aspect of the left mid-abdomen. **B.** A few days later the mass is to the right of the midline (*arrow*) at the head of L5.

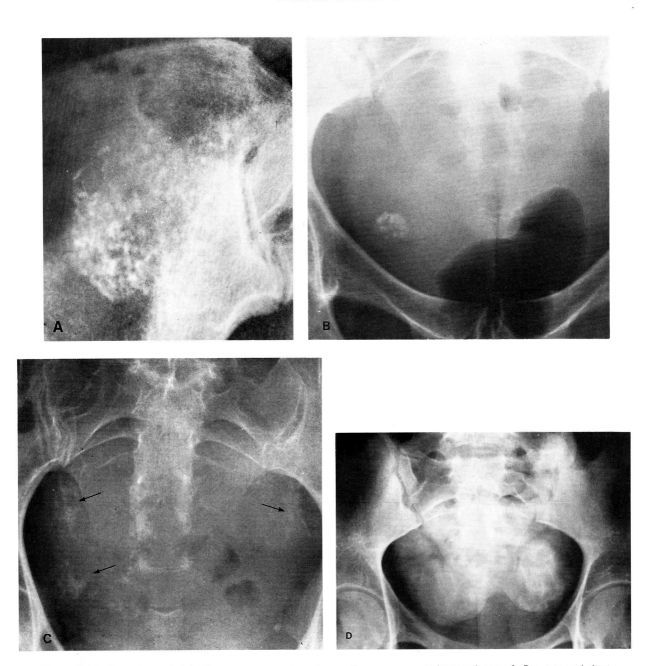

Figure 9–33. A spectrum of plain film appearances of ovarian papillary serous cystadenocarcinoma. **A.** Punctate and short linear densities are located in the peritoneal cavity overlying the right iliac fossa. **B.** A single cluster of densities less sharply outlined than lymph node calcification. **C.** Smudgy opacities scattered throughout the pelvis (*arrows*). **D.** A dense cloud of calcifications occupying much of the lower peritoneal cavity.

origin. Typically, evidence of the tumor is first noted in adolescence, with the onset of masculinizing signs accompanied by primary amenorrhea. Calcification appears either as a well-defined stippled density similar to lymph node calcification or a small dense focus that can be mistaken for a phlebolith (Fig 9–38). The radiographic appearance and age of presentation of this tumor are distinctly different from papillary serous cystadenocarcinoma.[44,45] Focal sclerosing stromal tumor of the ovary, another

rare benign tumor of young women with menstrual irregularities, also calcifies. The few cases reported have demonstrated a wide area of numerous discrete densities, each separable from the other, a pattern more reminiscent of uterine leiomyoma than an ovarian cystadenocarcinoma.[46,47]

Benign Cystadenoma

The older radiological literature makes frequent mention of psammomatous calcification in a cysta-

TABLE 9–2. SIMULATORS OF OVARIAN PSAMMOMATOUS CALCIFICATION IN THE PELVIS

Ovarian lesions
  Cystic teratoma
  Thecoma
  Brenner tumor
  Virilizing lipid-laden tumor
  Gonadoblastoma
  Focal sclerosing stromal tumor
Other pelvic tumors
  Carcinoma of the colon
  Chondrosarcoma
  Chordoma
  Leiomyoma of the uterus
  Leiomyosarcoma of the uterus
  Mixed malignant tumor of the uterus
  Bladder carcinoma
  Angiomatous lymphoid hamartoma
Intestinal intraluminal densities
  Retained barium
  Conjugated telepaque in the bowel
  Ingested bone meal
  Geophagy
Miscellaneous
  Tortuous uterine artery
  Subcutaneous parasite calcification—guinea worm

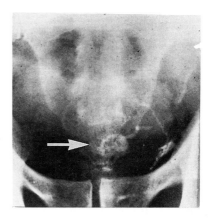

Figure 9–35. Dracunuclosis (guinea worm). Coiled worm in the soft tissues anterior to the pelvis (*arrow*).

denoma of the ovary. Yet, no case with roentgenographic–pathological correlation has been reported. It is prudent, therefore, to consider that cloudlike or diffuse densities in the pelvis and lower abdomen should never be regarded as a sign of a benign ovarian cyst. Occasionally, benign serous

cystadenomas have curvilinear calcifications (Fig 9–39). It should be included in the differential diagnosis of pelvic cystic lesions, along with aneurysm of the iliac artery (Figs 3–72, 9–40), peripheral uterine leiomyoma calcification, ovarian dermoid, mucocele of the appendix, and the rare echinococcal cyst of the pelvis.[48]

Mucinous Cystadenoma and Cystadenocarcinoma

Calcification is not usually featured in these neoplasms. Mucinous cystadenocarcinoma may rupture, however, with implantation of cell nests on the peritoneum resulting in pseudomyxoma peritonei. The accumulation of myxomatous material from these multiple implants can be associated with peripheral curvilinear calcification of cystic type (Fig 9–41)[32,49] or a combination of solid and cystic pat-

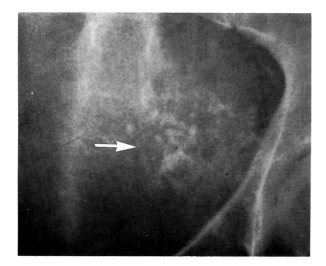

Figure 9–34. Chondrosarcoma of the left ischial bone. No evident bone destruction. A large soft tissue mass with calcification (*arrow*) occupied much of the pelvis. The tumor was entirely extraperitoneal.

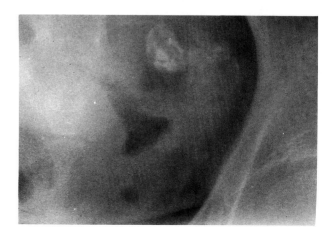

Figure 9–36. Amorphous and streaky calcification in a large ovarian fibroma.

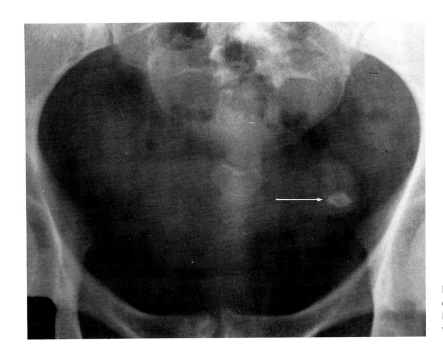

Figure 9–37. Marginally accentuated focus of calcification in a section of a small ovarian fibroma (*arrow*). The mass of the tumor is also visible because of abundant pelvic fat.

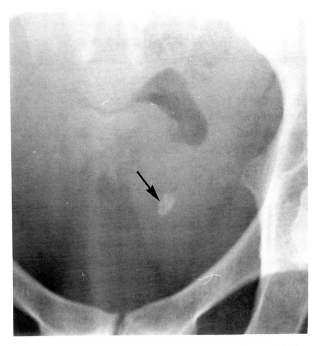

Figure 9–38. Gonadoblastoma. Calcification in this small lesion resembles a single phlebolith.

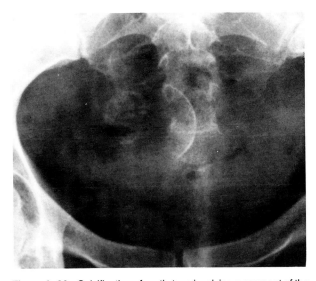

Figure 9–39. Calcification of cystic type involving a segment of the wall of benign serous cystadenoma. (*Courtesy of Dr. Paul Tartell.*)

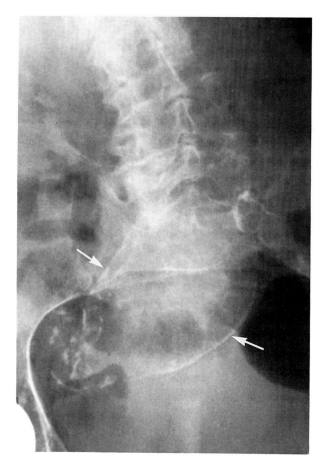

Figure 9–40. Aneurysm of the common iliac artery. This cystic calcification can be traced to the aorta superiorly and to iliac branches inferiorly, distinguishing it from a calcified ovarian lesion.

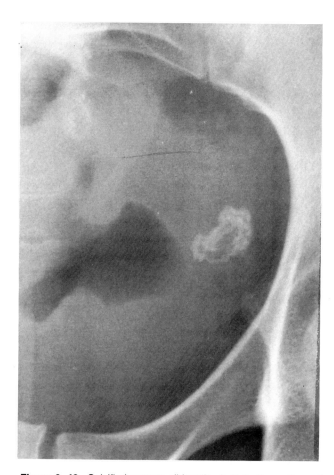

Figure 9–42. Calcified corpora albicantia. A distinctive pattern of calcification in a nonenlarged ovary. Note the pleated appearance of the continuous linear opacities.

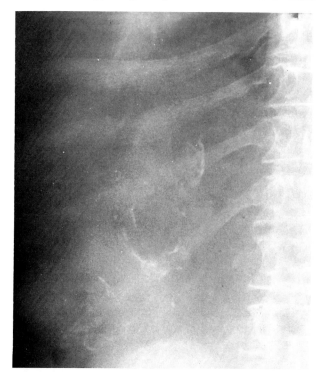

Figure 9–41. Pseudomyxoma peritoneii in a patient with mucinous cystadenocarcinoma of the ovary. There are linear and curvilinear calcifications at the periphery of the peritoneal myxomatous collections.

terns situated anywhere in the peritoneal cavity (Fig 3–42).

Miscellaneous Ovarian Calcifications

Rarely, radiographically demonstrable calcification is seen in corpora albicantia, the fibrous scar tissue found just under the ovarian capsule replacing the regressed corpora lutea. The calcifications that occur in a normal-sized ovary can be of popcorn configuration, resembling that of a uterine fibroid or roughly round clusters of sharply defined nodules, the clusters measuring a few centimeters in diameter and the individual nodules a few millimeters.[50] The individual calcific nodules may have lucent centers, simulating the appearance of small phleboliths.[51] Both of these patterns reflect discontinuous roentgenographically demonstrable calcification. More diffuse opacities have a corrugated contour conforming to the wavy borders of the corpora albicantia as seen on gross inspection (Fig 9–42). Among the handful of reported cases, a few have shown involvement of both ovaries with bilateral pelvic calcifications.

A rare cause of abdominal calcification is autoamputated ovary, ie, an ovary that has undergone

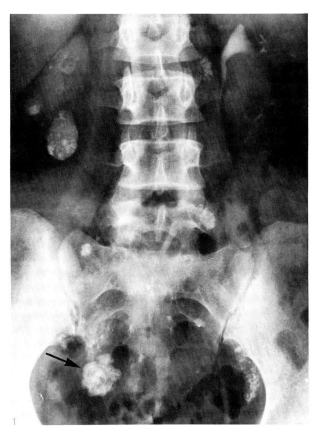

Figure 9–43. Calcification in genitourinary tuberculosis in a 62-year-old woman. Supine radiograph during urography shows a small, nonexcreting right kidney with mottled areas of calcification. The right ovary is calcified (*arrow*). The other calcifications are in abdominal and pelvic lymph nodes.

torsion, become infarcted, separated from its ligamentous moorings, and subsequently calcified. The typical radiographic appearance is that of a coarsely stippled oval pelvic mass, a few centimeters in greatest diameter.[52–54] Being freely mobile, the opacity can appear at different locations on serial films, sometimes in the pelvis and sometimes in the lower abdomen. It is usually an incidental radiological or surgical finding at any age group, although most often in children and young adults without a documented antecedent episode of abdominal pain. Pneumogynecography shows absence of one ovary and all or part of the ipsilateral fallopian tube.

Calcification of one or both ovaries, characteristically of mottled, solid mass type, can result from tuberculous infection.[55] The appearance resembles that of lymph node calcification (Fig 3–62), but the overall size is larger than that of the typical lymph node and the calcification is situated more medially than pelvic nodes (Fig 9–43). Associated findings, such as tuberculous calcifications of the urinary tract, help in the diagnosis.

MALE GENITAL TRACT

Vas Deferens

Calcification of the vas deferens is found most often in diabetic patients but sometimes occurs in nondiabetics as a manifestation of aging or as a result of infection. The relationship to diabetes mellitus was first reported by Marks and Ham[56] from a hospital with a large population of diabetic patients; of nine patients with vasal calcification, six had diabetes. In a later report from the same hospital, of 60 patients with vasal calcification, 56 had diabetes.[57] Even though many diabetic patients were seen at that hospital, non-diabetic patients comprised more than 80% of patients examined in the X-ray department. In the 56 patients with diabetes, the disease had been acquired at an average age of 33.4 years, and vasal calcification was first noted radiologically after an average duration of 18.3 years of diabetes. In general, it took longer for vasal calcification to develop in patients with discovery of diabetes at an early age than in those with onset later in life, 22 years being the average duration of diabetes in patients with recognition of the disease before age 40, and 13 years in patients whose illness was first noted after age 40. Other reports have confirmed the association of diabetes mellitus and calcification of the vas deferens.[58–60]

Calcification occurring in the elderly is located within the muscular wall of the vas deferens and is considered degenerative in nature. Vasal calcification resulting from infection is intraluminal; among the causative infections are tuberculosis, gonorrhea, syphilis, and chronic urinary tract infections. Usually it is not possible to distinguish radiologically the intramural from the intraluminal calcification.[61]

The vas deferens, ascending as the ductus deferens from the scrotum into the pelvic retroperitoneal space via the inguinal canal, may exhibit calcification of conduit type in any segment, but the most common site is its horizontal and descending ampullary segment (Fig 3–73). The calcification, most often bilateral and symmetrical, typically manifests as two horizontal calcific tramlines just cephalad to the empty bladder or posterior to the distended bladder (Figs 9–44, 9–45). On occasion the linear calcifications can be seen to continue toward the region of the inguinal canal (Fig 9–46) or even into the scrotum. Infrequently, the calcification can be seen only in that portion of the vas deferens close to the scrotum (Fig 9–47). Often the lines of calcific density are not continuous, there being very short intervening segments without visible calcification, suggesting that the calcification is laid down in plaques.

The radiological appearance of calcification of

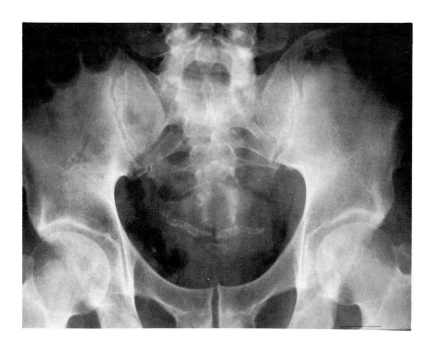

Figure 9–44. Calcification of the ampullary segments of the vasa deferentia in a 53-year-old diabetic man.

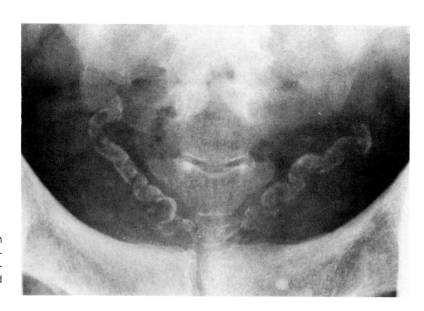

Figure 9–45. Prone projection of the abdomen of a 47-year-old diabetic man. There is calcification in the walls of the tortuous ampullary segments of the vasa deferentia as they descend toward the urethra.

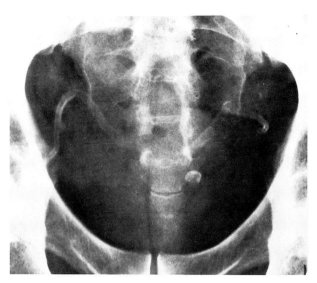

Figure 9–46. Bilateral calcification of the vasa deferentia in their ampullary segments as well as in the portions ascending from the inguinal canals, more pronounced on the patient's right.

the vas might be misinterpreted as calcification in an arterial wall. Vasal calcification is usually denser and thicker than arterial calcification, however (Fig 9–48), and in the usual location and direction of vasal calcification there are no sizable arteries in the male. The internal pudendal artery can parallel the vas as it traverses the obturator foramen, but unlike the vas the artery does not extend far inferiorly beyond the osseous borders of the foramen (Fig 9–49).

Seminal Vesicles

Calcification in the seminal vesicles is rare, occurring as small intraluminal concretions located posterior to the bladder and cephalad to the prostate. Very likely these calculi result from infection, such as tuberculosis and gonorrhea. The concretions may be so numerous as to produce a cloud of radiopacity defining the shape of the seminal vesicles. Calcification of the walls of the seminal vesicles may be superimposed on the ampulla of the vas. Usually, it has a wider diameter and is located slightly above the most medial vasal segment.[60]

Scrotum

Radiographically demonstrable calcification in the scrotum is infrequent. As already noted, calcification of the ductus deferens can occur in its intrascrotal portion. Hydroceles or spermatoceles can show curvilinear wall calcification of cyst type (Fig 9–50). A scrotal cystocele containing bladder calculi has been reported.[62] Dense, solid mass type calcification of oval shape can be due to tuberculosis of the testicle. A similar appearance can result from infarction of the testis secondary to torsion, reported most often in the newborn (Fig 9–51). Very uncommon is postinfarction calcification in an undescended testicle, resulting in the radiographic finding of an irregularly calcified mass, a few centimeters in diameter, in the mid or lower abdomen.[63] Hematoma in the scrotum, such as that following orchiectomy, can be the cause for the development of a roughly rounded

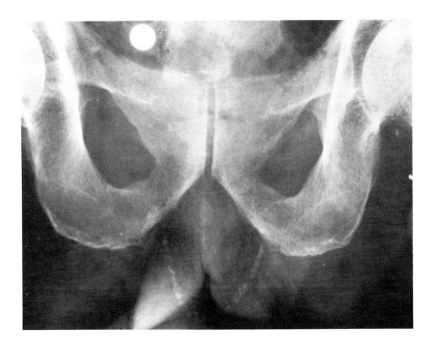

Figure 9–47. Calcification of each ductus deferens in the scrotum of a 77-year-old nondiabetic man. There was no radiographically demonstrable calcification in other portions of the vasa.

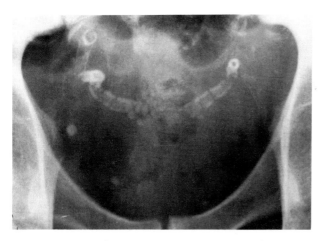

Figure 9–48. Calcification of the vasa deferentia in a 68-year-old diabetic man. Note the plaquelike appearance of the calcium deposition.

or oval dense calcification (Fig 9–52). Phleboliths can also be seen in the scrotum (Fig 3–76).

It is unusual for testicular tumors to show calcification. Streaky or lacelike calcification has been described in an occasional Leydig cell tumor, and fine punctate calcifications have been reported in teratoma.[64] Seminoma in the testicles does not calcify but metastatic deposits in iliac and paraaortic lymph nodes may become radiodense, especially after radiotherapy (Fig 9–53). A similar finding is seen with teratoma. Several instances of calcified steatomata (sebaceous cysts) of the skin of the scrotum have been reported, appearing radiographically as dense, well-defined, round, or oval calcifications of concretion type, a few millimeters to 1 cm or so in diameter.[65]

Prostatic Calcification

Prostatic calculi vary in size from a millimeter to several centimeters in diameter and vary in number from few to hundreds. Although found usually in men over 40 years old, they have been reported in young men and even children. The pathogenesis of these concretions is unknown; the most generally accepted theory is that they represent calcification of corpora amylacea, clumps of bacteria, blood clots, or pus. They may result from chronic prostatitis or, conversely, may act to cause an inflammatory process in the prostate. Prostatic calculi occur most commonly in the posterior and lateral lobes of the prostate, sometimes involving the gland diffusely and symmetrically but at other times being asymmetrical and localized.

They usually have a characteristic radiological appearance of many sharply defined homogeneous concretions clustered in the region of the symphysis pubis (Figs 9–54, 9–55), a midline location where pelvic phleboliths are uncommon. The location, size, and packing of the many concretions, sometimes faceted, are distinctive for prostatic calculi. Enlargement of the prostate upwards may displace calculi over the expected position of the vesicle shadow, where they can be mistaken for bladder concretions (Fig 9–56).

Tuberculosis can also produce calcification in the prostate gland, sometimes simulating the much more common nontuberculous calculous prostatis. The calcifications of tuberculosis are apt to be less well defined and smudgy, without the sharp borders of prostatic lithiasis.

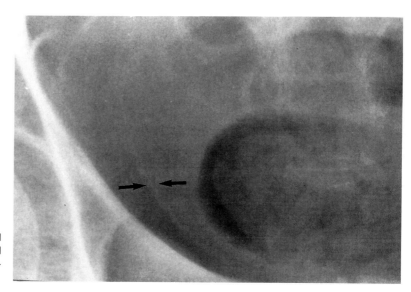

Figure 9–49. Calcification in the right pudendal artery in a diabetic patient (*arrows*). This vessel is generally thinner and more medially positioned than the vas deferens.

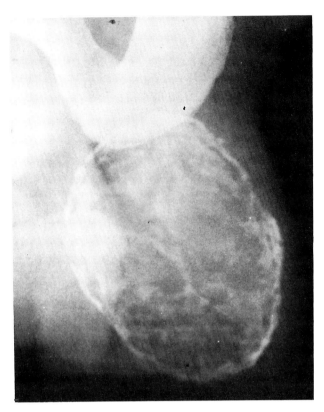

Figure 9–50. Hydrocele calcification of cyst type in a 69-year-old man with a hard scrotal mass.

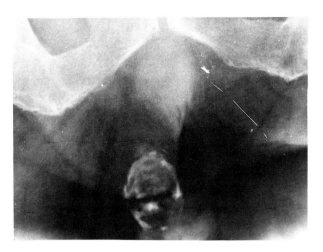

Figure 9–52. Most likely calcification of a hematoma in the scrotum. An elderly man had had bilateral orchiectomies several years before for treatment of carcinoma of the prostate. There are collections of amorphous calcification with an incomplete rim calcification of irregular thickness.

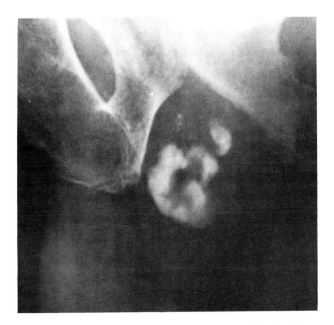

Figure 9–51. Testicular calcification presumably following infarction. An 86-year-old man with adenocarcinoma of the sigmoid was found to have a stony-hard left testicle, of which he was aware for at least 10 years. He recalled an episode of severe testicular pain as a young man. Very likely he had suffered torsion of the testicle. There are several clumps of dense amorphous calcification of solid mass type in the testis.

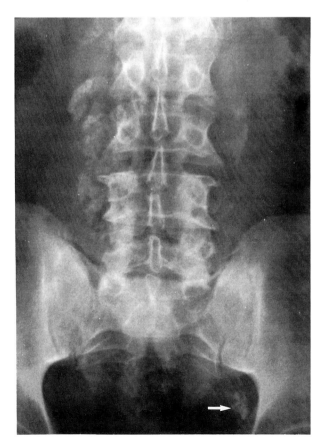

Figure 9–53. Testicular seminoma treated with radiotherapy. Diffuse calcification of paraaortic nodes more extensive on the right than the left. There is also calcification of a left external iliac node (*arrow*).

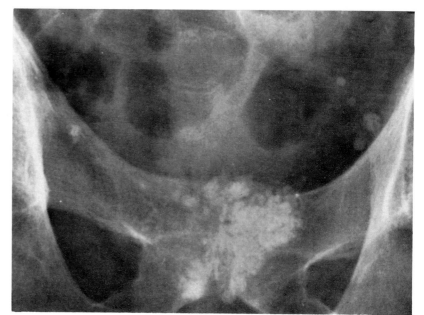

Figure 9–54. Prostatic calculi in asymmetrical distribution, being more pronounced in the left lobe. The concretions at the lateral aspects of the pelvis are phleboliths.

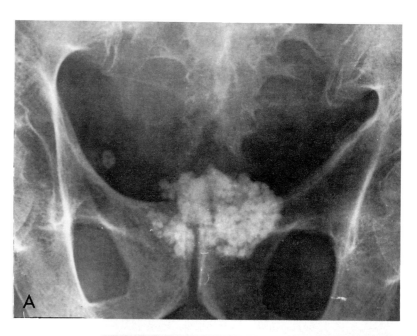

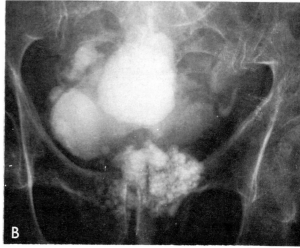

Figure 9–55. Prostatic calculi. **A.** Scout radiograph shows concretions of varying sizes involving an enlarged prostate, diffusely and symmetrically. The calcification near the right ischial spine is a phlebolith. **B.** Urography demonstrates the relation of the calcifications to the base of the bladder. Note the ureteral fishhooking and the vesical pseudodiverticula, secondary to bladder outlet obstruction due to the enlarged prostate.

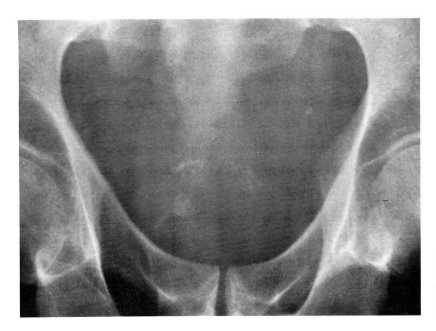

Figure 9–56. "Intravesical" prostatic stones. Marked expansion of the prostate has elevated the bladder. The relatively few calculi in the periphery of the prostate are situated far above the symphysis pubis.

REFERENCES

1. Wepfer JF, Sinsky TE. Roentgen manifestations of vaginitis emphysematosa. *Am J Roentgenol.* 1968; 102:946–950.
2. Seaman WB, Fleming RT. Pneumatosis of pelvic viscera. *Semin Roentgenol.* 1969;4:202–211.
3. Francke P Jr. Vaginitis emphysematosa. *Radiology.* 1961;77:114–116.
4. Whalen JP, Ziter F Jr. Emphysematous vaginitis. *Obstet Gynecol.* 1967;29:9–11.
5. Navani S. A primary vaginal stone. *Br J Radiol.* 1970; 43:222–223.
6. Dolan PA. Tumor calcification following therapy. *Am J Roentgenol.* 1963;89:166–174.
7. Hutcheson J, Page DL, Oldham RR. Calcified lymph node metastases from carcinoma of the cervix. *Cancer* 1973;32:266–269.
8. Deeths TM, Stanley RJ. Parametrial calcification in cervical carcinoma patients treated with radioactive gold. *Am J Roentgenol.* 1976;127:511–513.
9. Schabel SI, Burgener FA, Reynolds J. Radiographic manifestations of malignant mixed uterine tumors. *J Can Assoc Radiol.* 1975;26:176–183.
10. Hemley SD, Schwinger A. Lithopedion. Case report and survey. *Radiology.* 1952;58:235–238.
11. Oden PW, Lee HC. Lithopedion with calcified placenta. Case report. *Va Med Mon.* 1940;67:304–306.
12. Camiel MR, Berkan HS, Alexander LL. Roentgen visualization of uterine artery calcification. *Radiology.* 1967;88:138–139.
13. Fisher MD, Hamm R. Uterine artery calcification: Its association with diabetes. *Radiology.* 1975;117:537–538.
14. Poppel MH, Silverman M. Gas gangrene of uterus. *Radiology.* 1941;37:491–492.
15. Solomon A, Light S, Edelstein T. Gas forming organism invasion of a pregnant uterus. *Clin Radiol.* 1969; 20:105–106.
16. Holly LE II, Hartwell SW, McNair JN, et al. Mural emphysema of the uterus: A case report. *Am J Roentgenol.* 1960;84:913–922.
17. Kaufman BM, Cooper JM, Cookson P. Clostridium perfringens septicemia complicating degenerating uterine leiomyomas. *Am J Obstet Gynec.* 1974;118:877–878.
18. Weintraub RA, Tilos F. Gas abscess within a leiomyoma of the uterus. *Am J Roentgenol.* 1964;92:400–403.
19. Gross BH, Jafri SZH, Glazer GH. Significance of intrauterine gas demonstrated by computed tomography. *J Comput Assist Tomogr.* 1983;7:842–845.
20. Sloan RD. Cystic teratoma (dermoid) of the ovary. *Radiology.* 1963;81:847–853.
21. Peterson WF, Prevost EC, Edmonds FT, et al. Benign cystic teratoma of the ovary: Clinico-statistical study of 1007 cases with review of literature. *Am J Obstet Gynecol.* 1955;70:368–382.
22. Ounjian ZJ, Mani RL, Mani JR. Denovo development of teeth in a teratoma. *Br J Radiol.* 1980;53:40–41.
23. Wollin E, Ozonoff MB. Dermoid development of teeth in an ovarian teratoma. *N Engl J Med.* 1961;265:897–890.
24. Siegel MJ, McAlister WA, Shackelford LD. Radiographic findings in ovarian teratomas in children. *Am J Roentgenol.* 1978;131:613–615.
25. Cusmano JV. Dermoid cysts of the ovary. Roentgen features. *Radiology.* 1956;66:719–722.
26. Skaane P, Klott KJ. Fat–fluid level in a cystic ovarian teratoma. *J Comput Assist Tomogr.* 1981;5:577–579
27. Goldenberg NJ. Dermoid perforation of the colon. *Gastrointest Radiology.* 1978;3:221–222.

28. Tanner ML, Orron A, Baber JD, et al. Spontaneous rupture of an ovarian teratoid tumor (dermoid cyst) into the urinary bladder: Review of 11 cases and report of one new case. *Obstet Gynecol.* 1970;6:668–670.

29. Castro JR, Klein EW. The incidence and appearance of roentgenologically visible psammomatous calcification of papillary cystadenocarcinoma of the ovaries. *Am J Roentgenol.* 1962;88:886–891.

30. Teplick JG, Haskins ME, Alavi A. Calcified intraperitoneal metastases from ovarian carcinoma. *Am J Roentgenol.* 1976;127:1003–1006.

31. Lingley JR. The significance of psammoma calcification in the roentgen diagnosis of papillary tumors of the ovary. *Am J Roentgenol.* 1942;47:563–570.

32. Moncada R, Cooper RA, Garces M. Calcified metastases from malignant ovarian neoplasm. Review of the literature. *Radiology.* 1974;113:31–35.

33. Andress MR. A papillary cystadenocarcinoma of the ovary with peritoneal metastases diagnosed radiologically. *Br J Radiol.* 1970;43:143–146.

34. Fletcher BD, Morreels CL, Christian WH III, et al. Calcified adenocarcinoma of the colon. *Am J Roentgenol.* 1967;101:301–305.

35. Goodman K, Baim RS, Clair MR, et al. Angiomatous lymphoid hamartoma of the pelvis. *Radiology.* 1983;146:728.

36. Schabel SI, Rogers CJ. Opaque artifacts in a health food faddist simulating ovarian neoplasm. *Am J Roentgenol.* 1978;130:789–790.

37. Samuel E. Roentgenology of parasitic calcification. *Am J Roentgenol.* 1950;63:512–522.

38. Reddy CRRM, Sivaprasad MD, Parvathi G. Calcified guinea worm: Clinical, radiological and pathological study. *Ann Trop Med.* 1968;62:399–406.

39. Dockerty MB, Masson JC. Ovarian fibromas: A clinical and pathologic study of 283 cases. *Am J Obstet Gynecol.* 1944;47:741–752.

40. Clendenning WE, Hardt, JR, Block JB. Ovarian fibroma and mesenteric cysts. Their association with hereditary basal cell cancer of the skin. *Am J Obstet Gynecol.* 1963;87:1008–1012.

41. Mecca JT, Elguezabal A, Bryk D. Thecoma with extensive calcification. *Br J Radiol.* 1974;47:492–493.

42. Schultz SM, Curry TS III, Voet R. Psammomatous-like calcification in a Brenner tumor of the ovary. *Br J Radiol.* 1986;59:412–414.

43. Scully RE, Mark EJ, McNeely BU. Case 22-1982. Case records of the Massachusetts General Hospital. *N Engl J Med.* 1982;306:1348–1355.

44. Cooperman LR, Hamlin J, Ng E. Gonadoblastoma. A rare ovarian tumor related to the dysgerminoma with characteristic roentgen appearance. *Radiology.* 1968;90:322–324.

45. Seymour EQ, Hood JB, Underwood PB Jr. Gonadoblastoma: An ovarian tumor with characteristic pelvic calcifications. *Am J Roentgenol.* 1976;127;1001–1002.

46. Rosenberg RF, Hausner MM. Sclerosing stromal tumor of the ovary. *Radiology.* 1979;132:70.

47. Chalvaidjian A, Scully RE. Sclerosing stromal tumor of the ovary. *Cancer.* 1973;31:664–670.

48. Clements R, Bowyer FM. Hydatid disease of the pelvis. *Clin Radiol.* 1986;37;375–377.

49. Noonan CD. Primary and secondary malignancy of the female reproductive system. *Radiol Clin N Am.* 1965;3:375.

50. Buhrow CJ, Gary TM, Clark WE II. Ovarian corpora albicantia calcifications. A case report. *Radiology.* 1966;87:746–747.

51. Puckette SE Jr, Williamson HO, Seymour EQ. Calcification in an ovarian corpus albicans. *Radiology.* 1969;92:1105.

52. Lester PD, McAlister WH. A mobile calcified spontaneously amputated ovary. *J Can Assoc Radiol.* 1970;21:143–145.

53. Nixon GW, Condon VR. Amputated ovary: A cause of migratory abdominal calcification. *Am J Roentgenol.* 1977;128:1053–1055.

54. Kennedy LA, Pinckney LE, Currarino G, et al. Amputated calcified ovaries in children. *Radiology.* 1981;141:83–86.

55. Rozin S. The x-ray diagnosis of genital tuberculosis. *J Obstet Gynecol Br Emp.* 1952;59:59–63.

56. Marks JH, Ham DP. Calcification of vas deferens. *Am J Roentgenol.* 1942;47:859–863.

57. Wilson JL, Marks JH. Calcification of the vas deferens. Its relation to diabetes mellitus and arteriosclerosis. *N Engl J Med.* 1951;245:321–325.

58. Culver GJ, Tannenhaus J. Calcification of the vas deferens in diabetics. *JAMA.* 1960;173:648–651.

59. Camiel MR. Calcification of vas deferens associated with diabetes. *J Urol.* 1961;86:634–636.

60. Hafiz A, Melnick JC. Calcification of the vas deferens. *J Can Assoc Radiol.* 1968;19:56–60.

61. King JC Jr, Rosenbaum HD. Calcification of the vasa deferentia in nondiabetics. *Radiology.* 1971;100:603–606.

62. Postner MP, Smith RP. Scrotal cystocele with bladder calculi (case report). *Am J Roentgenol.* 1986;147:287–288.

63. Cho SK, Hamoudi AB, Clatworthy HW Jr. Infarction of an abdominal undescended testis presenting as a calcified abdominal mass in a newborn. *Radiology.* 1974;110:173–174.

64. Loveday BO, Price JL. Soft tissue radiography of the testes. *Clin Radiol.* 1978;29:685–689.

65. Phillips EW. Calcified steatomata of the scrotum. Report of a case. *Am J Roentgenol.* 1964;92:388–389.

CHAPTER TEN

The Radiology of Opaque Surgical Clips and Staples

Stephen R. Baker and Harry Delany

The plain film of the abdomen is usually obtained either for the evaluation of acute diseases or as a scout film before a contrast examination. In many cases, it is also a signpost of prior disorders and their treatments, some of which occurred many years ago. Careful assessment of bowel gas patterns on plain films can suggest previous resections of the intestine or stomach. The recognition of appliances on the skin such as colostomy bags gives added information about therapeutic responses to serious bowel or urinary abnormalities. More frequently seen are radiodense surgical clips and staples, which provide the roentgenologist with telling clinical evidence about the past. Many times an analysis of the location and pattern of these metallic densities can provide specific information, confirming data gathered from patient interview and a review of medical records. Occasionally, such plain film findings assume crucial diagnostic importance when the history is incomplete, unreliable, or unavailable.

There is no widely accepted policy governing use of these radiodense clips and sutures. Mostly, they are applied to bleeding sites to control intraoperative hemorrhage. In some cases, they are employed for identification purposes rather than for hemostasis. Their siting and distribution can provide roentgenographic confirmation of the performance of a surgical procedure. For example, nearly all surgeons place radiopaque clips on the severed main vagus trunks or branches as a marker of that type of operation. The margins or center of a mass or tumor bed may be outlined by clips to aid in positioning radiotherapy portals or to gauge response to treatment after completion of a course of radiation or chemotherapy. Displacement or migration of clips and disruption of staple lines can be significant clues to the existence of surgical error and its untoward complications. Moreover, a reliance on the use of clips in some operations and avoidance of them in others, as well as the number

and type deployed in various locations and surgical situations are all a matter of technical option. Collectively, they form a surgical signature identifying the operative patterns and preferences of individual practitioners.

The list of abdominal operative procedures is vast, and this chapter is not designed to be all encompassing. What follows is a survey or roentgenographic findings reflecting clip and staple patterns associated with some of the more common surgical procedures.

STOMACH

Interruption of the vagus nerve is a standard treatment for ulcer disease. A truncal vagotomy leads to hypomotility of the stomach muscles and stasis of gastric contents. Thus, it must be accompanied by a drainage procedure, either pyloroplasty or gastroenterostomy. Usually, only one or two clips identify the point of division of each trunk (Fig 10–1). Superselective vagotomy involves severing small vagal twigs on the proximal lesser curvature, including the nerve of Latterjee (Fig 10–2). An advantage of this operation is that pyloroplasty or gastroenterostomy is not required. It is a demanding procedure, however, requiring identification and interruption of small vagal branches connected to the stomach. Usually, at least ten metallic densities are introduced. Hence, in most instances, the number of clips seen near the esophogastric junction on plain films relates to the type of vagotomy rather than the occurrence of excessive bleeding at the operative site.

Radiodense clips or opaque staples inserted by stapling instruments are often used to secure an anastomosis during gastric resection. In Billroth II operations, they can be placed at the gastroenterostomy, the duodenal stump, or in both locations. In some cases, a combination of vagotomy

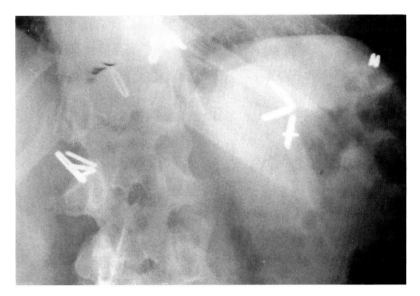

Figure 10–1. Vagotomy, Billroth II gastrectomy, and inadvertent splenectomy. This patient had a bilateral truncal vagotomy. A single clip overlying T12 and several clips more superiorlateral denote interruption of vagal trunks. Clips are also located at the gastroenterostomy site on the left and at the duodenal stump on the right. The two clips below the lateral (L) hemidiaphragm were placed to control bleeding after the spleen was accidentally lacerated.

and Billroth II resection appears on plain films as three foci of discrete metallic densities.

A complication of gastric surgery is an inadvertent laceration of the spleen sometimes leading to splenorrhaphy or emergency splenectomy. A plain film clue of the presence of this complication is recognition of one or several clips in the left upper quadrant, often accompanied by lateral deviation of the gastric pouch (Fig 10–1).

Occasionally, a clip falls into the peritoneal cavity either during an operation or sometime later as it

unclasps and then dislodges from its point of fixation. Usually, these errant clips are innocuous. Since they are situated within the peritoneal cavity, however, they may act as free foreign bodies and promote the development of adhesions and possible acute intestinal obstruction (Fig 10–3).

COLON

It is common for surgeons to apply staples or clips at the sites of anastomoses during colonic resections. The large bowel has great spatial variability as it traverses the lateral margins of the peritoneal cavity and crosses the midline below the stomach. Hence, the position of surgical metallic densities may be almost anywhere in the abdomen. Unless the anastamosis is performed using a ring of staples, only one or, at most, several clips are inserted at the resection line. A clue to left colon removal is the far peripheral position of a collection of clips applied to the lateral peritoneal reflection (Fig 10–4). Resection of the sigmoid colon can be identified on plain films by clips overlying the upper pelvis (Fig 10–5). Metallic densities confined to the pelvis are also a radiographic legacy of abdomino-perineal resections. Its hallmark is an irregular distribution of clips near the rectum (Fig 10–6), which is distinctly different from the pattern of radical resections of the uterus, bladder, or prostate gland, in which clips are aligned more laterally along the course of the iliac node chains.

Radiodense ring staple lines permit a plain film assessment not only of the point but also the integrity of a bowel reattachment. The radiographic collar of small opaque rings must be intact.

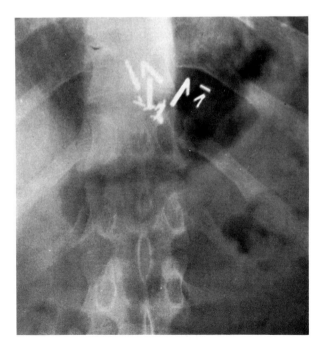

Figure 10–2. Superselective vagotomy. Numerous clips were placed to control bleeding associated with division of small branches of the vagus nerve along the proximal lesser curvature.

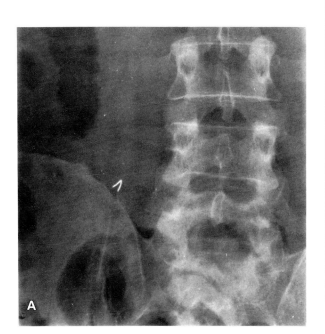

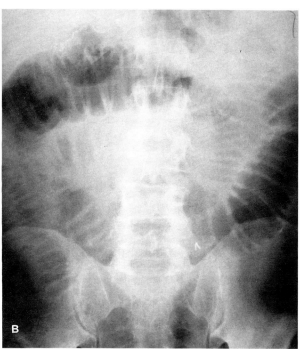

Figure 10–3. Loosened vagotomy clips in the peritoneal cavity. **A.** Incidental finding of an open clip. **B.** Ectopic vagotomy clip associated with an adhesive band which obstructed the small intestine.

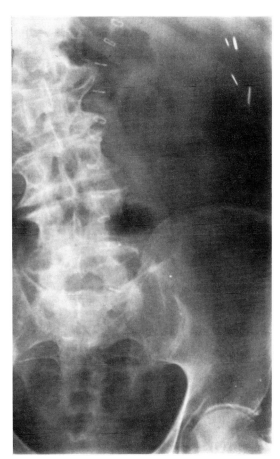

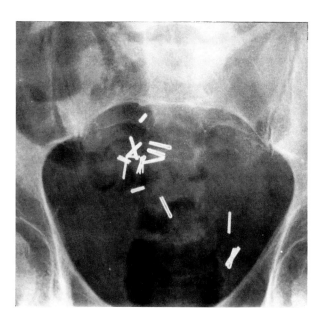

Figure 10–4. Left colon resection clips located peripheral to an intact left kidney.

Figure 10–5. Sigmoid resection. Large hemoclips were placed near both sides of the anastomosis. The more superior ones overlie the gas- and feces-filled colonic lumen.

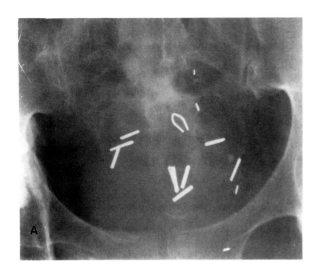
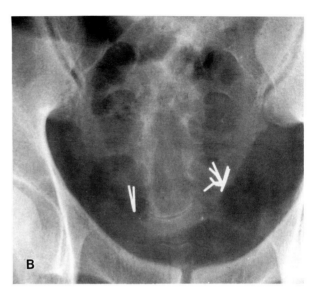

Figure 10–6. Abdominoperineal resections. **A.** Clips of varying sizes—proximal rectal tumor. **B.** Clips on both sides of the midline-distal rectal tumor.

Any interruption or displacement of a skein of staples should be viewed with suspicion because it can be suggestive for disruption of the anastomosis (Fig 10–7).

In recent years, many oncologic surgeons have taken a more aggressive approach toward the extirpation of metastatic deposits from colon cancer that are confined to one hepatic lobe. Often, clips are applied during the procedure, conveniently serving as a radiographic reminder of segmental resection of liver containing tumor. The coincidence of one set of metallic densities arrayed along the large bowel and another in the hepatic substance is a characteristic plain film pattern of an initial colonic resection and a subsequent operation for localized liver metastases (Fig 10–8).

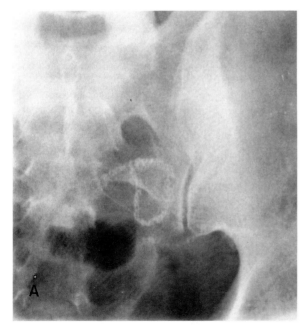
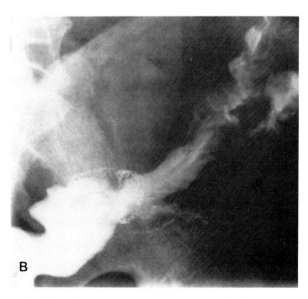

Figure 10–7. Suture disruption with leakage of colonic contents outside of bowel wall, 10 days after sigmoid resection for acute diverticulitis. **A.** Preliminary film before Hypaque enema shows interruptions of the staple ring at the anastomosis. **B.** Contrast passes through the bowel wall at the site of the sutures.

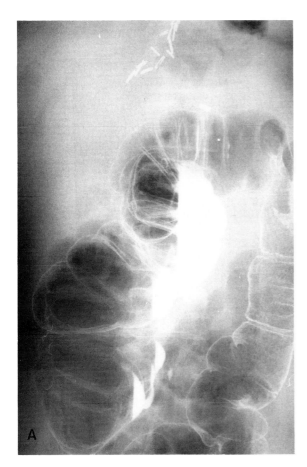
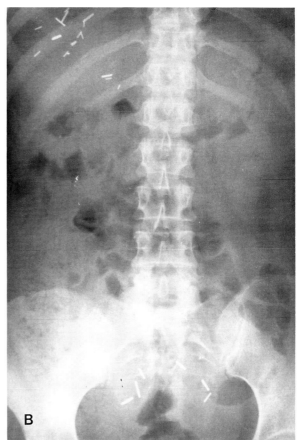

Figure 10–8. A. A frontal film from a double contrast barium enema. The large bowel is shortened after resection of a carcinoma of the proximal descending colon. Note two clips above the abbreviated transverse colon. The other clips are in the liver, placed there at the time of removal of a solitary metastasis to the left lobe. **B.** Two agglomerations of surgical clips. The pelvic clips were placed at sigmoid resection for carcinoma. The right upper quadrant clips denote a resection of a single metastasis to the liver.

LIVER AND BILIARY TRACT

Cholecystectomy, the most common operation of the biliary tract, is sometimes recognized on plain films by a single clip usually attached to the edge of the cystic duct remnant. The placement of many clips in the gallbladder bed may reflect the customary technique of some surgeons but more often it suggests a difficult operation complicated by the need to secure bleeding vessels in and around the site of resection (Fig 10–9).

Primary hepatic tumors are notoriously vascular and their surgical removal is often a bloody affair. Prompt hemostasis in a large operative field may be quickly achieved by the liberal use of hemostatic clips. Twenty or more of them closely packed in the upper abdomen is an expected finding after hepatectomy (Fig 10–10).

Shunts between large portal and systemic veins are identifiable by a particular arrangement of clips. In a portocaval shunt, these metallic densities are put along the margins of both veins near their point of anastamosis. Typically, this site overlies the right side of the L1 vertebral body (Fig 10–11). The plain

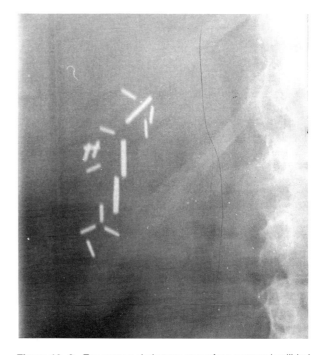

Figure 10–9. Emergency cholecystectomy for a ruptured gallbladder. Numerous clips were used to control bleeding.

411

412

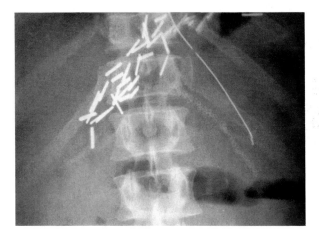

Figure 10–10. Upright film. Numerous clips were used to control hemorrhage during a left hepatectomy.

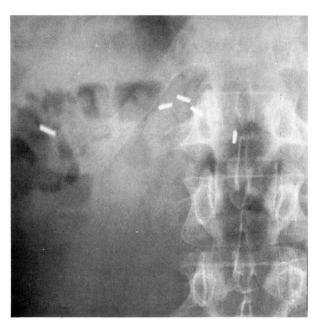

Figure 10–11. Portocaval shunt. The midline clip is on the inferior vena cava. The three nearby clips are on the portal vein at the anastomosis. The far lateral clip is on the cystic duct remnant inserted during a previous cholecystectomy.

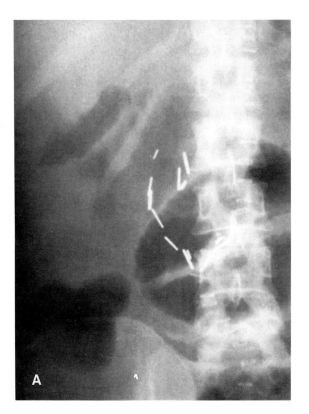

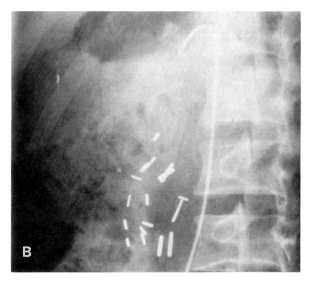

Figure 10–12. A. Mesocaval shunt in a patient with ascites. Arcuate distribution of clips at the anastomosis. **B.** Mesocaval shunt. Right posterior oblique view. The superior mesenteric vein clips are anterior to the inferior vena cava clips. A catheter has been placed in the superior mesenteric artery for infusion therapy to control bleeding esophageal varices.

film juxtaposition of clips with a mesocaval anastomosis is characteristic, appearing as a gently curving, vertically directed single or double row of densities located to the right of the midline along the course of the superior mesenteric vein at the level of L2 to L4. More medially, a few clips are also placed on the inferior vena cava (Fig 10–12).

THE URINARY TRACT

Adrenal carcinomas can become very large before evincing signs or symptoms of their presence. Like hepatic tumors, these lesions have a luxuriant blood supply and are apt to bleed during resection. A typical postoperative plain film appearance is a jumble of clips occupying a wide area in the right or left upper abdomen (Fig 10–13). In some adrenal tumor resections, clips are arranged around the edge of the tumor to help in radiotherapy treatment planning (Fig 10–14). Adrenal masses, even when huge, rarely extend over the midline. Thus, clip placement is almost always unilateral, with its medial extent delimited by the edge of the vertebral bodies. In contrast, clips inserted for removal of liver masses may be on both sides of the midline.

A renal malignancy that has not extended beyond the confines of the kidney, renal vein, and adjacent lymph nodes is often treated by nephrectomy. The operation entails ligation of feeding arteries and draining veins, dissection of adjacent lymph nodes, and en bloc removal of the kidney. A wide margin of normal tissue must be taken to en-

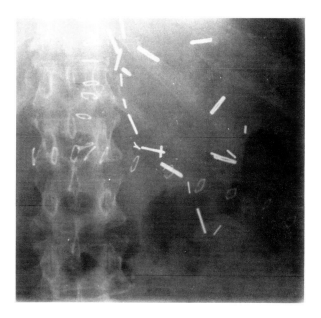

Figure 10–14. Left adrenal carcinoma. The clips were placed at the perimeter of the tumor.

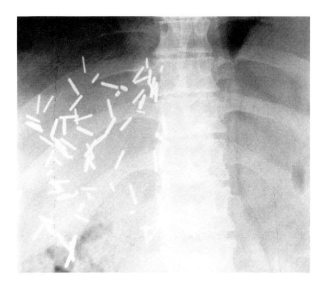

Figure 10–13. Hypervascular right adrenal carcinoma. Complete removal of the tumor was not achieved because it had extended to adjacent retroperitoneal structures and the liver.

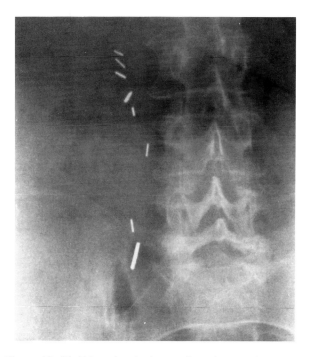

Figure 10–15. This patient had a very large hypernephroma extending inferiorly from the right kidney. At operation clips were used to control bleeding along the line of resection.

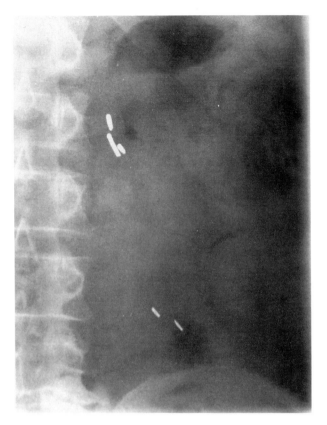

Figure 10–16. Left nephrectomy. Clips at the renal hilus and at the site of the tumor projecting from the inferior pole of the kidney.

Stage 0	no invasion
Stage A	invasion of submucosa
Stage B1	invasion of superficial muscle
Stage B2	invasion of deep muscle
Stage C	invasion of fat
Stage D	invasion of adjacent organs or distant metastases

Radical cystectomy is used most often for the treatment of well-differentiated, superficial but extensive lesions, most of which are classifiable as B1 tumors. The operation involves removal of the bladder, the seminal vesicles, the prostate, and the iliac lymph nodes and their adjacent lymphatic channels. Many urologists put clips at the site of the internal, external, and common iliac nodes (Fig 10–20). The line of resection inferiorly may also be marked with metallic densities. In some patients, nodal dissection extends to the paraaortic chain (Fig 10–21). In others, there may be only an ipsilateral resection of pelvic nodes confined to the side of the tumor (Fig 10–22).

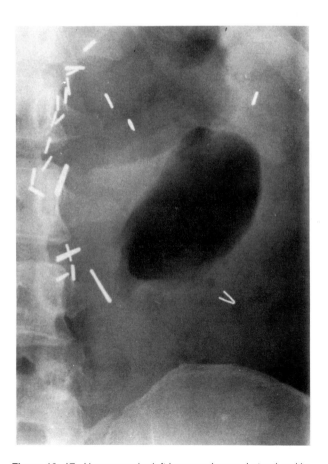

Figure 10–17. Hypervascular left hypernephroma. Lateral and inferior clips surround the tumor. Medial and superior clips were placed at the renal hilus and on adjacent lymph nodes.

sure a successful resection. A typical appearance is a row of clips along the spine (Fig 10–15). A few clips in the renal hilus and one or two others positioned more peripherally at the site of the tumor is a common variation (Fig 10–16). A third pattern is numerous clips placed medially and laterally (Fig 10–17).

Renal pelvic and ureteral tumors are often treated by nephroureterectomy. A clue to this procedure is the distribution of several clips along the course of the ureter. Generally, fewer metallic densities are seen than with resection of hypernephroma because these tumors are smaller and less vascular (Fig 10–18).

In renal transplants, the donated kidney is usually situated in the iliac fossa (Fig 10–19). Often, clips are placed at the margin of transplant and their spatial arrangement is monitored on successive films. A divergence of the clips indicates enlargement of the allograft, a helpful sign of impending transplant rejection.

Carcinoma of the urinary bladder can be staged according to the extent of penetration of the tumor through the vesical wall[1]:

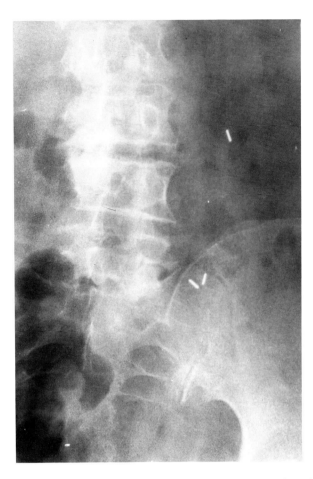

Figure 10–18. Several clips to the left of the midline are oriented along the course of the left ureter. This patient had a ureterone-phrectomy for transitional cell carcinoma of the proximal left ureter.

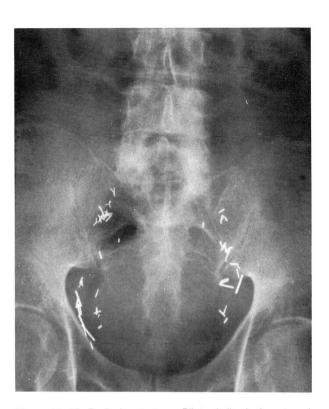

Figure 10–20. Radical cystectomy. Bilateral clips in the external, internal, and common iliac nodes.

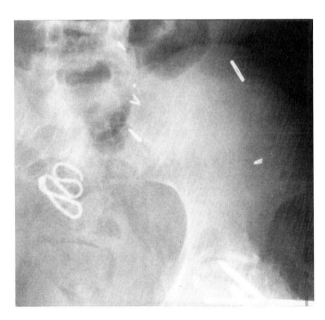

Figure 10–19. Clips were positioned at the periphery of a transplanted kidney during its placement into the recipient's left iliac fossa. Chronic renal failure and steroid treatment weakened the left femoral neck causing a fracture.

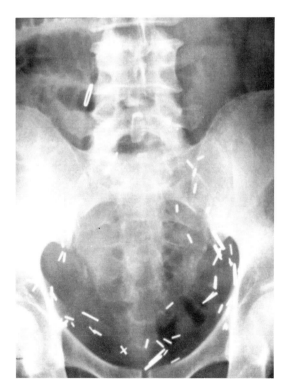

Figure 10–21. Radical cystectomy with surgical clips in iliac nodes and in one sampled distal para-aortic node. Clips in the lower pelvis were placed on the inferior wall of the bladder, the seminal vesicles, and the prostate gland.

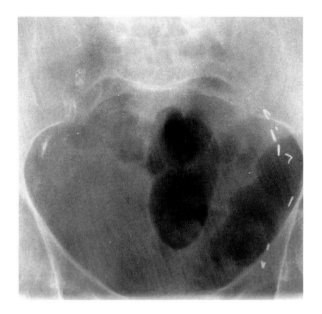

Figure 10–22. Carcinoma of the bladder. This patient had bilateral lymphangiography prior to surgery. Residual contrast remains in normal iliac nodes on the right. The left nodes were involved by tumor and were removed at cystectomy, as evidenced by lack of lymphangiographic contrast material and the presence of surgical clips along the expected course of the external iliac node chain.

Some surgeons remove only those groups of nodes shown to be replaced by tumor on lymphangiography.

The coexistence of isolated metallic clips and other radiopaque densities can provide additional information about the consequences of the operation. Impotence is an inevitable result of radical cystectomy. One method of treatment to maintain sexual function is the insertion of a permanent penile prosthesis. The prosthesis consists of metal rods that can be identified on plain films as it projects over the pelvis (Fig 10–23).

CARCINOMA OF THE PROSTATE

There are several approaches to carcinoma of the prostate. One option, observable on abdominal radiographs, is retropubic prostatectomy with pelvic lymph node dissection. Usually, the distribution of clips is indistinguishable from that seen with radical cystectomy. In some cases, additional clips are located within the prostatic bed near the midline overlying the upper edge of the symphysis pubis and in inguinal nodes (Fig 10–24).

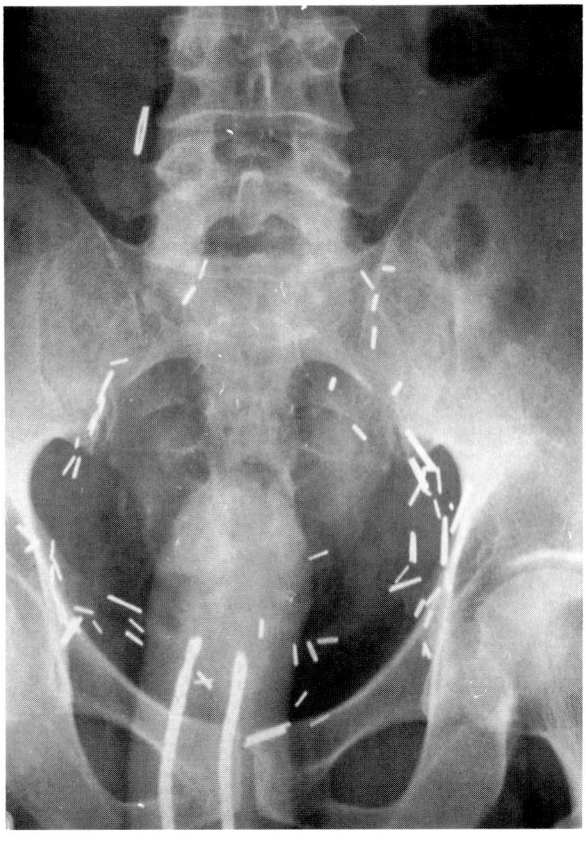

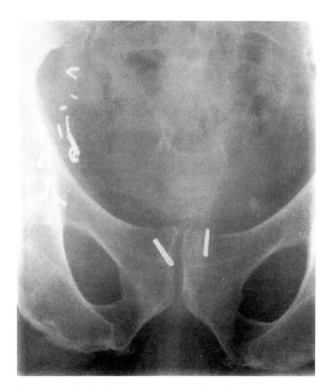

Figure 10–23. Radical cystectomy for stage B1 carcinoma of the bladder. Clips demarcate the bladder resection and bilateral lymph node dissection. Note the overlying shadow of the permanently rigid penis with two metallic rods that are part of the implanted prosthesis.

Figure 10–24. Radical prostatectomy. Two clips in the prostatic bed and a unilateral distribution of clips along the right inguinal and external iliac node chain.

CARCINOMA OF THE CERVIX

Radiation therapy for carcinoma of the cervix is facilitated by insertion of one to two metallic clips on the cervical lip. The clips serve to locate the center of the treatment field and aid in the positioning of radiation portals. The plain film finding of a solitary pelvic clip is indicative of uterine tumors and is, not seen after surgery for other malignancies (Figs 9–26, 10–25).

Radical hysterectomy consists of transabdominal removal of the uterus, bilateral salpingo-oophorectomy, and pelvic lymph node dissection. Less common today, it was popular in the past for the treatment of locally invasive cervical carcinoma. Clips oriented along the distribution of the iliac lymph nodes readily identify the operation on plain radiographs (Fig 10–26). In some patients, the dissection is extended superiorly to retroperitoneal nodes (Fig 10–27). A more diffuse assemblage of clips

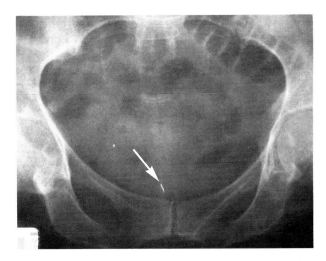

Figure 10–25. A single clip (*arrow*) affixed to the cervix to guide determination of location of treatment portals for radiotherapy for a patient with stage I carcinoma of the cervix.

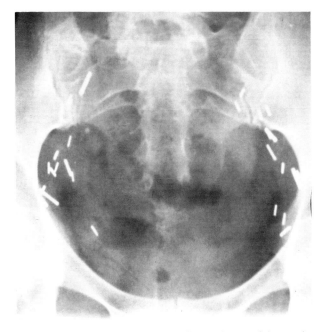

Figure 10–26. Radical hysterectomy for carcinoma of the cervix. Clips are arrayed along the course of the internal, external, and common iliac node chains on both sides of the pelvis.

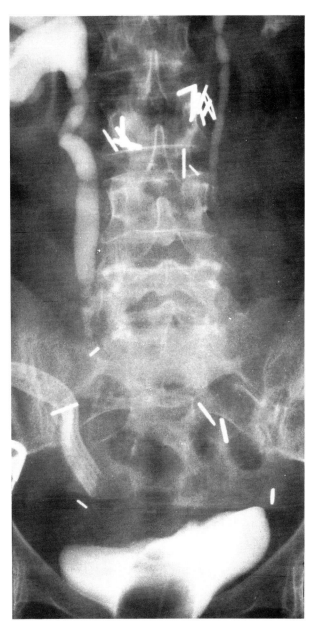

Figure 10–27. Retroperitoneal node sampling. A film from an intravenous urography in a patient who underwent a radical hysterectomy for carcinoma of the cervix. In addition to the pelvic clips there were two collections of clips overlying L3. These were placed at the site of retroperitoneal node biopsies.

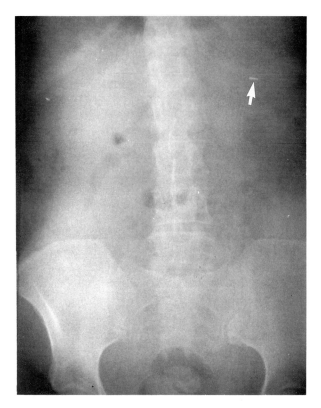

Figure 10–28. Ovarian carcinoma. A patient with intraperitoneal spread of disease and marked ascites. A single clip (*arrow*) was placed at the site of bleeding during a debulking procedure.

can be seen with pelvic exenteration for advanced cervical carcinoma.

Ovarian malignancies metastasize most often to the peritoneal cavity. A palliative procedure for extensive intra-abdominal spread of carcinoma is tumor debulking. Occasionally, clips are used to control bleeding at the site of resection of these masses. The association of ascites and an isolated metallic clip in the abdomen in a middle-aged or elderly female is strongly suggestive of metastatic ovarian cancer (Fig 10–28).

RETROPERITONEAL NODE DISSECTION

The dissection of para-aortic nodes is often evidenced on plain films by the distribution of clips in the lumbar spine at and near the midline. This procedure has been advocated for the treatment of malignancies of the pelvis, ie, carcinomas of the uterus, cervix, bladder, and prostate. Usually, there are also plain film findings of radical resection of the primary lesion and adjacent node-bearing areas.

Before recent advances in radiotherapy and chemotherapy, surgical excision of retroperitoneal nodes was considered a clinically worthy operation

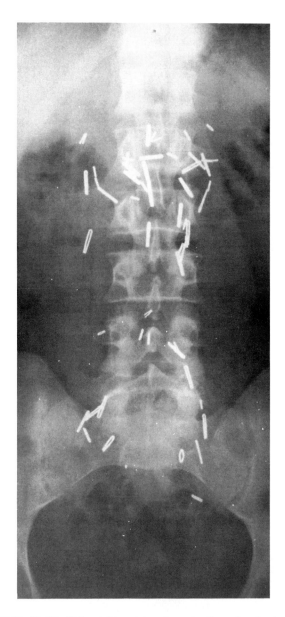

Figure 10–29. Retroperitoneal lymph node dissection for lymphoma. Numerous clips are located near and at the midline reflecting the distribution of retroperitoneal nodes. The common iliac nodes were also removed.

for lymphoma. Although primary surgical treatment is no longer used, the abdominal film of long time survivors has a distinctive appearance. The pelvis is free of metallic densities, but numerous clips are seen overlying and alongside the lumbar vertebral bodies. There is often a greater concentration of clips at the L1–L2 level where crossing lymphatic channels are most numerous (Fig 10–29).

RETROPERITONEAL VASCULAR OPERATIONS

Sympathectomy is another once common retroperitoneal operation that today is decreasing in popu-

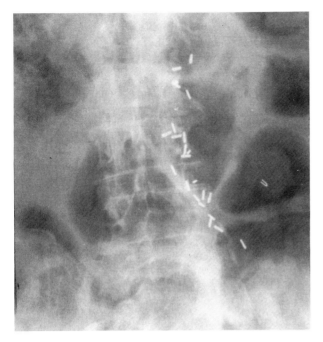

Figure 10–30. Left sympathectomy. Most of the clips are situated along the expected course of the left sympathetic trunk.

larity. The usual practice is placement of clips along the abdominal sympathetic chain, which runs astride the vertebral bodies along the lumbar spine. Unlike retroperitoneal node dissection, sympathectomy clips do not extend to the midline (Fig 10–30). Occasionally, arterial bypass grafts are secured by metallic clips. For example, aortoiliac bypasses can be recognized by clip densities grouped at both ends of the graft (Fig 10–31).

GROWTH OF MASSES

Not only can clips and staples identify the type and location of an operation, they also remain as a permanent radiopaque marker aiding assessment of response to treatment. Separation of clips on sequential plain films is a simple way to monitor the growth of masses. It must be remembered that movement of clips can be caused by both fibrosis and mass enlargement.[2] Thus, a change in position of one clip alone is not sufficient to assess growth. To be diagnosed on plain films. Tumor expansion should be accompanied by separation of the distance between clips (Fig 10–32).

SIMULATORS OF CLIPS

Not all short, linear metallic densities seen on abdominal films are introduced as part of an operative intervention. Clips or staples may be ingested inadvertently or may be the habitual practice of some demented people (Fig 10–33). Hari, a Japanese form of acupuncture, consists of the placement of many gold needles into the subcutaneous tissues.[3] They are cut off at the skin surface and remain in place permanently, usually causing no harm. With repeated treatments, the plain film demonstrates a bizarre pattern of curvilinear opaque fragments. Most often they are inserted in the back but can be situated anywhere on the abdominal wall. Such a spectacular appearance should not be confused with any other surgical procedure (Fig 10–34).

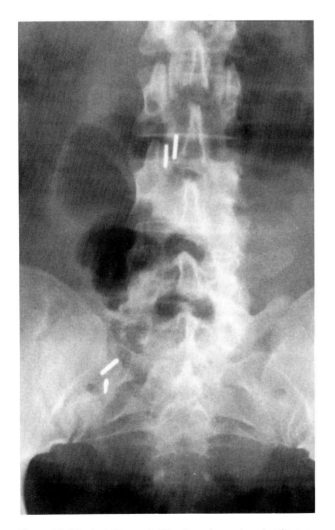

Figure 10–31. Aortoiliac graft. Clips have been placed at the proximal and distal margins of an aortoiliac graft. No clips were put on the anastomosis of the graft with the left common iliac artery.

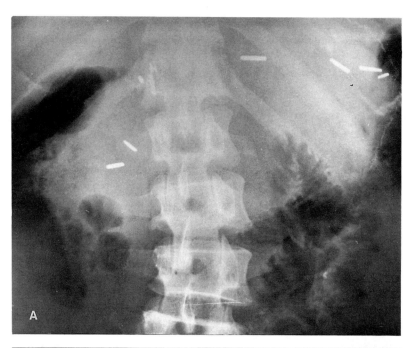

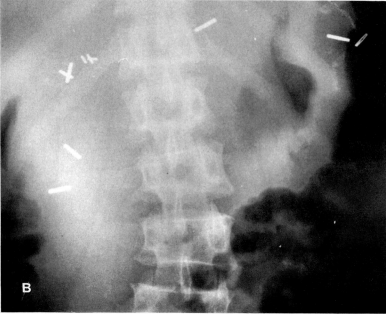

Figure 10–32. Moving clips. Rapid growth of a gastric lymphoma. **A.** At the initial operation four groups of clips were placed to assess the extent of tumor. **B.** Several months later progression of the tumor has caused the clips to migrate. The upper right clips have moved laterally, the two lower right clips were also pushed away from the midline, and have separated from each other. The single clip just to the left of T12 has been pushed medially and the left lateral clips have been deviated peripherally with two metallic densities superimposed on each other. Note also the deformity of the stomach bubble produced by the expanding lymphoma.

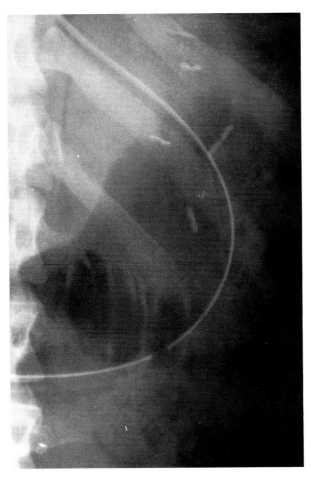

Figure 10–33. This patient has had no surgical procedures. The metallic densities are swallowed staples lying in the stomach.

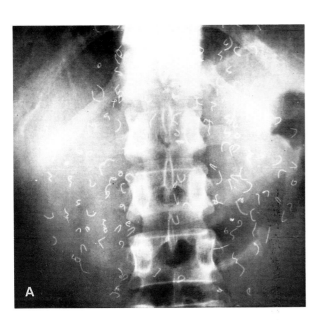

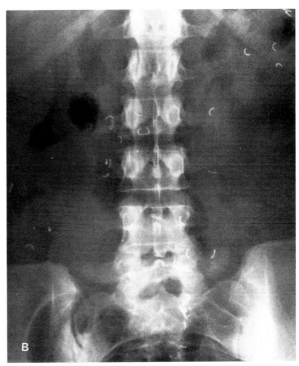

Figure 10–34. Acupuncture needles in two patients. The distribution of these densities depends on the clinical indication, which governs site of placement and on total treatments, which determines the aggregate number of needles inserted subcutaneously.

REFERENCES

1. Jewett HJ. Tumors of the bladder. In Campbell MF, Harrison JH (eds). *Urology,* 3rd ed. Philadelphia: WB Saunders; 1970.
2. Seymour EQ. Metallic clip displacement in evaluating tumor recurrence or enlargement. A source of error. *Radiology.* 1977;125:118.
3. Imray TJ, Hiramatsu Y. Radiographic manifestations of Japanese acupuncture. *Radiology.* 1975;115:625–626.

Index

Italicized letters following page numbers indicate figures (f)

Cysts (*cont.*)
  pneumatosis cystoides intestina-
    lis and, 211
  porcelain gallbladder and, 271–
    272
  pyelogenic, 336–338
  renal, 345f–349f
  splenic, 285, 287–289
  stones and, 55
  vaginitis emphysematosa and,
    379

Decubitus ulcers, gas and, 36, 37f
Dermoid cyst, 65, 66f, 390–394f
Diabetes
  aortic calcification and, 109
  calcification of the vas deferens
    and, 399
  colonic pseudo-obstruction and,
    177
  cystitis emphysematosa and, 365
  emphysematous pyelonephritis
    and, 331–333f
  gastric dilatation and, 129
  pancreatic lithiasis and, 310
  renal artery calcification and,
    344
  renal intraluminal gas and, 330–
    331, 332f
Diaphragm
  elevation of, abscesses and, 87
  retroperitoneal air vs. intraperi-
    toneal air, 88–91
Diaphragmatic hernia, pseudo-
    pneumoperitoneum and,
    84, 85f
Diverticula, 29–30
  abscesses and, 30
  colonic, 190–196f
  double-lucency sign and, 28
  duodenal, 149–151f, 260, 278
  jejunal, 213
  phleboliths and, 114
  pneumoretroperitoneum and,
    88, 89, 91
  ulcer and, 138, 140, 141f
  vesical, 370, 371f
Diverticulitis, 6f
  inflammatory adhesions and,
    180
  scout films and, 4–5
  small bowel obstruction and,
    169–170
  subphrenic abscesses and, 86
  ulcerative colitis and, 202
Dog ears, 94
Doge's cap sign, 82
Dolichocolon, 185

Double-bubble sign, 149
Double-lucency sign, 28, 134–137f
Double-wall sign. *See also* Bas-
    relief sign; Rigler's sign
Double-wall sign, pneumoperito-
    neum and, 75–76, 77f
Douching, pneumoperitoneum
    and, 73
Duodenal
  bulb, gallbladder and, 278
Duodenum, 148–150f
  diverticula of, 149–151f, 260, 278
  obstruction of
    gastric distension and, 132
  perforation of
    fat mimicking, 91
    pneumoretroperitoneum and,
      88, 89, 91
  signs of pancreatitis in, 302–304
Duplication of the colon, 192–193
Dystrophic calcification, 53

Echinococcal cyst
  adrenal, 322
  renal, 346, 349f
Echinococcus granulosus, 247, 252–
    253, 287, 322
Echinococcus multilocularis, 253
Ehlers-Danlos syndrome, 173
Embryonic omphalomesenteric
    duct, 192
Emphysema, pseudopneumoperi-
    toneum and, 85
Emphysematous
  cholecystitis, 5f, 277–279
    gas and, 34f
    hepatic abscess and, 260
    streaks and, 32
  cystitis, 194–195
  gastritis, 140–141
  pyelonephritis, 331–333f, 333,
    334f
Endoscopy, pneumoretroperito-
    neum and, 87–90f
Entamoeba histolytica, 204
Enteroliths, 218–219
  gallstones and, 275
  morphology of, 54
Epidural anesthesia, pseudopneu-
    moretroperitoneum and, 91
Evisceration, 47

Falciform ligament, pneumoperito-
    neum and, 78–79
Fallopian tubes, 389
Fasciola gigantica, 251

Fat, 2, 39–46
  calcified, 96–97f
  distended gallbladder and, 264
  intrarenal, 333, 334f
  liver and, 243
  perirenal, pancreatitis and, 305
  pseudopneumoperitoneum and,
    85–86
  pseudopneumoretroperitoneum
    and, 91
  radiodensity of the liver and,
    246
Fat-containing tumors, 45–46
Fatty liver, 255–256
Fecal impaction, 6f, 19f, 180, 202
Feces
  hepatic angle and, 93
  normal appearance of, 17
  preliminary studies and, 3–4
Female genital tract, 379–399
Fiber
  bowel size and, 185
  cecal volvulus and, 181–182
  small bowel obstruction and,
    170
Fistula
  biliary enteric, 273
  kidneys and, 329–330, 332f
  mobility and, 68–69
Fluid, bowel obstruction and, 160–
    161
Focal sclerosing stromal tumor of
    the ovary, 395
Football sign, 76
Foreign bodies, 220, 222f
  phleboliths and, 118–119
  scout film and, 5
  small bowel obstruction and,
    170

Gallbladder, 264–279
  appearance of gas in, 33–34f
  calcification in the wall of, 65
  calcified, 270–273
  enlargement of, 49, 50f, 264
  lucencies in, 273–277
Gallstones, 264–270f. *See also*
    Cholelithiasis
  efficacy of plain film and, 2
  enteroliths and, 218
  gastric opacities and, 146
  ileus, 5f, 170, 180, 273–277
  morphology of, 54, 55f, 56f
  movement of, 265–270
  renal artery aneurysm and,
    346
  survey roentgenograms and, 1
Gangrene, of the liver, 257–258

Italicized letters following page numbers indicate figures (*f*)

Italicized letters following page numbers indicate figures (*f*)